Probabilistic Risk Assessment and Management for Engineers and Scientists

IEEE Press
445 Hoes Lane, P.O. Box 1331
Piscataway, NJ 08855-1331

IEEE Reliability Society, *Sponsor*

RS-S Liaison to IEEE Press
Dev G. Raheja

Technical Reviewer
Yovan Lukic
Arizona Public Service Company

Probabilistic Risk Assessment and Management for Engineers and Scientists

second edition

Hiromitsu Kumamoto
Kyoto University

Ernest J. Henley
University of Houston

IEEE PRESS

IEEE Reliability Society, *Sponsor*

The Institute of Electrical and Electronics Engineers, Inc., New York

This book may be purchased at a discount from the publisher when ordered in bulk quantities. For more information contact:

IEEE PRESS Marketing
Attn: Special Sales
P.O. Box 1331
445 Hoes Lane
Piscataway, NJ 08855-1331
Fax: (908) 981-9334

Printed in the United States of America

10 9 8 7 6 5 4 3 2 1

ISBN 0-7803-1004-7

IEEE Order Number: PC3533

Library of Congress Cataloging-in-Publication Data

Kumamoto, Hiromitsu.
Probabilistic risk assessment and management for engineers and scientists / Hiromitsu Kumamoto, Ernest J. Henley. —2nd ed.
p. cm.
Rev. ed. of: Probabilistic risk assessment / Ernest J. Henley.
Includes bibliographical references and index.
ISBN 0-7803-1004-7
1. Reliability (Engineering) 2. Health risk assessment.
I. Henley, Ernest J. II. Henley, Ernest J. Probabilistic risk assessment. III. Title.
TS173.K86 1996 95-36502
620'.00452—dc20 CIP

Contents

Preface

Our previous IEEE Press book, *Probabilistic Risk Assessment*, was directed primarily at development of the mathematical tools required for reliability and safety studies. The title was somewhat a misnomer; the book contained very little material pertinent to the qualitative and management aspects of the factors that place industrial enterprises at risk.

This book has a different focus. The (updated) mathematical techniques material in our first book has been contracted by elimination of specialized topics such as variance reduction Monte Carlo techniques, reliability importance measures, and storage tank problems; the expansion has been entirely in the realm of management trade-offs of risk versus benefits. Decisions involving trade-offs are complex, and not easily made. Primitive academic models serve little useful purpose, so we decided to pursue the path of most resistance, that is, the inclusion of realistic, complex examples. This, plus the fact that we believe engineers should approach their work with a mathematical—not a trade school—mentality, makes this book difficult to use as an undergraduate text, even though all required mathematical tools are developed as appendices. We believe this book is suitable as an undergraduate plus a graduate text, so a syllabus and end-of-chapter problems are included. The book is structured as follows:

Chapter 1: Formal definitions of risk, individual and population risk, risk aversion, safety goals, and goal assessments are provided in terms of outcomes and likelihoods. Idealistic and pragmatic goals are examined.

Chapter 2: Accident-causing mechanisms are surveyed and classified. Coupling, dependency, and propagation mechanisms are discussed. Risk-management principles are described. Applications to preproduction quality assurance programs are presented.

Chapter 3: Probabilistic risk assessment (PRA) techniques, including event trees, preliminary hazard analyses, checklists, failure mode and effects analysis, hazard and operability studies, and fault trees, are presented, and staff requirements and management considerations are discussed. The appendix includes mathematical techniques and a detailed PRA example.

Chapter 4: Fault-tree symbols and methodology are explored. A new, automated, fault-tree synthesis method based on flows, flow controllers, semantic networks, and event development rules is described and demonstrated.

Chapter 5: Qualitative aspects of system analysis, including cut sets and path sets and the methods of generating them, are described. Common-cause failures, multistate variables, and coherency are treated.

Chapter 6: Probabilistic failure parameters such as failure and repair rates are defined rigorously and the relationships between component parameters are shown. Laplace and Markov analyses are presented. Statistical distributions and their properties are considered.

Chapter 7: Confidence limits of failure parameters, including classical and Bayesian approaches, form the contents of this chapter.

Chapter 8: Methods for synthesizing quantitative system behavior in terms of the occurrence probability of basic failure events are developed and system performance is described in terms of system parameters such as reliability, availability, and mean time to failure. Structure functions, minimal path and cut representations, kinetic-tree theory, and short-cut methods are treated.

Chapter 9: Inclusion-exclusion bounding, standby redundancy Markov transition diagrams, beta-factor, multiple Greek letter, and binomial failure rate models, which are useful tools for system quantification in the presence of dependent basic events, including common-cause failures, are given. Examples are provided.

Chapter 10: Human-error classification, THERP (techniques for human error-rate prediction) methodology for routine and procedure-following error, HCR (human cognitive reliability) models for nonresponse error under time pressure, and confusion models for misdiagnosis are described to quantitatively assess human-error contributions to system failures.

Chapter 11: Parametric uncertainty and modeling uncertainty are examined. The Bayes theorem and log-normal distribution are used for treating parametric uncertainties that, when propagated to system levels, are treated by techniques such as Latin hypercube Monte Carlo simulations, analytical moment methods, and discrete probability algebra.

Chapter 12: Aberrant behavior by lawyers and government regulators are shown to pose greater risks to plant failures than accidents. The risks are described and loss-prevention techniques are suggested.

In using this book as a text, the schedule and sequence of material for a three-credit-hour course are suggested in Tables 1 and 2. A solutions manual for all end-of-chapter problems is available from the authors. Enjoy.

Chapter 12 is based on the experience of one of us (EJH) as director of Maxxim Medical Inc. The author is grateful to the members of the Regulatory Affairs, Human Resources, and Legal Departments of Maxxim Medical Inc. for their generous assistance and source material.

TABLE 1. Undergraduate Course Schedule

Week	Chapter	Topic
1, 2, 3	4	Fault-Tree Construction
4, 5	5	Qualitative Aspects of System Analysis
6	3 (A1, A2)	Probabilities, Venn Diagrams, Boolean Operations
7, 8, 9	6	Quantification of Basic Events
10, 11	7	Confidence Intervals
12, 13	8	Quantitative Aspects of System Analysis

TABLE 2. Graduate Course Schedule

Week	Chapter	Topic
1, 2	1	Basic Risk Concepts
3, 4	2	Accident-Causing Mechanisms and Risk Management
5, 6, 7	3	Probabilistic Risk Assessment
8, 9	9	System Quantification for Dependent Basic Events
10	10	Human Reliability
11, 12	11	Uncertainty Quantification
13	12	Legal and Regulatory Risks

We are grateful to Dudley Kay, and his genial staff at the IEEE Press: Lisa Mizrahi, Carrie Briggs, and Valerie Zaborski. They provided us with many helpful reviews, but because all the reviewers except Charles Donaghey chose to remain anonymous, we can only thank them collectively.

HIROMITSU KUMAMOTO
Kyoto, Japan

ERNEST J. HENLEY
Houston, Texas

1

Basic Risk Concepts

1.1 INTRODUCTION

Risk assessment and risk management are two separate but closely related activities. The fundamental aspects of these two activities are described in this chapter, which provides an introduction to subsequent developments. Section 1.2 presents a formal definition of risk with focus on the assessment and management phases. Sources of debate in current risk studies are described in Section 1.3. Most people perform a risk study to avoid serious mishaps. This is called risk aversion, which is a kernel of risk management; Section 1.4 describes risk aversion. Management requires goals; achievement of goals is checked by assessment. An overview of safety goals is given in Section 1.5.

1.2 FORMAL DEFINITION OF RISK

Risk is a word with various implications. Some people define risk differently from others. This disagreement causes serious confusion in the field of risk assessment and management. The Webster's Collegiate Dictionary, 5th edition, for instance, defines risk as the chance of loss, the degree of probability of loss, the amount of possible loss, the type of loss that an insurance policy covers, and so forth. Dictionary definitions such as these are not sufficiently precise for risk assessment and management. This section provides a formal definition of risk.

1.2.1 Outcomes and Likelihoods

Astronomers can calculate future movements of planets and tell exactly when the next solar eclipse will occur. Psychics of the Delphi Temple of Apollo foretold the future by divine inspiration. These are rare exceptions, however. Just as a TV weatherperson, most people can only forecast or predict the future with considerable uncertainty. Risk is a concept attributable to future uncertainty.

Primary definition of risk. A weather forecast such as "30 percent chance of rain tomorrow" gives two outcomes together with their likelihoods: (30%, rain) and (70%, no rain). Risk is defined as a collection of such pairs of likelihoods and outcomes:*

$$\{(30\%, \text{rain}), (70\%, \text{no rain})\}.$$

More generally, assume n potential outcomes in the doubtful future. Then risk is defined as a collection of n pairs.

$$\text{Risk} \equiv \{(L_1, O_1), \ldots, (L_i, O_i), \ldots, (L_n, O_n)\} \tag{1.1}$$

where O_i and L_i denote outcome i and its likelihood, respectively. Throwing a dice yields the risk,

$$\text{Risk} \equiv \{(1/6, 1),\ (1/6, 2), \ldots, (1/6, 6)\} \tag{1.2}$$

where the outcome is a particular face and the likelihood is probability 1 in 6.

In situations involving random chance, each face involves a beneficial or a harmful event as an ultimate outcome. When the faces are replaced by these outcomes, the risk of throwing the die can be rewritten more explicitly as

$$\text{Risk} \equiv \{(1/6, O_1),\ (1/6, O_2), \ldots, (1/6, O_6)\} \tag{1.3}$$

Risk profile. The distribution pattern of the likelihood-outcome pair is called a risk profile (or a risk curve); likelihoods and outcomes are displayed along vertical and horizontal axes, respectively. Figure 1.1 shows a simple risk profile for the weather forecast described earlier; two discrete outcomes are observed along with their likelihoods, 30% rain or 70% no rain.

In some cases, outcomes are measured by a continuous scale, or the outcomes are so many that they may be continuous rather than discrete. Consider an investment problem where each outcome is a monetary return (gain or loss) and each likelihood is a density of experiencing a particular return. Potential pairs of likelihoods and outcomes then form a continuous profile. Figure 1.2 is a density profile $f(x)$ where a positive or a negative amount of money indicates loss or gain, respectively.

Objective versus subjective likelihood. In a perfect risk profile, each likelihood is expressed as an objective probability, percentage, or density per action or per unit time, or during a specified time interval (see Table 1.1). Objective frequencies such as two occurrences per year and ratios such as one occurrence in one million are also likelihoods; if the frequency is sufficiently small, it can be regarded as a probability or a ratio. Unfortunately, the likelihood is not always exact; probability, percentage, frequency, and ratios may be based on subjective evaluation. Verbal probabilities such as *rare*, *possible*, *plausible*, and *frequent* are also used.

---

*To avoid proliferation of technical terms, a *hazard* or a *danger* is defined in this book as a particular process leading to an undesirable outcome. Risk is a whole distribution pattern of outcomes and likelihoods; different hazards may constitute the risk "fatality," that is, various natural or man-made phenomena may cause fatalities through a variety of processes. The hazard or danger is akin to a causal scenario, and is a more elementary concept than risk.

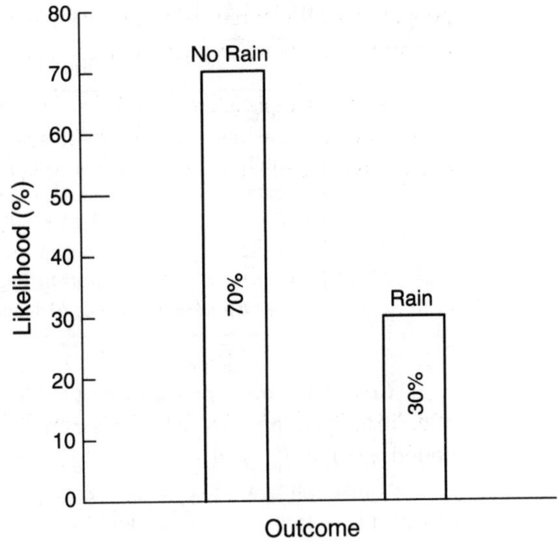

Figure 1.1. Simple risk profile from a weather forecast.

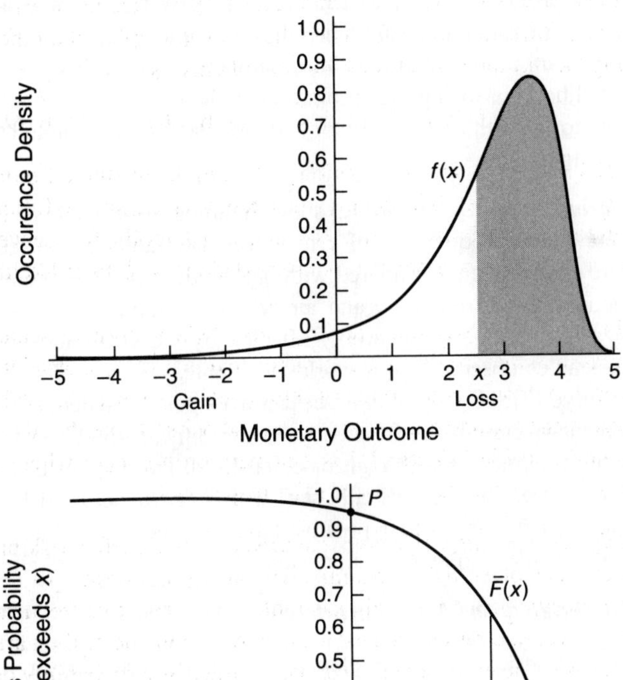

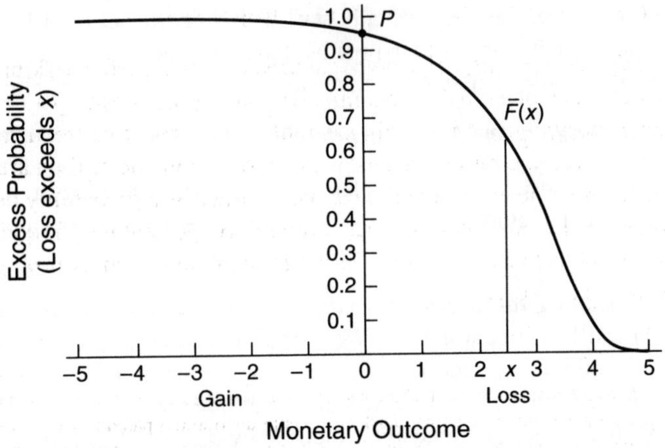

Figure 1.2. Occurrence density and complementary cumulative risk profile.

TABLE 1.1. Examples of Likelihood and Outcome

Likelihood		Outcome Category
Measure	Unit	
Probability Percentage Density Frequency Ratio Verbal Expression	Per Action Per Demand or Operation Per Unit Time During Lifetime During Time Interval Per Mileage	Physical Physiological Psychological Financial Time, Opportunity Societal, Political

Complementary cumulative profile. The risk profile (discrete or continuous) is often displayed in terms of complementary cumulative likelihoods. For instance, the likelihood $\bar{F}(x) = \int_x^\infty f(u)du$ of losing x or more money is displayed rather than the density $f(x)$ of just losing x. The second graph of Figure 1.2 shows a complementary cumulative risk profile obtained from the density profile shown by the first graph. Point P on the vertical axis denotes the probability of losing zero or more money, that is, a probability of not getting any profit. The complementary cumulative likelihood is a monotonously decreasing function of variable x, and hence has a simpler shape than the density function. The complementary representation is informative because decision makers are more interested in the likelihood of losing x or more money than in just x amount of money; for instance, they want to know the probability of "no monetary gain," denoted by point P in the second graph of Figure 1.2.

Farmer curves. Figure 1.3 shows a famous example from the Reactor Safety Study [1] where annual frequencies of x or more early fatalities caused by 100 nuclear power plants are predicted and compared with fatal frequencies by air crashes, fires, dam failures, explosions, chlorine releases, and air crashes. Nonnuclear frequencies are normalized by a size of population potentially affected by the 100 nuclear power plants; these are not frequencies observed on a worldwide scale. Each profile in Figure 1.3 is called a Farmer curve [2]; horizontal and vertical axes generally denote the accident severity and complementary cumulative frequency per unit time, respectively.

Only fatalities greater than or equal to 10 are displayed in Figure 1.3. This is an exceptional case. Fatalities usually start with unity; in actual risk problems, a zero fatality has a far larger frequency than positive fatalities. Inclusion of a zero fatality in the Farmer curve requires the display of an unreasonably wide range of likelihoods.

1.2.2 Uncertainty and Meta-Uncertainty

Uncertainty. A kernel element of risk is uncertainty represented by plural outcomes and their future likelihoods. This point is emphasized by considering cases without uncertainty.

Outcome guaranteed. No risk exists if the future outcome is uniquely known (i.e., $n = 1$) and hence guaranteed. We will all die some day. The probability is equal to 1, so there would be no fatal risk if a sufficiently long time frame is assumed. The rain risk does not exist if there was 100% assurance of rain tomorrow, although there would be other risks such as floods and mudslides induced by the rain. In a formal sense, any risk exists if and only if more than one outcome ($n \geq 2$) are involved with positive likelihoods during a specified future time interval. In this context, a situation with two opposite outcomes with

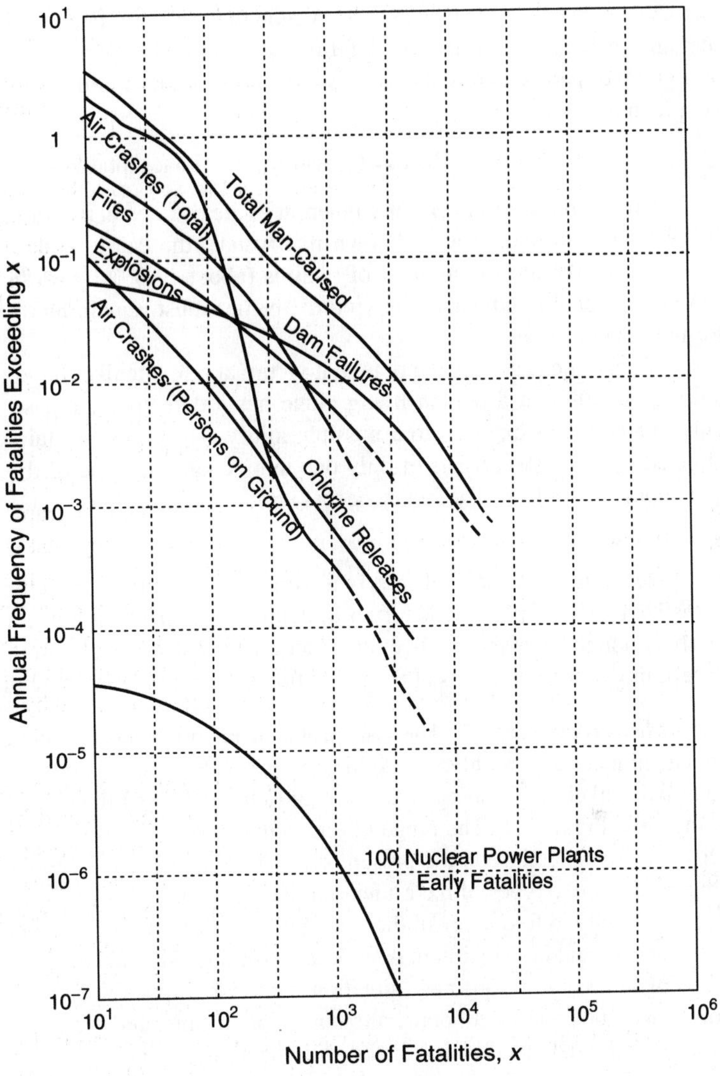

Figure 1.3. Comparison of annual frequency of x or more fatalities.

equal likelihoods may be the most risky one. In less formal usage, however, a situation is called more risky when severities (or levels) of negative outcomes or their likelihoods become larger; an extreme case would be the certain occurrence of a negative outcome.

Outcome localized. A 10^{-6} lifetime likelihood of a fatal accident to the U.S. population of 236 million implies 236 additional deaths over an average lifetime (a 70-year interval). The 236 deaths may be viewed as an acceptable risk in comparison to the 2 million annual deaths in the United States [3].

$$\text{Risk} = (10^{-6}, \text{fatality}): \quad \text{acceptable} \tag{1.4}$$

On the other hand, suppose that 236 deaths by cancer of all workers in a factory are caused, during a lifetime, by some chemical intermediary totally confined to the factory and never released into the environment. This number of deaths completely localized in the factory is not a risk in the usual sense. Although the ratio of fatalities in the U.S. population remains unchanged, that is, 10^{-6}/lifetime, the entire U.S. population is no longer suitable as a group of people exposed to the risk; the population should be replaced by the group of people in the factory.

$$\text{Risk} = (1, \text{fatality}) : \quad \text{unacceptable} \tag{1.5}$$

Thus a source of uncertainty inherent to the risk lies in the anonymity of the victims. If the names of victims were known in advance, the cause of the outcome would be a crime. Even though the number of victims (about 11,000 by traffic accidents in Japan) can be predicted in advance, the victims' names must remain unknown for risk problem formulation purposes.

If only one person is the potential victim at risk, the likelihood must be smaller than unity. Assume that a person living alone has a defective staircase in his house. Then only one person is exposed to a possible injury caused by the staircase. The population affected by this risk consists of only one individual; the name of the individual is known and anonymity is lost. The injury occurs with a small likelihood and the risk concept still holds.

Outcome realized. There is also no risk after the time point when an outcome is realized. The airplane risk for an individual passenger disappears after the landing or crash, although he or she, if alive, now faces other risks such as automobile accidents. The uncertainty in the risk exists at the prediction stage and before its realization.

Meta-uncertainty. The risk profile itself often has associated uncertainties that are called meta-uncertainties. A subjective estimate of uncertainties for a complementary cumulative likelihood was carried out by the authors of the Limerick Study [4]. Their result is shown in Figure 1.4. The range of uncertainty stretches over three orders of magnitude. This is a fair reflection on the present state of the art of risk assessment. The error bands are a result of two types of meta-uncertainties: uncertainty in outcome level of an accident and uncertainty in frequency of the accident. The existence of this meta-uncertainty makes risk management or decision making under risk difficult and controversial.

In summary, an ordinary situation with risk implies uncertainty due to plural outcomes with positive likelihoods, anonymity of victims, and prediction before realization. Moreover, the risk itself is associated with meta-uncertainty.

1.2.3 Risk Assessment and Management

Risk assessment. A principal purpose of risk assessment is the derivation of risk profiles posed by a given situation; the weatherman performed a risk assessment when he promulgated the risk profile in Figure 1.1. The Farmer curves in Figures 1.3 and 1.4 are final products of a methodology called probabilistic risk assessment (PRA), which, among other things, enumerates outcomes and quantifies their likelihoods.

For nuclear power plants, the PRA proceeds as follows: enumeration of sequences of events that could produce a core melt; clarification of containment failure modes, their probabilities and timing; identification of quantity and chemical form of radioactivity released if the containment is breached; modeling of dispersion of radionuclides in the atmosphere; modeling of emergency response effectiveness involving sheltering, evacuation, and medical treatment; and dose-response modeling in estimating health effects on the population exposed [5].

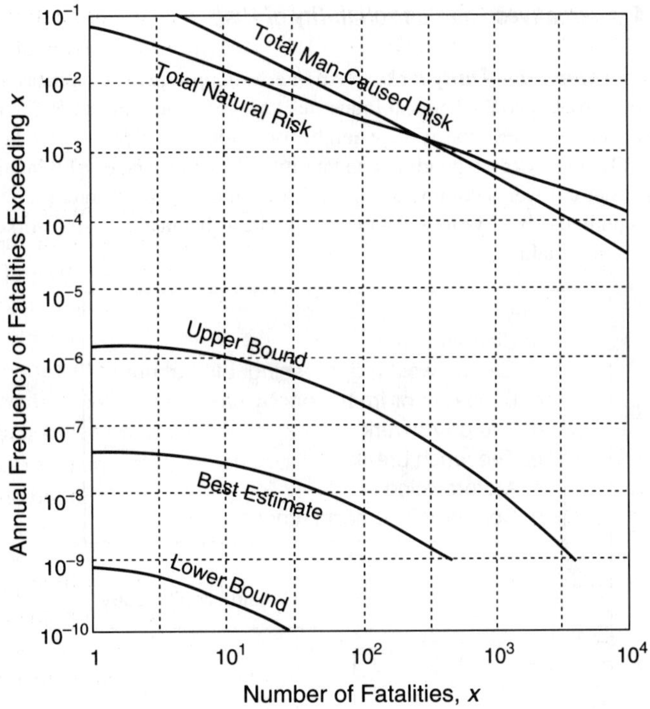

Figure 1.4. Example of meta-uncertainty of a complementary cumulative risk profile.

Risk management. Risk management proposes alternatives, evaluates (for each alternative) the risk profile, makes safety decisions, chooses satisfactory alternatives to control the risk, and exercises corrective actions.*

Assessment versus management. When risk management is performed in relation to a PRA, the two activities are called a probabilistic risk assessment and management (PRAM). This book focuses on PRAM.

The probabilistic risk assessment phase is more scientific, technical, formal, quantitative, and objective than the management phase, which involves value judgment and heuristics, and hence is more subjective, qualitative, societal, and political. Ideally, the PRA is based on objective likelihoods such as electric bulb failure rates inferred from statistical data and theories. However, the PRA is often compelled to use subjective likelihoods based on intuition, expertise, and partial, defective, or deceitful data, and dubious theories. These constitute the major source of meta-uncertainty in the risk profile.

Considerable efforts are being made to establish a unified and scientific PRAM methodology where subjective assessment, value judgment, expertise, and heuristics are dealt with more objectively. Nonetheless the subjective or human dimension does constitute one of the two pillars that support the entire conceptual edifice [3].

---

*Terms such as *risk estimation* and *risk evaluation* only cause confusion, and should be avoided.

1.2.4 Alternatives and Controllability of Risk

Example 1—Daily risks. An interesting perspective on the risks of our daily activity was developed by Imperial Chemical Industries Ltd. [6]. The ordinate of Figure 1.5 is the fatal accident frequency rate (FAFR), the average number of deaths by accidents in 10^8 hours of a particular activity. An FAFR of unity corresponds to one fatality in 11,415 years, or 87.6 fatalities per one million years. Thus a motor driver according to Figure 1.5 would, on the average, encounter a fatal accident if she drove continuously 17 years and 4 months, while a chemical industry worker requires more than 3000 years for his fatality. ■

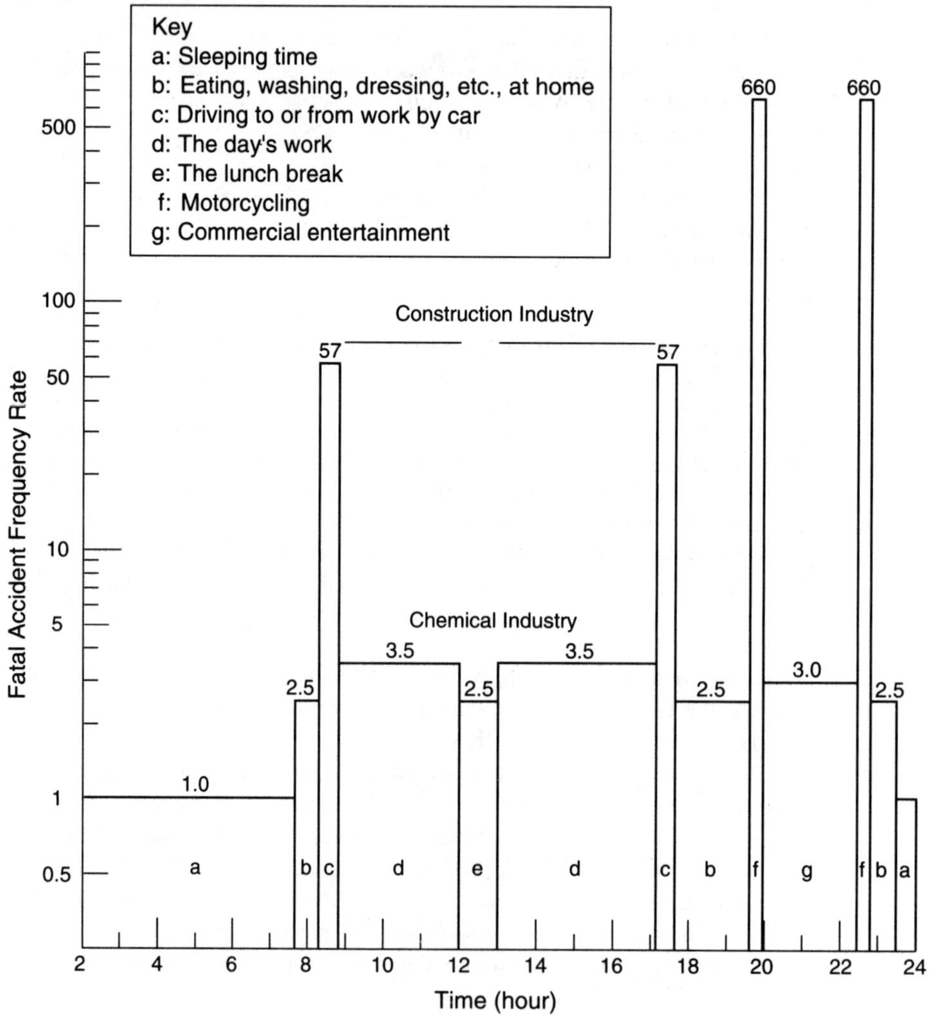

Figure 1.5. Fatal accident frequency rates of daily activities.

Risk control. The potential for plural outcomes and single realization by chance recur endlessly throughout our lives. This recursion is a source of diversity in human affairs. Our lives would be monotonous if future outcomes were unique at birth and there were no risks at all; this book would be useless too. Fortunately, enough or even an excessive amount of risk surrounds us. Many people try to assess and manage risks; some succeed and others fail.

Active versus passive controllability. Although the weatherperson performs a risk assessment, he cannot alter the likelihood, because rain is an uncontrollable natural phenomenon. However, he can perform a risk management together with the assessment; he can passively control or mitigate the rain hazard by suggesting that people take an umbrella; the outcome "rain" can be mitigated to "rain with umbrella."

Figure 1.5 shows seven sources (a to g) of the fatality risk. PRA deals with risks of human activities and systems found in engineering, economics, medicine, and so forth, where likelihoods of some outcomes can be controlled by active intervention, in addition to the passive mitigation of other outcomes.

Alternatives and controllability. Active or passive controllability of risks inherently assumes that each alternative chosen by a decision maker during the risk-management phase has a specific risk profile. A baseline decision or action is also an alternative. In some cases, only the baseline alternative is available, and no room is left for choice. For instance, if an umbrella is not available, people would go out without it. Similarly, passengers in a commercial airplane flying at 33,000 feet have only the one alternative of continuing the flight. In these cases, the risk is uncontrollable. Some alternatives have no appreciable effect on the risk profile, while others bring desired effects; some are more cost effective than others.

Example 2—Alternatives for rain hazard mitigation. Figure 1.6 shows a simple tree for the rain hazard mitigation problem. Two alternatives exist: 1) going out with an umbrella (A_1), and 2) going out without an umbrella (A_2). Four outcomes are observed: 1) O_{11} = rain, with umbrella; 2) O_{21} = no rain, with umbrella; 3) O_{12} = rain, without umbrella; and 4) O_{22} = no rain, without umbrella. The second subscript denotes a particular alternative, and the first a specific outcome under the alternative. In this simple example, the rain hazard is mitigated by the umbrella, though the likelihood (30%) of rain remains unchanged. Two different risk profiles appear, depending on the alternative chosen, where R_1 and R_2 denote the risks with and without the umbrella, respectively:

$$R_1 = \{(30\%, O_{11}), (70\%, O_{21})\} \tag{1.6}$$

$$R_2 = \{(30\%, O_{12}), (70\%, O_{22})\} \tag{1.7}$$

■

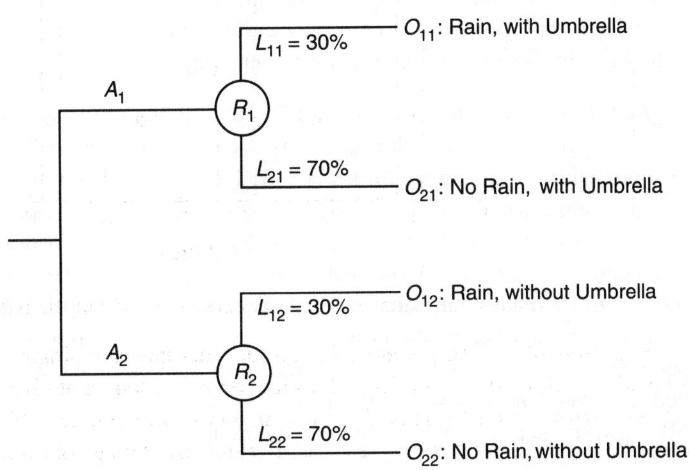

Figure 1.6. Simple branching tree for rain hazard mitigation problem.

In general, a choice of particular alternative A_j yields risk profile R_j where likelihood L_{ij}, outcome O_{ij}, and total number n_j of outcomes vary from alternative to alternative:

$$R_j = \{(L_{ij},\ O_{ij}) \mid i = 1, \ldots, n_j)\}, \qquad j = 1, \ldots, m \tag{1.8}$$

The subscript j denotes a particular alternative. This representation denotes an explicit dependence of the risk profile on the alternative.

Choices and alternatives exist in almost every activity: product design, manufacture, test, maintenance, personnel management, finance, commerce, health care, leisure, and so on. In the rain hazard mitigation problem in Figure 1.6, only outcomes could be modified. In risk control problems for engineering systems, both likelihoods and outcomes may be modified, for instance, by improving plant designs and operation and maintenance procedures. Operating the plant without modification or closing the operation are also alternatives.

Outcome matrix. A baseline risk profile changes to a new one when a different alternative is chosen. For the rain hazard mitigation problem, two sets of outcomes exist, as shown in Table 1.2. The matrix showing the relation between the alternative and outcome is called an outcome matrix. The column labeled *utility* will be described later.

TABLE 1.2. Outcome Matrix of Rain Hazard Mitigation Problem

Alternative	Likelihood	Outcome	Utility
A_1: With umbrella	$L_{11} = 30\%$	O_{11}: Rain, with umbrella	$U_{11} = 1$
	$L_{21} = 70\%$	O_{21}: No rain, with umbrella	$U_{21} = 0.5$
A_2: Without umbrella	$L_{12} = 30\%$	O_{12}: Rain, without umbrella	$U_{12} = 0$
	$L_{22} = 70\%$	O_{22}: No rain, without umbrella	$U_{22} = 1$

Lotteries. Assume that m alternatives are available. The choice of alternative A_j is nothing but a choice of lottery R_j among the m lotteries, the term *lottery* being used to indicate a general probabilistic set of outcomes. Two lotteries, R_1 and R_2, are available for the rain hazard mitigation problem in Figure 1.6; each lottery yields a particular statistical outcome. There is a one-to-one correspondence among risk, risk profile, lottery, and alternative; these terms may be used interchangeably.

Risk-free alternatives. Figure 1.7 shows another situation with two exclusive alternatives A_1 and A_2. When alternative A_1 is chosen, there is a fifty-fifty chance of losing \$1000 or nothing; the expected loss is $(1000 \times 0.5) + (0 \times 0.5) = \$500$. The second alternative causes a certain loss of \$500. In other words, only one outcome can occur when alternative A_2 is chosen; this is a risk-free alternative, as a payment for accident insurance to compensate for the \$1000 loss that occurs with probability 0.5. Alternative A_1 has two outcomes and is riskier than alternative A_2 because of the potential of the large \$1000 loss.

It is generally believed that most people prefer a certain loss to the same amount of expected loss; that is, they will buy insurance for \$500 to avoid lottery R_1. This attitude is called risk aversion; they would not buy insurance, however, if the payment is more than \$750, because the payment becomes considerably larger than the expected loss.

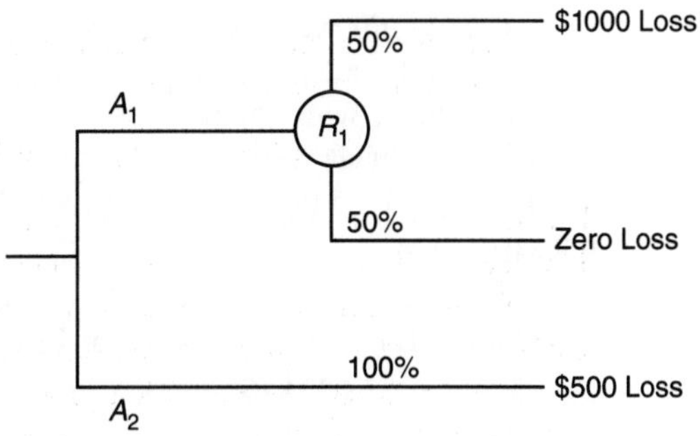

Figure 1.7. Risky alternative and risk-free alternative.

Some people seek thrills and expose themselves to the first lottery without buying the $500 insurance; this attitude is called *risk seeking* or *risk prone*. Some may buy insurance if the payment is, for instance, $250 or less, because the payment is now considerably smaller than the expected loss.

The risk-free alternative is often used as a reference point in evaluating risky alternatives like lottery R_1. In other words, the risky alternative is evaluated by how people trade it off with a risk-free alternative that has a fixed amount of gain or loss, as would be provided by an insurance policy.

Alternatives as barriers. The MORT (management oversight and risk tree) technique considers injuries, fatalities, and physical damage caused by an unwanted release of energy whose forms may be kinetic, potential, chemical, thermal, electrical, ionizing radiation, non-ionizing radiation, acoustic, or biologic. Typical alternatives for controlling the risks are called barriers in MORT [7] and are listed in Table 1.3.

TABLE 1.3. Typical Alternatives for Risk Control

Barriers	Examples
1. Limit the energy (or substitute a safer form)	Low voltage instruments, safer solvents, quantity limitation
2. Prevent build-up	Limit controls, fuses, gas detectors, floor loading
3. Prevent the release	Containment, insulation
4. Provide for slow release	Rupture disc, safety valve, seat belts, shock absorption
5. Channel the release away, that is, separate in time or space	Roping off areas, aisle marking, electrical grounding, lockouts, interlocks
6. Put a barrier on the energy source	Sprinklers, filters, acoustic treatment
7. Put a barrier between the energy source and men or objects	Fire doors, welding shields
8. Put a barrier on the man or object to block or attenuate the energy	Shoes, hard hats, gloves, respirators, heavy protectors
9. Raise the injury or damage threshold	Selection, acclimatization to heat or cold
10. Treat or repair	Emergency showers, transfer to low radiation job, rescue, emergency medical care
11. Rehabilitate	Relaxation, recreation, recuperation

Cost of alternatives. The costs of life-saving alternatives in dollars per life saved have been estimated and appear in Table 1.4 [5]. Improved medical X-ray equipment requires $3600, while home kidney dialysis requires $530,000. A choice of alternative is sometimes made through a risk-cost-benefit (RCB) or risk-cost (RC) analysis. For an automobile, where there is a risk of a traffic accident, a seat belt or an air bag adds costs but saves lives.

TABLE 1.4. Cost Estimates for Life-saving Alternatives in Dollars per Life Saved

Risk Reduction Alternatives	Estimated Cost (Dollars)
1. Improved medical X-ray equipment	3,600
2. Improved highway maintenance practices	20,000
3. Screening for cervical cancer	30,000
4. Proctoscopy for colon/rectal cancer	30,000
5. Mobile cardiac emergency unit	30,000
6. Road guardrail improvements	30,000
7. Tuberculosis control	40,000
8. Road skid resistance	40,000
9. Road rescue helicopters	70,000
10. Screening for lung cancer	70,000
11. Screening for breast cancer	80,000
12. Automobile driver education	90,000
13. Impact-absorbing roadside device	110,000
14. Breakaway signs and lighting posts	120,000
15. Smoke alarms in homes	240,000
16. Road median barrier improvements	230,000
17. Tire inspection	400,000
18. Highway rescue cars	420,000
19. Home kidney dialysis	530,000

1.2.5 Outcome Significance

Significance of outcome. The significance of each outcome from each alternative must be evaluated in terms of an amount of gain or loss if an optimal and satisfactory alternative is to be chosen. Significance varies directly with loss and inversely with gain. An inverse measure of the significance is called a utility, or value function (see Table 1.5).* In PRA, the outcome and significance are sometimes called a consequence and a magnitude, respectively, especially when loss outcomes such as property damage and fatality are considered.

Example 3—Rain hazard decision-making problem. Assume that the hypothetical outcome utilities in Table 1.2 apply for the problem of rain hazard mitigation. The two outcomes "O_{11}: rain, with umbrella" and "O_{22}: no rain, without umbrella" are equally preferable and scored as unity. A less preferable outcome is "O_{21}: no rain, with umbrella" scored as 0.5. Outcome "O_{12}: rain, without umbrella" is least preferable with a score of zero. These utility values are defined for

*The significance, utility, or value are formal, nonlinear measures for representing outcome severity. The significance of two fatalities is not necessarily equal to twice the single fatality significance. Proportional measures such as lost money, lost time, and number of fatalities are often used for practical applications without nonlinear value judgments.

TABLE 1.5. Examples of Outcome Severity and Risk Level Measure

Outcome Severity Measure	Risk Level Measure
Significance	Expected significance
Utility, value	Expected utility or value
Lost money	Expected money loss
Fatalities	Expected fatalities
Longevity loss	Expected longevity loss
Dose	Expected outcome severity
Concentration	Severity for fixed outcome
Lost time	Likelihood for fixed outcome

outcomes, not for the risk profile of each alternative. As shown in Figure 1.8, it is necessary to create a utility value (or a significance value) for each alternative or for each risk profile. Because the outcomes occur statistically, an expected utility for the risk profile becomes a reasonable measure to unify the elementary utility values for outcomes in the profile.

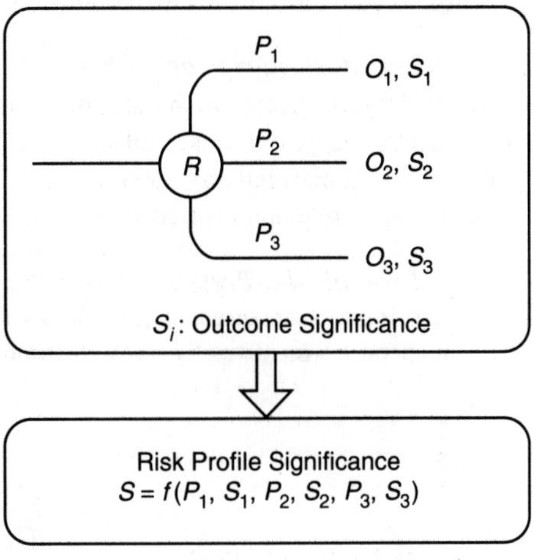

Figure 1.8. Risk profile significance derived from outcome significance.

The expected utility EU_1 for alternative A_1 is

$$EU_1 = (0.3 \times U_{11}) + (0.7 \times U_{21}) \tag{1.9}$$
$$= (0.3 \times 1) + (0.7 \times 0.5) = 0.65 \tag{1.10}$$

while the expected utility EU_2 for alternative A_2 is

$$EU_2 = (0.3 \times U_{12}) + (0.7 \times U_{22}) \tag{1.11}$$
$$= (0.3 \times 0) + (0.7 \times 1) = 0.7 \tag{1.12}$$

The second alternative, without the umbrella, is chosen because it has a larger expected utility. A person would take an umbrella, however, if elementary utility U_{21} is increased, for instance, to 0.9, which indicates that carrying the useless umbrella becomes a minor burden. A breakeven point for U_{21} satisfies $0.3 + 0.7U_{21} = 0.7$, that is, $U_{21} = (0.7 - 0.3)/0.7 = 0.57$.

Sensitivity analyses similar to this can be performed for the likelihood of rain. Assume again the utility values in Table 1.2. Denote by P the probability of rain. Then, a breakeven point for P satisfies

$$EU_1 = P \times 1 + (1 - P) \times 0.5 = P \times 0 + (1 - P) \times 1 = EU_2 \tag{1.13}$$

yielding $P = 0.5$. In other words, a person should not take the umbrella as long as the chance of rain is less than 50%. ■

The risk profile for each alternative now includes the utility U_i (or significance):

$$\text{Risk} \equiv \{(L_i, O_i, U_i) \mid i = 1, \ldots, n\} \tag{1.14}$$

This representation indicates an explicit dependence of a risk profile on outcome significance: the determination of the significance is a value judgment and is considered mainly in the risk-management phase. The significance is implicitly assumed when minor outcomes are screened out during the risk-assessment phase.

1.2.6 Causal Scenario

The likelihood as well as the outcome significance can be evaluated more easily when a causal scenario for the outcome is in place. Thus risk may be rewritten as

$$\text{Risk} \equiv \{(L_i, O_i, U_i, CS_i) \mid i = 1, \ldots, n\} \tag{1.15}$$

where CS_i denotes the causal scenario that specifies 1) causes of outcome O_i and 2) event propagations for the outcome. This representation expresses an explicit dependence of risk profile on the causal scenario identified during the risk-assessment phase.

Causal scenarios and PRA. PRA uses, among other things, event tree and fault tree techniques to establish outcomes and causal scenarios. A scenario is called an accident sequence and is composed of various deleterious interactions among devices, software, information, material, power sources, humans, and environment. These techniques are also used to quantify outcome likelihoods during the risk-assessment phase.

Example 4—Pressure tank PRA. The system shown in Figure 1.9 discharges gas from a reservoir into a pressure tank [8]. The switch is normally closed and the pumping cycle is initiated by an operator who manually resets the timer. The timer contact closes and pumping starts.

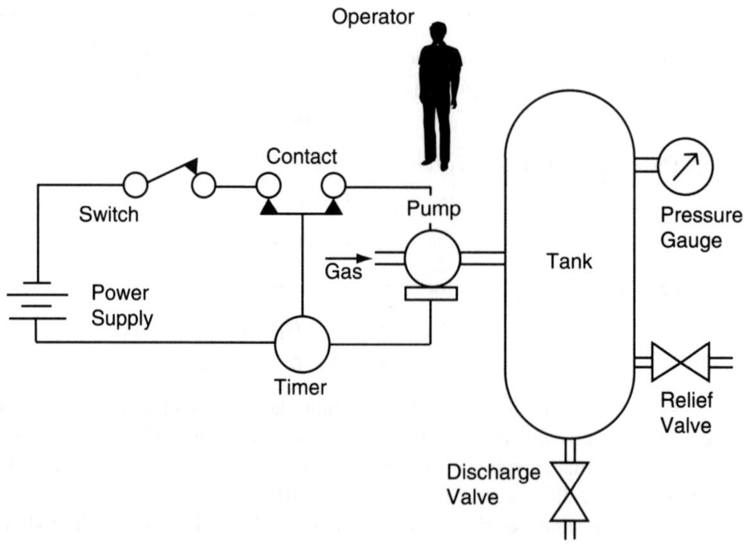

Figure 1.9. Schematic diagram of pressure tank system.

Well before any over-pressure condition exists the timer times out and the timer contact opens. Current to the pump cuts off and pumping ceases (to prevent a tank rupture due to overpressure). If the timer contact does not open, the operator is instructed to observe the pressure gauge and to open the manual switch, thus causing the pump to stop. Even if the timer and operator both fail, overpressure can be relieved by the relief valve.

After each cycle, the compressed gas is discharged by opening the valve and then closing it before the next cycle begins. At the end of the operating cycle, the operator is instructed to verify the operability of the pressure gauge by observing the decrease in the tank pressure as the discharge valve is opened. To simplify the analysis, we assume that the tank is depressurized before the cycle begins. An undesired event, from a risk viewpoint, is a pressure tank rupture by overpressure.

Note that the pressure gauge may fail during the new cycle even if its operability was correctly checked by the operator at the end of the last cycle. The gauge can fail before a new cycle if the operator commits an inspection error.

Figure 1.10 shows the event tree and fault tree for the pressure tank rupture due to overpressure. The event tree starts with an initiating event that initiates the accident sequence. The tree describes combinations of success or failure of the system's mitigative features that lead to desired or undesired plant states. In Figure 1.10, PO denotes the event "pump overrun," an initiating event that starts the potential accident scenarios. Symbol OS denotes the failure of the operator shutdown system, PP denotes failure of the pressure protection system by relief valve failure. The overbar indicates a logic complement of the inadvertent event, that is, successful activation of the mitigative feature. There are three sequences or scenarios displayed in Figure 1.10. The scenario labeled $PO \cdot OS \cdot PP$ causes overpressure and tank rupture, where symbol "·" denotes logic intersection, (AND). Therefore the tank rupture requires three simultaneous failures. The other two scenarios lead to safe results.

The event tree defines top events, each of which can be analyzed by a fault tree that develops more basic causes such as hardware or human faults. We see, for instance, that the pump overrun is caused by timer contact fails to open, or timer failure.* By linking the three fault trees (or their logic complements) along a scenario on the event tree, possible causes for each scenario can be enumerated. For instance, tank rupture occurs when the following three basic causes occur simultaneously: 1) timer contact fails to open, 2) switch contact fails to open, and 3) pressure relief valve fails to open. Probabilities for these three causes can be estimated from generic or plant-specific statistical data, and eventually the probability of the tank rupture due to overpressure can be quantified. ■

1.2.7 Population Affected

Final definition of risk. A population of a single individual is an exceptional case. Usually more than one person is affected anonymously by the risk. The population size is a factor that determines an important aspect of the risk. A comparison of risks using the Farmer curves in Figures 1.3 and 1.4 makes no sense unless the population is specified. The risk concept includes, as a final element, the population PO_i affected by outcome O_i.

$$\text{Risk} \equiv \{(L_i, O_i, U_i, CS_i, PO_i) \mid i = 1, \ldots, n\} \tag{1.16}$$

Populations are identified during the risk-assessment phase.

1.2.8 Population Versus Individual Risk

Definitions of two types of risks. The term *population risk* is used when a population as a whole is at risk. A population risk is also called a societal risk, a collective risk, or a societally aggregated risk. When a particular individual in the population is the risk recipient, then the risk is an individual risk and the population PO_i in the definition of risk reduces to a single person.

---

*Output event from an OR gate occurs when one or more input events occur; output event from an AND gate occurs when all input events occur simultaneously.

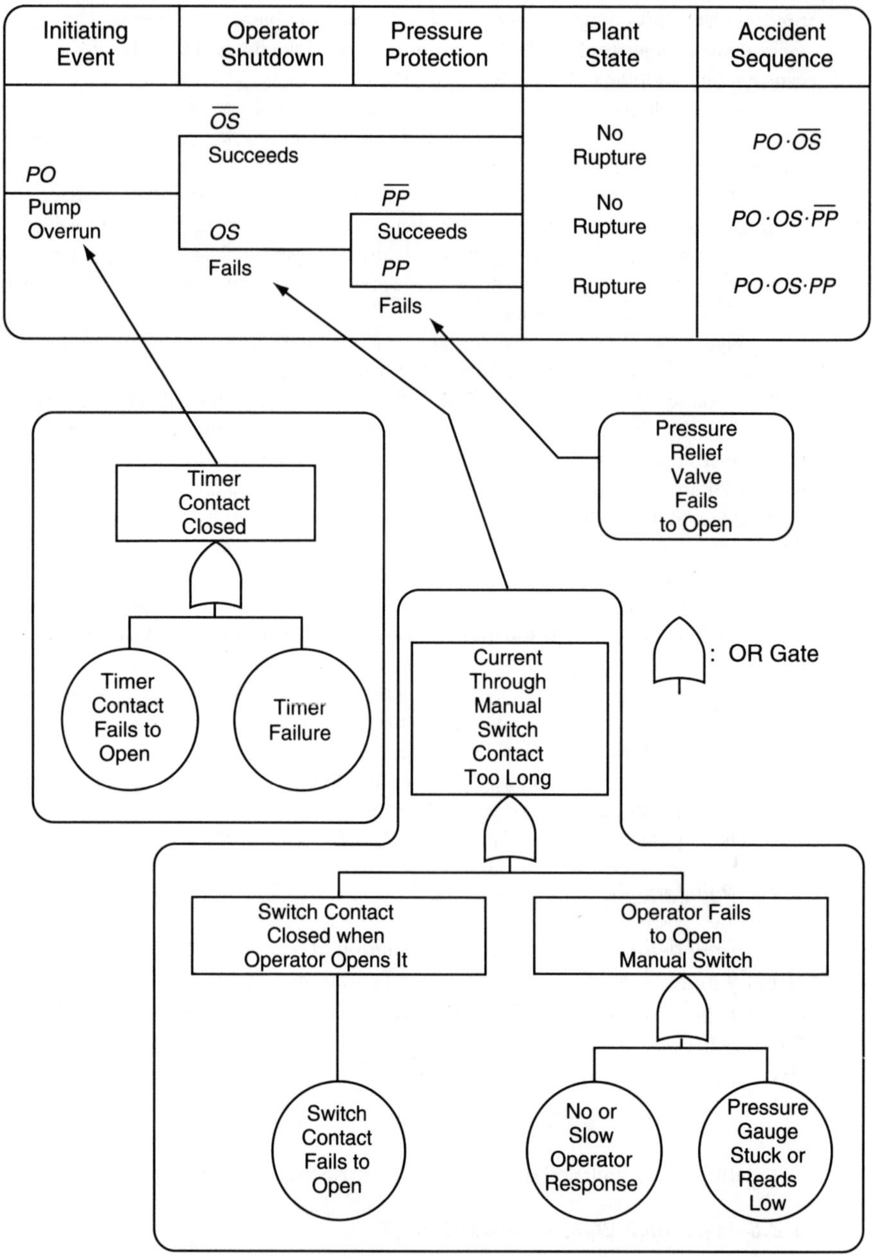

Figure 1.10. Event-tree and fault-tree analyses for pressure tank system.

Risk level measures. A risk profile is formally measured by an expected significance or utility (Table 1.5). A typical measure representing the level of individual risk is the likelihood or severity of a particular outcome or the expected outcome severity. Measures for the level of population risk are, for example, an expected number of people affected by the outcome or the sum of expected outcome severities.

If the outcome is a fatality, the individual risk level may be expressed by a fatal frequency (i.e., likelihood) per individual, and the population risk level by an expected number of fatalities. For radioactive exposure, the individual risk level may be measured by an individual dose (rem per person; expected outcome severity), and the population risk level by a collective dose (person rem; expected sum of outcome severities). The collective dose (or population dose) is the summation of individual doses over a population.

Population-size effect. Assume that a deleterious outcome brings an average individual risk of one fatality per million years, per person [9]. If 1000 people are affected by the outcome, the population risk would be 10^{-3} fatalities per year, per population. The same individual risk applied to the entire U.S. population of 235 million produces the risk of 235 fatalities per year. Therefore the same individual risk brings different societal risk depending on the size of the population (Figure 1.11).

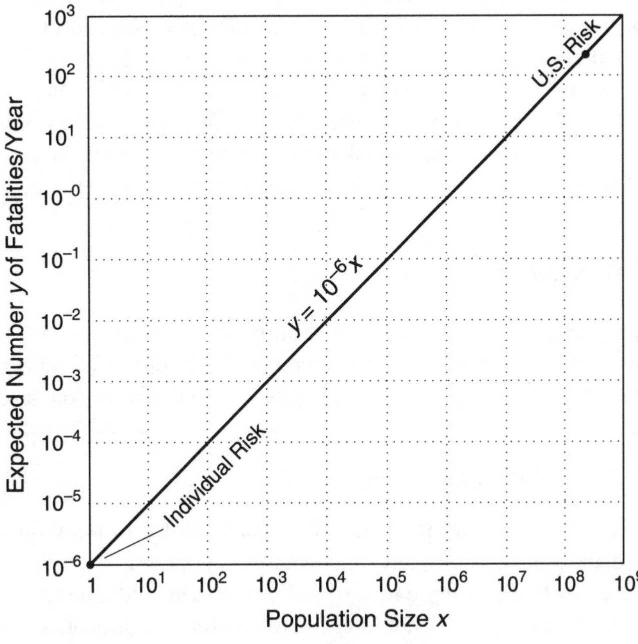

Figure 1.11. Expected number of annual fatalities under 10^{-6} individual risk.

Regulatory response (or no response) is likely to treat these two population risks comparably because the individual risk remains the same. However, there is a difference between the two population risks. There are severe objections to siting nuclear power plants within highly populated metropolitan centers; neither those opposed to nuclear power nor representatives from the nuclear power industry would seriously consider this option [3].

Individual versus population approach. An approach based on individual risk is appropriate in cases where a small number of individuals face relatively high risks; hence if the individual risk is reduced to a sufficiently small level, then the population risk also becomes sufficiently small. For a population of ten people, the population risk measured by the expected number of fatalities is only ten times larger than the individual risk measured by fatality frequency. But when a large number of people faces a low-to-moderate risk, then the individual risk alone is not sufficient because the population risk might be a large number [9].*

1.2.9 Summary

Risk is formally defined as a combination of five primitives: outcome, likelihood, significance, causal scenario, and population affected. These factors determine the risk profile. The risk-assessment phase deals with primitives other than the outcome significance, which is evaluated in the risk-management phase.

Each alternative for actively or passively controlling the risk creates a specific risk profile. The profile is evaluated using an expected utility to unify the outcome significance, and decisions are made accordingly. This point is illustrated by the rain hazard mitigation problem. One-to-one correspondences exist among risk, risk profile, lottery, and alternative. A risk-free alternative is often used as a reference point in evaluating risky alternatives. Typical alternatives for risk control are listed in Table 1.3.

The pressure tank problem illustrates some aspects of probabilistic risk assessment. Here, the fault-tree technique is used in combination with the event-tree technique.

Two important types of risk are presented: individual risk and population risk. The size of the population is a crucial parameter in risk management.

1.3 SOURCE OF DEBATES

The previous section presents a rather simplistic view of risks and associated decisions. In practice, risk-assessment and -management viewpoints differ considerably from site to site. These differences are a major source of debate, and this section describes why such debates occur.

1.3.1 Different Viewpoints Toward Risk

Figure 1.12 shows perspectives toward risk by an individual affected, a population affected, the public, a company that owns and/or operates a facility, and a regulatory agency. Each has a different attitude toward risk assessment and management.

The elements of risk are likelihood, outcome, significance, causal scenario, and population. Risk assessment determines the likelihood, outcome, causal scenario, and population. Determination of significance involves a value judgment and belongs to the risk-management phase. An important final product of the management phase is a decision that requires more than outcome significances; the outcome significances must be synthesized into a measure that evaluates a risk profile containing plural outcomes (see Figure 1.8).

In the following sections, differences in risk assessment are described first by focusing on all risk elements except significance. Then the significance and related problems such as risk aversion are discussed in terms of risk management.

---

*The Nuclear Regulatory Commission recently reduced the distance for computing the population cancer fatality risk to 10 mi from 50 mi [10]. The average individual risk for the 10-mi distance is larger than the value for the 50-mi distance because the risk to people beyond 10 mi will be less than the risk to the people within 10 mi. Thus it makes sense to make regulations based on the conservative 10-mi individual risk. However, the 50-mi population risk could be significantly larger than the 10-mi population risk unless individual risk or population density diminish rapidly with distance.

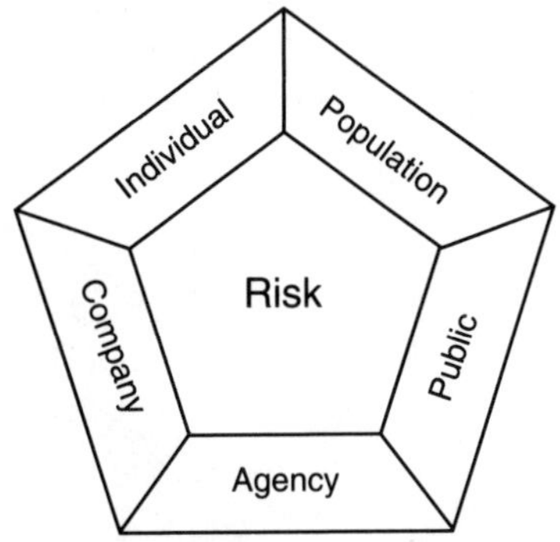

Figure 1.12. Five views of risk.

1.3.2 Differences in Risk Assessment

Outcome and causal scenario. Different people usually select different sets of outcomes because such sets are only obtainable through prediction. It is easy to miss novel outcomes such as, in the early 1980s, the transmission of AIDS by blood transfusion and sexual activity. Some question the basic premise of PRA—that is, the feasibility of enumerating all outcomes for new technologies and novel situations.

Event-tree and fault-tree techniques are used in PRA to enumerate outcomes and scenarios. However, each PRA creates different trees and consequently different outcomes and scenarios, because tree generation is an art, not a science. For instance, Figure 1.10 only analyzes tank rupture due to overpressure and neglects 1) a rupture of a defective tank under normal pressure, 2) an implosion due to low pressure, or 3) sabotage.

The nuclear power plant PRA analyzes core melt scenarios by event- and fault-tree techniques. However, these techniques are not the only ones used in the PRA. Containment capability after the core melt is evaluated by different techniques that model complicated physical and chemical dynamics occurring inside the containment and reactor vessels. Source terms (i.e., amount and types of radioactive materials released from the reactor site) from the containment are predicted as a result of such analyses. Different sets of assumptions and models yield different sets of scenarios and source terms.

Population affected. At intermediate steps of the PRA, only outcomes inside or on a boundary of the facility are dealt with. Examples of outcomes are chemical plant explosions, nuclear reactor core melts, or source terms. A technique called a consequence analysis is then performed to convert these internal or boundary outcomes into outside consequences such as radiation doses, property damage, and contamination of the environment. The consequence analysis is also based on uncertain assumptions and models. Figure 1.13 shows transport of the source term into the environment when a wind velocity is given.

Outcome chain termination. Outcomes engender new outcomes. The space shuttle schedule was delayed and the U.S. space market share reduced due to the Challenger accident. A manager of a chemical plant in Japan committed suicide after the explosion of his plant. Ultimately, outcome propagations terminate.

Likelihood. PRA uses event-tree and fault-tree techniques to search for basic causes of outcomes. It is assumed that these causes are so basic that historic statistical data are available to quantify the occurrence probabilities of these causes. This is feasible for simple hardware failures such as a pump failing to start and for simple human errors

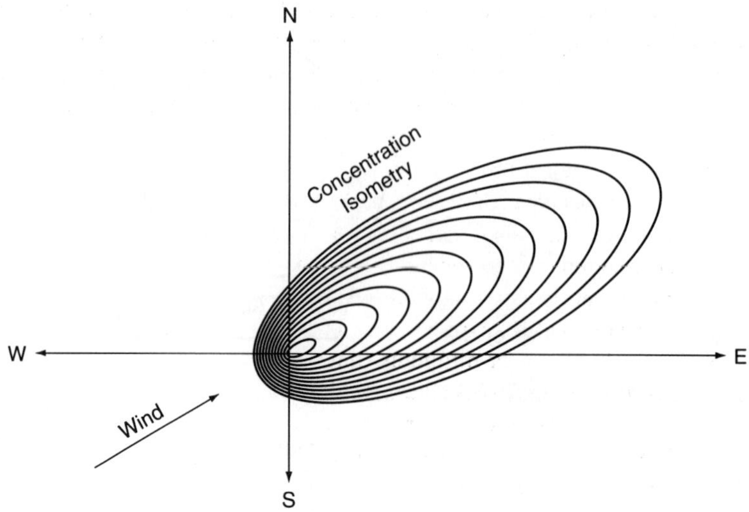

Figure 1.13. Schematic description of source term transport.

such as an operator inadvertently closing a valve. For novel hardware failures and for complicated cognitive human errors, however, available data are so sparse that subjective probabilities must be guesstimated from expert opinions. This causes discrepancies in likelihood estimates for basic causes.

Consider a misdiagnosis as the cognitive error. Figure 1.14 shows a schematic for a diagnostic task consisting of five activities: recollection of hypotheses (causes and their propagations) from symptoms, acceptance/rejection of a hypothesis in using qualitative or quantitative simulations, selection of a goal such as plant shutdown when the hypothesis is accepted, selection of means to achieve the goal, and execution of the means. A misdiagnosis occurs if an individual commits an error in any of these activities. Failure probabilities in the first four activities are difficult to quantify, and subjective estimates called *expert opinions* are often used.

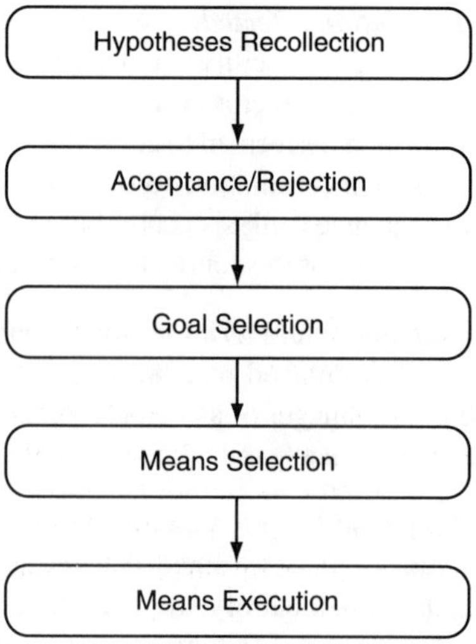

Figure 1.14. Typical steps of diagnosis task.

The subjective likelihood is estimated differently depending on whether the risk is controlled by individuals or systems. Most drivers believe in their driving skills and underestimate likelihoods of their involvement in automobile accidents in spite of the fact that the statistical accident rate is derived from a population that largely includes the skilled drivers.

Quantification of basic causes must be synthesized into the outcome likelihood through AND and OR causal propagation logic. Again, event- and fault-tree techniques are used. There are various types of dependencies, however, among the basic and intermediate causes of the outcome. For instance, several valves may have been simultaneously left closed if the same maintenance person incorrectly manipulated them. Evaluation of this dependency is crucial in that it causes significant differences in outcome likelihood estimates.

By a nuclear PRA consequence analysis, the source term is converted into a radiation dose in units of rems or millirems (mrems) per person in a way partly illustrated in Figure 1.13. The individual or collective dose must be converted into a likelihood of cancers when latent fatality risk is quantified; a conservative estimate is a ratio of 135 fatalities per million person-rems. Figure 1.15 shows this conversion [11], where the horizontal and vertical axes denote amount of exposure in terms of person-rems and probability of cancer, respectively. A linear, nonthreshold, dose-rate-independent model is typical. Many radiologists, however, believe that this model yields an incorrect estimate of cancer probability. Some people use a linear-quadratic form, while others support a pure quadratic form.

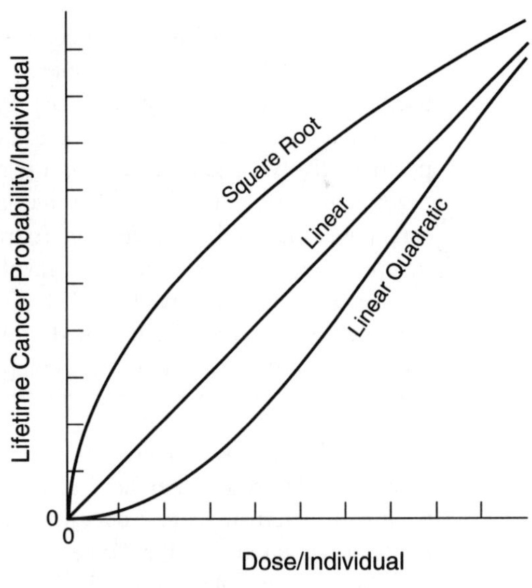

Figure 1.15. Individual dose and lifetime cancer probability.

The likelihood may not be a unique number. Assume the likelihood is ambiguous and somewhere between 3 in 10 and 7 in 10. A likelihood of likelihoods (i.e., meta-likelihood) must be introduced to deal with the meta-uncertainty of the likelihood itself. Figure 1.4 included a meta-uncertainty as an error bound of outcome frequencies. People, however, may have different opinions about this meta-likelihood; for instance, any of 90%, 95%, or 99% confidence intervals of the likelihood itself could be used. Furthermore, some people challenge the feasibility of assigning likelihoods to future events; we may be completely ignorant of some likelihoods.

1.3.3 Differences in Risk Management

The risk profile must be evaluated before decision making begins. Such an evaluation first requires an evaluation of profile outcomes. As described earlier, outcomes are evaluated in terms of significance or utility. The outcome significances must be synthesized into a unified measure to evaluate the risk profile. In this way, each alternative and its risk profile is evaluated. In particular, people are strongly sensitive to catastrophic outcomes. This attitude toward risk is called risk aversion and manifests itself when we buy insurance. As will be discussed in Section 1.4, decision making under risk requires an understanding of this attitude.

This section first discusses outcome significances, available alternatives, and risk-profile significance. Then other factors such as outcome incommensurability, risk/cost trade-off, equity value concepts, and risk/cost/benefit trade-offs for decision making under risk are discussed. Finally, bounded rationality concepts and risk homeostasis are presented.

Loss or gain classification. Each outcome should be classified as a gain or loss. The PRA usually focuses on outcomes with obvious negativity (fatality, property damage). For other problems, however, the classification is not so obvious. People have their own reference point below which an outcome is regarded as a loss. Some references are objective and others are subjective. For investment problems, for instance, these references may be very complex.

Outcome significance. Each loss or gain must be evaluated by a significance or utility scale. Verbal and ambiguous measures such as *catastrophic*, *severe*, and *minor* may be used instead of quantitative measures. People have difficulty in evaluating the significance of an outcome never experienced; a habitual smoker can evaluate his lung cancer only postoperatively. The outcome significance depends on pairs of fuzzy antonyms: voluntary/involuntary, old/new, natural/man-made, random/nonrandom, accidental/intentional, forgettable/memorable, fair/unfair. Extreme categories (e.g., a controllable, voluntary, old outcome versus an uncontrollable, involuntary, new one) differ by many orders of magnitude on a scale of perceived risk [3]. The significance also depends on cultural attributes, ethics, emotion, reconciliation, media coverage, context, or litigability. People estimate the outcome significance differently when population risk is involved in addition to individual risk.

Available alternatives. Only one alternative is available for most people; the risk is uncontrollable, and they have to face it. Some people understand problems better and have more alternatives to reduce the risks. Gambles and business ventures are different fields of risk taking. In the former, risks are largely uncontrollable; in the latter, the risks are often controllable and avoidable. Obviously, different decisions are made depending on how many alternatives are available.

Risk-profile significance. Individuals may reach different decisions even if common sets of alternatives and associated risk profiles are given. Recall in the rain hazard mitigation problem in Section 1.2 that each significance is related to a particular outcome, not to a total risk profile. Because each alternative usually has two or more outcomes, these elementary significances must be integrated into a scalar by a suitable procedure, if the alternatives are to be arranged in a linear order. In the rain hazard mitigation problem an expected utility is used to unify significances of two outcomes for each alternative. In other words, a risk-profile significance of an alternative is measured by the expected utility. The operation of taking an expected value is a procedure yielding the unified scalar significance. The alternative with a larger expected utility or a smaller expected significance is usually chosen.

Expected utility. The expected utility concept assumes that outcome significance can be evaluated independently of outcome likelihood. It also assumes that an impact of an outcome with a known significance decreases linearly with its occurrence probability when the outcome significance is given: [probability] × [significance]. The outcomes may be low likelihood–high loss (fatality), high likelihood–low loss (getting wet), or of intermediate severity. Some people claim that for the low-probability and high-loss events, the independence or the linearity in the expected utility is suspicious; one million fatalities with probability 10^{-6} may yield a more dreadful perception than one tenth of the perception of the same fatalities with probability 10^{-5}. This correlation between outcome and likelihood yields different evaluation approaches for risk-profile significance for a given alternative.

Incommensurability of outcomes. It is difficult to combine outcome significances even if a single-outcome category such as fatalities or monetary loss is being dealt with. Unfortunately, loss categories are more diverse, for instance, financial, functional, time and opportunity, physical (plant, environmental damage), physiological (injury and fatality), societal, political. A variety of measures are available for approximating outcome significances: money, longevity, fatalities, pollutant concentration, individual and collective doses, and so on. Some are commensurable, others are incommensurable. Unification becomes far more difficult for incommensurable outcomes because of trade-offs.

Risk/cost trade-off. Even if the risk level is evaluated for each alternative, the decisions may not be easy. Each alternative has a cost.

Example 5—Fatality goal and safety system expenditure. Figure 1.16 is a schematic of a cost versus risk-profile trade-off problem. The horizontal and vertical axes denote the unified risk-profile significance in terms of expected number of fatalities and costs of alternatives, respectively. A population risk is considered. The costs are expenditures for safety systems. For simplicity of description, an infinite number of alternatives with different costs are considered. The feasible region of alternatives is the shaded area. The boundary curve is a set of equivalent solutions called a *Pareto curve*. The risk homeostasis line will be discussed later in this section. When two alternatives on the Pareto curve are given, we cannot say which one is superior. Additional information is required to arrange the Pareto alternatives in a linear preference order.

Assume that G_1 is specified as a maximum allowable goal of the expected number of fatalities. Then point A in Figure 1.16 is the most economical solution with cost C_1. The marginal cost at point A indicates the cost to decrease the expected number of fatalities by one unit, that is, cost to save a life. People have different goals, however; for the more demanding goal G_2, the solution is point B with higher cost C_2. The marginal cost generally tends to increase as the consequences diminish. ■

Example 6—Monetary trade-off problem. When fatalities are measured in terms of money, the trade-off problem is illustrated by Figure 1.17. Assume a situation where an outcome with ten fatalities occurs with frequency or probability P during the lifetime of a plant. The horizontal axis denotes the probability or frequency. The expected number of fatalities during the plant lifetime thus becomes $10 \times P$. Suppose that one fatality cost A dollars. Then the expected lifetime cost C_O potentially caused by the accident is $10 \times A \times P$, which is denoted by the straight line passing through the origin. The improvement cost C_I for achieving the fatal outcome probability P is depicted by a hyperbolic-like curve where marginal cost increases for smaller outcome probabilities.

The total expected cost $C_T = C_O + C_I$ is represented by a unimodal curve with global minimal at TC. As a consequence, the improvement cost at point IC is spent and the outcome probability

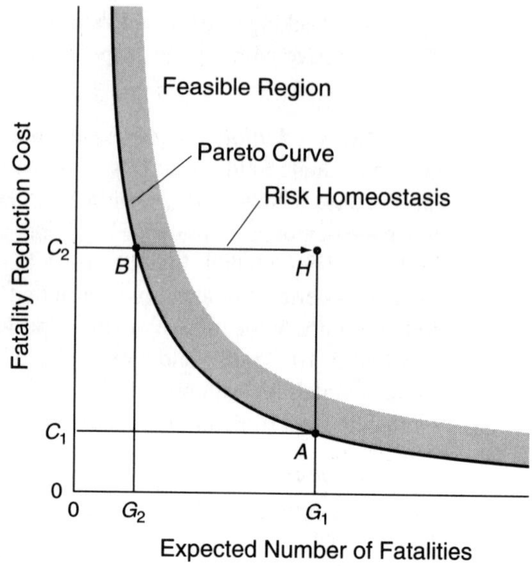

Figure 1.16. Trade-off problem between fatalities and reduction cost.

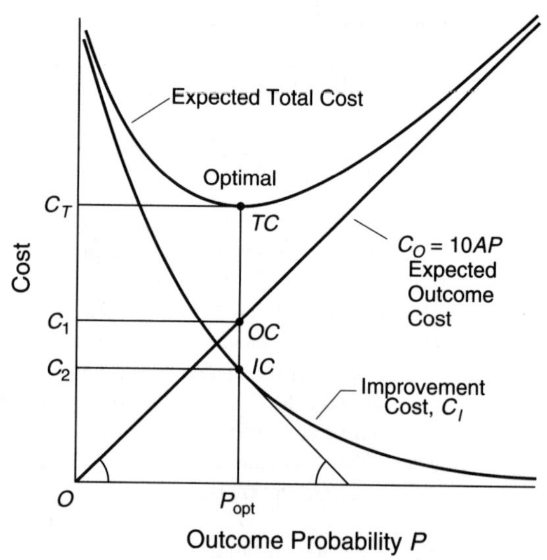

Figure 1.17. Trade-off problem when fatality is measured by monetary loss.

is determined. Point OC denotes the expected cost of the potential fatal outcome. The marginal improvement cost at point IC is equal to the slope $10 \times A$ of the straight line O–OC of expected fatal outcome cost. In other words, the optimal slope for the improvement cost is determined as the cost of ten fatalities. Theoretically, the safety investment increases so long as the marginal cost with respect to outcome likelihood P is smaller than the cost of ten fatalities. Obviously, the optimal investment cost increases when either fatality cost A or outcome size (ten fatalities in this example) increases.

In actual situations, the plant may cause multiple outcomes with different numbers of fatalities. For such cases, a diagram similar to Figure 1.17 is obtained with the exception that the horizontal axis now denotes the number of expected fatalities from all plant scenarios. The optimal marginal improvement cost with respect to the number of expected fatalities (i.e., the marginal cost for decreasing one expected fatality) is equal to the cost of one fatality.

The cost versus risk-level trade-offs in Figures 1.16 and 1.17 make sense if and only if the system yields risk and benefits; if no benefit is perceived, the trade-off problem is moot. ■

Equity value concept. Difficult problems arise in quantifying life in terms of dollars, and an "equity value of saving lives" has been proposed rather than "putting a price on human life" [5]. According to the equity value theory, an alternative that leads to greater expenditures per life saved than numerous other alternatives for saving lives is an inequitable commitment of society's resources that otherwise could have been used to save a greater number of lives. We have to stop our efforts at a certain slope of the risk-cost diagram of Figure 1.16 for any system we investigate [12], even if our risk unit consists of fatalities. This slope is the price we can pay for saving a life, that is, the equity value.

This theory is persuasive if the resources are centrally controlled and can be allocated for any purpose whatsoever. The theory becomes untenable when the resources are privately or separately owned: a utility company would not spend their money to improve automobile safety; people in advanced countries spend money to save people from heart diseases, while they spend far less money to save people from starvation in Africa.

Risk/cost/benefit (RCB) trade-off. According to Starr [13],

> the electricity generation options of coal, nuclear power, and hydroelectricity have been compared as to benefits and risks, and been persuasively defended by their proponents. In retrospect, the past decade has shown that the comparative risk perspective provided by such quantitative analysis has not been an important component of the past decisions to build any of these plants. Historically, initial choices have been made on the basis of performance economics and political feasibility, even in the nuclear power program.

Many technologies start with emphases on their positive aspects—their merits or benefits. After a while, possibly after a serious accident, people suddenly face the problem of choosing one of two alternatives, that is, accepting or rejecting the technology. Ideally, but not always, they are shown a risk profile of the alternative together with the benefits from the technology. Decision making of this type occurs daily at hospitals before or during a surgical operation; the risk profile there would be a Farmer curve with the horizontal axis denoting longevity loss or gain, while the vertical axis is an excess probability per operation.

Figure 1.18 shows another schematic relation between benefit and risk. The higher the benefit, the higher the risk. A typical example is a heart transplant versus an anticlotting drug.

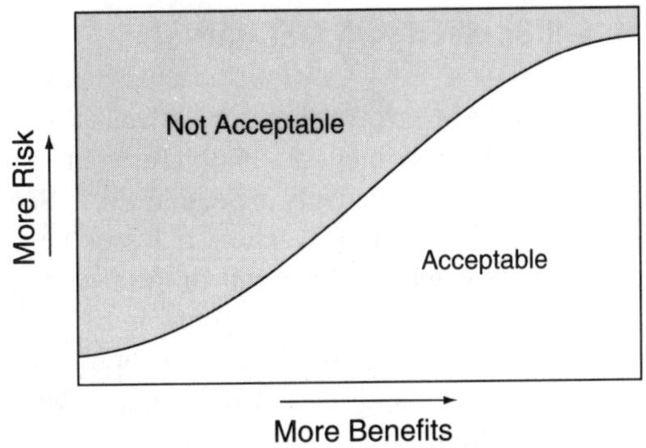

Figure 1.18. Schematic relation between benefits and acceptable risks.

Bounded rationality concept. Traditional decision-making theory makes four assumptions about decision makers.

1. They have a clearly defined utility value for each outcome.
2. They possess a clear and exhaustive view of the possible alternatives open to them.
3. They can create a risk profile for the future associated with each alternative.
4. They will choose between alternatives to maximize their expected utility.

However, flesh and blood decision making falls short of these Platonian assumptions. In short, human decision making is severely constrained by its keyhole view of the problem space that is called "bounded rationality" by Simon [14]:

> The capacity of the human mind for formulating and solving complex problems is very small compared with the size of the problems whose solutions are required for objectively rational behavior in the real world—or even for a reasonable approximation of such objective rationality.

The fundamental limitation in human information processing gives rise to "satisficing" behavior, that is, the tendency to settle for satisfactory rather than optimal courses of action.

Risk homeostasis. According to risk homeostasis theory [15], the solution with cost C_2 in Figure 1.16 tends to move to point H as soon as a decision maker changes the goal from G_1 to G_2; the former risk level G_1 is thus revisited. The theory states that people have tendencies to keep a constant risk level even if a safer solution is available. When a curved freeway is straightened to prevent traffic accidents, drivers tend to increase their speed, and thus incur the same risk level as before.

1.3.4 Summary

Different viewpoints toward risk are held by the individual affected, the population affected, the public, companies, and regulatory agencies. Disagreements arising in the risk-assessment phase encompass outcome, causal scenario, population affected, and likelihood, while in the risk-management phase disagreement exists in loss/gain classification, outcome significance, available alternatives, risk profile significances, risk/cost trade-off, and risk/cost/benefit trade-off.

The following factors make risk management difficult: 1) incommensurability of outcomes, 2) bounded rationality, and 3) risk homeostasis. An equity value guideline is proposed to give insight for the trade-off problem between monetary value and life.

1.4 RISK-AVERSION MECHANISMS

PRAM involves both objective and subjective aspects. A typical subjective aspect arising in the risk-management phase is an instinctive attitude called risk aversion, which is introduced qualitatively in Section 1.4.1. Section 1.4.2 describes three attitudes toward monetary outcomes: risk aversion, risk seeking, and risk neutral. Section 1.4.3 shows that the monetary approach can fail in the face of fatalities. Section 1.4.4 deals with an explanation of postaccident overestimation of outcome severity and likelihood. Consistent Bayesian explanations are given in Sections 1.4.5 and 1.4.6 with emphasis on a posteriori distribution. A public confidence problem with respect to the PRAM methodology is described in Section 1.4.7.

1.4.1 Risk Aversion

It is believed that people have an ambivalent attitude toward catastrophic outcomes; small stimuli distributed over time or space are ignored, while the sum of these stimuli, if exerted instantly and locally, cause a significant response. For instance, newspapers ignore ten single-fatality accidents but not one accident with ten fatalities. In order to avoid worst-case potential scenarios, people or companies buy insurances and pay amounts that are larger than the expected monetary loss. This attitude is called risk aversion.

One reason for the dispute about nuclear power lies in attitude toward risk. In spite of the high population risk, people pay less attention to automobile accidents, which cause more than ten thousand fatalities every year, because these accidents occur in an incremental and dispersed manner; however, people react strongly to a commercial airline accident where several hundred people die simultaneously. In addition to the individual- versus population-risk argument, the risk-aversive attitude is an unavoidable subject in the risk-management field.

1.4.2 Three Attitudes Toward Monetary Outcome

Risk-aversive, -neutral, and -seeking. People perceive the significance of money differently; its significance or utility is not necessarily proportional to the amount. Figure 1.19 shows three attitudes in terms of loss or value function curves: risk-aversive (convex), risk-seeking (concave), and risk-neutral (linear). For the loss function curves, the positive direction of the horizontal axis denotes more loss, and the negative direction more gain; the vertical axis denotes the loss significance of money. Each point on the monotonously increasing loss significance curve O–B–C–L in the upper-left-corner graph denotes a significance value for each insurance premium dollar spent, that is, a loss without uncertainty. The smaller the significance value, the lower the loss. Each point on the third quadrant curve, which is also monotonously increasing, denotes a significance value for a dollar gain.

Convex significance curve. A convex curve $s(x)$ is defined mathematically by the inequality holding for all x_1, x_2, and probability P.

$$s[Px_2 + (1 - P)x_1] \leq Ps(x_2) + (1 - P)s(x_1) \tag{1.17}$$

Insurance premium loss versus expected loss. Figure 1.20 shows an example of a convex significance curve $s(x)$. Consider the risk scenario as a lottery where x_1 and x_2 amounts of money are lost with probability $1 - P$ and P, respectively. As summarized in Table 1.6, the function on the left-hand side of the convex curve definition denotes the significance of the insurance premium $Px_2 + (1 - P)x_1$. This premium is equal to the expected amount of monetary loss from the lottery. Term $Ps(x_2) + (1 - P)s(x_1)$ on the right-hand side is the expected significance when two significances $s(x_1)$ and $s(x_2)$ for loss x_1 and x_2 occur with the same probabilities as in the lottery; thus the right-hand side denotes a significance value of the lottery itself. The convexity implies that the insurance premium loss is preferred to the lottery.

Avoidance of worse case. Because the insurance premium $Px_2+(1-P)x_1$ is equal to the expected loss of the lottery, one of the losses (say x_2) is greater than the premium loss, indicating that the risk-averse attitude avoids the worse case x_2 in the lottery; in other words, risk-averse people will pay the insurance premium to compensate for the potentially

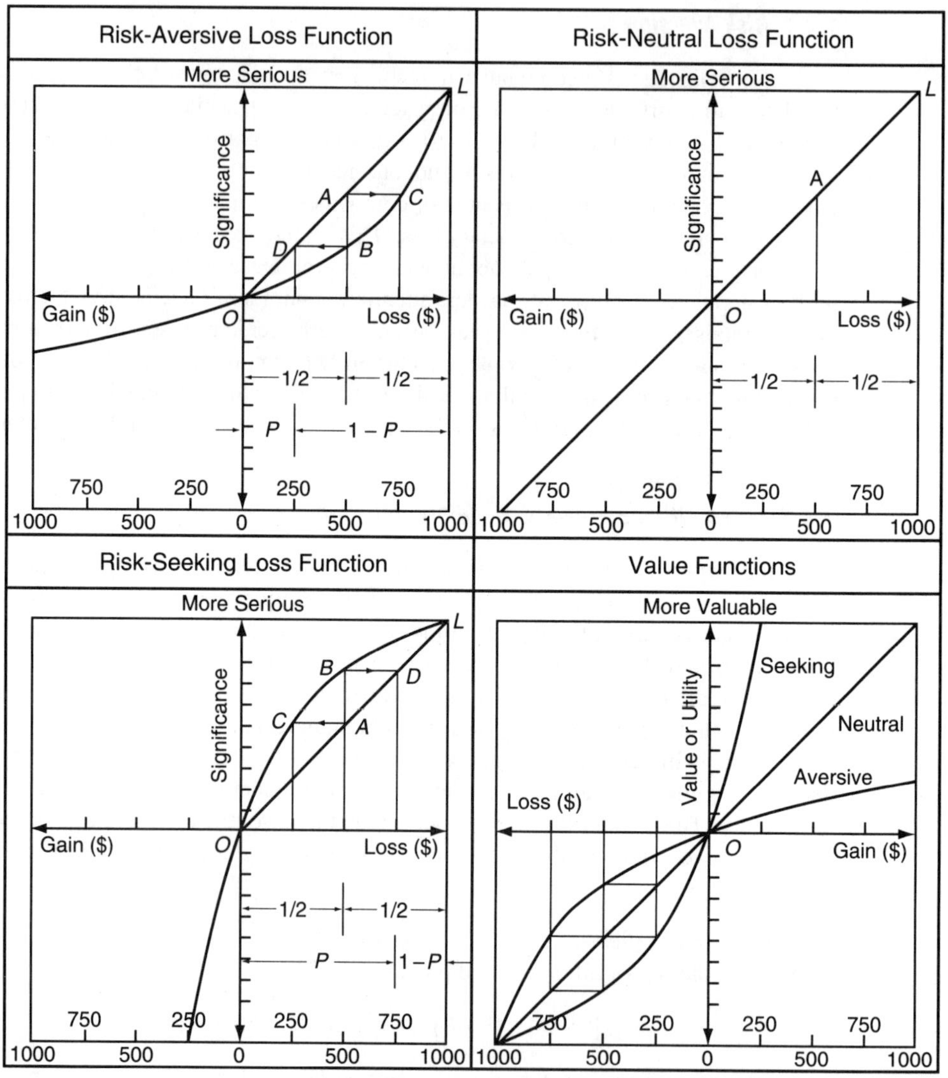

Figure 1.19. Risk-aversive, risk-neutral, and risk-seeking attitudes.

worse-loss outcome x_2. A concave curve for the risk-seeking attitude is defined by a similar inequality, but the inequality sign is reversed.

Example 7—A lottery and premium-paid. Point A in the upper-left-corner graph of Figure 1.19 is the middle point of a straight line segment between points O and L. The vertical coordinate of this point indicates a loss significance value of a lottery where getting \$1000 or nothing occurs with equal probabilities $P = 0.5$, respectively; the lottery is evaluated according to the expected significance, $0.5 \times s(0) + 0.5 \times s(1000) = s(1000)/2$. The horizontal coordinate of point A is a \$500 premium, which is equal to the expected loss of the lottery. Because the curve is convex, the line segment O–L is always above the nonlinear curve and we see that the premium loss of \$500 is preferred to the lottery with the same expected loss of money. ■

Example 8—Insurance premium and lottery range. Point C indicates an insurance payment with equivalent loss significance to the lottery denoted by point A. Thus the lottery can be

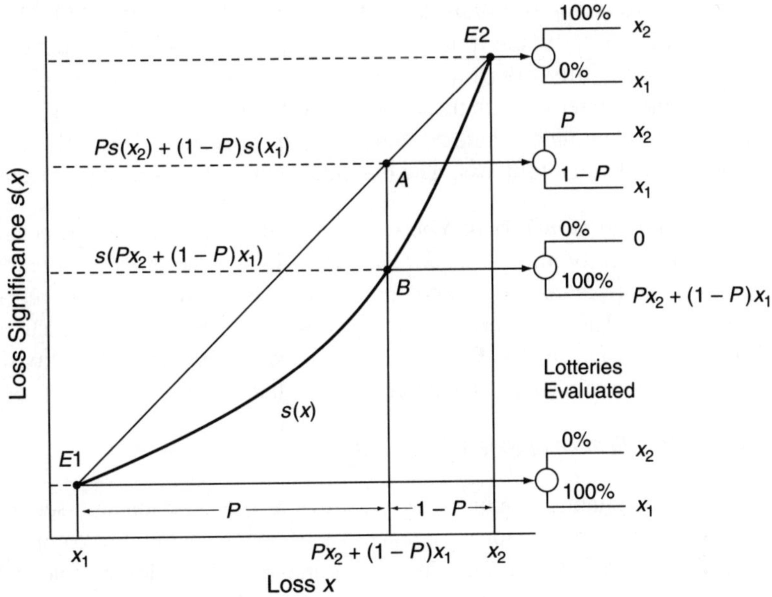

Figure 1.20. Convex significance curve (risk-aversive).

TABLE 1.6. Insurance Premium Significance and Expected Lottery Significance

Expression	Description
P	Probability of loss x_2
$1 - P$	Probability of loss x_1
$Px_2 + (1 - P)x_1$	Expected lottery loss
$Px_2 + (1 - P)x_1$	Insurance premium
$s(Px_2 + (1 - P)x_1)$	Insurance premium significance
$Ps(x_2) + (1 - P)s(x_1)$	Expected lottery significance

exchanged evenly for the sure loss of \$750, the horizontal axis of the point. The risk-aversive person will buy insurance as long as the payment is \$750, and thus avoid the larger potential loss of \$1000.

Point D, on the other hand, denotes a lottery with an equivalent significance to a premium loss of \$500; this is the lottery where losing \$1000 or nothing occurs with probability 1/4 or 3/4, respectively; the expected loss in the lottery is $\$1000/4 = \$250$, which is smaller than \$500. This person is paying \$500 to avoid the potential worst loss of \$1000 in the lottery, despite the fact that the expected loss \$250 is smaller than the \$500 payment. ■

Marginal significance. The significance curve is convex for the risk-aversive attitude and the marginal loss significance increases with the amount of lost money. According to the attitude, the \$1000 premium paid by a particular person is more serious than the \$100 premiums distributed among and paid by ten persons, provided that these persons have the same risk-aversion attitude. This is analogous to viewing a ten-fatality accident involving a single automobile as more serious than one-fatality accidents distributed over ten automobiles.

Risk-seeking and -neutral. For the risk-seeking attitude in the lower-left-corner graph of Figure 1.19, the straight line segment is below the nonlinear concave significance curve, and the fifty-fifty lottery is preferred to the premium loss of $500; the marginal significance decreases with the amount of lost money. The upper-right-corner graph shows a risk-neutral attitude, where a lottery with an expected loss of $500 is not distinguishable from the $500 premium loss. The marginal significance remains constant.

Utility of monetary outcome. When the horizontal and vertical axes are reversed, curves in terms of utility appear. The lower-right-corner graph of Figure 1.19 shows risk-aversive, risk-seeking, and risk-neutral utility curves that are concave, convex, and linear, respectively. The risk-aversion is represented by convex and concave curves for significance and utility, respectively. For the risk-aversive curve, marginal utility decreases with the increase of certain gain or the decrease of certain loss.

1.4.3 Significance of Fatality Outcome

When fatalities are involved, the previous risk-aversion and -seeking lottery problem described in terms of monetary outcomes becomes much more complicated. Figure 1.21 shows a case where one sure fatality is compared with a lottery that causes two and zero fatalities with equal probability 0.5. The expected number of fatalities in the lottery is just one. If a mother with two children is risk aversive, as is usually assumed, then she should choose certain death of one child to avoid the more serious potential death of two children. The choice is reversed if the mother is risk seeking.

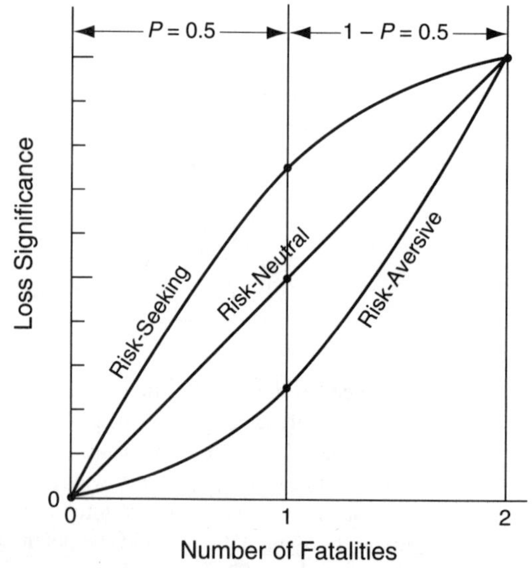

Figure 1.21. Comparison of one sure fatality with 50% chance of two fatalities.

The risk-seeking behavior is the intuitive outcome because, among other things, the sacrifice of one child is not justified ethically, emotionally, or rationally. However, this comparison of a certain death with potential deaths is totally sophomoric because only a sadist would pose such a question, and only a masochist would answer it. Another viewpoint is that the fatality has an infinite significance value, and we cannot compare one infinity with another when a sure fatality is involved.

1.4.4 Mechanisms for Risk Aversion

Overestimation of frequency and outcome. A more reasonable explanation of risk aversiveness for outcomes including fatalities was given by Bohnenblust and Schneider in Switzerland [12]. According to them, misestimations of risks after severe accidents are one of the major reasons for risk-aversive attitudes, which prefer ten single-fatality accidents to one accident with ten fatalities. Risks can be misestimated or overestimated with respect to size or likelihood of outcomes. This is similar to the error bands depicted in Figure 1.4, where the uncertainty is either due to errors of frequency or outcome severity estimation.

Overestimating outcome severity. Consider first the misestimation of an outcome severity such as the number of fatalities. Imagine a system that causes, on the average, one accident every one hundred years. Most of these accidents have relatively small consequences, say one fatality for each. Once in a while there may be a catastrophic event with ten fatalities. If the catastrophic event happens to occur, the public (or regulatory agencies) may believe that all accidents have catastrophic outcomes, thus they demand more safety measures than are justified by the actual damage expectation. Such a claim is not restricted to the particular facility that caused the accident; improvements are required for all other facilities of this type. As a consequence, all operators of this type of facility must adopt a risk-averse behavior to avoid the excessive consequences caused by the one large accident.

Overestimation of outcome likelihood. Suppose that at a plant there is a one chance in ten thousand years for a serious accident. After the occurrence of such an accident, however, the public perception is no longer that the installation has an accident interval of ten thousand years. The public might force the company to behave as if an accident occurred every thousand years, not every ten thousand years. This means that the risk and therefore the safety costs are overestimated by a factor of ten.

Erosion of public confidence. In the "Policy Statement on Safety Goals for the Operation of Nuclear Power Plants" published on August 4, 1986, the U.S. Nuclear Regulatory Commission (NRC) recognizes that, apart from their health and safety consequences, severe core damage accidents can erode public confidence in the safety of nuclear power and can lead to further instability and unpredictability for the industry. In order to avoid these adverse consequences, the Commission intends to continue to pursue a regulatory program with an objective of providing reasonable assurance, while giving appropriate consideration to the uncertainties involved [10].

1.4.5 Bayesian Explanation of Severity Overestimation

A priori distribution of defects. The public's and regulatory agencies' overestimation may not be a misestimation; it is consistent with a result from Bayesian statistics.* Assume that the accident occurs at a rate of once in one hundred years. Suppose that there is a debate about whether or not this type of facility poses a serious safety problem. The public believes a priori that the existence and nonexistence of the defect are equally probable, that is, $P = 0.5$; if the defect exists, the accident yields 10 fatalities with probability 0.99, and 1 fatality with probability 0.01; if the defect does not exist, these probabilities are reversed.

*The appendix of Chapter 3 describes the Bayes theorem for readers unfamiliar with Bayesian statistics.

A posteriori distribution of defects. Consider how the public belief about the defect changes when the first accident yields ten fatalities. According to the Bayes theorem, we have a posteriori probability of a defect conditioned by the occurrence of the ten-fatality accident.

$$\Pr\{\text{Defect} \mid 10\} = \Pr\{\text{Defect}, 10\}/\Pr\{10\} = \tag{1.18}$$

$$\frac{\Pr\{\text{Defect}\}\Pr\{10 \mid \text{Defect}\}}{\Pr\{\text{Defect}\}\Pr\{10 \mid \text{Defect}\} + \Pr\{\text{No defect}\}\Pr\{10 \mid \text{No defect}\}} = \tag{1.19}$$

$$\frac{0.5 \times 0.99}{0.5 \times 0.99 + 0.5 \times 0.01} = 0.99 \tag{1.20}$$

Even if the first accident was simply bad luck, the public does not think that way; public belief is that in this type of facility the probability of a serious defect increases to 0.99 from 0.5, yielding the belief that future accidents are almost certain to cause ten fatalities. An example is the Chernobyl nuclear accident. Experts alleviated the public postaccident shock by stating that the Chernobyl graphite reactor had a substantial defect that U.S. reactors do not have.

Gaps between experts and public. It can be argued that the public a priori distribution

$$\Pr\{\text{Defect}\} = \Pr\{\text{No defect}\} = 0.5 \tag{1.21}$$

is questionable in view of the PRA that gives a far smaller a priori defect probability. However, such a claim will not be persuasive to the public that has little understanding of the PRA, and who places more emphasis on the a posteriori information after the real accident, than on the a priori calculation before the accident. Spangler summarizes gaps in the treatment of technological risks by technical experts and the lay public, as given in Tables 1.7 and 1.8 [5,16].

1.4.6 Bayesian Explanation of Likelihood Overestimation

A priori frequency distribution. The likelihood overestimation can also be explained by a Bayesian approach. Denote by F the frequency of the serious accident. Before the accident the public accepted the following a priori distribution of the frequency: $\Pr\{F = 10^{-4}\} = 0.99$ and $\Pr\{F = 10^{-2}\} = 0.01$.

A posteriori distribution of frequency. Assume the first serious accident occurred after one year's operation of the facility. Then the a posteriori distribution of the frequency after accident A is

$$\Pr\{F = 10^{-2} \mid A\} = \Pr\{F = 10^{-2}, A\}/\Pr\{A\} = \tag{1.22}$$

$$\frac{\Pr\{F = 10^{-2}\}\Pr\{A \mid F = 10^{-2}\}}{\Pr\{F = 10^{-2}\}\Pr\{A \mid F = 10^{-2}\} + \Pr\{F = 10^{-4}\}\Pr\{A \mid F = 10^{-4}\}} = \tag{1.23}$$

$$\frac{0.01 \times 0.01}{0.01 \times 0.01 + 0.99 \times 0.0001} \simeq 0.5 >> 0.01 \tag{1.24}$$

An accident per one hundred years now becomes as plausible as an accident per ten thousand years. The public will not think that the first accident was simply bad luck.

TABLE 1.7. Treatment of Technological Risks by Technical Experts

Approach	Treatment Common to Experts
1. Criteria for risk acceptance	
a. Absolute vs relative risk	Risk judged in both absolute and relative terms
b. Risk-cost trade-offs	Essential to sound decision making because of finite societal resources for risk reduction and impractability of achieving zero risk; tends to ignore nondollar costs in such trade-offs
c. Risk-benefit comparisons of technological options	Emphasizes total (net) benefits to society, neglecting benefits that are difficult to quantify; also neglects indirect and certain long-term benefits
d. Equity consideration	Tends to treat shallowly without explicit decision criteria and structured analyses
2. Risk-assessment methods	
a. Expression mode	Quantitative
b. Logic mode	Computational • Risk = consequence × probability • Fault trees/event trees • Statistical calculation
c. Learning mode	Experimental • Laboratory animals • Clinical data for humans • Engineering test equipment and simulators
3. Basis for trusting information	
a. Source preference	Established institutions
b. Source reliability	Qualification of experts
c. Accuracy of information	Robustness/uncertainty of scientific knowledge
4. Risk-attribute evaluation	
a. Low-frequency risk	Objective, conservative assessment
b. Newness of risk	Broad range of high and low estimates
c. Catastrophic vs dispersed deaths	Gives equal weight
d. Immediate vs delayed deaths	Diverse views over treatment of incommensurables and discount rate
e. Statistical vs known deaths	Gives equal weight
f. Dreadfulness of risk	Generally ignores
g. Voluntary vs involuntary risk	Gives equal weight
5. Technological consideration	
a. Murphy's law (if anything can go wrong, it will)	Stimulus for redundancy and defense-in-depth in system design and operating procedures; margins of conservatism in design; quality assurance programs
b. Reports of technological failures and accidents	Valued source of data for technological fixes and prioritizing research; increased attention to consequence mitigation

TABLE 1.8. Treatment of Technological Risks by Lay Public

Approach	Treatment Common to the Public
1. Criteria for risk acceptance	
a. Absolute vs relative risk	Greater tendency to judge risk in absolute terms
b. Risk-cost trade-offs	Because human life is priceless, criteria involving risk-cost trade-offs are immoral; ignores risks of no-action alternatives to rejected technology; gives greater weight to nondollar costs
c. Risk-benefit comparisons of technological options	Emphasizes personal rather than societal benefits; includes both qualitative and quantitative benefits but tends to neglect indirect and long-term benefits
d. Equity consideration	Tends to distort equity considerations in favor of personal interests to the neglect of the interests of opposing parties or the common good of society
2. Risk-assessment methods	
a. Expression mode	Qualitative
b. Logic mode	Intuitive • Incomplete rationale • Emotional input to value judgments
c. Learning mode	Impressionistic • Personal experience/memory • Media accounts • Cultural exchange
3. Basis for trusting information	
a. Source preference	Nonestablishment sources
b. Source reliability	Limited ability to judge qualifications
c. Accuracy of information	Minimal understanding of strengths and limitations of scientific knowledge
4. Risk-attribute evaluation	
a. Low-frequency risk	Tends to exaggerate or ignore risk
b. Newness of risk	Tends to exaggerate or ignore risk
c. Catastrophic vs dispersed deaths	Gives greater weight to catastrophic deaths
d. Immediate vs delayed deaths	Gives greater weight to immediate deaths except for known exposure to cancer-producing agents
e. Statistical vs known deaths	Gives greater weight to known deaths
f. Dreadfulness of risk	Gives greater weight to dreaded risk
g. Voluntary vs involuntary risk	Gives greater weight to involuntary risk
5. Technological consideration	
a. Murphy's law (if anything can go wrong, it will)	Stimulus for what-if syndromes and distrust of technologies and technocrats; source of exaggerated views on risk levels using worst-case assumptions
b. Reports of technological failures and accidents	Confirms validity of Murphy's law; increased distrust of technocrats

1.4.7 PRAM Credibility Problem

In Japan some people believe that the engineering approaches such as PRA are relatively useless for gaining public acceptance of risky facilities. Perhaps credibilities gained by sharing a bottle of wine are more crucial to human relations. Clearly, the PRAM methodology requires more psychosocial research to gain public credit.

According to Chauncey Starr of the Electric Power Research Institute [13]:

> Science cannot prove safety, only the degree of existing harm. In the nuclear field emphasis on PRA has focused professional concern on the frequency of core melts. The arguments as to whether a core can melt with a projected probability of one in a thousand per year, or in a million per year, represent a misplaced emphasis on these quantitative outcomes. The virtue of the risk assessments is the disclosure of the system's causal relationships and feedback mechanisms, which might lead to technical improvements in the performance and reliability of the nuclear stations. When the probability of extreme events becomes as small as these analyses indicate, the practical operating issue is the ability to manage and stop the long sequence of events which could lead to extreme end results. Public acceptance of any risk is more dependent on public confidence in risk management than on the quantitative estimates of risk consequences, probabilities and magnitudes.

1.4.8 Summary

Risk aversion is defined as the subjective attitude that prefers a fixed loss to a lottery with the same amount of expected loss. When applied to monetary loss, risk aversion implies convex significance curves, monotonously increasing marginal significance, and insurance premiums larger than the expected loss. A risk-seeking or risk-neutral attitude can be defined in similar ways. The comparison approach between the fixed loss and expected loss, however, cannot apply to fatality losses.

Postaccident overestimation in outcome severity or in outcome frequency can be explained by the Bayes theorem. The public places more emphasis on the a posteriori distribution after an accident than on the a priori PRA calculation.

1.5 SAFETY GOALS

When goals are given, risk problems become more tractable; risk management tries to satisfy the goals, and the risk assessment checks the attainment of the goals. Goals for risk management can be specified in terms of various measures including availability, reliability, risk, and safety. Aspects of these measures are clarified in Section 1.5.1. A hierarchical arrangement of the goals is given in Section 1.5.2. Section 1.5.3 shows a three-layer decision structure with upper and lower bound goals. Examples of goals are given in Sections 1.5.4 and 1.5.5 for normal activities and catastrophic accidents, respectively. Differences between idealistic and pragmatic lower bound goals are described in Section 1.5.6, where the concept of regulatory cutoff level is introduced. The final section gives a model for varying the regulatory cutoff level as a function of population size.

1.5.1 Availability, Reliability, Risk, and Safety

Availability is defined as the characteristic of an item expressed by the probability that it will be operational at a future instant in time (IEEE Standard 352). In this context, a protection device such as a relief valve is designed to exhibit a high availability.

Reliability is defined as a probability that an item will perform a required function when used for its intended purpose, under the stated conditions, for a given period of time [4]. The availability is measured at an instant, and the reliability during a period of time.

Availability and reliability are independent of who is causing the loss outcome and who is exposed to it. On the other hand, risk depends on the gain/loss assignment of the outcome to people involved; shooting escaping soldiers is a gain for the guards, while being shot is a loss for the escapees. Safety is only applicable to the people subject to the potential loss outcome. That is, safety is originally a concept viewed from the aspect of people who are exposed to the potential loss.

Fortunately, this subtle difference among availability, reliability, risk, and safety is usually irrelevant to PRAM where the people involved are supposed to be honest enough to try to decrease potential losses to others. An alternative with less risk is thus considered safer; an instrument with a high availability or reliability is supposed to increase safety. Safety can thus be regarded as inversely proportional to the risk, and both terms are used interchangeably; it is, however, also possible for a company spending too much for safety to face another risk: bankruptcy.

1.5.2 Hierarchical Goals for PRAM

Systems subject to PRA have a hierarchical structure: components, units, subsystems, plant, and site. Safety goals also form a hierarchy. For a nuclear power plant, for instance, goals can be structured in the following way [17] (see Figure 1.22):

1. Initiating event level: occurrence frequency
2. Safety system level: unavailability
3. Containment: failure probability
4. Accident sequence level: sequence frequency
5. Plant: damage frequency, source term
6. Site and environment: collective dose, early fatalities, latent cancer fatalities, property damage

The safety goals at the top of the hierarchy are most important. For the nuclear power plant, the top goals are those on the site and environment level. When the goals on the top level are given, goals on the lower levels can, in theory, be specified in an objective and systematic way. If a hierarchical goal system is established in advance, the PRAM process is simplified significantly; the probabilistic risk-assessment phase, given alternatives, calculates performance indices for the goals on various levels, with error bands. The risk-management phase proposes the alternatives and evaluates the attainment of the goals.

To achieve goals on the various levels, a variety of techniques are proposed: suitable redundancy, reasonable isolation, sufficient diversity, sufficient independence, and sufficient margin [17]. Appendix A to Title 10 of the Code of Federal Regulations Part 50 (CFR Part 50) sets out 64 general design criteria for quality assurance; protection against fire, missiles, and natural phenomena; limitations on the sharing of systems; and other protective safety requirements. In addition to the NRC regulations, there are numerous supporting guidelines that contribute importantly to the achievement of safety goals. These include regulatory guides (numbering in the hundreds); the Standard Review Plan for reactor license applications, NUREG-75/087 (17 chapters); and associated technical positions and appendices in the Standard Review Plan [10].

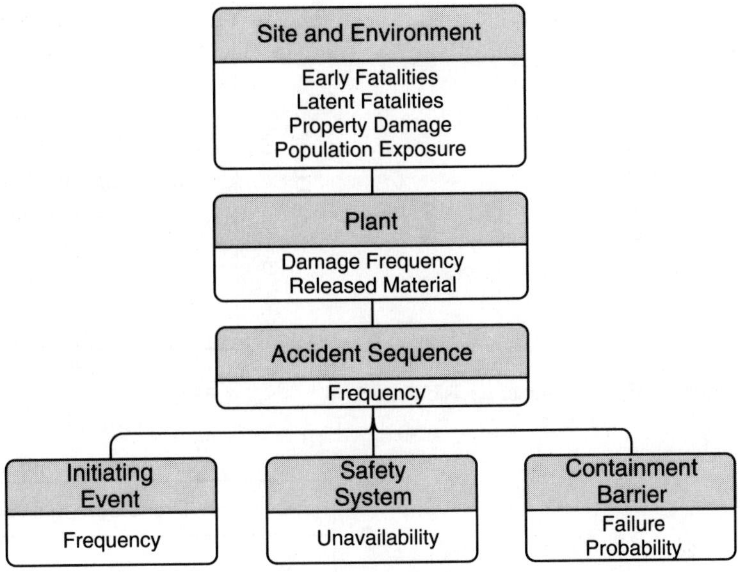

Figure 1.22. Hierarchy of safety goals.

1.5.3 Upper and Lower Bound Goals

Three-layer decision structure. Cyril Comar [18] proposed the following decision structure, as cited by Spangler [5]:

1. Eliminate any risk that carries no benefit or is easily avoided.
2. Eliminate any large risk $\geq U$ that does not carry clearly overriding benefits.
3. Ignore for the time being any small risk $\leq L$ that does not fall into category 1.
4. Actively study risks falling between these limits, with the view that the risk of taking any proposed action should be weighed against the risk of not taking that action.

Of course, upper bound level U is greater than lower bound level L. The shaded areas in Figure 1.23 show acceptable risk regions with an elimination level L. The easily avoided risk in the first statement can, by definition, be reduced below L regardless of the merits. The term *risk* is used mainly to denote a risk level in terms of outcome likelihood. The term *action* in the fourth statement means an alternative; thus action is not identical to a risk source such as a nuclear power plant or chemical plant; elimination of a particular action does not necessarily imply elimination of the risk source; the risk source may continue to exist when other actions or alternatives are introduced.

In Comar's second statement, the large risk $\geq U$ is reluctantly accepted if and only if it has overriding benefits such as risks incurred by soldiers at war (national security) or patients undergoing operations (rescue from a serious disease). Denote by R the risk level of an action. Then the decision structure described above can be as stated in Figure 1.24.

We see that only risks with moderate benefits are subject to the main decision structure, which consists of three layers separated by upper and lower limits U and L, respectively: $R \geq U$, $L < R < U$, and $R \leq L$. In the top layer $R \geq U$, the risk is first reduced below U;

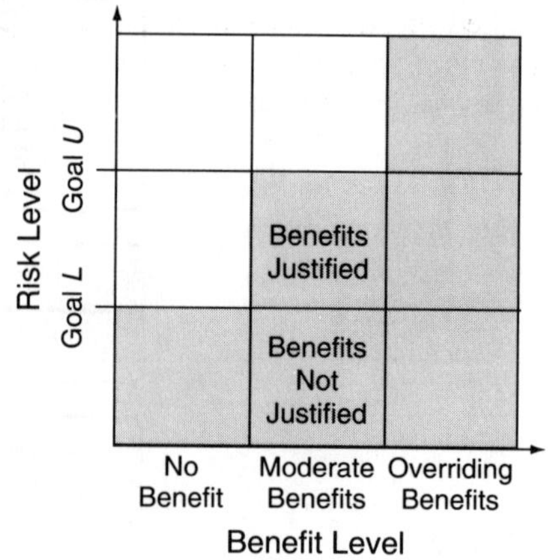

Figure 1.23. Three-layer decision structure.

```
Prescreening Structure

begin
if ( risk carries no benefit)
        reduce risk below L (inclusive);
if (risk has overriding benefits)
        reluctantly accept risk;
if (risk has moderate benefits)
        go to the main structure below;
end

Main Decision Structure

/* risk R has moderate benefits */
begin
if (R >= U)
        risk is unacceptable;
        reduce risk below U (exclusive)
            for justification or acceptance;
if (L < R < U)
        actively study risk for justification;
        begin
        if (risk is justified)
            reluctantly accept risk;
        if (risk is not justified)
            reduce risk until justified
              or below L (inclusive);
        end
if (R <= L)
        accept risk;
end
```

Figure 1.24. Algorithm for three-layer decision structure.

the resultant level may locate in the middle $L < R < U$ or the bottom layer $R \leq L$. In the middle layer, risk R is actively studied by risk-cost-benefit (RCB) analyses for justification; if it is justified, then it is reluctantly accepted; if it is not justified, then it is reduced until justification in the middle layer or inclusion in the bottom layer. In the bottom layer, the risk is automatically accepted even if it carries no benefits.

Note that the term *reduce* does not necessarily mean an immediate reduction; rather it denotes registration into a reduction list; some risks in the top layer or some risks not justified in the middle layer are difficult to reduce immediately but can be reduced in the future; some other risks such as background radiation, which carries no benefits, are extremely difficult to reduce in the prescreening structure, and would remain in the reduction list forever.

The lower bound L is closely related to the de minimis risk (to be described shortly), and its inclusion can be justified for the following reasons: 1) people do not pay much attention to risks below the lower bound even if they receive no benefits, 2) it becomes extremely difficult to decrease the risk below the lower bound, 3) there are almost countless and hence intractable risks below the lower bound, 4) above the lower bound there are many risks in need of reduction, and 5) without such a lower bound, all company profits could be allocated for safety [19].

Upper and lower bound goals. Comar defined the upper and lower bounds by probabilities of fatality of an individual per year of exposure to the risk.

$$U = 10^{-4}/(\text{year, individual}), \qquad L = 10^{-5}/(\text{year, individual}) \tag{1.25}$$

Wilson [20] defined the bounds for the individual fatal risk as follows.

$$U = 10^{-3}/(\text{year, individual}), \qquad L = 10^{-6}/(\text{year, individual}) \tag{1.26}$$

According to annual statistical data per individual, "being struck by lightning" is smaller than 10^{-6}, "natural disasters" stands between 10^{-6} and 10^{-5}, "industrial work" is between 10^{-5} and 10^{-4}, and "traffic accidents" and "all accidents" fall between 10^{-4} and 10^{-3} (see Table 1.9).

TABLE 1.9. Order of Individual Annual Likelihood of Early Fatality

Annual Likelihood	Activity
10^{-4} to 10^{-3}	All accidents
10^{-4} to 10^{-3}	Traffic accidents
10^{-5} to 10^{-4}	Industrial work
10^{-5}	Drowning
10^{-5}	Air travel
10^{-5}	Drinking five liters of wine
10^{-6} to 10^{-5}	Natural disasters
10^{-6}	Smoking three U.S. cigarettes
10^{-6}	Drinking a half liter of wine
10^{-6}	Visiting New York or Boston for two days
10^{-6}	Spending six minutes in canoe
$< 10^{-7}$	Lightning, tornadoes, hurricanes

Because the upper bound suggested by Comar is $U = 10^{-4}$, the current traffic accident risk level $R \geq U$ would imply the following: automobiles have overriding merits and are reluctantly accepted in the prescreening structure, or the risk level is in the reduction list of the main decision structure, that is, the risk has moderate benefits but should be reduced below U.

Wilson's upper bound $U = 10^{-3}$ means that the traffic accident risk level $R \leq U$ should be subject to intensive RCB study for justification; if the risk is justified, then it is reluctantly accepted; if the risk is not justified, then it must be reduced until another justification or until it is below the lower bound L.

Wilson showed that the lower bound $L = 10^{-6}$/(year, individual) is equivalent to the risk level of any one of the following activities: smoking three U.S. cigarettes (cancer, heart disease), drinking 0.5 liters of wine (cirrhosis of the liver), visiting New York or Boston for two days (air pollution), and spending six minutes in a canoe (accident). The lower bound $L = 10^{-5}$ by Comar can be interpreted in a similar way; for instance, it is comparable to drinking five liters of wine per year.

Spangler claims that the Wilson's annual lower bound $L = 10^{-6}$ is more acceptable than Comar's bound $L = 10^{-5}$ for the following situations [5]:

1. Whenever the risk is involuntary.
2. Whenever there is a substantial band of uncertainty in estimating risk at such low levels.
3. Whenever the risk has a high degree of expert and public controversy.
4. Whenever there is a reasonable prognosis that new safety information is more likely to yield higher-than-current best estimates of the risk level rather than lower estimates.

Accumulation problems for lower bound risks. The lower bound $L = 10^{-6}$/(year, individual) would not be suitable if the risk level were measured not per year but per operation. For instance, the same operation may be performed repetitively by a dangerous forging press. The operator of this machine may think that the risk per operation is negligible because there is only one chance in one million of an accident, so he removes safety interlocks to speed up the operation. However, more than ten thousand operations may be performed during a year, yielding a large annual risk level, say 10^{-2}, of injury. Another similar accumulation may be caused by multiple risk sources or by risk exposures to a large population; if enough negligible doses are added together, the result may eventually be significant [11]; if negligible individual risks of fatality are integrated over a large population, a sizable number of fatalities may occur.

ALARA—As low as reasonably achievable. A decision structure similar to the ones described above is recommended by ICRP (International Commission on Radiological Protection) Report No. 26 for individual-related radiological protection [10]. Note that population-related protection is not considered.

1. Justification of practice: No practice shall be adopted unless its introduction produces a positive net benefit.
2. Optimization of protection: All exposures shall be kept as low as reasonably achievable (i.e., ALARA), economic and social factors being taken into account.
3. The radiation doses to individuals shall not exceed the dose equivalent limits recommended for the appropriate circumstances by ICRP.

The third statement corresponds to upper bound U in the three-layer decision structure. The ICRP report lacks lower bound L, however, and there is a theoretical chance that the risk would be overreduced to any small number, as long as it is feasible to do so by ALARA.

The NRC adoption of ALARA radiation protection standards for the design and operation of light water reactors in May 1975 interpreted the term *as low as reasonably achievable* to mean as low as is reasonably achievable taking into account the state of technology and the economics of improvements, in relation to benefits, to public health and safety and other societal and socioeconomic considerations, and in relation to the utilization of atomic energy in the public interest [10]. Note here that the term *benefits* does not denote the benefits of atomic energy but reduction of risk levels; *utilization of atomic energy in the public interest* denotes the benefits in the usual sense for RCB analyses.

For population-related protection, the NRC proposed a conservative value of $1000 per total body person-rem (collective dose for population risk) averted for the risk/cost evaluations for ALARA [10]. The value of $1000 is roughly equal to $7.4 million per fatality averted if one uses the ratio of 135 lifetime fatalities per million person-rems. This ALARA value established temporarily by the commission is substantially higher than the equity value of $250,000 to $500,000 per fatality averted referenced by other agencies in risk-reduction decisions. (The lower equity values apply, of course, to situations where there is no litigation, i.e., to countries other than the United States.)

De minimis risk. The concept of de minimis risk is discussed in the book edited by Whipple [21]. A purpose of de minimis risk investigation is a justification of a lower bound L below which no active study of the risk, including ALARA or RCB analyses, is required. Davis, for instance, describes in Chapter 13 of the book how the law has long recognized that there are trivial matters that need not concern it; the maxim *de minimis non curat lex*, "the law does not concern itself with trifles," expresses that principle [11]. (In practice, of course, the instance of a judge actually dismissing a lawsuit on the basis of triviality is a very rare event.) She suggests the following applications of de minimis risk concepts [10].

1. For setting regulatory priorities
2. As a "floor" for ALARA considerations
3. As a cut-off level for collective dose assessments
4. For setting outer boundaries of geographical zones
5. As a floor for definition of low-level wastes
6. As a presumption of triviality in legal proceedings
7. To foster administrative and regulatory efficiency
8. To provide perspective for public understanding, including policy judgments

Some researchers of the de minimis say that 10^{-6}/(year, individual) risk is trivial, acceptable, or negligible and that no more safety investment or regulation is required at all for systems with the de minimis risk level. Two typical approaches for determining the de minimis radiation level are comparison with background radiation levels and detectability of radiation [11]. Radiation is presumed to cause cancers, and the radiation level can be converted to a fatal cancer level.

ALARA versus de minimis. Cunningham [10] noted:

> We have a regulatory scheme with upper limits above which the calculated health risk is generally unacceptable. Below these upper limits are various specific provisions and exemptions involving calculated risks that are considered acceptable based on a balancing of benefits and costs, and these need not be considered further. Regulatory requirements below the upper limits are based on the ALARA principle, and any risk involved is judged acceptable given not only the magnitude of the health risk presented but also various social and economic considerations. A de minimis level, if adopted, would provide a regulatory cutoff below which any health risk, if present, could be considered negligible. Thus, the de minimis level would establish a lower limit for the ALARA range of doses.

The use of ALARA-type procedures can provide a basis for establishing an explicit standard of de minimis risk beyond which no further analysis of costs and benefits need be employed to determine the acceptability of risk [10]; in this context, the de minimis risk is a dependent variable in the ALARA procedure. An example of such a procedure is the cost-benefit guideline of \$1000 per total person-rem averted (see Figure 1.25). Such a determination of the de minimis risk level by ALARA, however, would yield different lower bounds for different risk sources; this blurs the three-layer decision structure with a universal lower bound that says that no more ALARA is required below the constant bound even if a more cost-effective alternative than the \$1000 guideline is available.

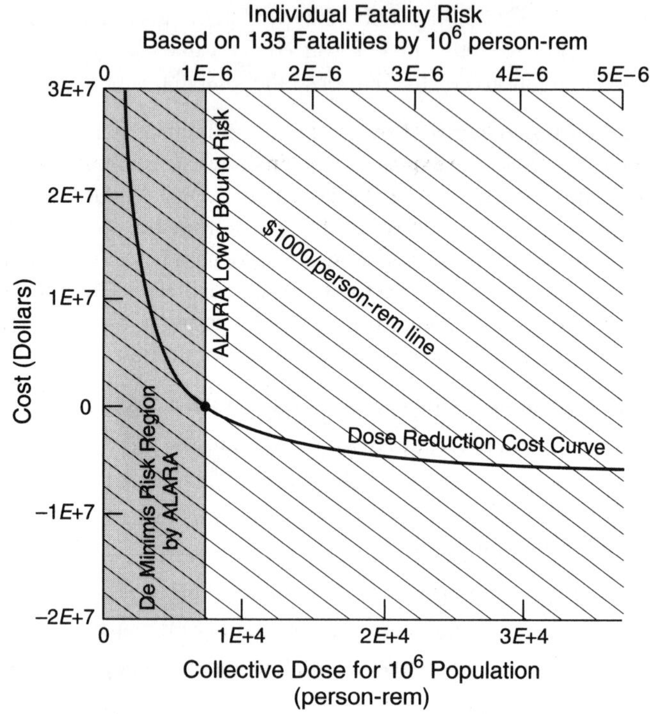

Figure 1.25. De minimis risk level determined by ALARA.

1.5.4 Goals for Normal Activities

Lower bound goals. Examples of quantitative design goals for lower bound L for a light-water-cooled power reactor are found in Title 10 of CFR Part 50, Appendix I [10]. They are expressed in terms of maximum permissible annual individual doses:

1. Liquid effluent radioactivity; 3 millirems for the whole body and 10 millirems to any organ.
2. Gaseous effluent radioactivity; 5 millirems to the whole body and 15 millirems to the skin.
3. Radioactive iodine and other radioactivity; 15 millirems to the thyroid.

If one uses the ratio of 135 lifetime fatalities per million person-rems, then the 3 mrems whole-body dose for liquid effluent radioactivity computes to a probability of four premature fatalities in 10 million. Similarly, 5 mrems of whole-body dose for gaseous effluent radioactivity yields a probability of 6.7×10^{-7}/(lifetime, individual) fatality per year of exposure. These values comply with the individual risk lower bound $L = 10^{-6}$/(year, individual) proposed by Wilson or by the de minimis risk.

Upper bound goals. According to the current radiation dose rate standard, a maximum allowable annual exposure to individuals in the general population is 500 mrems/year, excluding natural background and medical sources [11]. As a matter of fact, the average natural background in the United States is 100 mrem per year, and the highest is 310 mrem per year. The 500 mrems/year standard yields a probability for a premature fatality of 6.7×10^{-5}. This can be regarded as an upper bound U for an individual.

If the Wilson's bounds are used, the premature fatality likelihood lies in the middle layer, $L = 10^{-6} < 6.7 \times 10^{-5} < U = 10^{-3}$. Thus the risk must be justified; otherwise, the risk should be reduced below the lower bound. A possibility is to reduce the risk below the maximum allowable exposure by using a safety-cost trade-off value such as the \$1000 person-rem in the NRC's ALARA concept [10].

A maximum allowable annual exposure to radiological industrial workers is 5 rems per year [11], which is much less stringent than for individuals in the general population. Thus we do have different upper bounds U's for different situations.

Having an upper bound goal as a necessary condition is better than nothing. Some unsafe alternatives are rejected as unacceptable; the chance of such a rejection is increased by gradually decreasing the upper bound level. A similar goal for the upper bound has been specified for NO_2 concentrations caused by automobiles and factories. Various upper bound goals have been proposed for risks posed by airplanes, ships, automobiles, buildings, medicines, food, and so forth.

1.5.5 Goals for Catastrophic Accidents

Lower bound goals. Some lower bound goals for catastrophic accidents are stated qualitatively. A typical example is the qualitative safety goals proposed by the NRC in 1983 [22,10]. The first is related to individual risk, while the second is for population risk.

1. **Individual risk:** Individual members of the public should be provided a level of protection from the consequences of nuclear power plant operation such that individuals bear no significant additional risk to life and health.
2. **Population risk:** Societal risks to life and health from nuclear power plant operation should be comparable to or less than the risks of generating electricity by viable competing technologies and should not be a significant addition to other societal risks.

The NRC proposal also includes quantitative design objectives (QDOs).

1. **Prompt fatality QDO:** The risk to an average individual in the vicinity of a nuclear power plant of prompt fatalities that might result from reactor accidents should not exceed one-tenth of one percent (0.1 percent) of the sum of prompt fatality risks resulting from other accidents to which members of the U.S. population are generally exposed.
2. **Cancer fatality QDO:** The risk to the population in the area near a nuclear power plant of cancer fatalities that might result from nuclear power plant operation should not exceed one-tenth of one percent (0.1 percent) of the sum of cancer fatality risks resulting from all other causes.

3. **Plant performance objective:** The likelihood of a nuclear reactor accident that results in a large-scale core melt should normally be less than 1 in 10,000 per year of reactor operation.
4. **Cost-benefit guideline:** The benefit of an incremental reduction of societal mortality risks should be compared with the associated costs on the basis of $1000 per person-rem averted.

   The prompt (or accident) fatality rate from all causes in the United States in 1982 was 4×10^{-4} per year; 93,000 deaths in a population of 231 million. At 0.1% of this level, the prompt fatality QDO becomes 4×10^{-7} per year, which is substantially below the lower bound $L = 10^{-6}$ for an individual [10]. In 1983, the rate of cancer fatalities was 1.9×10^{-3}. At 0.1% of this background rate, the second QDO is 1.9×10^{-6}, which is less limiting than the lower bound.

   On August 4, 1986, the NRC left unchanged the two proposed qualitative safety goals (individual and population) and the two QDOs (prompt and cancer). It deleted the plant performance objective for the large-scale core melt. It also deleted the cost-benefit guideline. The following guideline was proposed for further examination:
5. **General performance guideline:** Consistent with the traditional defense-in-depth approach and the accident mitigation philosophy requiring reliable performance of containment systems, the overall mean frequency of a large release of radioactive materials to the environment from a reactor accident should be less than 10^{-6} per year of reactor operation.

The general performance guideline is also called an FP (fission products) large release criteria. Offsite property damage and erosion of public confidence by accidents are considered in this criteria in addition to the prompt and cancer fatalities.

The International Atomic Energy Agency (IAEA) recommended other quantitative safety targets in 1988 [23,24]:

1. For existing nuclear power plants, the probability of severe core damage should be below 10^{-4} per plant operating year. The probability of large offsite releases requiring short-term responses should be below 10^{-5} per plant operating year.
2. For future plants, probabilities lower by a factor of ten should be achieved.

The future IAEA safety targets are comparable with the plant performance objective and the NRC general performance guideline.

Risk-aversion goals. Neither the NRC QDOs nor the IAEA safety targets consider risk aversion explicitly in severe accidents; two accidents are treated equivalently if they yield the same expected numbers of fatalities, even though one accident causes more fatalities with a smaller likelihood. A Farmer curve version can be used to reflect the risk aversion. Figure 1.26 shows an example. It can be shown that a constant curve of expected number of fatalities is depicted by a straight line on a $\log f$ versus $\log x$ graph, where x is the number of fatalities and f is the frequency density around x.

Fatality excess curves have been proposed in the United States; more indirect curves such as dose excess have been proposed in other countries, although the latter can, in theory, be transformed into the former. The use of dose excess rather than fatality excess seems

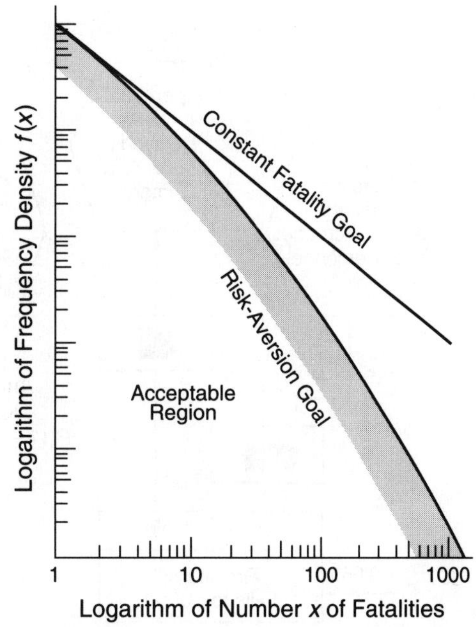

Figure 1.26. Constant fatality versus risk-aversion goal in terms of Farmer curves.

preferable in that it avoids the need to adopt a specific dose-risk correlation, to make extrapolations into areas of uncertainty, and to use upper limits rather than best estimates [11].

Risk profile obtained by cause-consequence diagram. Cause-consequence diagrams were invented at the RISϕ Laboratories in Denmark. This technology is a marriage of event trees (to show consequences) and fault trees (to show causes), all taken in their natural sequence of occurrence. Figure 1.27 shows an example. Here, construction starts with the choice of a critical initiating event, motor overheating.

The block labeled A in the lower left of Figure 1.27 is a compact way of showing fault trees that consist of component failure events (motor failure, fuse failure, wiring failure, power failure), logic gates (OR, AND), and state-of-system events (motor overheats, excessive current to motor, excessive current in circuit). An alternative representation (see Chapter 4) of block A is given in Figure 1.28.

The consequence tracing part of the cause-consequence analysis involves taking the initiating event and following the resulting chain of events through the plant. At various steps, the chains may branch into multiple paths. For example, the motor overheating event may or may not lead to a motor cabinet local fire. The chains of events may take alternative forms, depending on conditions. For example, the progress of a fire may depend on whether a traffic jam prevents the fire department from reaching the fire on time.

The procedure for constructing the consequence scenario is first to take the initiating event and each later event by asking:

1. Under what conditions does this event lead to further events?
2. What alternative plant conditions lead to different events?
3. What other components does the event affect? Does it affect more than one component?
4. What further event does this event cause?

The cause tracing part is represented by the fault tree. For instance, the event "motor overheating" is traced back to two pairs of concatenated causes: (fuse failure, wiring failure) and (fuse failure, power failure).

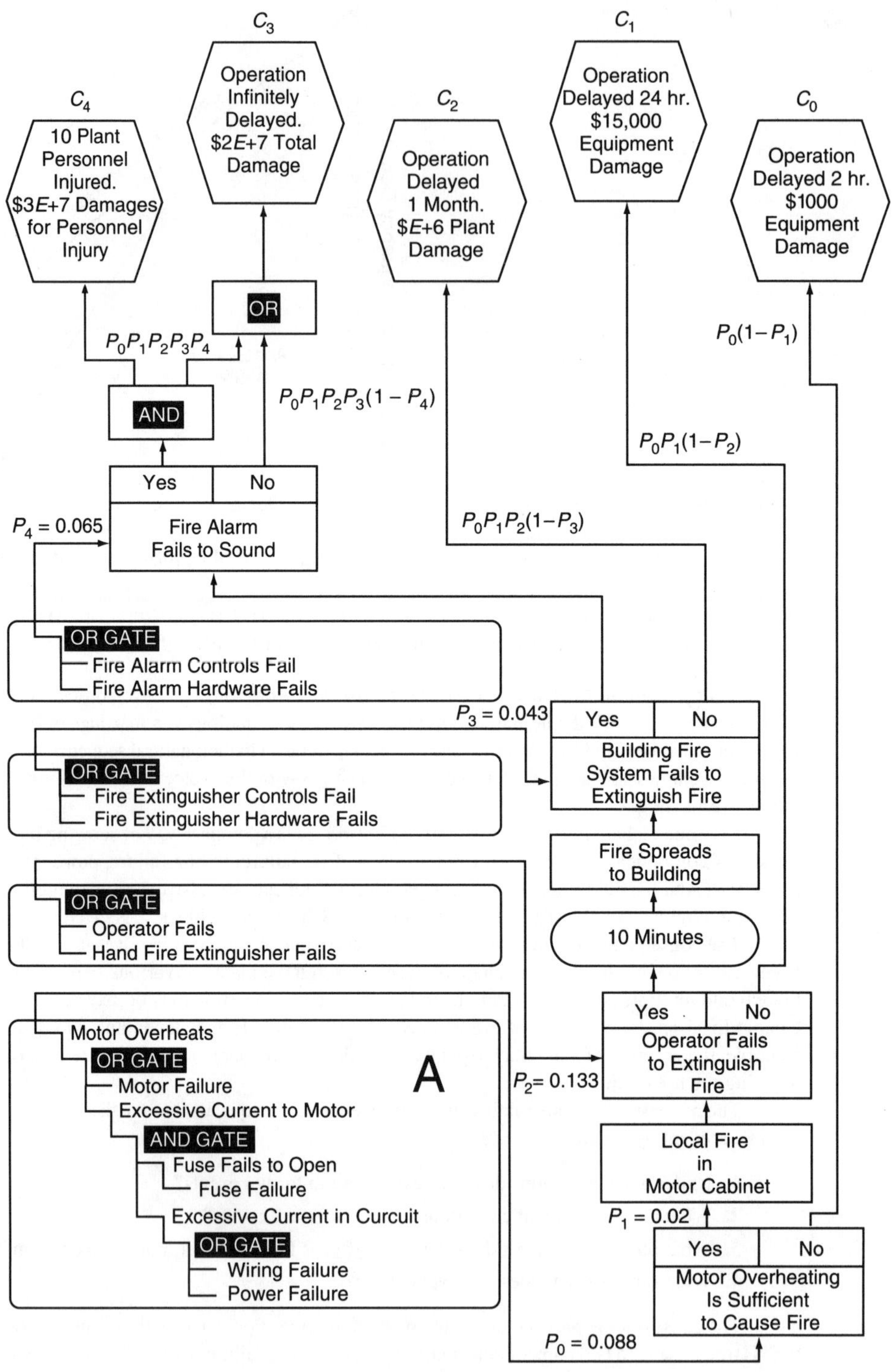

Figure 1.27. Example of cause-consequence diagram.

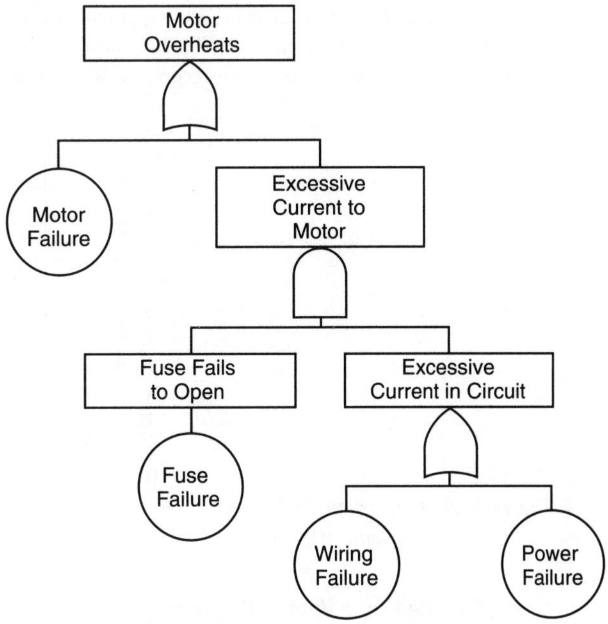

Figure 1.28. Alternative representation of "Motor Overheats" event.

We now show how the cause-consequence diagram can be used to construct a Farmer curve of the probability of an event versus its consequence. The fault tree corresponding to the top event, "motor overheats," has an expected number of failures of $P_0 = 0.088$ per 6 months, the time between motor overhauls. There is a probability of $P_1 = 0.02$ that the overheating results in a local fire in the motor cabinet. The consequences of a fire are C_0 to C_4, ranging from a loss of \$1000 if there is equipment damage with probability $P_0(1 - P_1)$ to $\$5 \times 10^7$ if the plant burns down with probability $P_0 P_1 P_2 P_3 P_4$. The downtime loss is estimated at \$1000 per hour; thus the consequences in terms of total loss are

$$C_0 = \$1000 + (2)(\$1000) = \$3000 \tag{1.27}$$

$$C_1 = \$15,000 + (24)(\$1000) = \$39{,}000, \text{ and so forth} \tag{1.28}$$

Assume the probabilities $P_0 = 0.088$, $P_1 = 0.02$, $P_2 = 0.133$, $P_3 = 0.043$, and $P_4 = 0.065$. Then a risk calculation is summarized as follows.

Event	Total Loss	Event Probability	Expected Loss
C_0	\$3000	$P_0(1 - P_1) = 0.086$	\$258
C_1	\$39,000	$P_0 P_1 (1 - P_2) = 1.53 \times 10^{-3}$	\$60
C_2	$\$1.744 \times 10^6$	$P_0 P_1 P_2 (1 - P_3) = 2.24 \times 10^{-4}$	\$391
C_3	$\$2 \times 10^7$	$P_0 P_1 P_2 P_3 (1 - P_4) = 9.41 \times 10^{-6}$	\$188
$C_3 + C_4$	$\$5 \times 10^7$	$P_0 P_1 P_2 P_3 P_4 = 6.54 \times 10^{-7}$	\$33

The total expected loss is thus

$$258 + 60 + 391 + 188 + 33 = \$930/6 \text{ months} = \$1860/\text{year} \tag{1.29}$$

Figure 1.29 shows the Farmer risk curve, including the \$300 expected risk-neutral loss line per event. This type of plot is useful for establishing design criteria for failure events such as "motor overheats," given their consequence and an acceptable level of risk. ■

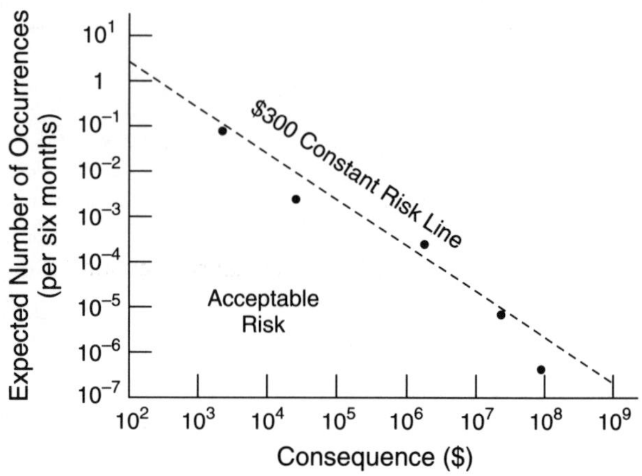

Figure 1.29. Risk profile with a \$300 constant risk line.

1.5.6 Idealistic Versus Pragmatic Goals

The Wilson's lower bound goal $L = 10^{-6}$/(year, individual) is reasonable either from idealistic or pragmatic viewpoints when a relatively small population is affected by the risk. A typical example of such a population would be a crew of the U.S. space shuttle. When a large number of people are exposed to the risk, however, the lower bound is not a suitable measure for the unconditional acceptance of the risk, that is, the Wilson's lower bound is not necessarily a suitable measure for the population risk (see Figure 1.11).

A randomized, perfect crime. Suppose that a decorative food additive* causes a 10^{-6} fatal cancer risk annually for each individual in the U.S. population, and that the number x of cancer fatalities over the population by the additive is distributed according to a binomial distribution.

$$\Pr\{x\} = \binom{n}{x} p^x (1-p)^{n-x}, \qquad p = 10^{-6}, \qquad n = 235 \times 10^6 \tag{1.30}$$

The expected number $E\{x\}$ of cancer fatalities per year is

$$E\{x\} = np = 235 \tag{1.31}$$

while the variance $V\{x\}$ of x is given by

$$V\{x\} = np(1-p) \simeq np = E\{x\} = 235 \tag{1.32}$$

By taking a 1.95 sigma interval, we see that it is 95% certain that the food additive causes from 205 to 265 fatalities. In other words, it is 97.5% certain that the annual cancer fatalities would exceed 205. The lower bound $L = 10^{-6}$ or the de minimis risk, when applied to the population risk, claims that this number is so small compared with two million annual deaths in the United States that it is negligible; $235/2{,}000{,}000 \simeq 0.0001$: among 10,000 fatalities, only one is caused by the additive.

---

*If the food additive saved human lives, we would have a different problem of risk-benefit trade-off.

In the de minimis theory, the size of the population at risk does not explicitly influence the selection of the level of the lower bound risk. Indeed, the argument has been made that it should not be a factor. The rationale for ignoring the size (or density) of the population at risk when setting standards should be examined in light of the rhetorical question posed by Milvy [3]:

> Why should the degree of protection that a person is entitled to differ according to how many neighbors he or she has? Why is it all right to expose people in lightly populated areas to higher risks than people in densely populated ones?

As a matter of fact, individual risk is viewed from the vantage point of a particular individual exposed; if the ratio of potential fatalities to the size of the population remains a constant, then the individual risk remains at the same level even if the population becomes larger and the potential fatalities increase. On the other hand, population risk is a view from a risk source or a society that is sensitive to the increase of fatalities.

Criminal murders, in any country, are crimes. The difference between the 205 food additive murders and criminal murders is that the former are performed statistically. A criminal murder requires that two conditions hold: intentional action to murder and evidence of causal relations between the action and the death. For the food additive case, the first condition holds with a statistical confidence level of 97.5%. However, the second condition does not hold because the causal relation is probabilistic—1 in 10,000 deaths in the United States. The 205 probabilistic deaths are the result of a perfect crime.

Let us now consider the hypothetical progress of a criminal investigation. Assume that the fatal effects of the food additive can be individually traced by autopsy. Then the food company using the additive would have to assume responsibility for the 205 cancer fatalities per year: there could even be a criminal prosecution. We see that for the food additive case there is no such concept as de minimis risk, acceptable risk level, or negligible level of risk unless the total number of fatalities caused by the food additive is made much smaller than 205.

Necessity versus sufficiency problem. A risk from an alternative is rejected when it exceeds the upper bound level U, which is all right because the upper bound goal is only a necessary condition for safety. Alternatives satisfying this upper bound goal would not be accepted if they neither satisfied the lower bound goal nor were justified by RCB analyses or ALARA. A risk level is subject to justification processes when it exceeds the lower bound level L, which is also all right because the lower bound goal is also regarded as a necessary condition for exemption from justification.

Many people in the PRA field, however, incorrectly think that considerably higher lower bound goals and even upper bound goals constitute sufficient conditions. They assume that safety goals are solutions for problems of how safe is safe enough, acceptable level of risks, and so forth. This failure to recognize the necessity feature of the lower and upper bound goals has caused confusion in PRA interpretations, especially for population risks.

Regulatory cutoff level. An individual risk of 10^{-6}/(year, individual) is sufficiently close to the idealistic, Platonic, lower bound sufficiency condition, that is, the de minimis risk. Such a risk level, however, is far from idealistic for risks to large populations. The lower bound L as a de minimis level for population risks must be a sufficiently small fractional number; less than one death in the entire population per year. If some risk level greater than this de minimis level is adopted as a lower bound, the reason must come from factors outside the risk itself. A pragmatic lower bound is called a regulatory cutoff level.

A pragmatic cutoff level is, in concept, different from the de minimis level: 1) the regulatory cutoff level is a level at or below which there are no regulatory concerns, and 2) a de minimis level is the lower bound level L at or below which the risks are accepted unconditionally. Some risks below the regulatory cutoff level may not be acceptable, although the risks are not regulated—the risks are only reluctantly accepted as a necessary evil. Consequently, the de minimis level for the population risk is smaller than the regulatory cutoff level currently enforced.

Containment structures with 100-foot-thick walls, population exclusion zones of hundreds of square miles, dozens of standby diesel generators for auxiliary feedwater systems, and so on are avoided by regulatory cutoff levels implicitly involving cost considerations [15].

Milvy [3] claims that a 10^{-6} *lifetime* risk to the U.S. population is a realistic and prudent regulatory cutoff level for the population risk. This implies 236 additional deaths over a 70-year interval (lifetime), and 3.4 deaths per year in the population of 236 million. This section briefly overviews a risk-population model as the regulatory cutoff level for chemical carcinogens.

Constant likelihood model. When the regulatory cutoff level is applied to an individual, or a discrete factory, or a small community population that is uniquely at risk, its consequences become extreme. A myriad of society's essential activities would have to cease. Certainly the X-ray technician and the short-order cook exposed to benzopyrene in the smoke from charcoal-broiled hamburgers are each at an individual cancer risk considerably higher than the lifetime risk of 10^{-6}. Indeed, even the farmer in an agricultural society is at a 10^{-3} to 10^{-4} lifetime risk of malignant melanoma from pursuing his trade in the sunlight. The 10^{-6} lifetime criterion may be appropriate when the whole U.S. population is at risk, but to enforce such a regulatory cutoff level when the exposed population is small is not a realistic option. Thus the following equation for regulatory cutoff level L_1 is too strict for a small population

$$L_1 = 10^{-6}/\text{lifetime} \tag{1.33}$$

Constant fatality model. On the other hand, if a limit of 236 deaths is selected as the criterion, the equation for cutoff level L_2 for a lifetime is

$$L_2 = (236/x)/\text{lifetime}, \qquad x\text{: population size} \tag{1.34}$$

This cutoff level is too risky for a small population size of several hundred.

Geometric mean model. We have seen that, for small populations, L_1 from the constant likelihood model is too strict and that L_2 from the constant fatality model is too risky. On the other hand, the two models give the same result for the whole U.S. population. Multiplying the two cutoff levels and taking the square root yields the following equation, which is based on a geometric mean of L_1 and L_2.

$$L = 0.015/\sqrt{x} \tag{1.35}$$

Using the equation with $x = 100$, the lifetime risk for the individual is 1.5×10^{-3} and the annual risk is 2.14×10^{-5}. This value is nearly equal to the lowest annual fatal occupational rate from accidents that occur in the finance, insurance, and real estate occupational category. The geometric mean risk-population model plotted in Figure 1.30 is deemed appropriate only for populations of 100 or more because empirical data suggest that smaller populations are not really relevant in the real world, in which environmental and occupational carcinogens almost invariably expose groups of more than 100 people. Figure 1.31 views the geometric mean model from expected number of lifetime fatalities rather than lifetime fatality likelihood.

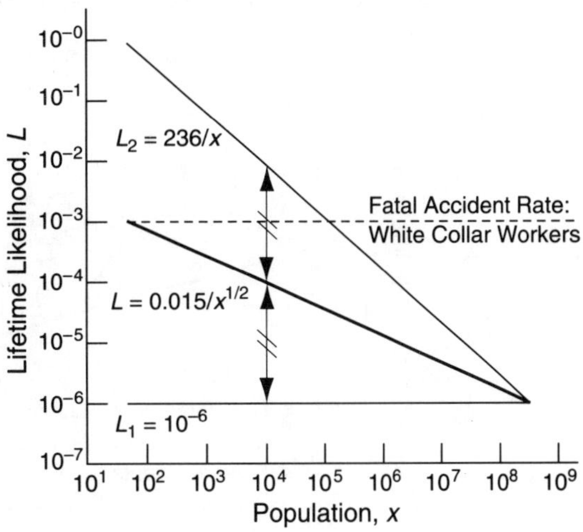

Figure 1.30. Regulatory cutoff level from geometric mean risk-population model.

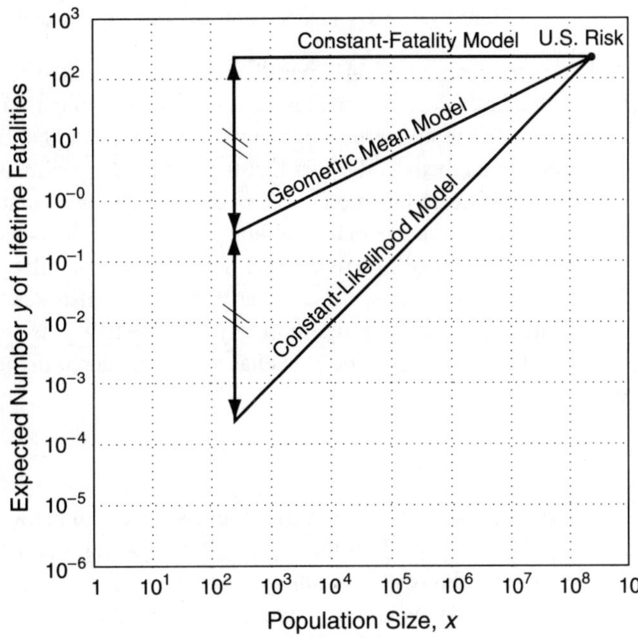

Figure 1.31. Geometric mean model viewed from lifetime fatalities.

Past regulatory decisions. Figure 1.32 compares the proposed cutoff level L with the historical data of regulatory decisions by the Environmental Protection Agency. Solid squares represent chemicals actively under study for regulation. Open circles represent the decision not to regulate the chemicals. The solid triangles provide fatal accident rates for: 1) private sector in 1982; 2) mining; 3) finance, insurance, and real estate; and 4) all. The solid line, $L = 0.28x^{-0.47}$, represents the best possible straight line that can be drawn through the solid squares. Its slope is very nearly the same as the slope of the geometric mean population-risk equation, $L = 0.015x^{-1/2}$, also shown in the figure.

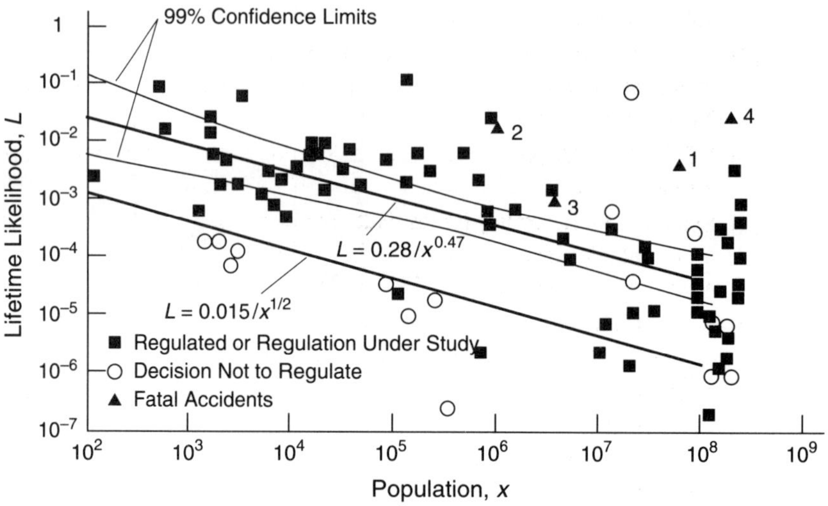

Figure 1.32. Regulatory cutoff level and historical decisions.

Although the lines are nearly parallel, the line generated from the data is displaced almost one and a half orders of magnitude above the risk-population model. This implies that these chemicals lie above the regulatory cutoff level and should be regulated. Also consistent with the analysis is the fact that ten of the 16 chemicals or data points that fall below the geometric mean line are not being considered for regulation. The six data points that lie above the geometric mean line, although not now being considered for regulation, in fact do present a sufficiently high risk to a sufficiently large population to warrant regulation.

The fact that the slopes are so nearly the same also seems to suggest that it is recognized—although perhaps only implicitly—by the EPA's risk managers that the size of the population at risk is a valid factor that has to be considered in the regulation of chemical carcinogens.

1.5.7 Summary

Risk goals can be specified on various levels of system hierarchy in terms of a variety of measures. The safety goal on the top level is a starting point for specifying the goals on the lower levels. PRAM procedures become more useful when a hierarchical goal system is established. A typical decision procedure with safety goals forms a three-layer structure. The ALARA principle or RCB analysis operates in the second layer. The de minimis risk gives the lower bound goal. The upper bound goal rejects risks without overriding benefits. Current upper and lower bound goals are given for normal activities and catastrophic accidents. When a risk to a large population is involved, the current lower bound goals should be considered as pragmatic goals or regulatory cutoff levels. The geometric mean model explains the behavior of the regulatory cutoff level as a function of population size.

REFERENCES

[1] USNRC. "Reactor safety study: An assessment of accident risk in U.S. commercial nuclear power plants." USNRC, NUREG-75/014 (WASH-1400), 1975.

[2] Farmer, F. R. "Reactor safety and siting: A proposed risk criterion." *Nuclear Safety*, vol. 8, no. 6, pp. 539–548, 1967.

[3] Milvy, P. "De minimis risk and the integration of actual and perceived risks from chemical carcinogens." In *De Minimis Risk*, edited by C. Whipple, ch. 7, pp. 75–86. New York: Plenum Press, 1987.

[4] USNRC. "PRA procedures guide: A guide to the performance of probabilistic risk assessments for nuclear power plants." USNRC, NUREG/CR-2300, 1983.

[5] Spangler, M. B. "Policy issues related to worst case risk analysis and the establishment of acceptable standards of de minimis risk." In *Uncertainty in Risk Assessment, Risk Management, and Decision Making*, pp. 1–26. New York: Plenum Press, 1987.

[6] Kletz, T. A. "Hazard analysis: A quantitative approach to safety." *British Insititution of Chemical Engineers Symposium, Ser.*, London, vol. 34, 75, 1971.

[7] Johnson, W. G. *MORT Safety Assurance Systems*. New York: Marcel Dekker, 1980.

[8] Lambert, H. E. "Case study on the use of PSA methods: Determining safety importance of systems and components at nuclear power plants." IAEA, IAEA-TECDOC-590, 1991.

[9] Whipple, C. "Application of the de minimis concept in risk management." In *De Minimis Risk*, edited by C. Whipple, ch. 3, pp. 15–25. New York: Plenum Press, 1987.

[10] Spangler, M. B. "A summary perspective on NRC's implicit and explicit use of de minimis risk concepts in regulating for radiological protection in the nuclear fuel cycle." In *De Minimis Risk*, edited by C. Whipple, ch. 12, pp. 111–143. New York: Plenum Press, 1987.

[11] Davis, J. P. "The feasibility of establishing a de minimis level of radiation dose and a regulatory cutoff policy for nuclear regulation." In *De Minimis Risk*, edited by C. Whipple, ch. 13, pp. 145–206. New York: Plenum Press, 1987.

[12] Bohnenblust, H. and T. Schneider. "Risk appraisal: Can it be improved by formal decision models?" In *Uncertainty in Risk Assessment, Risk Management, and Decision Making*, edited by V. T. Covello et al., pp. 71–87. New York: Plenum Press, 1987.

[13] Starr, C. "Risk management, assessment, and acceptability." In *Uncertainty in Risk Assessment, Risk Management, and Decision Making*, edited by V. T. Covello et al., pp. 63–70. New York: Plenum Press, 1987.

[14] Reason, J. *Human Error*. New York: Cambridge University Press, 1990.

[15] Pitz, G. F. "Risk taking, design, and training." In *Risk-Taking Behavior*, edited by J. F. Yates, ch. 10, pp. 283–320. New York: John Wiley & Sons, 1992.

[16] Spangler, M. "The role of interdisciplinary analysis in bringing the gap between the technical and human sides of risk assessment." *Risk Analysis*, vol. 2, no. 2, pp. 101–104, 1982.

[17] IAEA. "Case study on the use of PSA methods: Backfitting decisions." IAEA, IAEA-TECDOC-591, April, 1991.

[18] Comar, C. "Risk: A pragmatic de minimis approach." In *De Minimis Risk*, edited by C. Whipple, pp. xiii–xiv. New York: Plenum Press, 1987.

[19] Byrd III, D. and L. Lave. "Significant risk is not the antonym of de minimis risk." In *De Minimis Risk*, edited by C. Whipple, ch. 5, pp. 41–60. New York: Plenum Press, 1987.

[20] Wilson, R. "Commentary: Risks and their acceptability." *Science, Technology, and Human Values*, vol. 9, no. 2, pp. 11–22, 1984.

[21] Whipple, C. (ed.), *De Minimis Risk*. New York: Plenum Press, 1987.

[22] USNRC. "Safety goals for nuclear power plant operations," USNRC, NUREG-0880, Rev. 1, May, 1983.

[23] Hirsch, H., T. Einfalt, et al. "IAEA safety targets and probabilistic risk assessment." Report prepared for Greenpeace International, August, 1989.

[24] IAEA. "Basic safety principles for nuclear power plants." IAEA, Safety Series No. 75-INSAG-3, 1988.

PROBLEMS

1.1. Give a definition of risk. Give three concepts equivalent to risk.

1.2. Enumerate activities for risk assessment and risk management, respectively.

1.3. Explain major sources of debate in risk assessment and risk management, respectively.

1.4. Consider a trade-off problem when fatality is measured by monetary loss. Draw a schematic diagram where outcome probability and cost are represented by horizontal and vertical axes, respectively.

1.5. Pictorialize relations among risk, benefits, and acceptability.

1.6. Consider a travel situation where \$1000 is stolen with probability 0.5. For a traveler, a \$750 insurance premium is equivalent to the theft risk. Obtain a quadratic loss function $s(x)$ with normalizing conditions $s(0) = 0$ and $s(1000) = 1$. Calculate an insurance premium when the theft probability decreases to 0.1.

1.7. A Bayesian explanation of outcome severity overestimation is given by (1.19). Assume $\Pr\{10|\text{Defect}\} > \Pr\{10|\text{No defect}\}$. Prove:

(a) The a posteriori probability of a defect conditioned by the occurrence of a ten-fatality accident is larger than the a priori defect probability

$$\Pr\{\text{Defect}|10\} > \Pr\{\text{Defect}\}$$

(b) The overestimation is more dominant when the a priori probability is smaller, that is, the following ratio increases as the a priori defect probability decreases.

$$\Pr\{\text{Defect}|10\}/\Pr\{\text{Defect}\}$$

1.8. Explain the following concepts: 1) hierarchy of safety goals, 2) three-layer decision structure for risk acceptance, 3) ALARA, 4) de minimis risk, 5) geometric mean model for a large population risk exposure.

1.9. Give an example of qualitative and quantitative safety goals for catastrophic accidents.

2

Accident Mechanisms and Risk Management

2.1 INTRODUCTION

At first glance, hardware failures appear to be the dominant causes of accidents such as Chernobyl, Challenger, Bhopal, and Three Mile Island. Few reliability analysts support this conjecture, however. Some emphasize human errors during operation, design, or maintenance, others stress management and organizational factors as fundamental causes. Some emphasize a lack of safety culture or ethics as causes. This chapter discusses common accident-causing mechanisms.

To some, accidents appear inevitable because they occur in so many ways, but reality is more benign. The second half of this chapter presents a systematic risk-management approach for accident reduction.

2.2 ACCIDENT-CAUSING MECHANISMS

2.2.1 Common Features of Plants with Risks

Features common to plants with potentially catastrophic consequences are physical containment, stabilization of unstable phenomena, large size, new technology, component variety, complicated structure, large inertia, large consequence, and strict societal demand for safety.

Physical containment. A plant is usually equipped with physical barriers or containments to confine hazardous materials or shield hazardous effects. These containments are called physical barriers. For nuclear power plants, these barriers include fuel cladding, primary coolant boundary, and containment structure. For commercial airplanes, various portions of the airframe provide physical containment. Wells and banks vaults are simpler examples of physical containments. As long as these containment barriers are intact, no serious accident can occur.

Stabilization of unstable phenomena. Industrial plants create benefits by stabilizing unstable physical or chemical phenomena. Together with physical containment, these plants require normal control systems during routine operations, safety systems during emergencies, and onsite and offsite emergency countermeasures, as shown in Figure 2.1. Physical barriers, normal control systems, emergency safety systems, and emergency countermeasures correspond, for instance, to body skin, body temperature control, immune mechanism, and medical treatment, respectively.

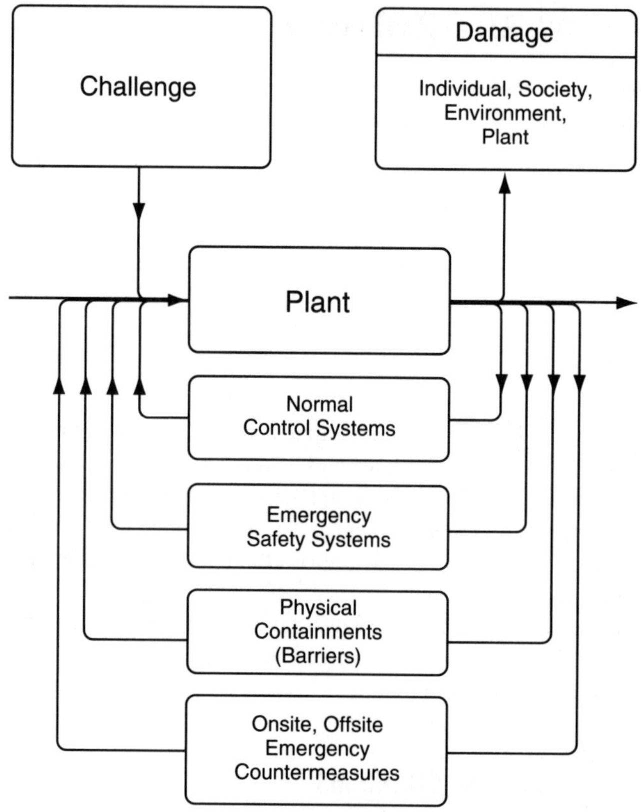

Figure 2.1. Protection configuration for plant with catastrophic risks.

If something goes wrong with the normal control systems, incidents occur; if emergency safety systems fail to cope with the incidents, plant accidents occur; if onsite emergency countermeasures fail to control the accident and the physical containment fails, the accident invades the environment; if offsite emergency countermeasures fail to cope with the invasion, serious consequences for the public and environment ensue.

The stabilization of unstable phenomena is the most crucial feature of systems with large risks. For nuclear power plants, the most important stabilization functions are power control systems during normal operation and safety shutdown systems during emergencies, normal and emergency core-cooling systems, and confinement of radioactive materials during operation, maintenance, engineering modification, and accidents.

Large size. Plants with catastrophic risks are frequently large in size. Examples include commercial airplanes, space rockets and shuttles, space stations, chemical plants, metropolitan power networks, and nuclear power plants. These plants tend to be large for the following reasons.

1. Economy of scale: Cost per product or service generally decreases with size. This is typical for ethylene plants in the chemical industry.
2. Demand satisfaction: Large commercial airplanes can better meet the demands of air travel over great distances.
3. Amenity: Luxury features can be amortized over a larger economic base, that is, a swimming pool on a large ship.

New technology. Size increases require new technologies. The cockpit of a large contemporary commercial airplane is as high as a three-story building. The pilots must be supported by new technologies such as autopilot systems and computerized displays to maneuver the airplane for landing and takeoff. New technologies reduce airplane accidents but may introduce pitfalls during initial burn-in periods.

Component variety. A large number of system components of various types are used. Components include not only hardware but also human beings, computer programs, procedures, instructions, specifications, drawings, charts, and labels. Large-scale systems consist of millions of components. Failures of some components might initiate or enable event propagations toward an accident. Human beings must perform tasks in this jungle of hardware and software.

Complicated structure. A plant and its operating organization form a complicated structure with various lateral and vertical interactions. A composite hierarchy is formed that encompasses the component, individual, unit, team, subsystem, department, facility, plant, corporation, and environment.

Inertia. An airplane cannot stop suddenly; it must remain in flight. A chemical plant or a nuclear power plant requires a long time to achieve a quiescent state after initiation of a plant shutdown. A long period is also required for resuming plant operations.

Large consequence. An accident can have direct effects on individuals, society, environment, and plant and indirect effects on research and development, schedules, share prices, public opposition, and company credibility.

Strict social demand for safety. Society demands that individual installations be far safer than, for example, automobiles, ski slopes, or amusement parks.

2.2.2 Negative Interactions Between Humans and the Plant

Human beings are responsible for the creation and improvement of plant safety and gain knowledge, abilities, and skills via daily operation. These are examples of positive interactions between human and plant. Unfortunately, as suggested by man-made accidents, most accidents are due to errors committed by humans [1]. It is thus necessary to investigate the negative interactions between humans and plants.

Figure 2.2 shows these negative interactions when the plant consists of physical components such as hardware and software. The humans and the plant form an operating organization. This organization, enclosed by a general environment, is the risk-management target. Each arrow in Figure 2.2 denotes a direction of an elementary one-step interaction labeled as follows:

1. Unsafe act—human injures herself. No damage or abnormal plant state ensues.
2. Abnormal plant states occur due to hardware or software failures.
3. Abnormal plant states are caused by human errors.
4. Human errors, injuries, or fatalities are caused by abnormal plant states.
5. Accidents have harmful consequences for the environment.
6. Negative environmental factors such as economic recessions or labor shortage have unhealthy effects on the plant operation.

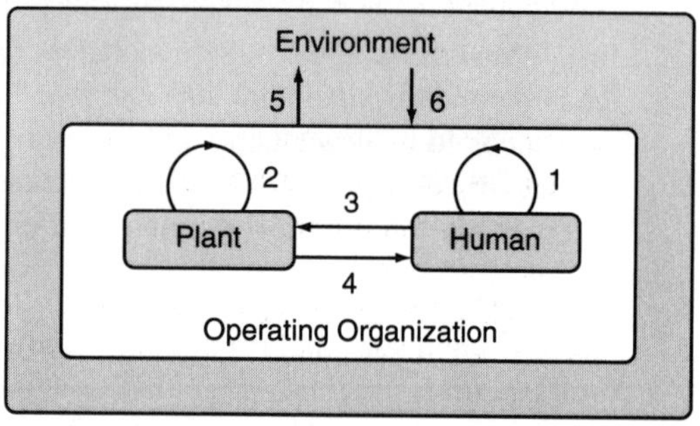

Figure 2.2. Negative one-step interactions between plant and human.

These interactions may occur concurrently and propagate in series and/or parallel, as shown in Figure 2.3.* Some failures remain latent and emerge only during abnormal situations. Event 6 in Figure 2.3 occurs if two events, 3 and B, exist simultaneously; if event B remains latent, then event 6 occurs by single event 3.

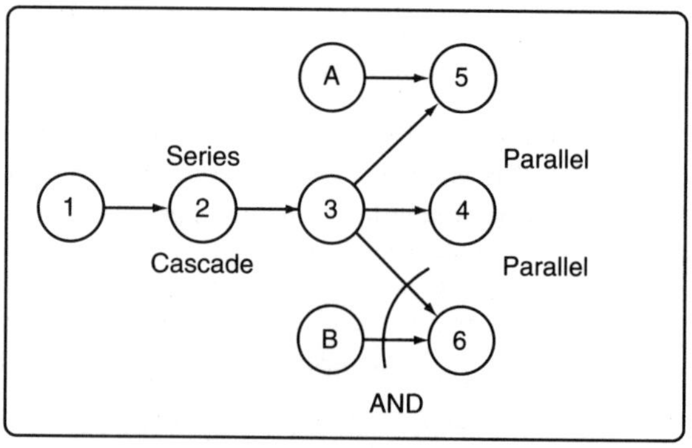

Figure 2.3. Parallel and series event propagations.

2.2.3 A Taxonomy of Negative Interactions

A description of accident-causing mechanisms involves a variety of negative interactions. Some of these interactions are listed here from four points of view: why, how, when, and where. The why-classification emphasizes causes of failures and errors; the how-classification is based on behavioral observable aspects; the when-classification is based on the time frame when a failure occurs; the where-classification looks at places where failures or errors occur.

---

*An arc crossing arrows denotes logic AND.

2.2.3.1 Why-Classification

Mechanical, functional, and interface failures. In *mechanical failures*, a device becomes unusable and fails to perform its function because some of its components fail. For *functional failures*, a device is usable, but fails to perform its function because of causes not attributable to the device or its components; a typical example is a perfect TV set when a TV station has a transmission problem. When devices interface, a failure of this interface is called an *interface failure*; this may cause a functional failure of one or two of the devices interfaced; a computer printer fails if its device driver has a bug.

Primary, secondary, and command failures. A *primary failure* is defined as the component being in a nonworking state for which the component is held accountable, and repair action on the component is required to return the component to the working state. A primary failure occurs under causes within the design envelope, and component natural aging (wearout or random) is responsible for the failure. For example, "tank rupture due to metal fatigue" is a primary failure. The failure probability is usually time dependent.

A *secondary failure* is the same as a primary failure except that the component is not held accountable for the failure. Past or present excessive stresses beyond the design envelope are responsible for the secondary failure. These stresses involve out-of-tolerance conditions of amplitude, frequency, duration, or polarity, and energy inputs from thermal, mechanical, electrical, chemical, magnetic, or radioactive energy sources. The stresses are caused by neighboring components or the environment, which includes meteorological or geological conditions and other engineering systems.

Human beings such as operators and inspectors can cause secondary failures if they break component. Examples of secondary failures are "maintenance worker installs wrong circuit breaker," "valve is damaged by earthquake," and "stray bullet cracks storage tank." Note that disappearance of the excessive stresses does not guarantee the working state of the component because the stresses have damaged the component that must be repaired.

A *command failure* is defined as the component being in a nonworking state due to improper control signals or noise, and repair action is not required to return the component to the working state; the component will function normally when a correct command is fed. Examples of command failures are "power is applied, inadvertently, to the relay coil," "switch fails to open because of electrical noise," "noisy input to safety monitor randomly generates spurious shutdown signals," and "operator fails to push panic button" (command failure for the panic button).

Secondary and command failures apply to human errors when the human is regarded as a device. Thus if an operator opens a valve because of an incorrect instruction, his failure is a command failure.

Basic and intermediate failures. A *basic failure* is a lowest-level, highest resolution failure for which failure-rate (occurrence-likelihood) data are available. An example is a mechanically stuck-closed failure of an electrical switch. Failures caused by a propagation of basic failures are called *intermediate*. An example is a lack of electricity caused by a switch failure. A primary or mechanical failure is usually considered a basic failure; occurrence-likelihood data are often unavailable for a secondary failure. When occurrence data are guesstimated for secondary failures, these are treated as basic failures. Causes of command failure such as "area power failure" are also treated as basic failures when occurrence data are available.

Parallel and cascade failures. Two or more failures may result from a single cause. This parallel or fanning-out propagation is called a *parallel failure*. Two or more failures may occur sequentially starting from a cause. This sequential or consecutive propagation is called a *cascade* or *sequential failure*. These propagations are shown in Figure 2.3. An accident scenario usually consists of a mixture of parallel and cascade failures.

Direct, indirect, and root causes. A *direct cause* is a cause most adjacent in time to a device failure. A *root cause* is an origin of direct causes. Causes between a direct and a root cause are called *indirect*. Event 3 in Figure 2.3 is a direct cause of event 4; event 1 is a root cause of event 4; event 2 is an indirect cause of event 4.

Main cause and supplemental causes. A failure may occur by simultaneous occurrence of more than one cause. One cause is identified as a *main cause*, all others are *supplemental causes;* event 3 in Figure 2.3 is a main cause of event 6 and event B is a supplemental cause.

Inducing factors. Some causes do not necessarily yield a device failure; they only increase chances of failures. These causes are called *inducing factors*. Smoking is an inducing factor for heart failure. Inducing factors are also called *risk factors*, *background factors*, *contributing factors*, or *shaping factors*. Management and organizational deficiencies are regarded as inducing factors.

Hardware-induced, human-induced, and system-induced failures. This classification is based on what portions of a system trigger or facilitate failures. A human error caused by an erroneous indicator is *hardware induced*. Hardware failures caused by incorrect operations are *human induced*. Human and hardware failures caused by improper management are termed *system induced*.

2.2.3.2 How-Classification

Random, wearout, and initial failures. A *random failure* occurs with a constant rate of occurrence; an example is an automobile water pump failing after 20,000 miles. A *wearout failure* occurs with an increasing rate of occurrence; an old automobile in a burn-out period suffers from wearout failures. An *initial failure* occurs with a decreasing rate of occurrence; an example is a brand-new automobile failure in a burn-in period.

Demand and run failure. A *demand failure* is a failure of a device to start or stop operating when it receives a start or stop command; this failure is called a *start* or a *stop failure*. An example is a diesel generator failing to start upon receipt of a start signal. A *run failure* is one where a device fails to continue operating. A diesel generator failing to continue operating is a typical example of a run failure.

Persistent and intermittent failures. A *persistent failure* is one where a device failure continues once it has failed. For an *intermittent failure*, a failure only exists sporadically. A relay may fail intermittently while closed. A typical cause of an intermittent failure is electromagnetic circuit noise.

Active and latent failures. *Active failures* are felt almost immediately; as for *latent failures*, their adverse consequences lie dormant, only becoming evident when they combine with other factors to breach system defenses. Latent failures are most likely caused by designers, computer software, high-level decision makers, construction workers, managers, and maintenance personnel.

One characteristic of latent failures is that they do not immediately degrade a system, but in combination with other events—which may be active human errors or random hardware failures—they cause catastrophic failure. Two categories of latent failures can be identified: operational and organizational. Typical operational latent failures include maintenance errors, which may make a critical system unavailable or leave the system in a vulnerable state. Organizational latent failures include design errors, which yield intrinsically unsafe systems, and management or policy errors, which create conditions inducing active human errors. The latent failure concept is discussed more fully in Reason [1] and Wagenaar et al. [2].

Omission and commission errors. When a necessary action is not performed, this failure is an *omission error*. An example is an operator forgetting to read a level indicator or to manipulate a valve. A *commission error* is one where a necessary step is performed, but in an incorrect way.

Independent and dependent failures. Failures A and B are *independent* when the product law of probability holds:

$$\Pr\{A \text{ and } B\} = \Pr\{A\}\Pr\{B\} \tag{2.1}$$

Failures are *dependent* if the probability of A depends on B, or vice versa:

$$\Pr\{A \text{ and } B\} \neq \Pr\{A\}\Pr\{B\} \tag{2.2}$$

Independent failures are sometimes called *random failures;* this is misleading because failures with a constant occurrence rate are also called random in some texts.

2.2.3.3 When-Classification

Recovery failure. Failure to return from an abnormal device state to a normal one is called a *recovery failure*. This can occur after maintenance, test, or repair [3].

Initiating and enabling events. *Initiating events* cause system upsets that trigger responses from the system's mitigative features. *Enabling events* cause failure of the system's mitigative features' ability to respond to initiating events; enabling events facilitate serious accidents, given occurrence of the initiating event [4].

Routine and cognitive errors. Errors in carrying out known, routine procedures are called *routine* or *skill-based errors*. Errors in thinking and nonroutine tasks are *cognitive errors*, which generate incorrect actions. A typical example of a cognitive error is an error in diagnosis of a dangerous plant state.

Lapse, slip, and mistake. Suppose that specified, routine actions are known. A *lapse* is the failure to recall one of the required steps, that is, a lapse is an omission error. A *slip* is a failure to correctly execute an action when it is recalled correctly. An example is a driver's inadvertently pushing a gas pedal when he intended to step on the brake. Lapses and slips are two types of routine errors. A *mistake* is a cognitive error, that is, it is a judgment or analysis error.

2.2.3.4 Where-Classification

Internal and external events. An *internal event* occurs inside the system boundary, while an *external event* takes place outside the boundary. Typical examples of external events include earthquakes and area power failures.

Active and passive failures. A device is called active when it functions by changing its state; an example is an emergency shutdown valve that is normally open. A device without a state change is called passive; a pipe or a wire are typical examples. An *active failure* is an active device failure, while a *passive failure* is a passive device failure.

LOCA and transient. A *LOCA* (loss of coolant accident) is a breach in a coolant system that causes an uncontrollable loss of water. *Transients* are other abnormal conditions of a plant that require that the plant be shut down temporarily [4]. A loss of offsite power is an example of a transient. Another example is loss of feedwater to a steam generator. A common example is shutdown because of government regulatory action.

2.2.4 Chronological Distribution of Failures

Different types of failures occur at various chronological stages in the life of a plant.

1. **Siting.** A site is an area within which a plant is located [5]. Local characteristics, including natural factors and man-made hazards, can affect plant safety. Natural factors include geological and seismological characteristics and hydrological and meteorological disturbances. Accidents take place due to an unsuitable plant location.
2. **Design.** This includes prototype design activities during research, development, and demonstration periods, and product or plant design. Design errors may be committed during scaleup because of insufficient budgets for pilot plant studies or truncated research, development, and design. Key technologies sometimes remain black boxes due to technology license contracts. Designers are given proprietary data but do not know where it came from. This can cause inadvertent design errors, especially when black boxes are used or modified and original specifications are hidden. Black box designs are the rule in the chemical industry where leased or rented process simulations are widely used.

   In monitoring device recalls, the Food and Drug Administration (FDA) has compiled data that show that from October 1983 to November 1988 approximately 45% of all recalls were due to preproduction-related problems. These problems indicate that deficiencies had been incorporated into the device design during a preproduction phase [6].
3. **Manufacturing and construction.** Defects may be introduced during manufacturing and construction; a plant could be fabricated and constructed with deviations from original design specifications.
4. **Validation.** Errors in design, manufacturing, and construction stages may persist after plant validations that demonstrate that the plant is satisfactory for service. A simple example of validation failures is a software package with bugs.
5. **Operation.** This is classified into normal operation, operation during anticipated abnormal occurrences, operation during complex events below the design basis, and operation during complex events beyond the design basis.

   (5-1) Normal operation. This stage refers to a period where no unusual challenge is posed to plant safety. The period includes start-up, steady-state, and shutdown. Normal operations include daily operation, maintenance, testing, inspection, and minor engineering modifications.

Tight operation schedules and instrumentation failures may induce operator errors. Safety features may inadvertently be left nullified after maintenance because some valves may be incorrectly set; these types of maintenance failures typically constitute latent failures. Safety systems are frequently intentionally disabled to avoid too many false alarms. Safety systems become unavailable during a test interval.

(5-2) Anticipated abnormal occurrences. These occurrences are handled in a straightforward manner by appropriate control systems response as depicted in Figure 2.1. The term *anticipated* means such an event occurs more than once in a plant life. If normal control systems fail, anticipated abnormal occurrences could develop into the complex events described below.

(5-3) Complex events below the design basis. System designers assume that hardware, software, and human failures are possible, and can lead to minor abnormal disturbances or highly unlikely accident sequences. Additional protection can be achieved by incorporating engineered features into the plant. These features consist of passive features such as physical barriers and active features such as emergency shutdown systems, standby electric generators, and water-tank systems.

Active systems are called *engineered safety systems*, and their performance is measured by on-demand performance and duration performance. The simplest forms of safety systems include circuit breakers and rupture disks. As shown in Figure 2.1, these safety features are required to supplement protection afforded by normal control systems.

Design parameters of each engineered safety feature are defined by classic, deterministic analyses that evaluate their effectiveness against complex events. The event in a spectrum of events that has the most extreme design parameters is used as the design basis. The engineering safety features are provided to halt progress of an undesirable event occurring below the design basis and, when necessary, to mitigate its consequences.

Safety features may fail to respond to complex events below the design basis because something is wrong with the features themselves. High-stress conditions after a plant upset may induce human errors, and cause events that occur below the design basis to propagate complex events beyond the design basis.

(5-4) Complex events beyond the design basis. Attention is directed to events of low likelihood but that are more severe than those explicitly considered in the design. An event beyond the design basis can result in a severe accident because some safety features have failed. For a chemical plant, these severe accidents could cause a toxic release or a temperature excursion. These accidents have a potential for major environmental consequences if chemical materials are not adequately confined.

The classification of events into normal operation, anticipated abnormal occurrences, complex events below design basis, and complex events beyond design basis is taken from IAEA No. 75-INSAG-3 [5]. It is useful for large nuclear power plants where it has been estimated that as much as

90% of all costs relate to safety. It is too complicated and costly to apply to commercial manufacturing plants. Some of the concepts, however, are useful.

2.2.5 Safety System and Its Malfunctions

As shown in Figure 2.1, safety systems are key elements for ensuring plant safety. A malfunctioning safety system is important because it either nullifies a plant safety feature or introduces a plant upset condition.

2.2.5.1 Nuclear reactor shutdown system. Figure 2.4 is a schematic diagram of a pressurized water reactor. Heat is continuously removed from the reactor core by primary coolant loops whose pressure is maintained at about 1500 psi by the pressurizers. Several pumps circulate the coolant. The secondary coolant loops remove heat from the primary loops via the heat exchangers, which, in turn, create the steam to drive the turbines that generate electricity.

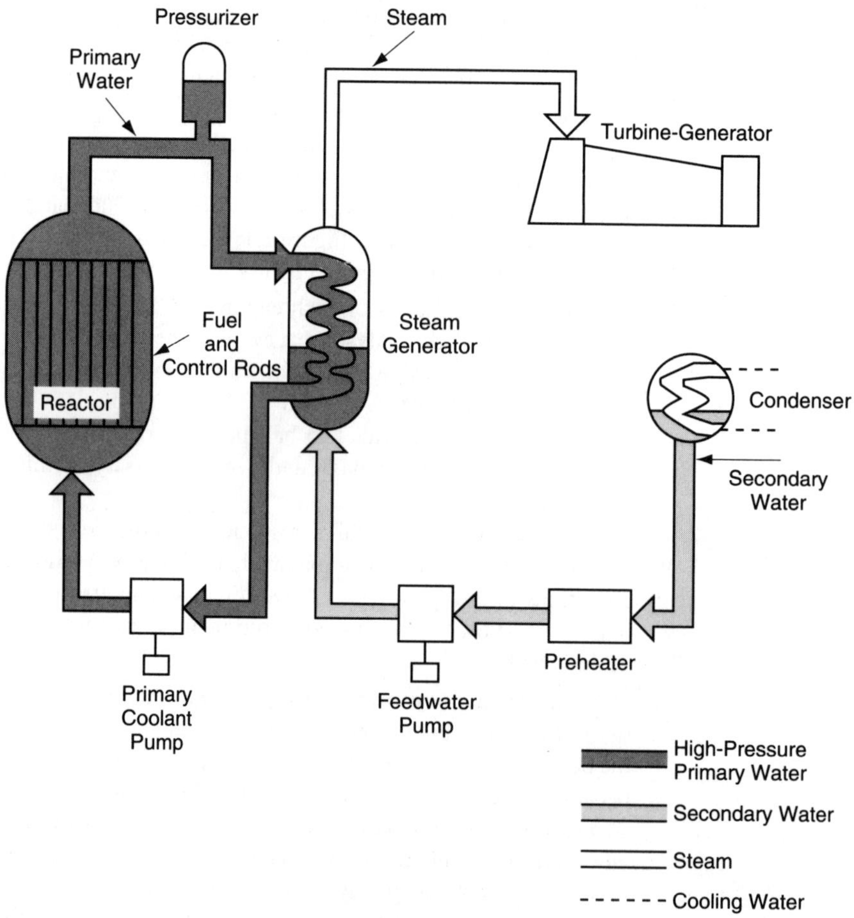

Figure 2.4. Simplified diagram of pressurized water reactor.

The control rods regulate the nuclear fission chain reaction in the reactor core. As more rods are inserted into the core, fewer fissions occur. The chain reaction stops when a critical number of control rods are fully inserted.

When unsafe events in the reactor are detected, the shutdown system must drop enough control rods into the reactor to halt the chain reaction. This insertion is a *reactor scram* or *reactor trip*. The reactor monitoring system has sensors that continuously measure the following: neutron flux density, coolant temperature at the reactor core exit (outlet temperature), coolant temperature at the core entrance (inlet temperature), coolant flow rate, coolant level in pressurizer, and on-off status of coolant pumps.

An inadvertent event is defined as a deviation of a state variable from its normal trajectory. The simplest is an event where one of the measured variables goes out of a specified range. A more complicated event is a function of one or more of the directly measured variables.

Figure 2.5 shows a diagram of a reactor shutdown system. Five features of the system are listed.

1. Inadvertent events are monitored by four identical channels, A, B, C, and D.
2. Each channel is physically independent of the others. For example, every channel has a dedicated sensor and a voting unit, a voting unit being defined as an action taken when m out of n sensors give identical indications.
3. Each channel has its own two-out-of-four:G voting logic. Capital G, standing for *good*, means that the logic *can* generate the trip signal if two or more sensors successfully detect an inadvertent event. The logic unit in channel A has four inputs, x_A, x_B, x_C, x_D, and one output, T_A. Input x_A is a signal from a channel A sensor. This input is zero when the sensor detects no inadvertent events, and unity when it senses one or more events. Inputs x_B, x_C, and x_D are defined similarly. Note that a channel also receives sensor signals from other channels. Output T_A represents a decision by the voting logic in channel A; zero values of T_A indicate that the reactor should not be tripped; a value of 1 implies a reactor trip. The voting logic in channel B has the same inputs, x_A, x_B, x_C, and x_D, but it has output T_B specific to the channel. Similarly, channels C and D have output T_C and T_D, respectively.
4. A one-out-of-two:G twice logic with input T_A, T_B, T_C, and T_D is used to initiate control rod insertion, which is controlled by magnets energized by two circuits. The two circuits must be cut off to deenergize the magnets; $(T_A, T_C) = (1, 1)$, or $(T_A, T_D) = (1, 1)$, or $(T_B, T_C) = (1, 1)$, or $(T_B, T_D) = (1, 1)$. The rods are then released by the magnets and dropped into the reactor core by gravity. ■

2.2.5.2 *Operating range and trip actions* For nuclear power plants, important neutron and thermal-hydraulic variables are assigned operating ranges, trip setpoints, and safety limits. The safety limits are extreme values of the variables at which conservative analyses indicate undesirable or unacceptable damage to the plant. The trip setpoints are at less extreme values of variables that, if attained as a result of an anticipated operational occurrence or an equipment malfunction or failure, would actuate an automatic plant protective action such as a programmed power reduction, or plant shutdown. Trip setpoints are chosen such that plant variables will not reach safety limits. The operating range, which is the domain of normal operation, is bounded by values of variables less extreme than the trip setpoints.

It is important that trip actions not be induced too frequently, especially when they are not required for protection of the plant or public. A trip action could compromise safety by sudden and precipitous changes, and it could induce excessive wear that might impair safety systems reliability [5].

Figure 2.6 shows a general configuration of a safety system. The monitoring portion monitors plant states; the judgment portion contains threshold units, voting units, and other logic devices; the actuator unit drives valves, alarms, and so on. Two types of failures occur in the safety system. ■

2.2.5.3 *Failed-Safe failure.* The safety system is activated when no inadvertent event exists and the system should not have been activated. A smoke detector false alarm or a reactor spurious trip is a typical failed-safe (FS) failure. It should be noted, however, that FS failures are not necessarily safe.

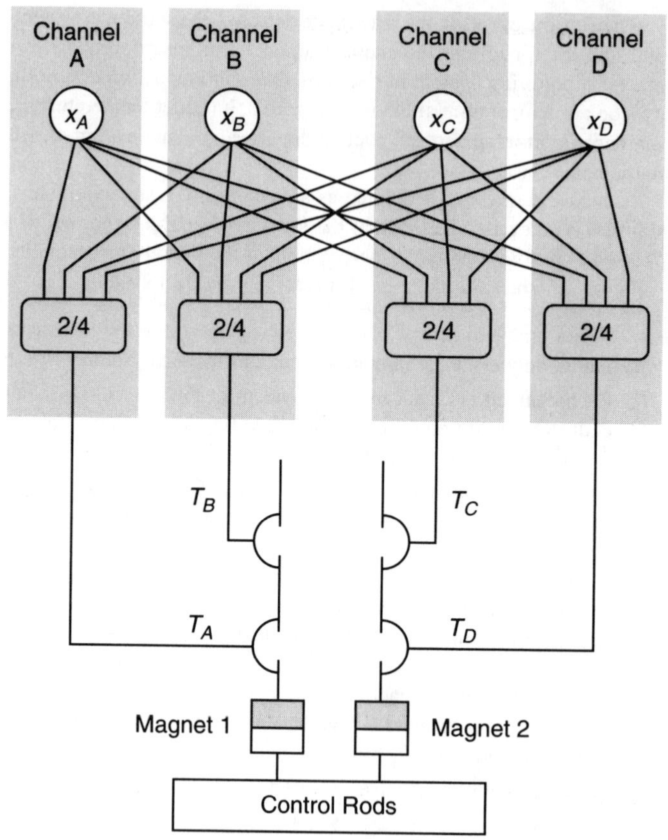

Figure 2.5. Four-channel configuration of nuclear reactor shutdown system.

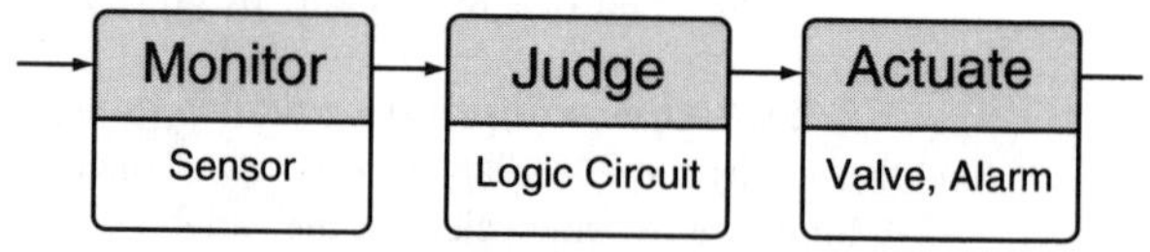

Figure 2.6. Three elements of emergency safety systems.

Example 1—Unsafe FS failure. Due to a gust of wind, an airplane safety system incorrectly detects airplane speed and decreases thrust. The airplane falls 5000 m and very nearly crashes. ■

Example 2—Unsafe FS failure. An airplane engine failed immediately after takeoff. The airplane was not able to climb rapidly, and the safety system issued the alarm, "Pull up." This operation could stall the airplane, so the pilot neglected the alarm and dropped the airplane to gain speed, avoiding a stall. ■

2.2.5.4 Failed-Dangerous failure. The safety system is not activated when inadvertent events exist and the system should have been activated. A typical example is "no alarm" from a smoke detector during a fire. A variety of causes yield failed-dangerous (FD) failures.

Example 1—Incorrect sensor location. Temperature sensors were spaced incorrectly in a chemical reactor. A local temperature excursion was not detected. ■

Example 2—Sensing secondary information. Valve status was detected by monitoring an actuator signal to the valve. A mechanically stuck-closed failure was not detected because the valve-open signal correctly reached the valve. ■

Example 3—Sensor failure. Train service incorrectly resumed after a severe earthquake due to a seismic sensor biased low. ■

Example 4—Excessive information load. A mainframe computer at a flood-warning station crashed due to excessive information generated by a typhoon. ■

Example 5—Sensor diversion. Sensors for normal operations were used for a safety system. A high temperature could not be detected because the normal sensors went out of range. Similar failures can occur if an inadvertent event is caused by sensor failures of plant controllers. ■

Example 6—Insufficient capacity. A large release of water from a safety water tank washed poison materials into the Rhine due to insufficient capacity of the catchment basin. ■

Example 7—Reputation. Malodorous gas generated by abnormal chemical reactions was not released to the environment because a company was nervous about lawsuits from neighbors. The chemical plant exploded. ■

Example 8—Too many alarms. At the Three Mile Island accident, alarm panels looked like Christmas trees, inducing operator errors, and eventually causing FD failures of safety systems. ■

Example 9—Too little information. A pilot could not understand the alarms when his airplane lost lift power. He could not cope with the situation. ■

Example 10—Intentional nullification. It has been charged that a scientist nullified vital safety systems to perform his experiment in the Chernobyl accident. ■

Example 11—One-time activation. It is difficult to validate rupture disks and domestic fire extinguishers because they become useless once they are activated. ■

Example 12—Simulated validation. Safety systems based on artificial intelligence technologies are checked only for hypothetical accidents, not for real situations. ■

2.2.6 Event Layer and Likelihood Layer

Given event trees and fault trees, various computer codes are available to calculate probabilistic parameters for accident scenarios. However, risk assessment involves more than a simple manipulation of probability formulas. Attention must be paid to evaluating basic occurrence probabilities used by these computer codes.

2.2.6.1 Event layer. Consider the event tree and fault tree in Figure 1.10. We observe that the tank rupture due to overpressure occurs if three events occur simultaneously: pump overrun, operator shutdown system failure, and pressure protection relief valve failure. The pump-overrun event occurs if either of two events occurs: timer contact fails to open, or timer itself fails. These causal relations described by the event and fault trees are on an event layer level.

Event layer descriptions yield explicit causes of accident in terms of event occurrences. These causes are hardware or software failures or human errors. Fault trees and the event trees explicitly contain these failures. Failures are analyzed into their ultimate resolution by a fault-tree analysis and basic events are identified. However, these basic events are not the ultimate causes of the top event being analyzed, because occurrence likelihoods of the basic events are shaped by the likelihood layer described below.

2.2.6.2 Likelihood layer. Factors that increase likelihoods of events cause accidents. Event and fault trees only describe causal relations in terms of a set of if-then statements. Occurrence probabilities of basic events, statistical dependence of event occurrences, simultaneous increase of occurrence probabilities, and occurrence probability uncertainties are greatly influenced by shaping factors in the likelihood layer. This point is shown in Figure 2.7.

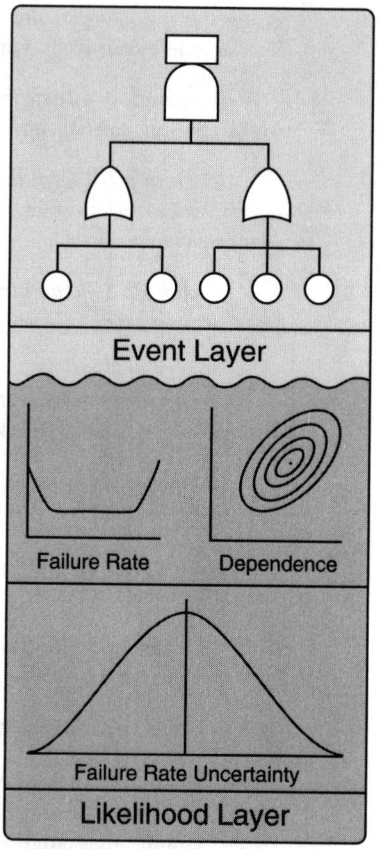

Figure 2.7. Event layer and likelihood layer for accident causation.

The likelihood layer determines, for instance, device failure rates, statistical dependency of device failures, simultaneous increase of failure rates, and failure rate uncertainties. These shaping factors do not appear explicitly in fault or event trees; they can affect accident-causation mechanisms by changing the occurrence probabilities of events in the trees. For instance, initiating events, operator actions, and safety system responses in event trees are affected by the likelihood layer. Similar influences exist for fault-tree events.

2.2.6.3 Event-likelihood model. Figure 2.8 shows a failure distribution in the event layer and shaping factors in the likelihood layer, as proposed by Embrey [3]. When an accident such as Chernobyl, Exxon Valdez, or Clapham Junction is analyzed in depth it appears at first to be unique. However, certain generic features of such accidents become

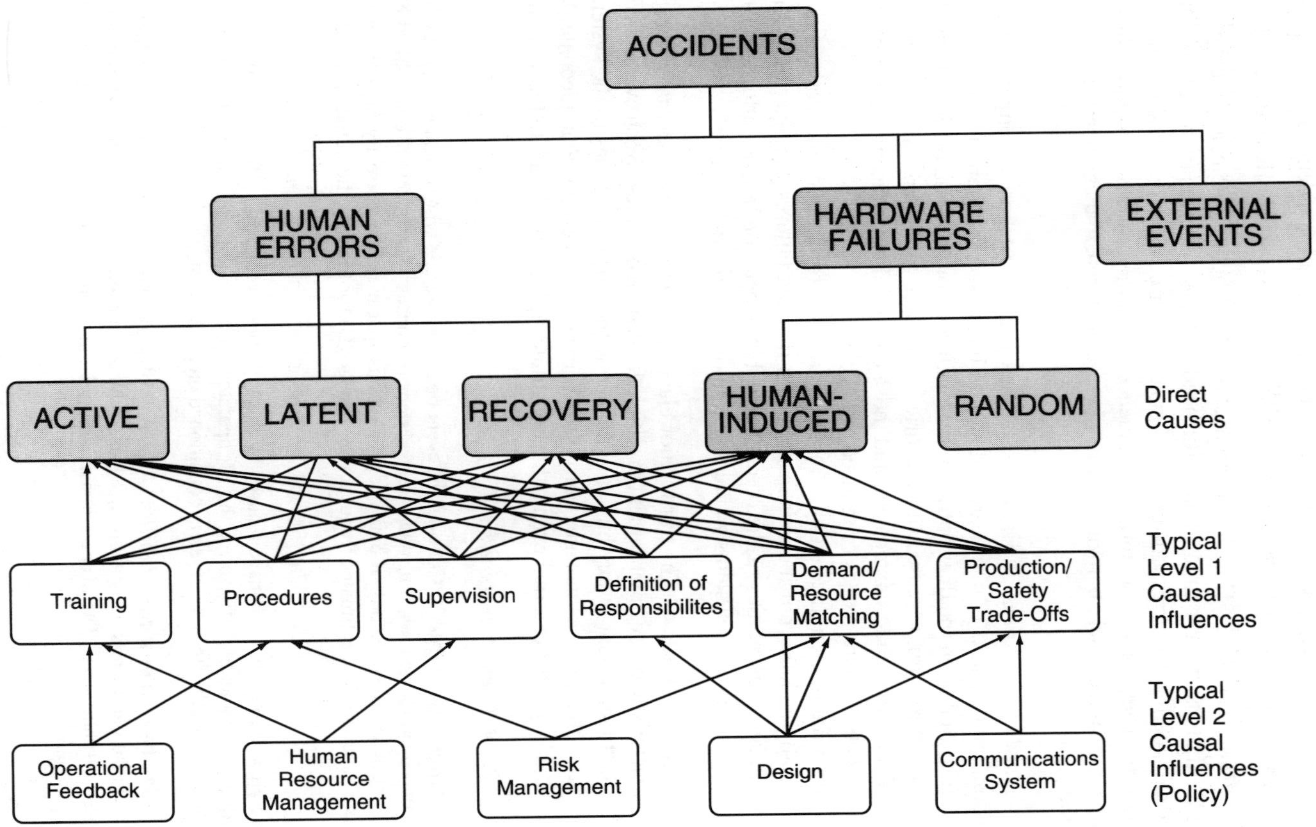

Figure 2.8 Generic model of accident causation.

apparent when a large number of cases are examined. Figure 2.8 is intended to indicate, in a simplified manner, how such a generic model might be represented. The generic model is called MACHINE (model of accident causation using hierarchical influence network elicitation). The direct causes, in the event layer, of all accidents are combinations of human errors, hardware failures, and external events.

Human errors. Human errors are classified as active, latent, and recovery failures. The likelihoods of these failures are influenced by factors such as training, procedures, supervision, definition of responsibilities, demand/resource matching, and production/safety trade-offs. These factors, in turn, are influenced by some of the higher-policy factors such as operational feedback, human resource management, risk management, design, and communications system.

Hardware failures. Hardware failures can be categorized under two headings. Random (and wearout) failures are ordinary failures used in reliability models. Extensive data are available on the distribution of such failures from test and other sources. Human-induced failures comprise two subcategories, those due to human actions in areas such as assembly, testing, and maintenance, and those due to inherent design errors that give rise to unpredicted failure modes or reduced life cycle.

As reliability engineers know, most failure rates for components derived from field data actually include contributions from human-induced failures. To this extent, such data are not intrinsic properties of the components, but depend on human influences (management, organization) in systems where the components are employed.

External events. The third major class of direct causes is external events. These are characteristic of the environment in which the system operates. Such events are considered to be independent of any human influence within the boundaries of the system being analyzed, although risk-management policy is expected to ensure that adequate defenses are available against external events that constitute significant threats to the system.

2.2.6.4 Event-tree analysis

Simple event tree. Consider the event tree in Figure 2.9, which includes an initiating event (IE), two operator actions, and two safety system responses [7]. In this oversimplified example, damage can be prevented only if both operator actions are carried out correctly and both plant safety systems function. The estimated frequency of damage (D) for this specific initiating event is

$$f_D = f_{IE} \times [1 - (1 - p_1)(1 - q_1)(1 - p_2)(1 - q_2)] \tag{2.3}$$

where f_D = frequency of damage (caused by this initiating event); f_{IE} = frequency of the initiating event; p_i = probability of error of the ith operator action conditioned on prior events; and q_i = unavailability of the ith safety system conditioned on prior events.

Safety-system unavailability. Quality of organization and management should be reflected in the parameters f_{IE}, p_i, and q_i. Denote by $\overline{q}_i$ an average unavailability during an interval between periodic tests. The average unavailability is an approximation to time-dependent unavailability q_i, and is given by*

$$\overline{q}_i = \frac{T_0}{T} + \gamma + Q + \frac{1}{2}\lambda T \tag{2.4}$$

*The time-dependent unavailability is fully described in Chapter 6.

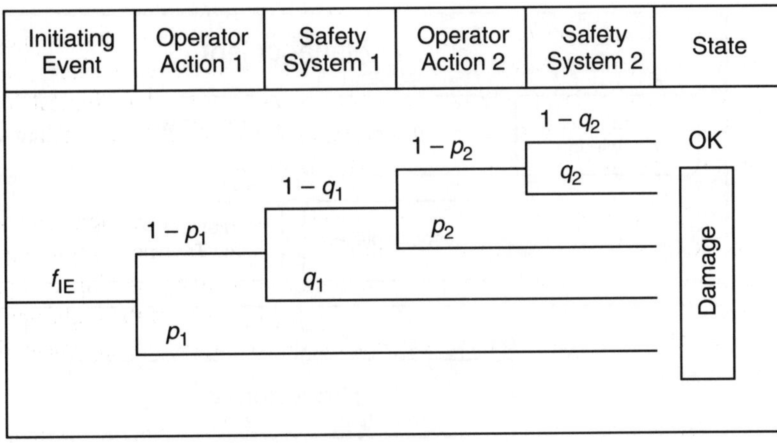

Figure 2.9. Simple event tree with two operator actions and two safety systems.

where T = interval between tests,
T_0 = duration of test,
γ = probability of failure due to testing,
Q = probability of failure on demand,
λ = expected number of random failures per unit time between tests.

Thus contributing to the average unavailability are T_0/T = test contribution while the safety system is disabled during testing; γ = human error in testing; Q = failure on demand; and $\frac{1}{2}\lambda T$ = random failures between tests while the safety system is on standby.

Likelihood layer contributions. As shown in Figure 2.10, these contributions are affected by maintenance activities. These activities are, in turn, affected by the quality of all maintenance procedures. Quality of various procedures is determined by overall factors such as safety knowledge, attitude toward plant operation and maintenance, choice of plant performance goals, communication, responsibilities, and level of intelligence and training. This figure is a simplified version of the one proposed by Wu, Apostolakis, and Okrent [7].

Safety knowledge. Safety knowledge refers to everyone who possesses knowledge of plant behavior, severe accident consequences, and related subjects, and whose combined knowledge leads to a total and pervasive safety ambiance.

Attitude. Uneventful, routine plant operation often makes the work environment boring rather than challenging. Plant personnel may misinterpret stagnation for safety. A team with a slack and inattentive attitude toward plant operation will experience difficulty in bringing the plant back to normal operation after an abnormal occurrence.

Plant performance goal. Plant performance goals are set by plant managers at a high organizational level and influence plant personnel in making decisions during plant operation. For example, if an operating team constantly receives pressure and encouragement from high-level managers to achieve high plant availability and to increase the production during daily operations, operators weigh production consequences higher than safety consequences. Another extreme is a corporate policy that plant safety will help achieve efficiency and economy.

Communication and responsibility. It is not uncommon to find a situation where supervisors know operators sleep during their shifts but take no action (lack of responsibility). Some supervisors do not have sufficient time to be in the plant to observe and supervise the efforts of the work force (lack of communication). Some companies tend to rely solely on written communication

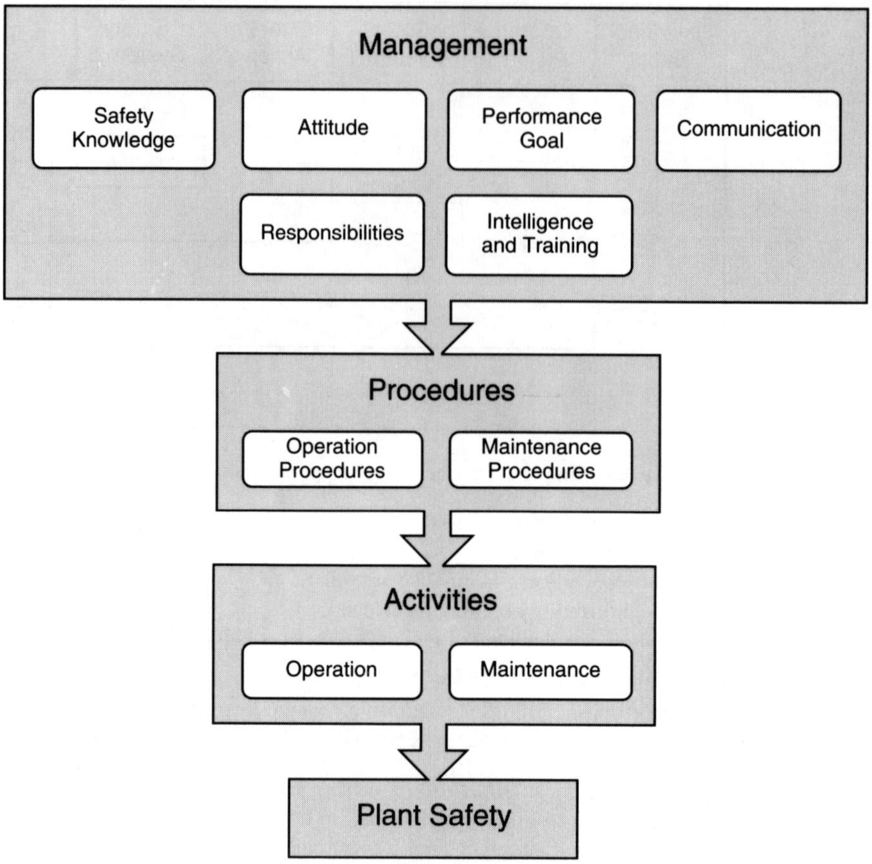

Figure 2.10. Operation and maintenance affected by management.

rather than verbal face-to-face communication. Lessons learned at other plants in the industry are frequently not utilized. ■

2.2.7 Dependent Failures and Management Deficiencies

Risks would be much lower if there were no dependencies; redundant configurations alone would provide reasonable protection. Dependence is a serious challenge to plant safety. All important accident sequences that can be postulated for nuclear reactor systems involve failures of multiple components, systems, and containment barriers [8]. This section describes various types of dependent failures.

2.2.7.1 Coupling mechanisms. Four types of coupling mechanisms yield dependencies, as shown in Figure 2.11: functional coupling, common-unit coupling, proximity coupling, and human coupling.

Functional coupling. If a window is fully open on a hot summer day, an air-conditioner cannot cool the room. Air-conditioner design specifications assume that the window is closed. Functional coupling between devices A and B is defined as a situation where device A gives boundary conditions under which device B can perform its function. In other words, if device A fails, device B cannot achieve its function because the operating

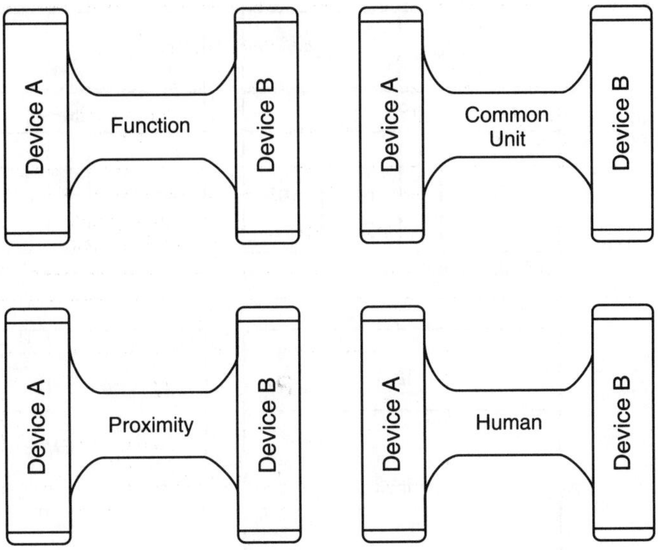

Figure 2.11. Four coupling mechanisms of dependent failures.

environment is outside the scope of device B's design specifications. Devices A and B fail sequentially due to functional coupling.

An example is a case where systems A and B are a scram system and an emergency core-cooling system (ECCS), respectively, for a nuclear power plant. Without terminating chain reactions by insertion (scram) of control rods, the ECCS cannot achieve its function even if it operates successfully. A dependency due to functional coupling is called a functional dependency [8].

Common-unit coupling. Imagine a situation where devices A and B have a common unit, for instance, a common power line. If the common unit fails, then the two devices fail simultaneously. This type of dependency is called a shared-equipment dependency [8].

Proximity coupling. Several devices may fail simultaneously because of proximity. Assume a floor plan with room numbers in Figure 2.12(a). Figures 2.12(b), (c), and (d) identify rooms influenced by five sources of impact, two sources of vibration, and two sources of temperature increase. Impact-susceptible devices in rooms 102 and 104 may fail due to impact source IMP-1.

The proximity coupling is activated either by external events or internal failures. External events usually result in severe environmental stresses on components and structures. Failures of one or more systems within a plant (internal failures) can create extreme environmental stresses. For instance, sensors in one system might fail due to an excessive temperature resulting from a second system's failure to cool a heat source [8]. The simultaneous sensor failures are due to a proximity coupling triggered by a functional dependency on the cooling system.

Human coupling. These are dependencies introduced by human activities, including errors of omission and commission. Persons involved can be anyone associated with a plant-life-cycle activity, including designers, manufacturers, constructors, inspectors, operators, and maintenance personnel. Such a dependency emerges, for example, when an operator turns off a safety system when she fails to diagnose the plant condition—an event

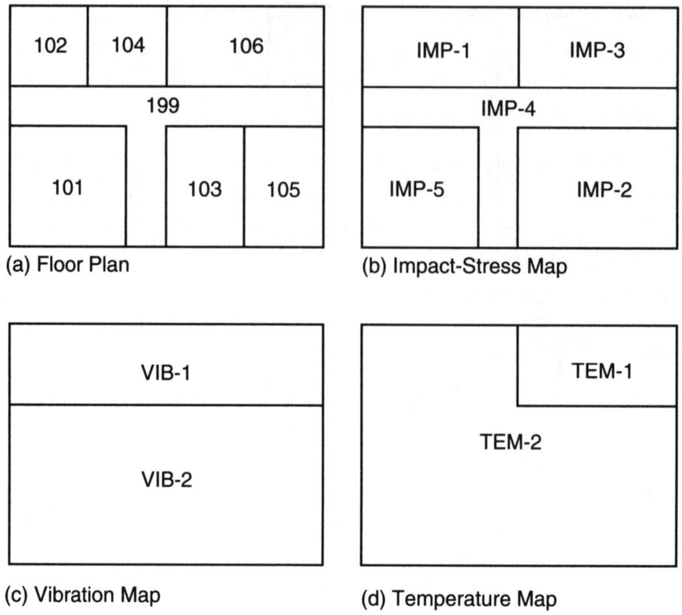

Figure 2.12. Proximity coupling by impact-stress, vibration, and temperature.

that happened during the Three Mile Island accident when an operator turned off an emergency core-cooling system [8]; the operator introduced a dependency between the cooling system and an accident initiator. Valves were simultaneously left closed by a maintenance error.

2.2.7.2 Parallel versus cascade propagation

Common-cause failure. This is a failure of multiple devices due to shared causes [8, 9]. Failed devices or failure modes may not be identical.

Some common-cause events have their origin in occurrences internal to the plant. These include common-unit coupling such as depletion of fuel for diesel generators and proximity coupling such as fire, explosion, or projectiles from the failure of rotating or pressurized components. Human coupling, such as failure due to undetected flaws in manufacture and construction, is also considered here [5].

Common-cause events external to the plant include natural events such as earthquakes, high winds, and floods, as well as such man-made hazards as aircraft crashes, fires, and explosions, which could originate from activities not related to the plant. For a site with more than one plant unit, events from one unit are considered as additional external initiating events for the other units.

A so-called *common-cause analysis* deals with common causes other than the dependencies already modeled in the logic model (see Chapter 9).

Common-mode failure. This is a special case of common-cause failures. The common-mode failure is a multiple, concurrent, and dependent failure of identical devices that fail *in the same mode* [8]. Causes of common-mode failure may be single or multiple; for instance, device A fails due to a mechanical defect, but devices B and C fail due to external vibrations. Devices from the same manufacturer may fail in a common mode.

Propagating failure. This occurs when equipment fails in a mode that causes sufficient changes in operating conditions, environment, or requirements to cause other items of equipment to fail. The propagating failure (cascade propagation) is a way of causing common-cause failures (parallel propagation).

2.2.7.3 Management deficiency dependencies. Dependent-failure studies usually assume that multiple failures occur within a short time interval, and that components affected are of the same type. Organizational and managerial deficiencies, on the other hand, can affect various components during long time intervals. They not only introduce dependencies between failure occurrences but also increase occurrence probabilities [7].

2.2.8 Summary

Features common to plants with catastrophic risks are presented: confinement by physical containment and stabilization of unstable phenomena are important features. These plants are protected by physical barriers, normal control systems, emergency safety systems, and onsite and offsite emergency countermeasures.

Various failures, errors, and events occur in hazardous plants, and these are seen as series and parallel interactions between humans and plant. Some of these interactions are listed from the points of view of why, how, when, and where. It is emphasized that these negative interactions occur during any time in the plant's life: siting, design, manufacturing/construction, validation, and operation. The plant operation period is divided into four phases: normal operation, anticipated abnormal occurrences, complex events below the design basis, and complex events beyond the design basis.

A nuclear reactor shutdown system is presented to illustrate emergency safety systems that operate when plant states reach trip setpoints below safety limits, but above the operating range. Safety systems fail in two failure modes, failed-safe and failed-dangerous, and various aspects of these failures are given through examples.

Accident-causing mechanisms can be split into an event layer and a likelihood layer. Event and fault trees deal with the event layer. Recently, more emphasis has been placed on the likelihood layer, where management and organizational qualities play crucial roles for occurrence probabilities, dependence of event occurrences and dependent increases of probabilities, and uncertainties of occurrence probabilities. Four types of coupling mechanisms that cause event dependencies are presented: functional coupling, common-unit coupling, proximity coupling, and human coupling. Events can propagate in series or in parallel by these coupling mechanisms. Management deficiencies not only introduce dependencies but also increase occurrence probabilities.

2.3 RISK MANAGEMENT

2.3.1 Risk-Management Principles

Figure 2.13 shows risk-management principles according to IAEA document No. 75-INSAG-3 [5]. The safety culture is at the base of risk management. Procedures are established and all activities are performed with strict adherence to these procedures. This, in turn, establishes the company's safety culture, because employees become aware of management's commitment.

The term *procedure* must be interpreted in a broad sense. It includes not only operation, maintenance, and training procedures but also codes, standards, formulas, speci-

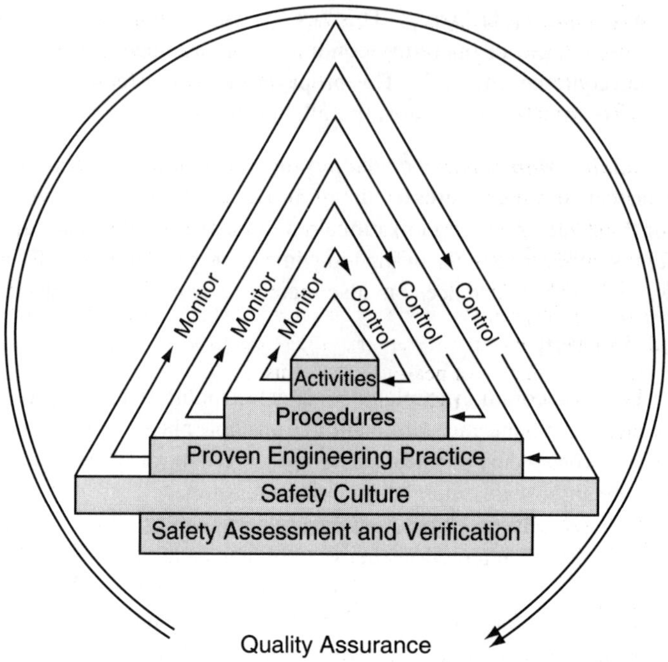

Figure 2.13. Risk management principles based on safety culture.

fications, instructions, rules, and so forth. The activities include plant-life-cycle activities ranging from siting to operation.

Change is inevitable and this results in deviations from previously proven practice. These deviations must be monitored and controlled. The term *monitor* implies verbs such as review, verify, survey, audit, test, inspect. Similarly, the term *control* covers verbs such as correct, modify, repair, maintain, alarm, enforce, regulate, and so on. The multilayer monitor/control system in Figure 2.13 is called a *quality assurance program.*

Safety culture. The IAEA document defines the safety culture in the following way:

> The phrase *safety culture* refers to a very general matter, the personal dedication and accountability of all individuals engaged in any activity which has a bearing on plant safety. The starting point for the necessary full attention to safety matters is with the senior management of all organizations concerned. Policies are established and implemented which ensure correct practices, with the recognition that their importance lies not just in the practices themselves but also in the environment of safety consciousness which they create. Clear lines of responsibility and communication are established; sound procedures are developed; strict adherence to these procedures is demanded; internal reviews of safety related activities are performed; above all, staff training and education emphasize reasons behind the safety practices established, together with the consequences of shortfalls in personal performance.
>
> These matters are especially important for operating organizations and staff directly engaged in plant operation. For the latter, at all levels, training emphasizes significance of their individual tasks from the standpoint of basic understanding and knowledge of the plant and equipment at their command, with special emphasis on reasons underlying safety limits and safety consequences of violations. Open attitudes are required in such staff to ensure that information relevant to plant safety is freely communicated; when errors are committed,

their admission is particularly encouraged. By these means, an all pervading safety thinking is achieved, allowing an inherently questioning attitude, prevention of complacency, commitment to excellence, and fostering of both personal accountability and corporate self-regulation in safety matters.

Small group activities. Japanese industries make the best use of small-group activities to increase productivity and safety. From a safety point of view, such activities stimulate the safety culture of a company. Small-group activities improve safety knowledge by small-group brainstorming, bottom-up proposal systems to uncover hidden causal relations and corresponding countermeasures, safety meetings involving people from various divisions (R&D, design, production, and marketing), branch factory inspections by heads of other branches, safety exchanges between operation and maintenance personnel, participation of future operators in the plant construction and design phase, and voluntary elicitation of near-miss incidents.

The small-group activities also boost morale by voluntary presentation of illustrations about safety matters, voluntary tests involving knowledge of plant equipment and procedures, inventing personal nicknames for machines, and Shinto purification ceremonies.

The safety culture is further strengthened by creating an environment that decreases rush jobs, and encourages revision, addition, miniaturization, simplification, and systematization of various procedures. The culture is supported by management concepts such as 1) rules should be changed if violated, 2) learning from model cases rather than accidents, 3) permission of small losses, and 4) safety is fundamental for existence and continuation of the company. ■

Proven engineering practices. Devices are designed, manufactured, and constructed by technologies that are proven by tests and experience, which are reflected in approved codes and standards and other appropriately documented statements, and that are implemented by proper selection and training of qualified workers. The use of proven engineering methods should continue throughout the plant's life. GMP (good manufacturing practices) must be vigilantly maintained.

Quality assurance. Quality assurance programs (QA) are a component of modern management. They complement the quality control (QC) programs that normally reside in the production department. Quality assurance is broader than quality control and has as its goal that all items delivered and services and tasks performed meet specified requirements. Organizational arrangements should provide a clear definition of the responsibilities and channels of communication and coordination for quality assurance. These arrangements are founded on the principle that the responsibility for achieving quality in a task rests with those performing it, others verify that the task has been properly performed, and yet others audit the entire process. The authority of the quality assurance staff is established firmly and independently within the organization.

When repairs and modifications are made, analyses are conducted and reviews made to ensure that the system is returned to a configuration covered in the safety analysis and technical specifications. Engineering change orders must be QC and QA monitored. If opportunities for advancement or improvement over existing practices are available and seem appropriate, changes are applied cautiously only after demonstration that the alternatives meet the requirements.

Quality assurance practices thus cover validation of designs; supply and use of materials; approval of master device files and manufacturing, inspection, and testing methods; and operational and other procedures to ensure that specifications are met. The associated documents are subject to strict procedures for verification, issue, amendment, and withdrawal.

The relationships between, and the existence of, separate QA, QC, loss prevention, and safety departments vary greatly between industries, large and small companies, and frequently depend on government regulation. The FDA, the NRC, and the DoD (Department of Defense) all license and inspect plants, and each has very detailed and different QA, QC, and safety protocol requirements. Unregulated companies that are not self-insured are usually told what they must do about QA, QC, and safety by their insurance companies' inspectors.

Ethnic and educational diversity; employee lawsuits; massive interference and threats of closure, fines, and lawsuits by armies of government regulatory agencies (Equal Employment Opportunity Commission, Occupational Safety & Health Administration, Environmental Protection Agency, fire inspectors, building inspectors, State Water and Air Agencies, etc.); and adversarial attorneys given the right by the courts to disrupt operations and interrogate employees have made it difficult for American factory managers to implement, at reasonable cost, anything resembling the Japanese safety and quality programs. Ironically enough, the American company that in 1990 was awarded the prestigious Malcom Baldridge Award for the best total quality control program in the country declared bankruptcy in 1991 (see Chapter 12).

Safety assessment and verification. Safety assessments are made before construction and operation of a plant. The assessment should be well documented and independently reviewed. It is subsequently updated in the light of significant new safety information.

Safety assessment includes systematic critical reviews of the ways in which structures, systems, and components fail and identifies the consequences of such failures. The assessment is undertaken expressly to reveal any underlying design weaknesses. The results are documented in detail to allow independent audit of scope, depth, and conclusions.

2.3.2 Accident Prevention and Consequence Mitigation

Figure 2.14 shows the phases of accident prevention and accident management. Accident prevention (upper left-hand box) is divided into failure prevention and propagation prevention, while accident management (lower left-hand box) focuses on onsite consequence mitigation and offsite consequence mitigation.

In medical terms, failure prevention corresponds to infection prevention, propagation prevention to outbreak prevention, and consequence mitigation to treatment and recovery after outbreak.

As shown in the upper right portion of Figure 2.14, neither anticipated disturbances nor events below the design basis yield accidents if the propagation prevention works successfully. On the other hand, if something is wrong with the propagation prevention or if extreme initiating events are involved, these disturbances or events would develop to events beyond the design basis, which raises three possibilities: the onsite consequence mitigation works and prevents containment failures and hence offsite releases, the offsite consequence mitigation works and minimizes offsite consequences, or all features fail and large consequences occur.

2.3.3 Failure Prevention

The first means of preventing failures is to strive for such high quality in design, manufacture, construction, and operation of the plant that deviations from normal operations

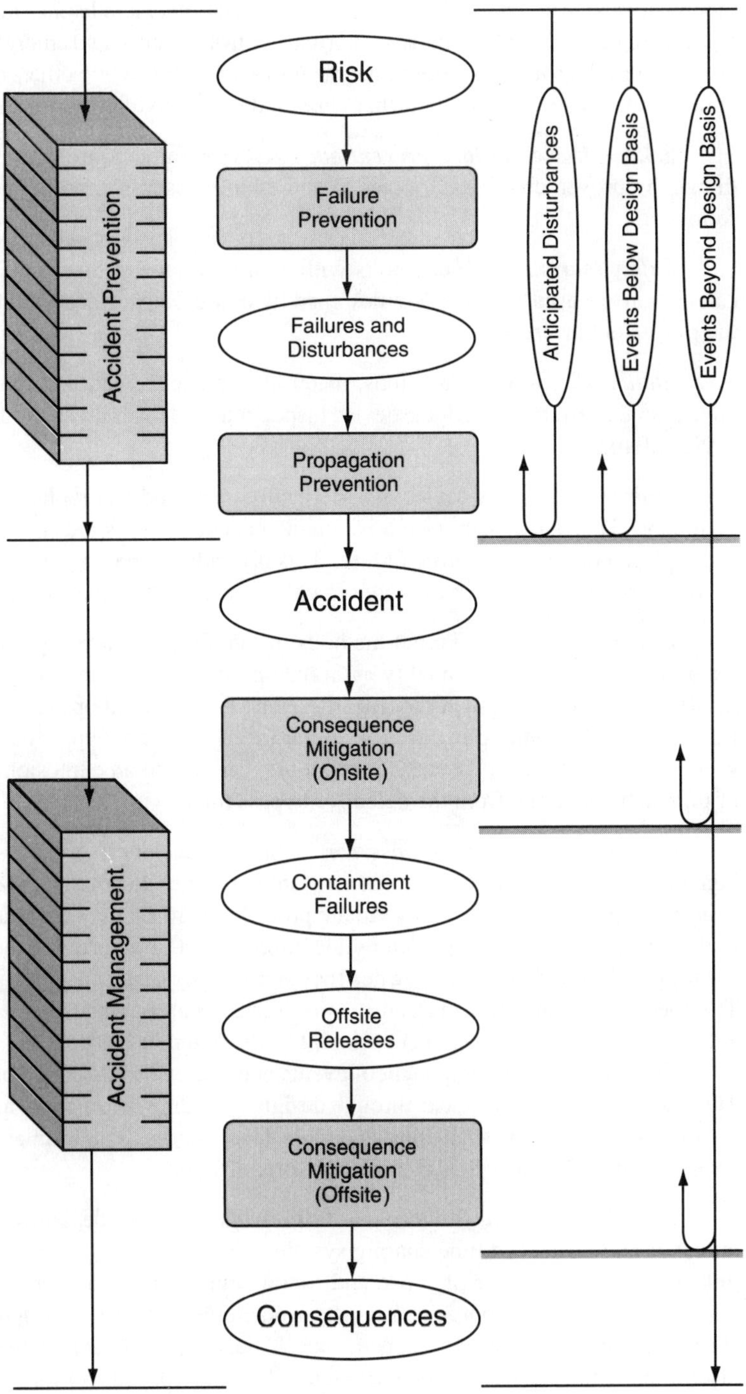

Figure 2.14. Risk-management process.

are infrequent and quality products are produced. A deviation may occur from two sources: inanimate device and human. Device-related deviations include ones not only for the plant equipment but also physical barriers, normal control systems, and emergency safety systems (see Figure 2.1); some deviations become initiating events while others are enabling events. Human-related deviations are further classified into individual, team, and organization.*

2.3.3.1 Device-failure prevention. Device failures are prevented, among other things, by proven engineering practice and quality assurance programs. Some examples follow.

Safety margins. Metal bolts with a larger diameter than predicted by theoretical calculation are used. Devices are designed by conservative rules and criteria according to the proven engineering practice.

Standardization. Functions, materials, and specifications are standardized to decrease device failure, to facilitate device inspection, and to facilitate prediction of remaining device lifetime.

Maintenance. A device is periodically inspected and replaced or renewed before its failure. This is periodic preventive maintenance. Devices are continuously monitored, and replaced or renewed before failure. This is condition-based maintenance. These types of monitor-and-control activities are typical elements of the quality assurance program.

Change control. Formal methods of handling engineering and material changes are an important aspect of quality assurance programs. Failures frequently occur due to insufficient review of system modification. The famous Flixborough accident occurred in England in 1974 when a pipeline was temporarily installed to bypass one of six reactors that was under maintenance. Twenty-eight people died due to an explosion caused by ignition of flammable material from the defective bypass line.

2.3.3.2 Human-prevention error. Serious accidents often result from incorrect human actions. Such events occur when plant personnel do not recognize the safety significance of their actions, when they violate procedures, when they are unaware of conditions in the plant, when they are misled by incomplete data or incorrect mindset, when they do not fully understand the plant, or when they consciously or unconsciously commit sabotage. The operating organization must ensure that its staff is able to manage the plant satisfactorily according to the risk-management principles illustrated in Figure 2.13.

The human-error component of events and accidents has, in the past, been too great. The remedy is a twofold attack: through design, including automation, and through optimal use of human ingenuity when unusual circumstances occur. This implies education. Human errors are made by individuals, teams, and organizations.

2.3.3.3 Preventing failures due to individuals. As described in Chapter 10, the human is an unbalanced time-sharing system consisting of a slow brain, life-support units linked to a large number of sense and motor organs and short- and long-term memory units. The human-brain bottleneck results in phenomena such as "shortcut," "perseverance," "task fixation," "alternation," "dependence," "naivety," "queuing and escape," and "gross discrimination," which are fully discussed in Chapter 10. Human-machine systems should be designed in such a way that machines help people achieve their potential by giving them

---

*Human reliability analysis is described in Chapter 10.

support where they are weakest, and vice versa. It should be easy to do the right thing and hard to do the wrong thing [16].

If personnel are trained and qualified to perform their duties, correct decisions are facilitated, wrong decisions are inhibited, and means for detecting, correcting, or compensating errors are provided.

Humans are physiological, physical, pathological, and pharmaceutical beings. A pilot may suffer from restricted vision due to high acceleration caused by high-tech jet fighters. At least three serious railroad accidents in the United States have been traced by DOT (Department of Transportation) investigations to the conductors having been under the influence of illegal drugs.

2.3.3.4 Team-failure prevention. Hostility, subservience, or too much restraint among team members should be avoided. A copilot noticed a dangerous situation. He hesitated to inform his captain about the situation, and an airplane accident occurred.

Effective communication should exist between the control-room and operating personnel at remote locations who may be required to take action affecting plant states. Administrative measures should ensure that actions by operators at remote locations are first cleared with the control room.

2.3.3.5 Preventing organizationally induced failures. A catechism attributed to W. E. Deming is that the worker wants to do a good job and is thus never responsible for the problem. Problems, when they arise, are due to improper organization and systems. He was, of course, referring only to manufacturing and QC problems. Examples of organizationally induced safety problems include the following.

Prevention of excessive specialization. A large-scale integrated (LSI) chip factory neutralized base with acid, thus producing salts. As a result, a pipe was blocked, eventually causing an explosion. Electronic engineers at the LSI factory did not know chemical-reaction mechanisms familiar to chemical engineers.

Removal of horizontal barriers. In the 1984 Bhopal accident in India, a pressure increase in a chemical tank was observed by an operator. However, this information was not relayed to the next shift operators. Several small fires at a wooden escalator had occurred before the 1987 King's Cross Underground fire. Neither the operating nor the engineering division of the railroad tried to remove the hazard because one division held the other responsible.

Removal of vertical barriers. In the Challenger accident in 1986, a warning from a solid-rocket-propellant manufacturer did not reach the upper-level management of the National Aeronautics and Space Administration (NASA). A fire started when a maintenance subcontractor noticed oil deposits on an air-conditioning filter, but did not transmit this information to the company operating the air conditioner.

2.3.4 Propagation Prevention

The second accident-prevention step is to ensure that a perturbation or incipient failure will not develop into a serious situation. In no human endeavor can one ever guarantee that failure prevention will be totally successful. Designers must assume that component, system, and human failures are possible, and can lead to abnormal occurrences, ranging from minor disturbances to highly unlikely accident sequences. These occurrences will not cause serious consequences if physical barriers, normal control systems, and emergency safety features remain healthy and operate correctly.

Physical barriers. Physical barriers include safety glasses and helmets, firewalls, trenches, empty space, and—in the extreme case of a nuclear power plant—concrete bunkers enclosing the entire plant. Every physical barrier must be designed conservatively, its quality checked to ensure that margins against failure are retained, and its status monitored.

This barrier itself may be protected by special measures; for instance, a containment structure at a nuclear power plant is equipped with devices that control pressure and temperature due to accident conditions; such devices include hydrogen ignitors, filtered vent systems, and area spray systems [5]. Safety-system designers ensure to the extent practicable that the different safety systems protecting physical barriers are functionally independent under accident conditions.

Normal control systems. Minor disturbances (usual disturbances and anticipated abnormal occurrences) for the plant are dealt with through normal feedback control systems to provide tolerance for failures that might otherwise allow faults or abnormal conditions to develop into accidents. This reduces the frequency of demand on the emergency safety systems. These controls protect the physical barriers by keeping the plant in a defined region of operating parameters where barriers will not be jeopardized. Care in system design prevents runaways that might permit small deviations to precipitate grossly abnormal plant behavior and cause damage.

Engineered safety features and systems. High reliability in these systems is achieved by appropriate use of fail-safe design, by protection against common-cause failures, by independence between safety systems (inter-independence) and between safety systems and normal control systems (outer-independence), and by monitor and recovery provisions. Proper design ensures that failure of a single component will not cause loss of function of the safety system (a single-failure criterion).

Inter-independence. Complete safety systems can make use of redundancy, diversity, and physical separations of parallel components, where appropriate, to reduce the likelihood of loss of vital safety functions. For instance, both diesel-driven and steam-driven generators are installed for emergency power supply if the need is there and money permits; different computer algorithms can be used to calculate the same quantity.

The conditions under which equipment is required to perform safety functions may differ from those to which it is normally exposed, and its performance may be affected adversely by aging or by maintenance conditions. The environmental conditions under which equipment is required to function are identified as part of a design process. Among these are conditions expected in a wide range of accidents, including extremes of temperature, pressure, radiation, vibration, humidity, and jet impingement. Effects of external events such as earthquakes should be considered.

Because of the importance of fire as a source of possible simultaneous damage to equipment, design provisions to prevent and combat fires in the plant should be given special attention. Fire-resistant materials are used when possible. Fire-fighting capability is included in the design specifications. Lubrication systems use nonflammable lubricants or are protected against initiation and effects of fires.

Outer-independence. Engineered safety systems should be independent of normal process control systems. For instance, the safety shutdown systems for a chemical plant should be independent from the control systems used for normal operation. Common sensors or devices should only be used if reliability analysis indicates that this is acceptable.

Recovery. Not only the plant itself but also barriers, normal control systems, and safety systems should be inspected and tested regularly to reveal any degradation that might lead to abnormal operating conditions or inadequate performance. Operators should be trained to recognize the onset of an accident and to respond properly and in a timely manner to abnormal conditions.

Automatic actuation. Further protection is available through automatic actuation of process control and safety systems. Any onset of abnormal behavior will be dealt with automatically for an appropriate period, during which the operating staff can assess systems and decide on a subsequent course of action. Typical decision intervals for operator action range from 10 to 30 min or longer depending on the situation.

Symptom-based procedures. Plant-operating procedures generally describe responses based on the diagnosis of an event (event-based procedures). If the event cannot be diagnosed in time, or if further evaluation of the event causes the initial diagnosis to be discarded, symptom-based procedures define responses to symptoms observed rather than plant conditions deduced from these symptoms.

Other topics relating to propagation prevention are fail-safe design, fail-soft design, and robustness.

Fail-safe design. According to fail-safe design principles, if a device malfunctions, it puts the system in a state where no damage can ensue. Consider a drive unit for withdrawing control rods from a nuclear reactor. Reactivity increases with the withdrawal, thus the unsafe side is an inadvertent activation of the withdrawal unit. Figure 2.15 shows a design without a fail-safe feature because the dc motor starts withdrawing the rods when short circuit occurs. Figure 2.16 shows a fail-safe design. Any short-circuit failure stops electricity to the dc motor. A train braking system is designed to activate when actuator air is lost.

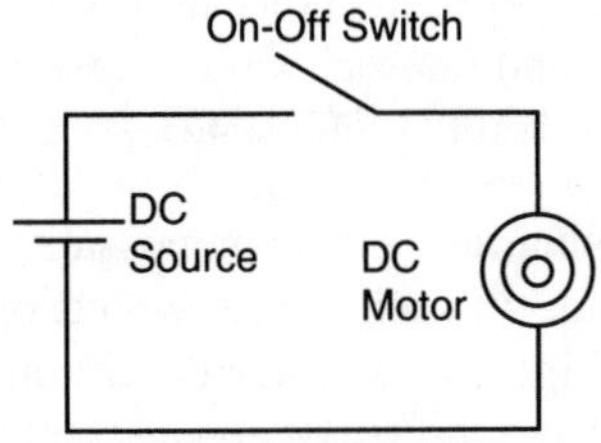

Figure 2.15. Control rod withdrawal circuit without fail-safe feature.

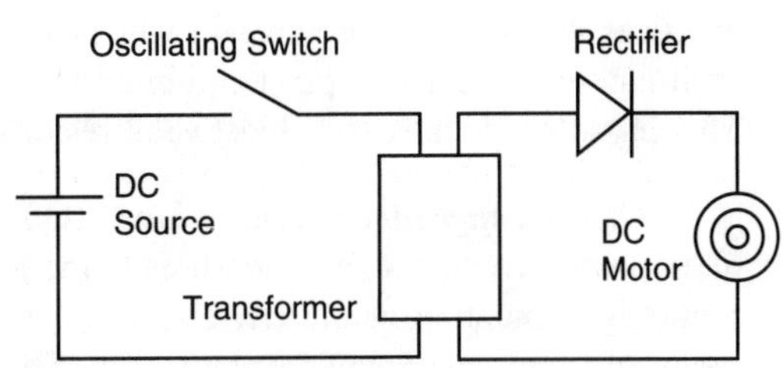

Figure 2.16. Control rod withdrawal circuit with fail-safe feature.

Fail-soft design. According to fail-soft design principles, failures of devices result only in partial performance degradations. A total shutdown can be avoided. This feature is also called a graceful degradation. Examples of the fail-soft design feature are given below.

1. **Traffic control system:** Satellite computers control traffic signals along a road when main computers for the area fail. Local controllers at an intersection control traffic signals when the satellite computer fails.

2. **Restructurable flight-control system:** If a rudder plate fails, the remaining rudders and thrusts are restructured as a new flight-control system, allowing continuation of the flight.
3. **Animals:** Arteries around open wounds contract and blood flows change, maintaining blood to the brain.
4. **Metropolitan water supply:** A water supply restriction is enforced during a drought, thus preventing rapid decrease of ground-water levels.

Robustness. A process controller is designed to operate successfully under uncertain environment and unpredictable changes in plant dynamics. Robustness generally means the capability to cope with events not anticipated.

2.3.5 Consequence Mitigation

Consequence mitigation covers the period after occurrence of an accident. The occurrence of an accident means that events beyond a design basis occurred; events below the design basis, by definition, could never develop into the accident because normal control systems or engineered safety features are assumed to operate as intended.

Because accidents occur, procedural measures must be provided for managing their course and mitigating their consequences. These measures are defined on the basis of operating experience, safety analysis, and the results of safety research. Attention is given to design, siting, procedures, and training to control progressions and consequences of accidents. Limitation of accident consequences are based on safe shutdown, continued availability of utilities, adequate confinement integrity, and offsite emergency preparedness. High-consequence, severe accidents are extremely unlikely if they are effectively prevented or mitigated by defense-in-depth philosophy.

As shown in Figure 2.14, consequence mitigation consists of onsite consequence mitigation and offsite consequence mitigation.

Onsite consequence mitigation. This includes preplanned and ad hoc operational practices that, in circumstances in which plant design specifications are exceeded, make optimum use of existing plant equipment in normal and unusual ways to restore control. This phase would have the objective of restoring the plant to a safe state.

Offsite consequence mitigation. Offsite countermeasures compensate for the remote possibility that safety measures at the plant fail. In such a case, effects on the surrounding population or the environment can be mitigated by protective actions such as sheltering or evacuation of the population. This involves closely coordinated activities with local authorities.

Accident management. Onsite and offsite consequence mitigation after occurrence of an accident is called *accident management* (Figure 2.14). For severe accidents beyond the design basis, accident management would come into full play, using normal plant systems, engineered safety features, special design features, and offsite emergency measures in mitigation of the effects of events beyond the design basis.

Critique of accident management. Events beyond the design basis may, however, develop in unpredictable ways. A Greenpeace International document [10], for instance, evaluates accident management in the following.

The concept of accident management has been increasingly studied and developed in recent years, and is beginning to be introduced into PRA's. The idea is that even after vital safety systems have failed, an accident can still be "managed" by improvising the use of other systems for safety purposes, and/or by using safety systems in a different context than originally planned. The aim is to avoid severe core damage whenever possible; or, failing that, at least to avoid early containment failure.

Accident management places increased reliance on operator intervention, since accident management strategies must be implemented by plant personnel. The possibilities of simulator training, however, are limited. Hence, there is large scope for human errors. This is enhanced by a serious pressure of time in many cases, which will create high psychological stress. For this reason alone, the significant reductions in severe core damage frequency and early containment failure probability which have been claimed in PRA's (for example, in the German Risk Study, Phase B) appear completely unrealistic.

Furthermore, accident management, even if performed as planned, might prove ineffective, leading from one severe accident sequence to another just as hazardous. In some cases, it can even be counter-productive.

Many questions still remain in connection with accident management. In the case of the German Risk Study, certain accident management measures are considered which cannot be performed in present-day German reactors, and require complicated and expensive backfitting of safety systems.

2.3.6 Summary

Risk management consists of four phases: failure prevention, propagation prevention, onsite consequence mitigation, and offsite consequence mitigation. The first two are called *accident prevention*, and the second two *accident management*. Risk-management principles are embedded in proven engineering practice and quality assurance, built on a nurtured safety culture. Quality assurance consists of multilayer monitor/control provisions that remove and correct deviations, and safety assessment and verification provisions that evaluate deviations.

Failure prevention applies not only to failure of inanimate devices but also human failures by individuals, teams, and organizations. One strives for such high quality in design, manufacture, construction, and operation of a plant that deviations from normal operational states are infrequent. Propagation prevention ensures that a perturbation or incipient failure would not develop into a more serious situation such as an accident. Consequence mitigation covers the period after occurrence of an accident and includes management of the course of the accident and mitigating of its consequences.

2.4 PREPRODUCTION QUALITY ASSURANCE PROGRAM

Figure 2.13 showed an overview of a quality assurance program based on monitor/control provisions together with a safety assessment and verification program. This section describes in detail how such programs can be performed for a preproduction design period that focuses on the medical equipment manufacturing industry [6]. In the United States and Europe, manufacturers of medical devices are required to have documented PQA (preproduction quality assurance) programs and are subject to onsite GMP inspections.

The previous discussions were focused largely on risk reduction from accidents at large facilities such as chemical, nuclear, or power plants. From the following, much of the same methodology is seen to apply to reducing the risk of product failures. Much of this material is adapted from FDA regulatory documents [6,11], which explains the ukase prose.

2.4.1 Motivation

Design deficiency cost. A design deficiency can be very costly once a device design has been released to production and a device is manufactured and distributed. Costs may include not only replacement and redesign costs, with resulting modifications to manufacturing procedures and retraining (to enable manufacture of the modified device), but also liability costs and loss of customer faith in the market [6].

Device-failure data. Analysis of recall and other adverse experience data available to the FDA from October 1983 to November 1988 indicates one of the major causes of device failures is deficient design; approximately 45% of all recalls were due to preproduction-related problems.

Object. Quality is the composite of all the characteristics, including performance, of an item or product (MIL-STD-109B). Quality assurance is a planned and systematic pattern of all actions necessary to provide adequate confidence that the device, its components, packaging, and labeling are acceptable for their intended use (MIL-STD-109B). The purpose of a PQA program is to provide a high degree of confidence that device designs are proven reliable, safe, and effective prior to releasing designs to production for routine manufacturing. No matter how carefully a device may be manufactured, the inherent safety, effectiveness, and reliability of a device cannot be improved except through design enhancement. It is crucial that adequate controls be established and implemented during the design phase to assure that the safety, effectiveness, and reliability of the device are optimally enhanced prior to manufacturing. An ultimate purpose of the PQA program is to enhance product quality and productivity, while reducing quality costs.

Applicability. The PQA program is applicable to the development of new designs as well as to the adaptation of existing designs to new or improved applications.

2.4.2 Preproduction Design Process

The preproduction design process proceeds in the following sequence: 1) establishment of specifications, 2) concept design, 3) detail design, 4) prototype production, 5) pilot production, and 6) certification (Figure 2.17). This process is followed by a postdesign process consisting of routine production, distribution, and use.

Specification. Design specifications are a description of physical and functional requirements for an article. In its initial form, the design specification is a statement of general functional requirements. The design specification evolves through the R&D phase to reflect progressive refinements in performance, design, configuration, and test requirements.

Prior to the actual design activity, the design specifications should be defined in terms of desired characteristics, such as physical, chemical, and performance. The performance characteristics include safety, durability/reliability, precision, stability, and purity. Acceptable ranges or limits should be provided for each characteristic to establish allowable variations and these should be expressed in terms that are readily measurable. For example, the pulse-amplitude range for an external pacemaker could be established as 0.5 to 28mA at an electrical load of 1000 ohms, and pulse duration could be 0.1 to 9.9ms.

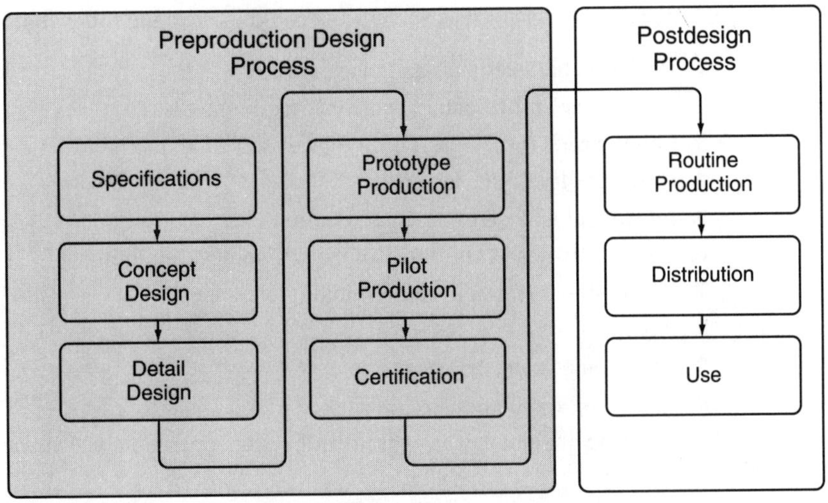

Figure 2.17. Preproduction design process followed by postdesign process.

The design aim should be translated into written design specifications. The expected use of the device, the user, and user environment should be considered.

Concept and detail design. The actual device evolves from concept to detail design to satisfy the specifications. In the detail design, for instance, suppliers of parts and materials (P/M) used in the device; software elements developed in-house; custom software from contractors; manuals, charts, inserts, panels, display labels; packaging; and support documentation such as test specifications and instructions are determined.

Prototype production. Prototypes are developed in the laboratory or machine shop. During this production, conditions are typically better controlled and personnel more knowledgeable about what needs to be done and how to do it than production personnel. Thus the prototype production differs in conditions from pilot and routine productions.

Pilot production. Before the specifications are released for routine production, actual-finished devices should be manufactured using the approved specifications, the same materials and components, the same or similar production and quality control equipment, and the methods and procedures that will be used for routine production. This type of production is essential for assuring that the routine manufacturing process will produce the intended devices without adversely affecting the devices. The pilot production is a necessary part of process validation [11].

2.4.3 Design Review for PQA

The design review is a planned, scheduled, and documented audit of all pertinent aspects of the design that can affect safety and effectiveness. Such a review is a kernel of the PQA program. Each manufacturer should establish and implement an independent review of the design at each stage as the design matures. The design review assures conformance to design criteria and identifies design weaknesses. The objective of design review is the early detection and remedy of design deficiencies. The earlier design review is initiated, the sooner problems can be identified and the less costly it will be to implement corrective action.

Checklist. A design review checklist could include the following.

1. Physical characteristics and constraints
2. Regulatory and voluntary standards requirements
3. Safety needs for the user, need for fail-safe characteristics
4. Producibility of the design
5. Functional and environmental requirements
6. Inspectability and testability of the design, test requirements
7. Permissible maximum and minimum tolerances
8. Acceptance criteria
9. Selection of components
10. Packaging requirements
11. Labeling, including warnings, identification, operation, and maintenance instructions
12. Shelf-life, storage, stability requirements
13. Possible misuse of the product that can be anticipated, elimination of human-induced failures
14. Product serviceability/maintainability

Specification changes. Changes made to the specifications during R&D should be documented and evaluated to assure that they accomplish the intended result and do not compromise safety or effectiveness. Manufacturers should not make unqualified, undocumented changes during preproduction trials in response to suggestions or criticism from users. In the manufacturer's haste to satisfy the user, changes made without an evaluation of the overall effect on the device could result in improving one characteristic of the device while having an unforeseen adverse effect on another.

Concept and detail design. A device's compatibility with other devices in the intended operating system should be addressed in the design phase, to the extent that compatibility is necessary to assure proper functioning of the system. The full operating range of within-tolerance specifications for the mating device(s) should be considered, not merely nominal values.

A disposable blood tubing set was designed and manufactured by Company A for use with Company B's dialysis machine. The tubing was too rigid, such that when the air-embolism occlusion safety system on the dialysis machine was at its lowest within-specification force, the tubing would not necessarily occlude and air could be passed to the patient. The tubing occluded fully under the nominal occlusion force.

Quick fixes should be prohibited. These include adjustments that may allow the device to perform adequately for the moment, but do not address the underlying cause. All design defects should be corrected in a manner that will assure the problem will not recur.

Identification of design weakness. Potential design weakness should be identified by FMECA (failure mode effects criticality analysis) or FTA (fault-tree analysis). FMECA is described in MIL-STD-1629A [12].*

---

*See Chapter 3 of this book for FMEA and FMECA. See Chapter 4 for FTA.

FMEA (failure mode and effects analysis) is a process of identifying potential design weaknesses through reviewing schematics, engineering drawings, and so on, to identify basic faults at the part/material level and determine their effect at finished or subassembly level on safety and effectiveness. FTA is especially applicable to medical devices because human/device interfaces can be taken into consideration, that is, a particular kind of adverse effect on a user, such as electrical shock, can be assumed as a top event to be analyzed. The design weakness is expressed in terms of a failure mode, that is, a manner or a combination of basic human/component failures in which a device failure is observed.

FMEA, FMECA, or FTA should include an evaluation of possible human-induced failures or hazardous situations. For example, battery packs were recalled because of an instance when the battery pack burst while being charged. The batteries were designed to be trickle charged, but the user charged the batteries using a rapid charge. The result was a rapid build-up of gas that could not be contained by the unvented batteries.

For those potential failure modes that cannot be corrected through redesign effort, special controls such as warning labels, alarms, and so forth, should be provided. For example, if a warning label had been provided for the burst batteries pack, or the batteries vented, the incident probably would not have happened. As another example, one possible failure mode for an anesthesia machine could be a sticking valve. If the valve's sticking could result in over- or underdelivery of the desired anesthesia gas, a fail-safe feature should be incorporated into the design to prevent the wrong delivery, or if this is impractical, a suitable alarm system should be included to alert the user in time to take corrective action.

When a design weakness is identified, consideration should be made of other distributed devices in which the design weakness may also exist. For example, an anomaly that could result in an incorrect output was discovered in a microprocessor used in a blood-analysis diagnostic device at a prototype-testing stage. This same microprocessor was used in other diagnostic machines already in commercial distribution. A review should have been made of the application of the microprocessor in the already-distributed devices to assure that the anomaly would not adversely affect performance.

Reliability assessment. Prior to commercial distribution, reliability assessment may be initiated by theoretical and statistical methods by first determining the reliability of each component, then progressing upward, establishing the reliability of each subassembly and assembly, until the reliability of the entire device or device system is established. References [13] and [14] apply to predicting the reliability of electronic devices. Component reliability data sources are well reviewed in [15].*

This type of reliability assessment does not simulate the actual effect of interaction of system parts and the environment. To properly estimate reliability, complete devices and device systems should be tested under simulated-use conditions.

Parts and materials quality assurance. Parts and materials should be selected on the basis of their suitability for the chosen application, compatibility with other P/M and the environment, and proven reliability. Conservative choices in selection of P/M are characteristic of reliable devices. Standard proven P/M should be used as much as possible in lieu of unproven P/M.

For example, a manufacturer used an unproven plastic raw material in the initial production of molded connectors. After distribution, reports were received that the tubing

---

*See Chapters 6 and 7 for quantification of component reliability. Chapters 8 and 9 describe quantification of system reliability parameters.

was separating from the connectors. Investigation and analysis by the manufacturer revealed that the unproven plastic material used to mold the connectors deteriorated with time, causing a loss of bond strength. The devices were subsequently recalled.

The P/M quality assurance means not only assuring P/M will perform their functions under normal conditions but that they are not unduly stressed mechanically, electrically, environmentally, and so on. Adequate margins of safety should be established when necessary. A whole-body image device was recalled because screws used to hold the upper detector head sheared off, allowing the detector head to fall to its lowest position. The screws were well within their tolerances for all specified attributes under normal conditions. However, the application was such that the screws did not possess sufficient shear strength for the intended use.

When selecting P/M previously qualified, attention should be given to the currentness of the data, applicability of the previous qualification to the intended application, and adequacy of the existing P/M specification. Lubricant seals previously qualified for use in an anesthesia gas circuit containing one anesthesia gas may not be compatible with another gas. These components should be qualified for each specific environment.

Failure of P/M during qualification should be investigated and the result described in written reports. Failure analysis, when deemed appropriate, should be conducted to a level such that the failure mechanism can be identified.

Software quality assurance. Software quality assurance (SQA) should begin with a plan, which can be written using a guide such as ANSI/IEEE Standard 730-1984, IEEE Standard for Software Quality Assurance Plans. Good SQA assures quality software from the beginning of the development cycle by specifying up front the required quality attributes of the completed software and the acceptance testing to be performed. In addition, the software should be written in conformance with a company standard using structured programming. When device manufacturers purchase custom software from contractors, the SQA should assure that the contractors have an adequate SQA program.

Labeling. Labeling includes manuals, charts, inserts, panels, display labels, test and calibration protocols, and software for CRT display. A review of labeling should assure that it is in compliance with applicable laws and regulations and that adequate directions for the product's intended use are easily understood by the end-user group. Instructions contained in the labeling should be verified.

After commercial distribution, labeling had to be corrected for a pump because there was danger of overflow if certain flow charts were used. The problem existed because an error was introduced in the charts when the calculated flow rates were transposed onto flow charts.

Manufacturers of devices that are likely to be used in a home environment and operated by persons with a minimum of training and experience should design and label their products to encourage proper use and to minimize the frequency of misuse. For example, an exhalation valve used with a ventilator could be connected in reverse position because the inlet and exhalation ports were the same diameter. In the reverse position the user could breathe spontaneously but was isolated from the ventilator. The valve should have been designed so that it could be connected only in the proper position.

Labeling intended to be permanently attached to the device should remain attached and legible through processing, storage, and handling for the useful life of the device. Maintenance manuals should be provided where applicable and should provide adequate instructions whereby a user or service activity can maintain the device in a safe and effective condition.

Simulated testing for prototype production. Use testing should not begin until the safety of the device from the prototype production has been verified under simulated-use conditions, particularly at the expected performance limits. Simulated-use testing should address use with other applicable devices and possible misuse. Devices in a home environment should typically anticipate the types of operator errors most likely to occur.

Extensive testing for pilot production. Devices from the pilot production should be qualified through extensive testing under actual- or simulated-use conditions and in the environment, or simulated environment, in which the device is expected to be used.

Proper qualification of devices that are produced using the same or similar methods and procedures as those to be used in routine production can prevent the distribution and subsequent recall of many unacceptable products. A drainage catheter using a new material was designed, fabricated, and subsequently qualified in a laboratory setting. Once the catheter was manufactured and distributed, however, the manufacturer began receiving complaints that the bifurcated sleeve was separating from the catheter shrink base. Investigation found the separation was due to dimensional shrinkage of the material and leeching of the plasticizers from the sleeve due to exposure to cleaning solutions during manufacturing. Had the device been exposed to actual production conditions during fabrication of the prototypes, the problem may have been detected before routine production and distribution.

When practical, testing should be conducted using devices produced from the pilot production. Otherwise, the qualified device will not be truly representative of production devices. Testing should include stressing the device at its performance and environmental specification limits.

Storage conditions should be considered when establishing environmental test specifications. For example, a surgical staple device was recalled because it malfunctioned. Investigation found that the device malfunctioned because of shrinkage of the plastic cutting ring due to subzero conditions to which the device was exposed during shipping and storage.

Certification. The certification is defined as a documented review of all qualification documentation prior to release of the design for production. The qualification here is defined as a documented determination that a device (and its associated software), component, packaging, or labeling meet all prescribed design and performance requirements. The certification should include a determination of the

1. resolution of any difference between the procedures and standards used to produce the design while in R&D and those approved for production
2. resolution of any differences between the approved device specifications and the actual manufactured product
3. validity of test methods used to determine compliance with the approved specifications
4. adequacy of specifications and specification change control program
5. adequacy of the complete quality assurance plan

Postproduction quality monitoring. The effort to ensure that the device and its components have acceptable quality and are safe and effective must be continued in the manufacturing and use phase, once the design has been proven safe and effective and devices are produced and distributed.

2.4.4 Management and Organizational Matters

Authorities and responsibilities. A PQA program should be sanctioned by upper management and should be considered a crucial part of each manufacturer's overall effort to produce only reliable, safe, and effective products. The organizational elements and authorities necessary to establish the PQA program, to execute program requirements, and to achieve program goals, should be specified in formal documentation. Responsibility for implementing the overall program and each program element should also be formally assigned and documented. The SQA representative or department should have the authority to enforce implementation of SQA policies and recommendations.

Implementation. The design review program should be established as a permanent part of the PQA and the design review should be conducted periodically throughout the preproduction life-cycle phase as the design matures to assure conformance to design criteria and to identify design weaknesses. The PQA program including the design review should be updated as experience is gained and the need for improvement is noted.

Design reviews should, when appropriate, include FMECA and FTA to identify potential design weaknesses. When appropriate and applicable, the reliability assessment should be made for new and modified designs and acceptable failure rates should be established. The review of labeling should be included as part of the design review process.

Each manufacturer must have an effective program for identification of failure patterns or trends and analysis of quality problems, taking appropriate corrective actions to prevent recurrence of these problems, and the timely internal reporting of problems discovered either in-house or in the field. Specific instructions should be established to provide direction about when and how problems are to be investigated, analyzed, and corrected, and to provide responsibility for assuring initiation and completion of these tasks.

Procedures. Device design should progress through clearly defined and planned stages, starting with the concept design and ending in the pilot production. A detailed, documented description of the design-review program should be established, including organizational units involved, procedures used, flow diagrams of the process, identification of documentation required, a schedule, and a checklist of variables to be considered and evaluated. The SQA program should include a protocol for formal review and validation of device software to ensure overall functional reliability.

Testing should be performed according to a documented test plan that specifies the performance parameters to be measured, test sequence, evaluation criteria, test environment, and so on. Once the device is qualified, all manufacturing and quality assurance specifications should be placed under formal change control.

Staffing. Reviews should be objective, unbiased examinations by appropriately trained, qualified personnel, which should include individuals other than those responsible for the design. For example, design review should be conducted by representatives of Manufacturing, Quality Assurance, Engineering, Marketing, Servicing, and Purchasing, as well as those responsible for R&D.

Change control. When corrective action is required, the action should be appropriately monitored, with responsibility assigned to assure that a follow-up is properly conducted. Schedules should be established for completing corrective action. Quick fixes should be prohibited.

When problem investigation and analysis indicate a potential problem in the design, appropriate design improvements must be made to prevent recurrence of the problem. Any design changes must undergo sufficient testing and preproduction evaluation to assure that the revised design is safe and effective. This testing should include testing under actual- or simulated-use conditions and clinical testing as appropriate to the change.

Documentation and communication. Review results should be well documented in report form and signed by designated individuals as complete and accurate. All changes made as a result of review findings should be documented. Reports should include conclusions and recommended follow-up and should be disseminated in a timely manner to appropriate organizational elements, including management.

Failure reports of P/M should be provided to management and other appropriate personnel in a timely manner to assure that only qualified P/M are used.

A special effort should be made to assure that failure data obtained from complaint and service records that may relate to design problems are made available and reviewed by those responsible for design.

2.4.5 Summary

A preproduction quality assurance program is described to illustrate quality assurance features based on monitor/control loops and safety assessment and verification activities. The program covers a preproduction design process consisting of design specifications, concept design, detail design, prototype production, pilot production, and certification. The PQA program contains design review, which deals with checklist, specification, concept and detail design, identification of design weaknesses, reliability assessment, parts and materials quality assurance, software quality assurance, labeling, prototype production testing, pilot production testing, and so forth. The PQA ensures smooth and satisfactory design transfer to a routine production. Management and organizational matters are presented from the points of view of authorities and responsibilities, PQA program implementation, procedures, staffing requirements, documentation and communication, and change control.

REFERENCES

[1] Reason, J. *Human Error*. New York: Cambridge University Press, 1990.

[2] Wagenaar, W. A., P. T. Hudson, and J. T. Reason. "Cognitive failures and accidents." *Applied Cognitive Psychology*, vol. 4, pp. 273–294, 1990.

[3] Embrey, D. E. "Incorporating management and organizational factors into probabilistic safety assessment." *Reliability Engineering and System Safety*, vol. 38, pp. 199–208, 1992.

[4] Lambert, H. E. "Case study on the use of PSA methods: Determining safety importance of systems and components at nuclear power plants." IAEA, IAEA-TECDOC-590, 1991.

[5] International Nuclear Safety Advisory Group. "Basic safety principles for nuclear power plants." IAEA, Safety series, No. 75-INSAG-3, 1988.

[6] FDA. "Preproduction quality assurance planning: Recommendations for medical device manufacturers." The Food and Drug Administration, Center for Devices and Radiological Health, Rockville, MD, September 1989.

[7] Wu, J. S., G. E. Apostolakis, and D. Okrent. "On the inclusion of organizational and managerial influences in probabilistic safety assessments of nuclear power plants." In *The Analysis, Communication, and Perception of Risk*, edited by B. J. Garrick and W. C. Gekler, pp. 429–439. New York: Plenum Press, 1991.

[8] USNRC. "PRA procedures guide: A guide to the performance of probabilistic risk assessments for nuclear power plants." USNRC, NUREG/CR-2300, 1983.

[9] Mosleh, A., et al. "Procedures for treating common cause failures in safety and reliability studies." USNRC, NUREG/CR-4780, 1988.

[10] Hirsch, H., T. Einfalt, O. Schumacher, and G. Thompson. "IAEA safety targets and probabilistic risk assessment." Report prepared for Greenpeace International, August, 1989.

[11] FDA. "Guideline on general principles of process validation." The Food and Drug Administration, Center for Drugs and Biologies and Center for Devices and Radiological Health, Rockville, MD, May, 1987.

[12] Department of Defense. "Procedures for performing failure mode, effects, and criticality analysis." MIL-STD-1629A.

[13] Department of Defense. "Reliability prediction of electronic equipment." Department of Defense. MIL-HDBK-217B.

[14] Department of Defense. "Reliability program for systems and equipment development and production." Department of Defense, MIL-STD-785B.

[15] Villemeur, A. *Reliability, Availability, Maintainability and Safety Assessment*, vol. 1. New York: John Wiley & Sons, 1992.

[16] Evans, R. A. "Easy & hard." *IEEE Trans. on Reliability*, Editorial, vol. 44, no. 2, p. 169, 1995.

PROBLEMS

2.1. Draw a protection configuration diagram for a plant with catastrophic risks. Enumerate common plant features.

2.2. Explain the following concepts: 1) active and latent failures; 2) lapse, slip, and mistakes; 3) LOCA; 4) common-cause failure.

2.3. Give chronological stages for failure occurrence.

2.4. Give examples of failed-safe and failed-dangerous failures of safety systems.

2.5. Draw a diagram explaining how operation and maintenance are affected by management.

2.6. Describe four types of dependent failures coupling mechanisms.

2.7. Pictorialize a quality assurance program.

2.8. Pictorialize a risk-management process consisting of accident prevention and accident management.

2.9. Explain six steps for a preproduction design process. Describe major activities for design reviews.

3

Probabilistic Risk Assessment

3.1 INTRODUCTION TO PROBABILISTIC RISK ASSESSMENT

3.1.1 Initiating-Event and Risk Profiles

Initiating events. From a risk-analysis standpoint there can be no bad ending if there is a good beginning. There are, regrettably, a variety of bad beginnings. In probabilistic risk assessment, bad beginnings are called initiating events or accident initiators. Without initiating events, no accident can occur. PRA is a methodology that transforms initiating events into risk profiles.

A plant with four risk-mitigation features was shown in Figure 2.1. They are physical barriers, normal control systems, emergency safety systems, and onsite and offsite emergency countermeasures. Initiating events are denoted as a "challenge." Risk profiles for the plant result from correlating the damage done with the frequency of accident occurrence.

Onsite and offsite consequences can be prevented or mitigated by a risk-management process consisting of the four phases shown in Figure 2.14. An initiating event is a failure. Thus the four phases are initiating-event prevention, initiating-event-propagation prevention, onsite consequence mitigation, and offsite consequence mitigation. Occurrence likelihoods of initiating events are decreased by prevention actions. An initiating event, once it occurs, is subject to initiating-event-propagation prevention. If an initiating event develops into an accident, then onsite and offsite consequence mitigations to halt accident progression and to mitigate consequences take place.

For consequences to occur, an initiating event must occur; this event must progress to an accident, and this accident must progress sufficiently to yield onsite and offsite consequences. This chain is similar to an influenza outbreak. Contact with the virus is an initiating event; an outbreak of flu is an accident; patient death is an onsite consequence; airborne infections have offsite consequences. Initiating events are transformed into risk profiles that depend on the relevant risk-management process. PRA provides a systematic approach for clarifying the transformation of an initiating event into a risk profile.

It should be noted that risk profiles are not the only products of a risk study. The PRA process and data identify vulnerabilities in plant design and operation. PRA predicts general accident scenarios, although some specific details might be missed. No other approach has superior predictive abilities [1].

3.1.2 Plants without Hazardous Materials

PRA is not restricted to a plant containing hazardous materials; PRA applies to all engineered systems or plants, with or without material hazards. The PRA approach is simpler for plants without hazardous materials. Additional steps are required for plants with material hazards because material releases into the environment must be analyzed. Using the medical analogy, both infectious and noninfectious diseases can be dealt with.

Passenger railway. As an example of a system without material hazards, consider a single track passenger railway consisting of terminals A and B and a spur between the terminals (Figure 3.1). An unscheduled departure from terminal A that follows failure to observe red departure signal 1 is an initiating event. This type of departure occurred in Japan when the departure signal was stuck red because of a priority override from terminal B. This override was not communicated to terminal A personnel, who assumed that the red signal was not functioning. The traffic was heavy and the terminal A train conductor neglected the red signal and started the train.

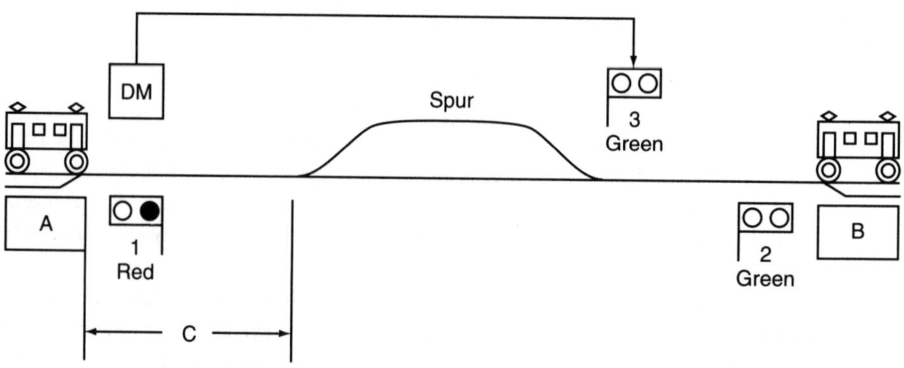

Figure 3.1. A single track railway with departure-monitoring device.

The railway has a departure-monitoring device (DM), designed to prevent accidents due to unscheduled departures by changing traffic signal 3 at the spur entrance to red, thus preventing a terminal B train from entering region C between the spur and terminal A. However, this monitoring device was not functioning because it was under maintenance when the departure occurred. A train collision occurred in region C, and 42 people died.

The unscheduled departure as an initiating event would not have yielded a train collision in region C if the departure monitoring device had functioned, and the terminal B train had remained on the main track between B and the spur until the terminal A train had entered the spur.

Two cases are possible—collision and no collision. Suppose that the terminal B train has not passed the spur signal when the terminal A train commits the unscheduled departure: this defines a particular type of initiating event. Another type of initiating event would be an unscheduled departure after the terminal B train crosses the spur signal. Suppose also that the railway has many curves and that a collision occurs whenever there are two trains moving in opposite directions in region C.

The first type of initiating event develops into a collision if the departure-monitoring device fails, or if the terminal B train driver neglects the red signal at the spur area, when correctly set by the monitoring device. These two collision scenarios are displayed as an event tree in Figure 3.2. Likelihood of collision is a function of initiating-event frequency, that is, unscheduled departure frequency, and failure probabilities of two mitigation features, that is, the departure-monitoring device and the terminal B train conductor who should watch spur signal 3.

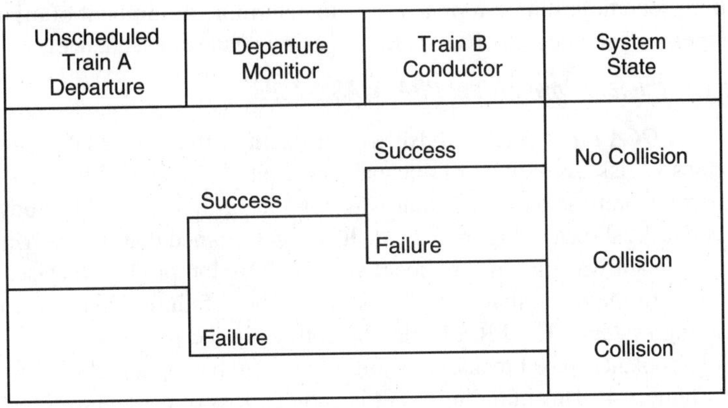

Figure 3.2. A simplified event tree for a single track railway.

It should be noted that the collision does not necessarily have serious consequences. It only marks the start of an accident. By our medical analogy, the collision is like an outbreak of a disease. The accident progression after a collision varies according to factors such as relative speed of two trains, number of passengers, strength of the train chassis, and train movement after the collision. The relative speed depends on deceleration before the collision. Factors such as relative speed, number of passengers, or strength of chassis would determine fatalities. Most of these factors can only be predicted probabilistically. This means that the collision fatalities can only be predicted as a likelihood. A risk profile, which is a graphical plot of fatality and fatality frequency, must be generated.

3.1.3 Plants with Hazardous Materials

Transforming initiating events into risk profiles is more complicated if toxic, flammable, or reactive materials are involved. These hazardous materials can cause offsite and onsite consequences.

Freight railway. For a freight train carrying a toxic gas, an accident progression after collision must include calculation of hole diameters in the gas container. Only then can the amount of toxic gas released from the tank be estimated. The gas leak is called a *source term* in PRA terminology. Dispersion of this source term is then analyzed and probability distributions of onsite and/or offsite fatalities are then calculated. The dispersion process depends on meteorological conditions such as wind directions and weather sequences; offsite fatalities also depend on population density around the accident site.

Ammonia storage facility. Consider, as another example, an ammonia storage facility where ammonia for a fertilizer plant is transported to tanks from a ship [2]. Potential initiating events include ship-to-tank piping failure, tank failure due to earthquakes, tank overpressure, tank-to-plant piping failure, and tank underpressure. Onsite and offsite risk profiles can be calculated by a procedure similar to the one used for the railway train carrying toxic materials.

Oil tanker. For an oil tanker, an initiating event could be a failure of the marine engine system. This can lead to a sequence of events, that is, drifting, grounding, oil leakage, and sea pollution. A risk profile for the pollution or oil leakage can be predicted from information about frequency of engine failure as an accident initiator; initiating-event propagation to the start of the accident, that is, the grounding; accident-progression analysis after grounding; source-term analysis to determine the amount of oil released; released oil dispersion; and degree of sea pollution as an offsite consequence.

3.1.4 Nuclear Power Plant PRA: WASH-1400

LOCA event tree. Consider as an example the reactor safety study, WASH-1400, an extensive risk assessment of nuclear power plants sponsored by the United States Atomic Energy Commission (AEC) that was completed in 1974. This study includes the seven basic tasks shown in Figure 3.3 [3]. It was determined that the overriding risk of a nuclear power plant was that of a radioactive (toxic) fission product release, and that the critical portion of the plant, that is, the subsystem whose failure initiates the risk, was the reactor cooling system. The PRA begins by following the potential course of events beginning with (coolant) "pipe breaks," this initiating event having a probability or a frequency of P_A in Figure 3.4. This initiating event is called a loss of coolant accident. The second phase begins, as shown in Figure 3.3, with the task of identifying the accident sequences: the different ways in which a fission product release might occur.

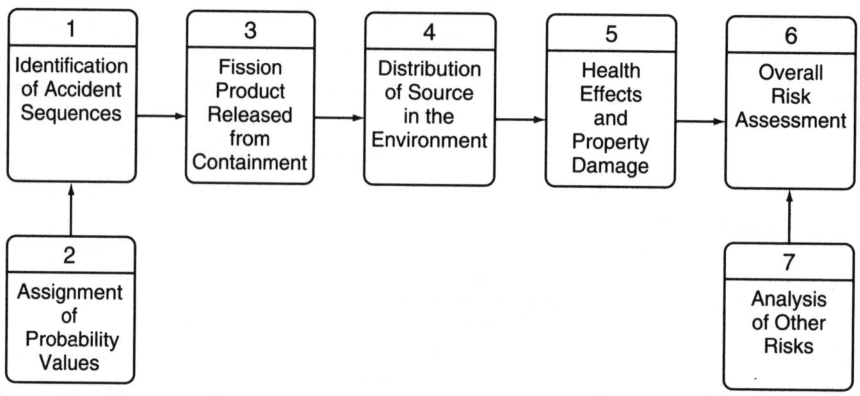

Figure 3.3. Seven basic tasks in a reactor safety study.

Fault-tree analysis. FTA was developed by H. A. Watson of the Bell Telephone Laboratories in 1961 to 1962 during an Air Force study contract for the Minuteman Launch Control System. The first published papers were presented at the 1965 Safety Symposium sponsored by the University of Washington and the Boeing Company, where a group including D. F. Haasl, R. J. Schroder, W. R. Jackson, and others had been applying and extending the technique. Fault trees (FTs) were used with event trees (ETs) in the WASH-1400 study.

Since the early 1970s when computer-based analysis techniques for FTs were developed, their use has become very widespread.* Indeed, the use of FTA is now mandated by a number of governmental agencies responsible for worker and/or public safety. Risk-as-

*Computer codes are listed and described in reference [4].

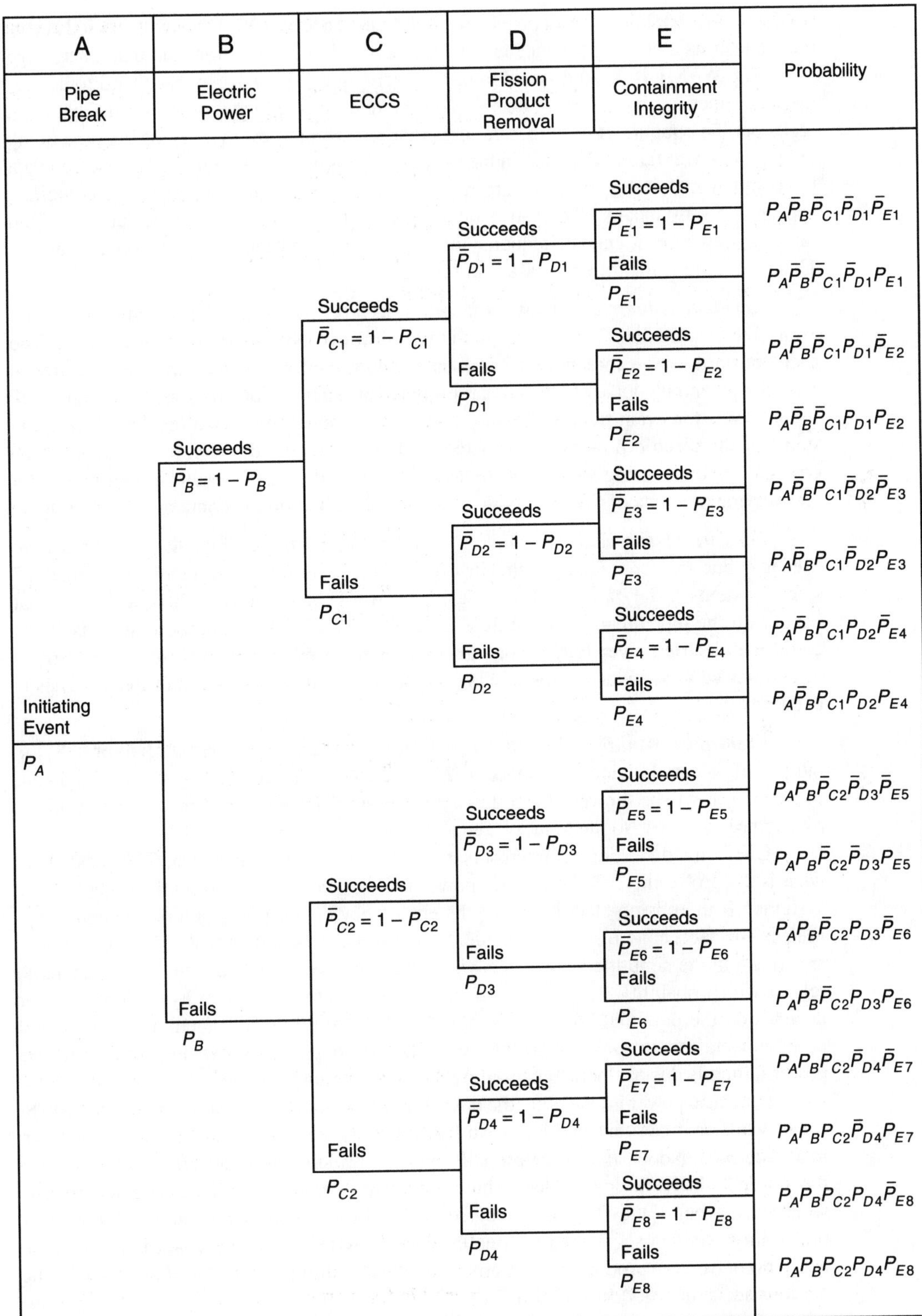

Figure 3.4. An event tree for a pipe-break initiating event.

sessment methodologies based on FTs and ETs (called a level 1 PRA) are widely used in various industries including nuclear, aerospace, chemical, transportation, and manufacturing.

The WASH-1400 study used fault-tree techniques to obtain, by backward logic, numerical values for the P's in Figure 3.4. This methodology, which is described in Chapter 4, seeks out the equipment or human failures that result in top events such as the pipe break or electric power failure depicted in the headings in Figure 3.4. Failure rates, based on data for component failures, operator error, and testing and maintenance error are combined appropriately by means of fault-tree quantification to determine the unavailability of the safety systems or an annual frequency of each initiating event and safety system failure. This procedure is identified as task 2 in Figure 3.3.

Accident sequence. Now let us return to box 1 of Figure 3.3, by considering the event tree (Figure 3.4) for a LOCA initiating event in a typical nuclear power plant. The accident starts with a coolant pipe break having a probability (or frequency) of occurrence P_A. The potential course of events that might follow such a pipe break are then examined. Figure 3.4 is the event tree, which shows all possible alternatives. At the first branch, the status of the electric power is considered. If it is available, the next-in-line system, the emergency core-cooling system, is studied. Failure of the ECCS results in fuel meltdown and varying amounts of fission product release, depending on the containment integrity.

Forward versus backward logic. It is important to recognize that event trees are used to define accident sequences that involve complex interrelationships among engineered safety systems. They are constructed using forward logic: We ask the question "What happens if the pipe breaks?" Fault trees are developed by asking questions such as "How could the electric power fail?" Forward logic used in event-tree analysis and FMEA is often referred to as inductive logic, whereas the type of logic used in fault-tree analysis is deductive.

Event-tree pruning. In a binary analysis of a system that either succeeds or fails, the number of potential accident sequences is 2^N, where N is the number of systems considered. In practice, as will be shown in the following discussion, the tree of Figure 3.4 can be pruned, by engineering logic, to the reduced tree shown in Figure 3.5.

One of the first things of interest is the availability of electric power. The question is, what is the probability, P_B, of electric power failing, and how would it affect other safety systems? If there is no electric power, the emergency core-cooling pumps and sprays are useless—in fact, none of the postaccident functions can be performed. Thus, no choices are shown in the simplified event tree when electric power is unavailable and a very large release with probability $P_A \times P_B$ occurs. In the event that the unavailability of electric power depends on the pipe that broke, the probability P_B should be calculated as a conditional probability to reflect such a dependency.* This can happen, for example, if the electric power failure is due to flooding caused by the piping failure.

If electric power is available, the next choice for study is the availability of the ECCS. It can work or it can fail, and its unavailability, P_{C1}, would lead to the sequence shown in Figure 3.5. Notice that there are still choices available that can affect the course of the accident. If the fission product removal systems operate, a smaller radioactive release would result than if they failed. Of course, their failure would in general produce a lower probability accident sequence than one in which they operated. By working through the entire event tree, we produce a spectrum of release magnitudes and their likelihoods for the various accident sequences (Figure 3.6).

---

*Conditional probabilities are described in Appendix A.1 to this chapter.

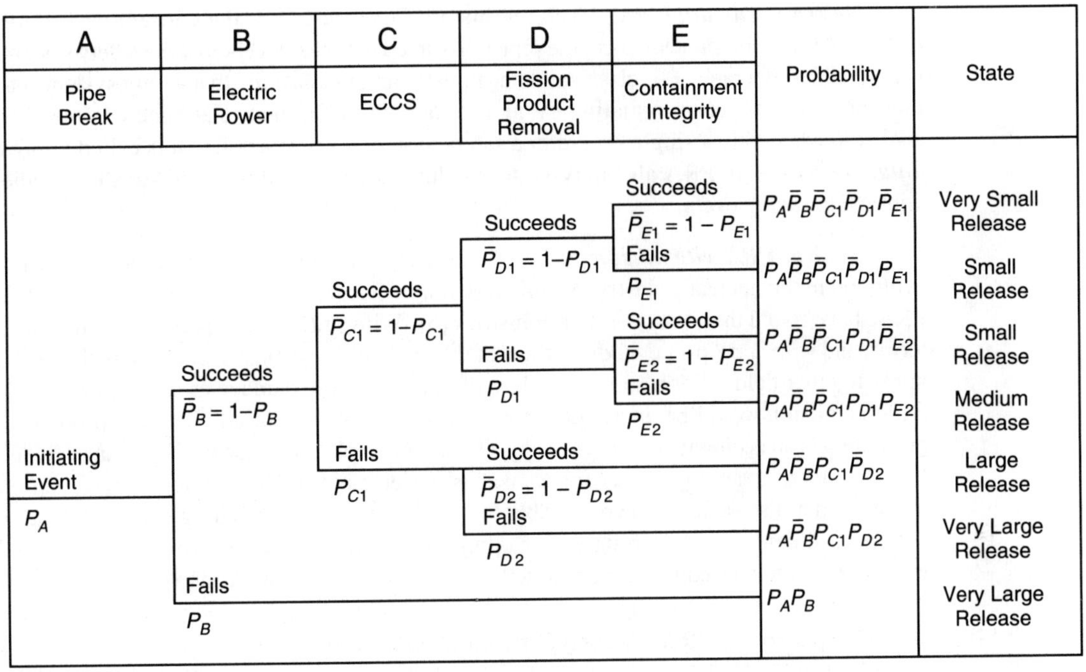

Figure 3.5. Simplifying the event tree in Figure 3.4.

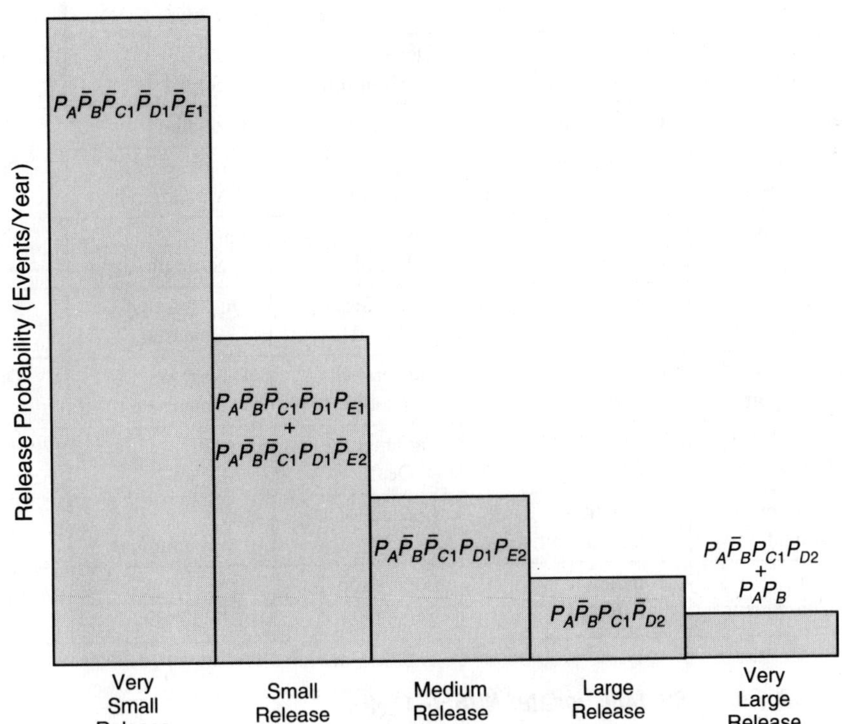

Figure 3.6. Frequency histogram for release magnitude.

Deterministic analysis. The top line of the event tree is the conventional design basis for LOCA. In this sequence, the pipe is assumed to break but each of the safety systems is assumed to operate. The classical deterministic method ensures that safety systems can prevent accidents for an initiating event such as LOCA. In more elaborate deterministic analyses, when only a single failure of a safety system is considered, that is called a *single failure criterion.* In PRA all safety-system failures are assessed probabilistically together with the initiating event.

Nuclear PRA with modifications. There are many lessons to be learned from PRA evolution in the nuclear industry. Sophisticated models and attitudes developed for nuclear PRAs have found their way to other industries [5]. With suitable interpretation of technical terms, and with appropriate modifications of the methodology, most aspects of nuclear PRA apply to other fields. For instance, nuclear PRA defines core damage as an accident, while a train collision would be an accident for a railway problem. For an oil tanker problem, a grounding is an accident. For a medical problem, outbreak of disease would be an accident. Correspondences among PRAs for a nuclear power plant, a single track railway, an oil tanker, and a disease are shown in Table 3.1 for terms such as initiating event, mitigation system, accident, accident progression, progression factor, source term, dispersion and transport, onsite consequence, consequence mitigation, and offsite consequence.

TABLE 3.1. Comparison of PRAs Among Different Applications

Concept	Nuclear PRA	Railway PRA	Oil Tanker	Disease Problem
Initiating Event	LOCA	Unscheduled Departure	Engine Failure	Virus Contact
Mitigation System	ECCS	Departure Monitoring	SOS Signal	Immune System
Accident	Core Damage	Collision	Grounding	Flu
Accident Progression	Progression via Core Damage	Progression via Collision	Progression via Grounding	Progression via Flu
Progression Factor	Reactor Pressure	Collision Speed	Ship Strength	Medical Treatment
Source Term	Radionuclide Released	Toxic Gas Released	Oil Released	Virus Released
Dispersion, Transport	Dispersion, Transport	Dispersion, Transport	Dispersion, Transport	Dispersion, Transport
Onsite Consequence	Personnel Death	Passenger Death	Crew Death	Patient Death
Consequence Mitigation	Evacuation, Decontamination	Evacuation	Oil Containment	Vaccination, Isolation
Offsite Consequence	Population Affected	Population Affected	Sea Pollution	Population Infected

3.1.5 WASH-1400 Update: NUREG-1150

Five steps in a PRA. According to the most recent study, NUREG-1150, PRA consists of the five steps shown in Figure 3.7: accident-frequency analysis, accident-progression

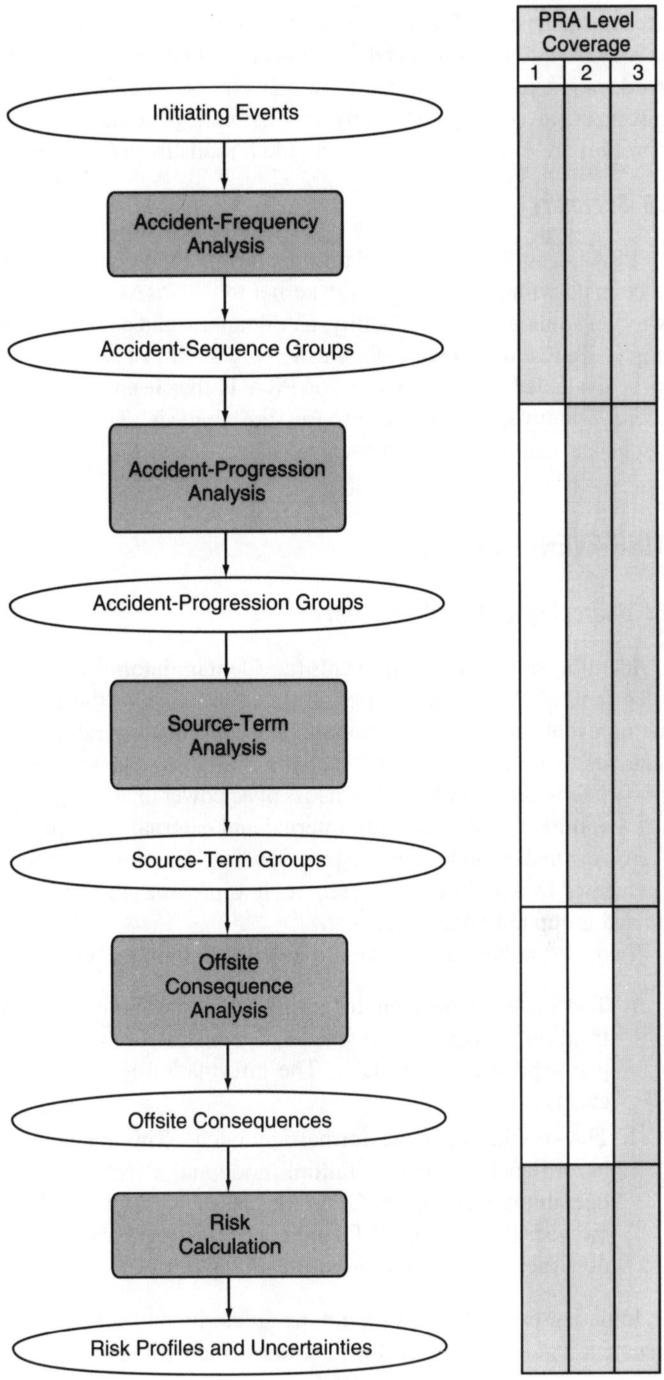

Figure 3.7. Five steps for PRA (NUREG-1150).

analysis, source-term analysis, offsite consequence analysis, and risk calculation [6]. This figure shows how initiating events are transformed into risk profiles via four intermediate products: accident-sequence groups, accident-progression groups, source-term groups, and offsite consequences.* Some steps can be omitted, depending on the application, but other steps may have to be introduced. For instance, a collision accident scenario for passenger trains does not require a source-term analysis or offsite consequence analysis, but does require an onsite consequence analysis to estimate passenger fatalities. Uncertainties in the risk profiles are evaluated by sampling likelihoods from distributions.†

3.1.6 Summary

PRA is a systematic method for transforming initiating events into risk profiles. Event trees coupled with fault trees are the kernel tools. PRAs for a passenger railway, a freight railway, an ammonia storage facility, an oil tanker, and a nuclear power plant are presented to emphasize that this methodology can apply to almost any plant or system for which risk must be evaluated. A recent view of PRA is that it consists of five steps: 1) accident-frequency analysis, 2) accident-progression analysis, 3) source-term analysis, 4) offsite consequence analysis, and 5) risk calculation.

3.2 INITIATING-EVENT SEARCH

3.2.1 Searching for Initiating Events

Identification of initiating events (accident initiators) is an important task because risk profiles can only be obtained through transformation of these events into consequences. Initiating events are any disruptions to normal plant operation that require automatic or manual activation of plant safety systems. Initiating events due to failures of active and support systems are included. Thus a loss of ac power or cooling water becomes an initiating event. A full PRA deals with both internal and external initiating events.

A clear understanding of the general safety functions and features in the plant design, supplemented by a preliminary system review, provides the initial information necessary to select and group initiating events [7].

Two approaches can be taken to identify initiating events.

1. The first is a general engineering evaluation, taking into consideration information from previous risk assessments, documentation reflecting operating history, and plant-specific design data. The information is evaluated and a list of initiating events is compiled.
2. The second is a more formal approach. This includes checklists: preliminary hazard analysis (PHA), failure mode and effects analysis (FMEA), hazard and operability study (HAZOPS), or master logic diagrams (MLD). Although these methods (except for MLD) are not exclusively used for initiating-event identification, they are useful for identification purposes.

Initiating-event studies vary among industries and among companies. Unless specific government regulations dictate the procedure, industrial practice and terminology will vary widely.

---

*In nuclear power plant PRAs, accident-sequence groups and accident-progression groups are called *plant-damage states* and *accident-progression bins*, respectively.

†Uncertainty quantifications are described in Chapter 11.

3.2.2 Checklists

The only guideposts in achieving an understanding of initiators are sound engineering judgment and a detailed grasp of the environment, the process, and the equipment. A knowledge of toxicity, safety regulations, explosive conditions, reactivity, corrosiveness, and flammabilities is fundamental. Checklists such as the one used by Boeing Aircraft (shown in Figure 3.8) are a basic tool in identifying initiating events.

Hazardous Energy Sources	
1. Fuels	11. Gas Generators
2. Propellants	12. Electrical Generators
3. Initiators	13. Rapid-Fire Energy Sources
4. Explosive Charges	14. Radioactive Energy Sources
5. Charged Electrical Capacitors	15. Falling Objects
6. Storage Batteries	16. Catapulted Objects
7. Static Electrical Charges	17. Heating Devices
8. Pressure Containers	18. Pumps, Blowers, Fans
9. Spring-Loaded Devices	19. Rotating Machinery
10. Suspension Systems	20. Actuating Devices
	21. Nuclear Devices, etc.

Hazardous Process and Events	
1. Acceleration	10. Moisture
2. Contamination	High Humidity
3. Corrosion	Low Humidity
4. Chemical Dissociation	11. Oxidation
5. Electricity	12. Pressure
Shock	High Pressure
Inadvertent Activation	Low Pressure
Power Source Failure	Rapid Pressure Changes
Electromagnetic Radiation	13. Radiation
6. Explosion	Thermal
7. Fire	Electromagnetic
8. Heat and Temperature	Ionizing
High Temperature	Ultraviolet
Low Temperature	14. Chemical Replacement
9. Leakage	15. Mechanical Shock, etc.

Figure 3.8. Checklists of hazardous sources.

Initiating events lead to accidents in the form of uncontrollable releases of energy or toxic materials. Certain parts of a plant are more likely to pose risks than others. Checklists are used to identify uncontrollable releases (toxic release, explosion, fire, etc.) and to decompose the plant into subsystems to identify sections or components (chemical reactor, storage tank, etc.) that are likely sources of an accident or initiating event.

In looking for initiating events, it is necessary to bound the plant and the environment under study. It is not reasonable, for example, to include the probability of an airplane crashing into a distillation column. However, airplane crashes, seismic risk, sabotage, adversary action, war, public utility failures, lightning, and other low-probability initiators do enter into calculations for nuclear power plant risks because one can afford to protect against them and, theoretically, a nuclear power plant can kill more people than can a distillation column.

3.2.3 Preliminary Hazard Analysis

Hazards. An initiating event coupled with its potential consequence forms a hazard. If the checklist study is extended in a more formal (qualitative) manner to include consideration of the event sequences that transform an initiator into an accident, as well as corrective measures and consequences of the accident, the study is a preliminary hazard analysis.

In the aerospace industry, for example, the initiators, after they are identified, are characterized according to their effects. A common ranking scheme is

Class I Hazards:	Negligible effects
Class II Hazards:	Marginal effects
Class III Hazards:	Critical effects
Class IV Hazards:	Catastrophic effects

In the nuclear industry, Holloway classifies initiating events and consequences according to their annual frequencies and severities, respectively [8]. The nth initiator groups usually result in the nth consequence group if mitigation systems function successfully; a less frequent initiating event implies a more serious consequence. However, if mitigations fail, the consequence group index may be higher than the initiator group index.

Initiator groups. These groups are classified according to annual frequencies.

1. IG1: 0.1 to 10 events per year.
2. IG2: 10^{-3} to 10^{-1} events per year. These initiators are expected to be reasonably likely in a plant lifetime.
3. IG3: 10^{-5} to 10^{-3} events per year. These initiators often require reliably engineered defenses.
4. IG4: 10^{-6} to 10^{-5} events per year. These initiators include light aircraft crashes and require some assurance of mitigation.
5. IG5: 10^{-7} to 10^{-6} events per year. These initiators include heavy aircraft crashes or primary pressure vessel failure. Defenses are not required because of the low probabilities of occurrence.

Consequence groups. These groups, classified by severity of consequence, are

1. CG1: Trivial consequences expected as part of normal operation
2. CG2: Minor, repairable faults without radiological problems
3. CG3: Major repairable faults possibly with minor radiological problems
4. CG4: Unrepairable faults possibly with severe onsite and moderate offsite radiological problems
5. CG5: Unrepairable faults with major radiological releases

PHA tables. A common format for a PHA is an entry formulation such as shown in Tables 3.2 and 3.3. These are partially narrative in nature, listing both the events and the corrective actions that might be taken. During the process of making these tables, initiating events are identified.

Column entries of Table 3.2 are defined as

1. Subsystem or function: Hardware or functional element being analyzed.
2. Mode: Applicable system phase or modes of operation.

TABLE 3.2. Suggested Format for Preliminary Hazard Analysis

1	2	3	4	5	6	7
Subsystem or Function	Mode	Hazardous Element	Event Causing Hazardous Condition	Hazardous Condition	Event Causing Potential Accident	Potential

8	9	10			11
		Accident Prevention Measures			
Effect	Hazard Class	10A1 Hardware	10A2 Procedures	10A3 Personnel	Validation

TABLE 3.3. Format for Preliminary Hazard Analysis

	Hazardous Element	Triggering Event 1	Hazardous Condition	Triggering Event 2	Potential Accident	Effect	Corrective Measures
1	Alkali metal perchlorate	Alkali metal perchlorate is contaminated with lube oil	Potential to initiate strong reaction	Sufficient energy present to initiate reaction	Explosion	Personnel injury; damage to surrounding structures	Keep metal perchlorate at a suitable distance from all possible contaminants
2	Steel tank	Contents of steel tank contaminated with water vapor	Rust forms inside pressure tank	Operating pressure not reduced	Pressure tank rupture	Personnel injury; damage to surrounding structures	Use stainless steel pressure tank; locate tank at a suitable distance from equipment and personnel

3. Hazardous element: Elements in the subsystem or function being analyzed that are inherently hazardous. Element types are listed as "hazardous energy sources" in Figure 3.8. Examples include gas supply, water supply, combustion products, burner, and flue.
4. Event causing hazardous condition: Events such as personnel error, deficiency and inadequacy of design, or malfunction that could cause the hazardous element to become the hazardous condition identified in column 5. This event is an initiating-event candidate and is called triggering event 1 in Table 3.3.
5. Hazardous condition: Hazardous conditions that could result from the interaction of the system and each hazardous element in the system. Examples of hazardous conditions are listed as "hazardous process and events" in Figure 3.8.

6. Event causing potential accident: Undesired events or faults that could cause the hazardous condition to become the identified potential accident. This event is called triggering event 2 in Table 3.3.
7. Potential accident: Any potential accidents that could result from the identified hazardous conditions.
8. Effect: Possible effects of the potential accident, should it occur.
9. Hazard class: Qualitative measure of significance for the potential effect on each identified hazardous condition, according to the following criteria:

    Class I (Safe)—Potential accidents in column 7 will not result in major degradation and will not produce equipment damage or personnel injury.

    Class II (Marginal)—Column 7 accidents will degrade performance but can be counteracted or controlled without major damage or any injury to personnel.

    Class III (Critical)—The accidents will degrade performance, damage equipment, or result in a hazard requiring immediate corrective action for personnel or equipment survival.

    Class IV (Catastrophic)—The accidents will severely degrade performance and cause subsequent equipment loss and/or death or multiple injuries to personnel.
10. Accident-prevention measures: Recommended preventive measures to eliminate or control identified hazardous conditions and/or potential accidents. Preventive measures to be recommended should be hardware design requirements, incorporation of safety devices, hardware design changes, special procedures, personnel requirements.
11. Record validated measures and keep aware of the status of the remaining recommended preventive measures. "Has the recommended solution been incorporated?" and "Is the solution effective?" are the questions answered in validation. ■

Support-system failures. Of particular importance in a PHA are equipment and subsystem interface conditions. The interface is defined in MIL-STD-1629A as the systems, external to the system being analyzed, that provide a common boundary or service and are necessary for the system to perform its mission in an undegraded mode (i.e., systems that supply power, cooling, heating, air services, or input signals are interfaces). Thus, an interface is nothing but a support system for the active systems. This emphasis on interfaces is consistent with inclusion of initiating events involving support-system failures. Lambert [9] cites a classic example that occurred in the early stages of ballistic missile development in the United States. Four major accidents occurred as the result of numerous interface problems. In each accident, the loss of a multimillion-dollar missile/silo launch complex resulted.

The failure of Apollo 13 was due to a subtle initiator in an interface (oxygen tank). During prelaunch, improper voltage was applied to the thermostatic switches leading to the heater of oxygen tank #2. This caused insulation on the wires to a fan inside the tank to crack. During flight, the switch to the fan was turned on, a short circuit resulted, it caused the insulation to ignite and, in turn, caused the oxygen tank to explode.

In general, a PHA represents a first attempt to identify the initiators that lead to accidents while the plant is still in a preliminary design stage. Detailed event analysis is commonly done by FMEA after the plant is fully defined.

3.2.4 Failure Mode and Effects Analysis

This is an inductive analysis that systematically details, on a component-by-component basis, all possible failure modes and identifies their resulting effects on the plant [10]. Possible single modes of failure or malfunction of each component in a plant are identified and analyzed to determine their effect on surrounding components and the plant.

Failure modes. This technique is used to perform single-random-failure analysis as required by IEEE Standard 279-1971, 10 CFR 50, Appendix K, and regulatory guide 1.70, Revision 2. FMEA considers every mode of failure of every component. A relay, for example, can fail by [11]:

contacts stuck closed
contacts slow in opening
contacts stuck open
contacts slow in closing
contact short circuit
  to ground
  to supply
  between contacts
  to signal lines
contacts chattering
contacts arcing, generating noise
coil open circuit
coil short circuit
  to supply
  to contacts
  to ground
  to signal lines
coil resistance
  low
  high
coil overheating
coil overmagnetized or excessive hysteresis (same effect as contacts stuck closed or slow in opening)

Generic failure modes are listed in Table 3.4 [12].

TABLE 3.4. Generic Failure Modes

No.	Failure Mode	No.	Failure Mode
1	Structural failure (rupture)	19	Fails to stop
2	Physical binding or jamming	20	Fails to start
3	Vibration	21	Fails to switch
4	Fails to remain (in position)	22	Premature operation
5	Fails to open	23	Delayed operation
6	Fails to close	24	Erroneous input (increased)
7	Fails open	25	Erroneous input (decreased)
8	Fails closed	26	Erroneous output (increased)
9	Internal leakage	27	Erroneous output (decreased)
10	External leakage	28	Loss of input
11	Fails out of tolerance (high)	29	Loss of output
12	Fails out of tolerance (low)	30	Shorted (electrical)
13	Inadvertent operation	31	Open (electrical)
14	Intermittent operation	32	Leakage (electrical)
15	Erratic operation	33	Other unique failure condition as applicable to the system characteristics, requirements and operational constraints
16	Erroneous indication		
17	Restricted flow		
18	False actuation		

Checklists. Checklists for each category of equipment must also be devised. For tanks, vessels, and pipe sections, a possible checklist is

1. Variables: flow, quantity, temperature, pressure, pH, saturation.
2. Services: heating, cooling, electricity, water, air, control, N_2.
3. Special states: maintenance, start-up, shutdown, catalyst change.
4. Changes: too much, too little, none, water hammer, nonmixing, deposit, drift, oscillation, pulse, fire, drop, crash, corrosion, rupture, leak, explosion, wear, opening by operator, overflow.
5. Instrument: sensitivity, placing, response time.

Table 3.5 offers a format for the FMEA. This format is similar to those used in a preliminary hazard analysis, the primary difference being the greater specificity and degree of resolution of the FMEA (which is done after initial plant designs are completed).

3.2.5 FMECA

Criticality analysis (CA) is an obvious next step after an FMEA. The combination is called an FMECA—failure mode and effects and criticality analysis. CA is a procedure by which each potential failure mode is ranked according to the combined influence of severity and probability of occurrence.

Severity and criticality. In both Tables 3.3 and 3.5, each effect is labeled with respect to its critical importance to mission operation. According to MIL-STD-1629A, *severity* and *criticality* are defined as follows [10,13].

1. Severity: The consequences of a failure mode. Severity considers the worst potential consequence of a failure, determined by the degree of injury, property damage, or system damage that ultimately occurs.
2. Criticality: A relative measure of the consequences of a failure mode *and* its frequency of occurrences.

As with the consequence groups for the PHA used to rank initiating events, severity for FMECA is rated in more than one way and for more than one purpose.

Severity classification. MIL-STD-1629A recommends the following severity classification.

1. Category 1: Catastrophic—A failure that may cause death or weapon system loss (i.e., aircraft, tank, missile, ship, etc.)
2. Category 2: Critical—A failure that may cause severe injury, major property damage, or major system damage that results in mission loss.
3. Category 3: Marginal—A failure that may cause minor injury, minor property damage, or minor system damage that results in delay or loss of availability or mission degradation.
4. Category 4: Minor—A failure not serious enough to cause injury, property damage, or system damage, but that results in unscheduled maintenance or repair.

Multiple-failure-mode probability levels. Denote by P a single-failure-mode probability for a component during operation. Denote by P_0 an overall component failure probability during operation. Note that the overall probability includes all failure modes.

TABLE 3.5. Failure Modes and Effects Analysis [14]

Item	Failure Modes	Cause of Failure	Possible Effects	Probability	Criticality	Possible Action to Reduce Failure Rate or Effects
Motor case	Rupture	a. Poor workmanship b. Defective materials c. Transportation damage d. Handling damage e. Overpressurization	Damage by missile	0.0006	Critical	Manufacturing process control for workmanship to meet standards. Quality control of basic materials to eliminate defectives. Inspection and testing of completed cases. Suitable packaging to protect motor during transportation.
Propellant grain	a. Cracking b. Voids c. Bond separation	a. Abnormal stress b. Excessively low temperature c. Aging effects	Excessive burning rate; overpressurization; motor case rupture during operation	0.0001	Critical	Controlled production. Storage and operation only within temperature limits. Formulation to resist effects of aging.
Liner	a. Separation from motor case b. Separation from motor grain or insulation	a. Inadequate cleaning of motor case b. Use of unsuitable bonding material c. Inadequate bonding process control	Case rupture	0.0001	Critical	Strict observance of proper cleaning procedures. Strict inspection after cleaning of motor case to ensure that all contaiminants have been removed.

Qualitative levels for probability P are dependent on what fraction of P_0 the failure mode occupies. In other words, each level reflects a conditional probability of a failure mode, given a component failure.

1. Level A—Frequent: $0.20P_0 < P$
2. Level B—Reasonably probable: $0.10P_0 < P \leq 0.20P_0$
3. Level C—Occasional: $0.01P_0 < P \leq 0.10P_0$
4. Level D—Remote: $0.001P_0 < P \leq 0.01P_0$
5. Level E—Extremely unlikely: $P \leq 0.001P_0$

Failure-mode criticality number. Consider a particular severity classification sc for system failures. A ranking of failure mode m for severity classification purposes can be achieved by computing *criticality* number $C_{m,sc}$ (see Figure 3.9). This criticality number $C_{m,sc}$ is the number of system failures falling in severity classification sc per hour or trial caused by component failure mode m.

$$C_{m,sc} = \beta_{sc}\alpha\lambda_p \tag{3.1}$$

$$= \beta_{sc}\alpha\lambda_b\pi_A\pi_E \tag{3.2}$$

where

1. $C_{m,sc}$ = criticality number for failure mode m, given severity classification sc for system failure.
2. β_{sc} = failure effect probability. The β_{sc} values are the conditional probabilities that the failure effect results in the identified severity classification sc, given that the failure mode occurs. Values of β_{sc} are selected from an established set of ranges:

Analyst's Judgment	Typical Value of β_{sc}
Actual effect	$\beta_{sc} = 1.00$
Probable effect	$0.01 < \beta_{sc} < 1.00$
Possible effect	$0.00 < \beta_{sc} \leq 0.01$
None	$\beta_{sc} = 0.00$

3. α = failure mode ratio. This is the probability expressed as a decimal fraction that the component fails in the identified mode. If all potential failure modes of a component are listed, the sum of the α values for that component equals one.
4. λ_p = component failure rate in failures per hour or trial.
   Component failure rate λ_p is calculated by

$$\lambda_p = \lambda_b\pi_A\pi_E \tag{3.3}$$

   where

5. λ_b = component basic failure rate in failures per hour or trial that is obtained, for instance, from MIL-HDBK-217.
6. π_A = application factor that adjusts λ_b for the difference between operating stresses under which λ_b was measured and the operating stresses under which the component is used.
7. π_E = environmental factor that adjusts λ_b for differences between environmental stresses under which λ_b was measured and the environmental stresses under which the component is going to be used.

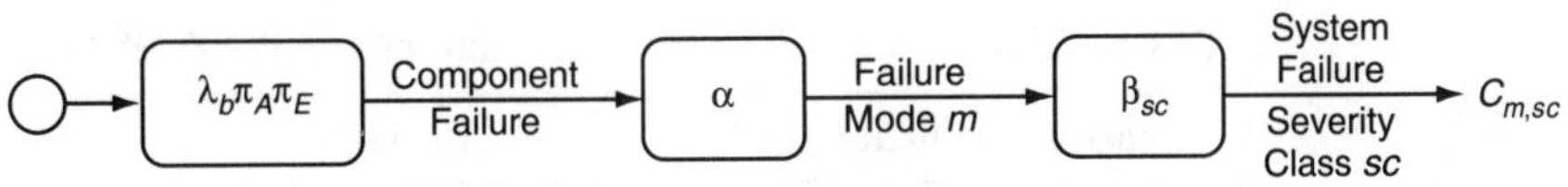

Figure 3.9. Calculation of criticality number $C_{m,sc}$.

As a result, the failure-mode criticality number $C_{m,sc}$ is represented by:

$$C_{m,sc} = \beta_{sc}\alpha\lambda_b\pi_A\pi_E \tag{3.4}$$

Component criticality number. Assume a total number of n failure modes for a component. For each severity classification sc, component criticality number C_{sc} is

$$C_{sc} = \sum_{m=1}^{m=n} C_{m,sc} \tag{3.5}$$

The component criticality number C_{sc} is the number of system failures in severity classification sc per hour or trial caused by the component. Note that m denotes a particular component failure mode, sc is a specific severity classification for system failures, and n is a total number of failure modes for the component.

Note that this ranking method places value on possible consequences or damage through severity classification sc. Besides being useful for initiating event identification as a component failure mode, criticality analysis is useful for achieving system upgrades by identifying [14]

1. which components should be given more intensive study for elimination of the hazard, and for fail-safe design, failure-rate reduction, or damage containment.
2. which components require special attention during production, require tight quality control, and need protective handling at all times.
3. special requirements to be included in specifications for suppliers concerning design, performance, reliability, safety, or quality assurance.
4. acceptance standards to be established for components received at a plant from subcontractors and for parameters that should be tested intensively.
5. where special procedures, safeguards, protective equipment, monitoring devices, or warning systems should be provided.
6. where accident prevention efforts and funds could be applied most effectively. This is especially important, since every program is limited by the availability of funds.

3.2.6 Hazard and Operability Study

Guide words. In identifying subsystems of the plant that give rise to an accident initiator, it is useful to list guide words that stimulate the exercise of creative thinking. A HAZOPS [15–19] suggests looking at a process to see how it might deviate from design intent by applying the following guide words.

More of	Less of
None of	Part of
Later than	Sooner than
Reverse	Wrong Address
Other than	As well as

Examples of process parameter deviations are listed in Table 3.6 [18].

TABLE 3.6. Process Parameter Deviations for HAZOP

Process Parameter	Deviation
Flow	**No** flow **Reverse** flow **More** flow **Extra** flow **Change** in flow proportions Flow to **wrong place**
Temperature	**Higher** temperature **Lower** temperature
Pressure	**Higher** pressure **Lower** pressure
Volume	**Higher** level (in a tank) **Lower** level (in a tank) Volume rate changes **faster** than expected **Proportion** of volumes is **changed**
Composition	**More** component A **Less** component B **Missing** component C **Composition changed**
pH	**Higher** pH **Lower** pH **Faster** change in pH
Viscosity	**Higher** viscosity **Lower** viscosity
Phase	**Wrong** phase **Extra** phase

HAZOPS and FMEA. In a sense, a HAZOPS is an extended FMEA technique, the extension being in the direction of including process parameter deviations in addition to equipment failure modes. Any potential hazards or operability problems (e.g., loss of automatic control) are explored as consequences of such deviations. This can also be used for initiating-event identification.

The use of HAZOPS technique at the Imperial Chemical Industries is described as follows.

> HAZOPS is a detailed failure mode and effect analysis of the Piping and Instrument (P & I) line diagram. A team of four or five people study the P & I line diagram in formal and systematical manner. The team includes the process engineer responsible for the chemical engineering design; the project engineer responsible for the mechanical engineering design and having control of the budget; the commissioning manager who has the greatest commitment to making the plant a good one and who is usually appointed at a very early stage of the project design; a hazard analyst who guides the team through the hazard study and quantifies any risks as necessary.

> This team studies each individual pipe and vessel in turn, using a series of guide words to stimulate creative thinking about what would happen if the fluid in the pipe were to deviate from the design intention in any way. The guide words which we use for continuous chemical plants include high flow, low flow, no flow, reverse flow, high and low temperature and pressure and any other deviation of a parameter of importance. Maintenance, commissioning, testing, start-up, shutdown and failure of services are also considered for each pipe and vessel.
>
> This in-depth investigation of the line diagram is a key feature of the whole project and obviously takes a lot of time—about 200 man hours per $2,000,000 capital. It is very demanding and studies, each lasting about 2.5 hours, can only be carried out at a rate of about two or three per week. On a multimillion dollar project, therefore, the studies could extend over many weeks or months. Problems identified by the hazard study team are referred to appropriate members of team or to experts in support groups. If, during the course of this study, we uncover a major hazard which necessitates some fundamental redesign or change in design concept, the study will be repeated on the redesigned line diagram. Many operability, maintenance, start-up and shutdown problems are identified and dealt with satisfactorily.

Computerized versions of HAZOPS and FMEA are described in [19,20].

3.2.7 Master Logic Diagram

A fault-tree-based PRA uses a divide-and-conquer strategy, where an accident is decomposed into subgroups characterized by initiating events, and this is further decomposed into accident sequences characterized by the event-tree headings. For each initiating event or event-tree heading, a fault tree is constructed. This divide-and-conquer strategy is less successful if some initiating events are overlooked. An MLD uses the fault trees to search for accident initiators.

An example of an MLD for a nuclear power plant is shown in Figure 3.10 [7]. The top event on the first level in the diagram represents the undesired event for which the PRA is being conducted, that is, an excessive offsite release of radionuclides. This top event is successively refined by levels. The OR gate on level 2 answers the question, "How can a release to the environment occur?" yielding "Release of core material" and "Release of noncore material." The AND gate on level 3 shows that a release of radioactive material requires simultaneous core damage and containment failure. The OR gate on level 4 below "Core damage" answers the question, "How can core damage occur?" After several more levels of "how can" questions, the diagram arrives at a set of potential initiating events, which are hardware or people failures.

A total of 59 internal initiating events were eventually found by MLD for the scenario partly shown in Figure 3.10. These events are further grouped according to mitigating system requirements. The NUREG-1150 PRA was able to reduce the number of initiating-event categories by combining several that had the same plant response. For example, the loss of steam inside and outside the containment was collapsed into loss of steam, resulting in a reduction of the initiating event categories for the NUREG-1150 analysis.

3.2.8 Summary

Initiating-event identification is a most important PRA task because accidents have initiators. The following approaches can be used for identification: checklists; preliminary

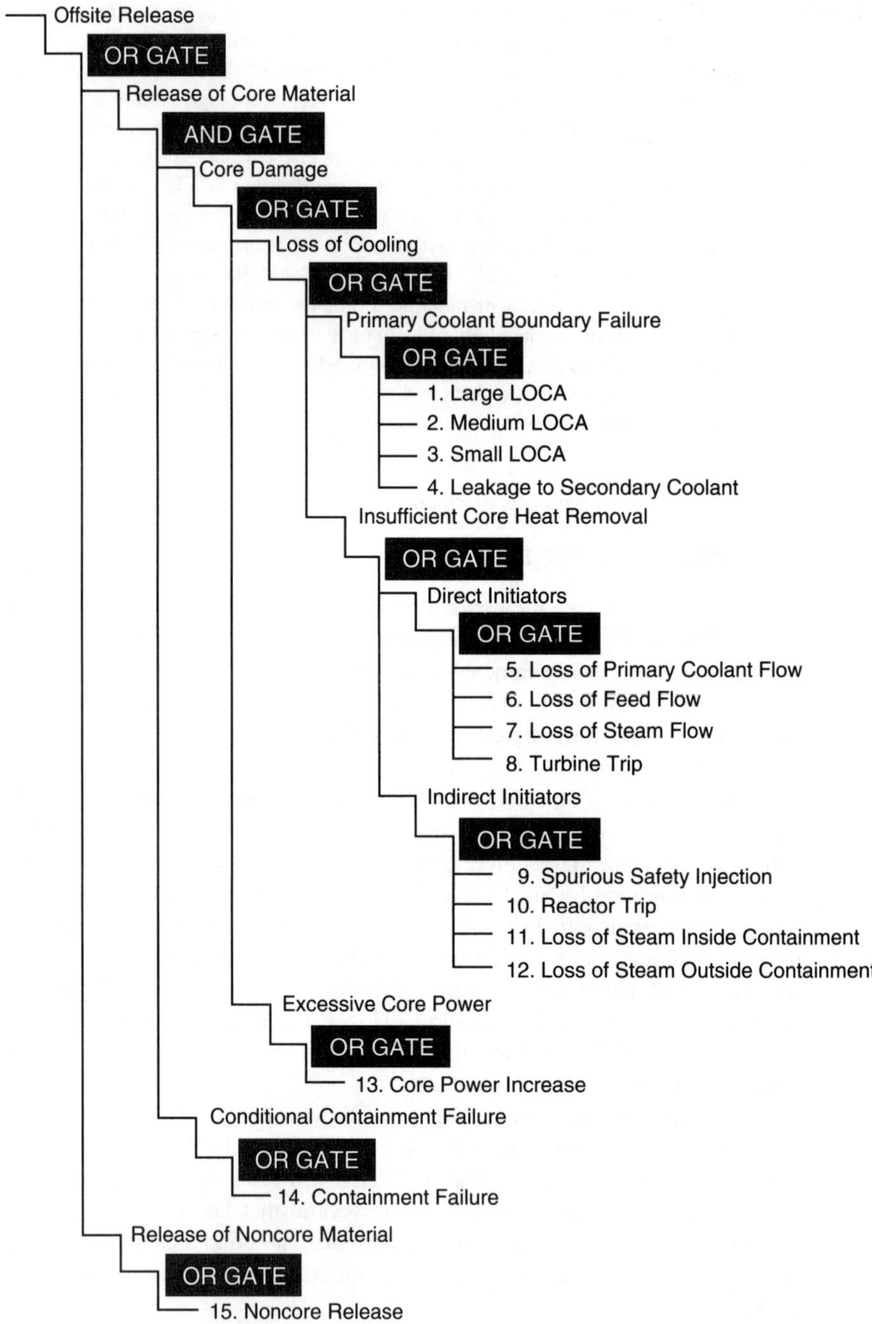

Figure 3.10. Master logic diagram for searching for initiating events.

hazard analysis; failure modes and effects analysis; failure mode, effects, and criticality analysis; hazard and operability study; and master logic diagrams.

3.3 THE THREE PRA LEVELS

As shown by the "PRA Level Coverage" in Figure 3.7, a level 1 PRA consists of the first and last of the five PRA steps, that is, accident-frequency analysis and risk calculation. A level 2 PRA performs accident-progression and source-term analyses *in addition to* the level 1 PRA analyses. A level 3 PRA performs a total of five analyses, that is, an offsite consequence analysis *and* level 2 PRA analyses. Each PRA performs risk calculations. Level 1 risk profiles refer to accident occurrence, level 2 profiles to material release magnitudes, and level 3 profiles to consequence measures such as fatalities.

3.3.1 Level 1 PRA—Accident Frequency

This PRA mainly deals with accident frequencies, that is, frequencies of core damage, train collisions, oil tanker groundings, and so forth. Accident sequences and their groups are identified in a level 1 PRA. The plant states associated with these accident-sequence groups are core damage by melting, train damage by collision, oil tanker damage by grounding, and so on. These accident-sequence groups are used as inputs to a level 2 PRA.

3.3.1.1 Accident-frequency analysis. A level 1 PRA analyzes how initiating events develop into accidents. This transformation is called an accident-frequency analysis in PRA terminology. Level 1 PRAs identify combinations of events that can lead to accidents and then estimate their frequency of occurrence. The definition of *accident* varies from application to application. Some applications involve more than one accident. For instance, for a railway it may include collision and derailment. Initiating events also differ for different applications. A loss of coolant is an initiating event for a nuclear power plant, while an unscheduled departure is an accident initiator for a railway collision.

A level 1 PRA consists of the activities shown in Figure 3.11.

1. Initiating-event analysis (see Section 3.3.1.3).
2. Event-tree construction (see Section 3.3.1.4).
3. Fault-tree construction (see Section 3.3.1.5).
4. Accident-sequence screening (see Section 3.3.1.6).
5. Accident-sequence quantification (see Section 3.3.1.6).
6. Grouping of accident sequences (see Section 3.3.1.10).
7. Uncertainty analysis (see Section 3.3.1.11).

These activities are supported by the following analyses.

1. Plant-familiarization analysis (see Section 3.3.1.2).
2. Dependent-failure analysis (see Section 3.3.1.7).
3. Human-reliability analysis (see Section 3.3.1.8).
4. Database analysis (see Section 3.3.1.9).

This section overviews these activities.

3.3.1.2 Plant-familiarization analysis. An initial PRA task is to gain familiarity with the plant under investigation, as a foundation for subsequent tasks. Information is assembled from such sources as safety analysis reports, piping and instrumentation diagrams,

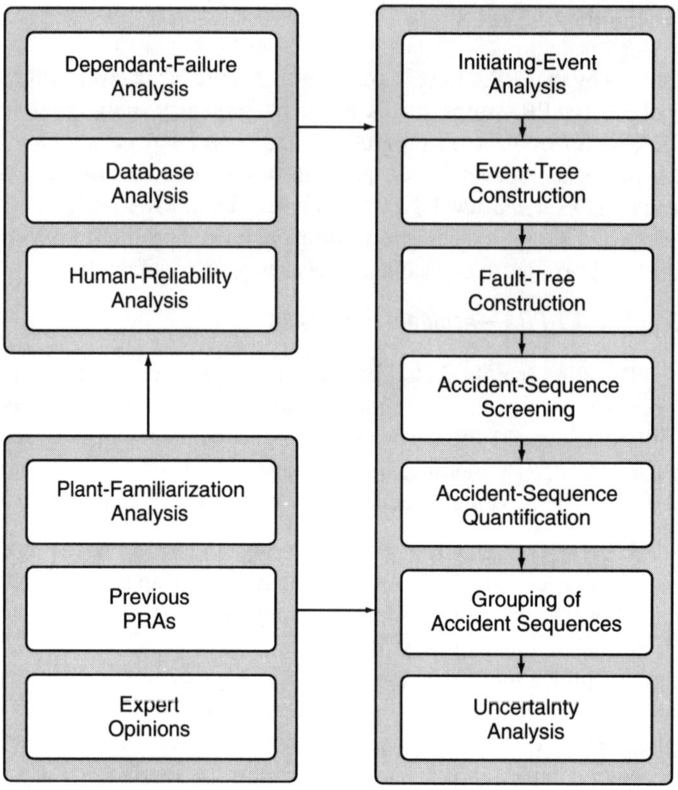

Figure 3.11. A level 1 PRA.

technical specifications, and operating and maintenance procedures and records. A plant site visit to inspect the facility and gather information from plant personnel is part of the process. Typically, one week is spent in the initial visit to a large plant. At the end of the initial visit, much of the information needed to perform the remaining tasks will have been collected and discussed with plant personnel. The PRA team should now be familiar with plant design and operation, and be able to maintain contact with the plant staff throughout PRA to verify information and to identify plant changes that occur during the PRA [6].

3.3.1.3 Initiating-event analysis. The initiating events are analyzed in a stepwise manner. The first step is the most important, and was described in detail in Section 3.2.

1. Identification of initiating events by review of previous PRAs, plant data, and other information
2. Elimination of very low frequency initiating events
3. Identification of safety functions required to prevent an initiating event from developing into an accident
4. Identification of active systems performing a function
5. Identification of support systems necessary for operation of the active systems
6. Delineation of success criteria (e.g., two-out-of-three operating) for each active system responding to an initiating event
7. Grouping of initiating events, based on similarity of safety system response

Initiating-event and operation mode. For a nuclear power plant, a list of initiating events is available in NUREG-1150. These include LOCA, support-system initiators, and other transients. Different sets of initiating events may apply to modes of operation such as full power, low power (e.g., up to 15% power), start-up, and shutdown. The shutdown mode is further divided into cold shutdown, hot shutdown, refueling, and so on. An inadvertent power increase at low power may produce a plant response different from that at full power [21].

Grouping of initiating events. For each initiating event, an event tree is developed that details the relationships among the systems required to respond to the event, in terms of potential system successes and failures. For instance, the event tree of Figure 3.2 considers an unscheduled departure of terminal A train when another train is between terminal B and spur signal 3. If more than one initiating event is involved, these events are examined and grouped according to the mitigation system response required. An event tree is developed for each group of initiating events, thus minimizing the number of event trees required.

3.3.1.4 Event-tree construction

Event trees coupled with fault trees. Event trees for a level 1 PRA are called *accident-sequence event trees.* Active systems and related support systems in event-tree headings are modeled by fault trees. Boolean logic expressions, reliability block diagrams, and other schematics are sometimes used to model these systems. A combination of event trees and fault trees is illustrated in Figure 1.10 where the initiating event is a pump overrun and the accident is a tank rupture. Figure 3.2 is another example of an accident-sequence event tree where the unscheduled departure is an initiating event. This initiator can also be analyzed by a fault tree that should identify, as a cause of the top event, the human error of neglecting a red departure signal because of heavy traffic. The departure-monitoring system failure can be analyzed by a fault tree that deduces basic causes such as an electronic interface failure because of a maintenance error. The cause-consequence diagram described in Chapter 1 is an extension of this marriage of event and fault trees.

Event trees enumerate sequences leading to an accident for a given initiating event. Event trees are constructed in a step-by-step process. Generally, a function event tree is created first. This tree is then converted into a system event tree. Two approaches are available for the marriage of event and fault trees: large ET/small FT approach, and small ET/large FT approach.

Function event trees. Initiating events are grouped according to safety system responses; therefore, construction focuses on safety system functions. For the single track railway problem, the safety functions include departure monitoring and spur signal watching. The first function is performed either by an automatic departure monitoring device or by a human.

A nuclear power plant has the following safety functions [7]. The same safety function can be performed by two or more safety systems.

1. Reactivity control: shuts reactor down to reduce heat production.
2. Coolant inventory control: maintains a coolant medium around the core.
3. Coolant pressure control: maintains the coolant in its proper state.
4. Core-heat removal: transfers heat from the core to a coolant.
5. Coolant-heat removal: transfers heat from the coolant.

6. Containment isolation: closes openings in containment to prevent radionuclide release.
7. Containment temperature and pressure control: prevents damage to containment and equipment.
8. Combustible-gas control: removes and redistributes hydrogen to prevent explosion inside containment.

It should be noted that the coolant inventory control can be performed by low-pressure core spray systems or high-pressure core spray systems.

1. High-pressure core spray system: provides coolant to reactor vessel when vessel pressure is high or low.
2. Low-pressure core spray system: provides coolant to reactor vessel when vessel pressure is low.

Each event-tree heading except for the initiating event refers to a mitigation function or physical systems. When all headings except for the initiator are described on a function level rather than a physical system level, then the tree is called a function event tree. Function event trees are developed for each initiator group because each group generates a distinctly different functional response. The event-tree headings consist of the initiating-event group and the required safety functions.

The LOCA event tree in Figure 3.5 is a function event tree because ECCS, for instance, is a function name rather than the name of an individual physical system. Figure 3.2 is a physical system tree.

System event trees. Some mitigating systems perform more than one function or portions of several functions, depending on plant design. The same safety function can be performed by two or more mitigation systems. There is a many-to-many correspondence between safety functions and accident-mitigation systems.

The function event tree is not an end product; it is an intermediate step that permits a stepwise approach to sorting out the complex relationships between accident initiators and the response of mitigating systems. It is the initial step in structuring plant responses in a temporal format. The function event tree headings are eventually decomposed by identification of mitigation systems that can be measured quantitatively [7]. The resultant event trees are called system event trees.

Large ET/small FT approach. Each mitigation system consists of an active system and associated support systems. An active system requires supports such as ac power, dc power, start signals, or cooling from the support systems. For instance, a reactor shutdown system requires a reactor-trip signal. This signal may also be used as an input to actuate other systems. In the large ET/small FT approach, a special-purpose tree called a support system event tree is constructed to represent states of different support systems. This support system event tree is then assessed with respect to its impact on the operability of a set of active systems [22]. This approach is also called an explicit method, event trees with boundary conditions, or small fault tree models with support system states. Fault tree size is reduced, but the total number of fault trees increases because there are more headings in the support system event tree.

Figure 3.12 is an example of a support system event tree. Four types of support systems are considered: ac power, dc power, start signal (SS), and component cooling

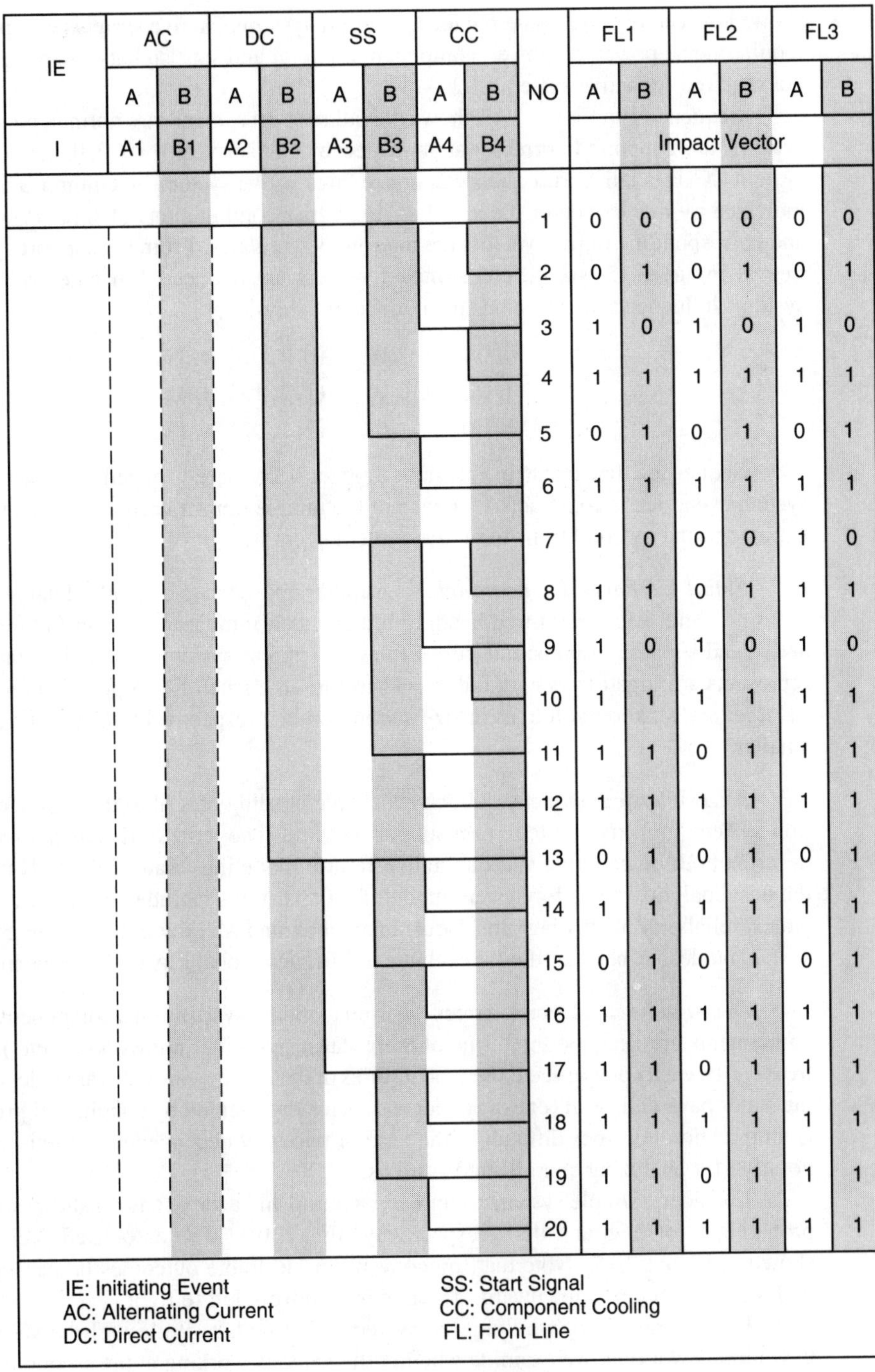

NO	FL1 A	FL1 B	FL2 A	FL2 B	FL3 A	FL3 B
1	0	0	0	0	0	0
2	0	1	0	1	0	1
3	1	0	1	0	1	0
4	1	1	1	1	1	1
5	0	1	0	1	0	1
6	1	1	1	1	1	1
7	1	0	0	0	1	0
8	1	1	0	1	1	1
9	1	0	1	0	1	0
10	1	1	1	1	1	1
11	1	1	0	1	1	1
12	1	1	1	1	1	1
13	0	1	0	1	0	1
14	1	1	1	1	1	1
15	0	1	0	1	0	1
16	1	1	1	1	1	1
17	1	1	0	1	1	1
18	1	1	1	1	1	1
19	1	1	0	1	1	1
20	1	1	1	1	1	1

Figure 3.12. Support system event tree.

(CC). Three kinds of active systems exist: FL1, FL2, and FL3. Each of these support or active systems is redundantly configured, as shown by columns A and B. Figure 3.13

shows how active systems are related to support systems. Active systems except for FL2_A require the ac power, dc power, component cooling, and start signals. Start signal SS_A is not required for active system FL2_A.

Sequence 1 in Figure 3.12 shows that all support systems are normal, hence all active systems are supported correctly as indicated by impact vector $(0, 0, 0, 0, 0, 0)$. Support system CC_B is failed in sequence 2, hence three active systems in column B are failed, as indicated by impact vector $(0, 1, 0, 1, 0, 1)$. Other combinations of support system states and corresponding impact vectors are interpreted similarly. From the support system event tree of Figure 3.12, six different impact vectors are deduced. In other words, support systems influence active systems in six different ways.

$$
\begin{array}{ll}
(0, 0, 0, 0, 0, 0), & (0, 1, 0, 1, 0, 1) \\
(1, 0, 1, 0, 1, 0), & (1, 1, 1, 1, 1, 1) \\
(1, 0, 0, 0, 1, 0), & (1, 1, 0, 1, 1, 1)
\end{array}
$$

Sequences that result in the same impact vector are grouped together. An active system event tree is constructed for each of the unique impact vectors. Impact vectors give explicit boundary conditions for active system event trees.

Small ET/Large FT approach. Another approach is a small ET/large FT configuration. Here, each event-tree heading represents a mitigation system failure, including active and support systems; failures of relevant support systems appear in a fault tree that represents a mitigation system failure. Therefore, the small ET/large FT approach results in larger and smaller fault trees in size and in number, respectively; the event trees become smaller.

3.3.1.5 System models. Each event-tree heading describes the failure of a mitigation system, an active system, or a support system. The term *system modeling* is used to describe both quantitative and qualitative failure modeling. Fault-tree analysis is one of the best analytical tools for system modeling. Other tools include decision trees, decision tables, reliability block diagrams, Boolean algebra, and Markov transition diagrams. Each system model can be quantified to evaluate occurrence probability of the event-tree heading.

Decision tree. Decision trees are used to model systems on a component level. The components are described in terms of their states (working, nonworking, etc.). Decision trees can be easily quantified if the probabilities of the component states are independent or if the states have unilateral (one-way) dependencies represented by conditional probabilities. Quantification becomes difficult in the case of two-way dependencies. Decision trees are not used for analyzing complicated systems.

Consider a simple system comprising a pump and a valve having successful working probabilities of 0.98 and 0.95, respectively (Fig. 3.14). The associated decision tree is shown in Figure 3.15. Note that, by convention, desirable outcomes branch upward and undesirable outcomes downward. The tree is read from left to right.

If the pump is not working, the system has failed, regardless of the valve state. If the pump is working, we examine whether the valve is working at the second nodal point. The probability of system success is $0.98 \times 0.95 = 0.931$. The probability of failure is $0.98 \times 0.05 + 0.02 = 0.069$; the total probability of the system states add up to one.

Truth table. Another way of obtaining this result is via a truth table, which is a special case of decision tables where each cell can take a value from more than two candidates. For the pump and valve, the truth table is

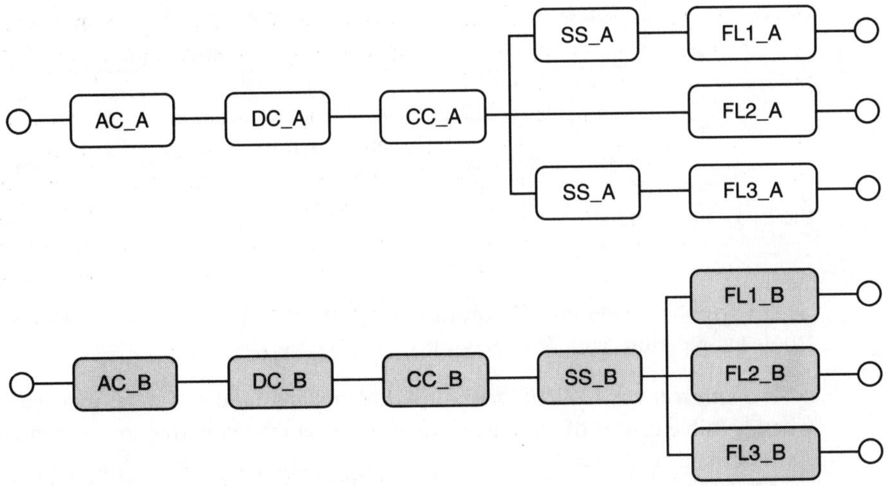

Figure 3.13. Dependency of front-line systems on support systems.

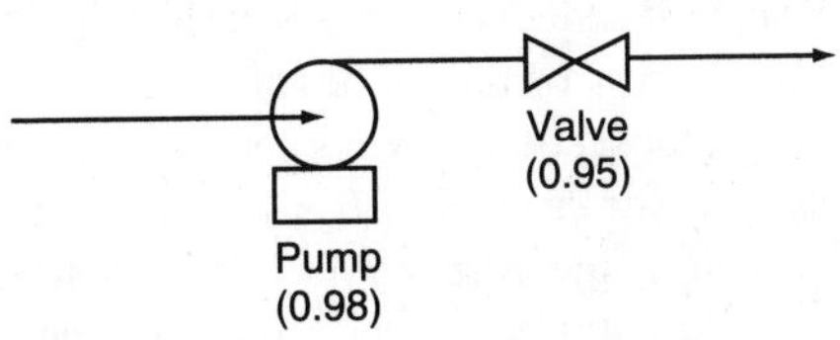

Figure 3.14. A two-component series system.

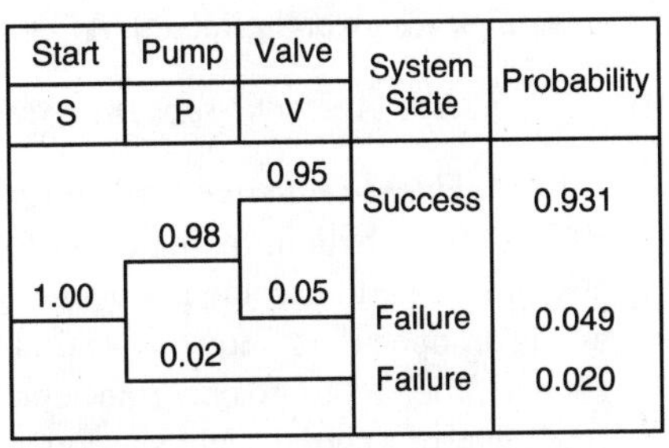

Figure 3.15. Decision tree for two component series system.

Pump State	**Valve State**	**System Success Probability**	**System Failure Probability**
Working	Working	0.98×0.95	0.0
Failed	Working	0.0	0.02×0.95
Working	Failed	0.0	0.98×0.95
Failed	Failed	0.0	0.02×0.05
		Total: 0.931	0.069

Reliability block diagram. A reliability block diagram for the system of Figure 3.14 is shown as Figure 3.16. The system functions if and only if input node I and output node O are connected. A component failure implies a disconnect at the corresponding block.

Boolean expression. Consider a Boolean variable X_1 defined by $X_1 = 1$ if the pump is failed and $X_1 = 0$ if the pump is working. Denote the valve state in a similar way by variable X_2. The system state is denoted by variable Y; $Y = 1$ if the system is failed, and $Y = 0$ otherwise. Then, we have a Boolean expression for the system state in terms of

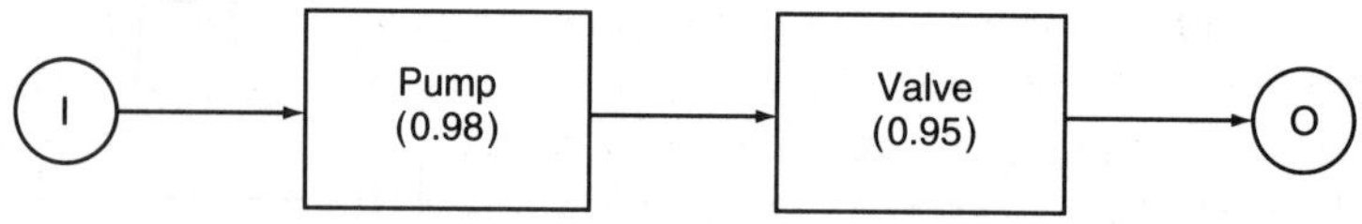

Figure 3.16. Reliability block diagram for two component series system.

the two component states:

$$Y = X_1 \vee X_2 \tag{3.6}$$

where symbol $\vee$ denotes a Boolean OR operation. Appendix A.2 provides a review of Boolean operations and Venn diagrams.

Fault tree as AND/OR tree. Accidents and failures can be reduced significantly when possible causes of abnormal events are enumerated during the system design phase. As described in Section 3.1.4, an FTA is an approach to cause enumeration. An FT is an AND/OR tree that develops a top event (the root) into more basic events (leaves) via intermediate events and logic gates. An AND gate requires that the output event from the gate occur only when input events to the gate occur simultaneously, while an OR gate requires that the output event occur when one or more input events occur. Additional examples are given in Section A.3.4.

3.3.1.6 Accident-sequence screening and quantification

Accident-sequence screening. An accident sequence is an event-tree path. The path starts with an initiating event followed by success or failure of active and/or support systems. A partial accident sequence containing a subset of failures is not processed further and is dropped if its frequency estimate is less than, for instance, 1.0×10^{-9} per year, since each additional failure occurrence probability reduces the estimate further. However, if the frequency of a partial accident sequence is above the cutoff value, the sequence is developed and recovery actions pertaining to specific situations are applied to the appropriate remaining sequences.

Accident-sequence quantification. A Boolean reduction, when performed for fault trees (or decision trees, reliability block diagrams, etc.) along an accident sequence, reveals a combination of failures that can lead to the accident. These combinations are called cut sets. This was demonstrated in Chapter 1 for Figure 1.10. Once important failure events are identified, frequencies or probabilities are assigned to these events and the accident-sequence frequency is quantified. Dependent failures and human reliability as well as hardware databases are used in the assignment of likelihoods.

3.3.1.7 Dependent-failure analysis

Explicit dependency. System analysts generally try to include explicit dependencies in the basic plant logic model. Functional and common-unit dependencies arise from the reliance of active systems on support systems, such as the reliance of emergency coolant injection on service water and electrical power. Dependent failures are usually modeled as integral parts of fault and event trees. Interaction among various components within systems, such as common maintenance or test schedules, common control or instrumentation circuitry, and location within plant buildings (common operating environments), are often included as basic events in system fault trees.

Implicit dependency. Even though the fault- and event-tree models explicitly include major dependencies, in some cases it is not possible to identify the specific mechanisms of a common-cause failure from available databases. In other cases, there are many different types of common-cause failures, each with a low probability, and it is not practical to model them separately. Parametric models (see Chapter 9) can be used to account for the collective contribution of *residual* common-cause failures to system or component failure rates.

3.3.1.8 Human-reliability analysis. Human-reliability analysis identifies human actions in the PRA process.* It also determines the human-error rates to be used in quantifying these actions. The NUREG-1150 analysis considers pre-initiator human errors that occur before an initiating event (inclusive), and post-initiator human errors after the initiating event. The post-initiator errors are further divided into accident-procedure errors and recovery errors.

Pre-initiator error. This error can occur because of equipment miscalibrations during test and maintenance or failure to restore equipment to operability following test and maintenance. Calibration, test, and maintenance procedures and practices are reviewed for each active and support system to evaluate pre-initiator faults. The evaluation includes identification of improperly calibrated components and those left in an inoperable state following test or maintenance activities. An initiating event may be caused by human errors, particularly during start-ups or shutdowns when there is a maximum of human intervention.

Accident-procedure error. This includes failure to diagnose and respond appropriately to an accident sequence. Procedures expected to be followed in responding to each accident sequence modeled by the event trees are identified and reviewed for possible sources of human errors that could affect the operability or function of the responding systems.

Recovery error. Recovery actions may or may not be stated explicitly in emergency operating procedures. These actions that are taken in response to a failure include restoring electrical power, manually starting a pump, and refilling an empty water storage tank. A recovery error represents failure to carry out a recovery action.

Approaches. Pre-initiator errors are usually incorporated into system models. For example, a cause of the departure-monitoring failure of Figure 3.2 is included in the fault tree as a maintenance error before the unscheduled departure. Accident-procedure errors are typically included at the event-tree level as a heading or a top event because they are an expected plant/operator response to the initiating event. The event tree of Figure 3.2 includes a train B conductor human error after the unscheduled departure. Accident procedure errors are included in the system models if they impact only local components. Recovery actions are included either in the event trees or the system models. Recovery actions are usually considered when a relevant accident sequence without recovery has a nonnegligible likelihood.

To support eventual accident-sequence quantification, estimates are required for human-error rates. These probabilities can be evaluated using THERP techniques [23] and plant-specific characteristics.

---

*This topic is discussed in Chapter 10.

3.3.1.9 Database analysis. This task involves the development of a database for quantifying initiating-event frequencies and basic event probabilities for event trees and system models [6]. A generic database representing typical initiating-event frequencies as well as plant-component failure rates and their uncertainties are developed. Data for the plant being analyzed may differ significantly, however, from averaged industry-wide data. In this case, the operating history of the plant is reviewed to develop plant-specific initiating-event frequencies and to determine whether any plant components have unusually high or low failure rates. Test and maintenance practices and plant experiences are also reviewed to determine the frequency and duration of these activities and component service hours. This information is used to supplement the generic database via a Bayesian update analysis (see Chapter 11).

3.3.1.10 Grouping of accident sequences. There may be a variety of accident progressions even if an accident sequence is given; a chemical plant fire may or may not result in a storage tank explosion. On the other hand, different accident sequences may progress in a similar way. For instance, all sequences that include delayed fire department arrival would yield a serious fire.

Accident sequences are regrouped into sequences that result in similar accident progressions. A large number of accident sequences may be identified and their grouping facilitates accident-progression analyses in a level 2 PRA. This is similar to the grouping of initiating events prior to accident-frequency analysis.

3.3.1.11 Uncertainty analysis. Statistical parameters relating to the frequency of an accident-sequence or an accident-sequence group can be accomplished by Monte Carlo calculations that sample basic likelihoods. Uncertainties in basic likelihoods are represented by distributions of frequencies and probabilities that are sampled and combined along an accident-sequence or accident sequence group levels. Statistical parameters such as median, mean, 95% upper bound, and 5% lower bound are thus obtained.*

3.3.1.12 Products from a level 1 PRA. An accident-sequence analysis (level 1 PRA) typically yields the following products.

1. Definition and estimated frequency of accident sequences
2. Definition and estimated frequency of accident-sequence groups
3. Total frequency of abnormal accident frequencies

3.3.2 Level 2 PRA—Accident Progression and Source Term

A level 2 PRA consists of accident progression and source-term analysis in addition to the level 1 PRA.

Accident-progression analysis. This investigates physical processes for accident-sequence groups. For the single track railway problem, physical processes before and after a collision are investigated; for the oil tanker problem, grounding scenarios are investigated; for plant fires, propagation is analyzed.

The principal tool for an accident-progression analysis is an accident-progression event tree (APET). Accident-progression scenarios are identified by this extended version

*Uncertainty analysis is described in Chapter 11.

of event trees. In terms of the railway problem, an APET may include branches with respect to factors such as relative collision speed, number of passengers, toxic gas inventory, train position after collision, and hole size in gas containers. The output of an APET is a listing of different outcomes for the accident progression. Unless hazardous materials are involved, onsite consequences such as passenger fatalities by a railway collision are investigated together with their likelihoods. When hazardous materials are involved, outcomes from APET are grouped into accident-progression groups (APGs) as shown in Figure 3.7. Each outcome of an APG has similar characteristics, and becomes the input for the next stage of analysis, that is, source-term analysis.

Accident-progression analyses yield the following products.

1. Accident-progression groups
2. Conditional probability of each accident progression group, given an accident-sequence group

Source-term analysis. This is performed when there is a release of toxic, reactive, flammable, or radioactive materials. A source-term analysis yields the fractions of the inventory of toxic material released. The amount of material released is the inventory multiplied by a release fraction. In the nuclear industry, source terms are grouped in terms of release initiation time, duration of release, and contributions to immediate and latent health problems, since different types of pollutants are involved.

3.3.3 Level 3 PRA—Offsite Consequence

A level 3 PRA considers, in addition to a level 2 PRA, the full range of consequences caused by dispersion of hazardous materials into the environment. An offsite consequence analysis yields a set of consequence measure values for each source-term group. For NUREG-1150, these measures include early fatalities, latent cancer fatalities, population dose (within 50 miles and total), and two measures for comparison with NRC's safety goals (average individual early fatality probability within 1 mi and average individual latent fatality probability within 10 mi). The nuclear industry, of course, is unique. It has been estimated that 90% of every construction dollar spent is safety related.

3.3.4 Summary

There are three PRA levels. A level 1 PRA is principally an accident-frequency analysis. This PRA starts with plant-familiarization analysis followed by initiating-event analysis. Event trees are coupled with fault trees. System event trees are obtained by elaborating function event trees. Two approaches are available for event-tree construction: large ET/small FT, and small ET/large FT. System modeling is usually performed using fault trees. Decision trees, truth tables, reliability block diagrams, and other techniques can be used for system modeling. Accident-sequence quantification requires dependent-failure analysis, human-reliability analysis, and an appropriate database. Uncertainty analyses are performed for the sequence quantification by sampling basic likelihoods from distributions. Grouping of accident sequences yields input to accident-progression analysis for the next PRA level.

A level 2 PRA includes an accident-progression analysis and source-term analysis in addition to the level 1 PRA. A level 3 PRA is an offsite consequence analysis in addition to a level 2 PRA. One cannot do a level 3 PRA without doing a level 2.

3.4 RISK CALCULATIONS

3.4.1 The Level 3 PRA Risk Profile

The final result of a PRA is the risk profiles produced by assembling the results of all three PRA risk-analysis studies.

Consequence measure. Consider a particular consequence measure denoted by CM divided into m small intervals $I_l, l = 1, \ldots, m$.

Frequency and probability. Define the following frequencies and conditional probabilities (see Figure 3.17):

1. $f(\mathrm{IE}_h)$: Annual frequency of initiating event h.
2. $P(\mathrm{ASG}_i|\mathrm{IE}_h)$: Conditional probability of accident-sequence group i, given occurrence of initiating event h. This is obtained by an accident-frequency analysis using accident-sequence event and fault trees.
3. $P(\mathrm{APG}_j|\mathrm{ASG}_i)$: Conditional probability of accident-progression group j, given occurrence of accident-sequence group i. This is obtained by accident-progression analysis using APETs.
4. $P(\mathrm{STG}_k|\mathrm{APG}_j)$: Conditional probability of source-term group k, given occurrence of accident-progression group j. This is usually a zero–one probability. In other words, the matrix element for given values of j and k is 1.0 if APG_j is

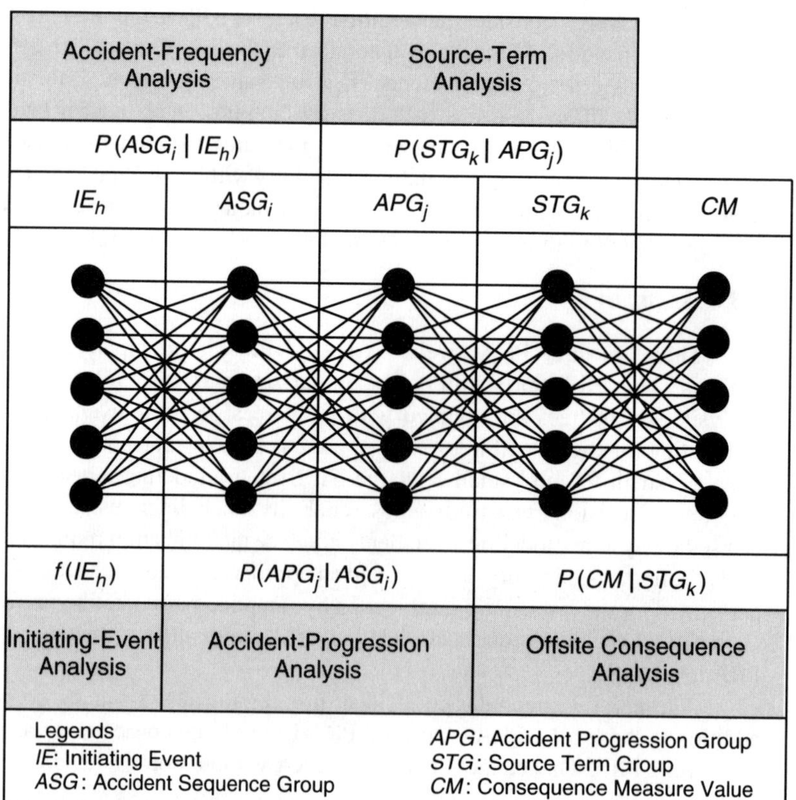

Figure 3.17. Frequency and conditional probabilities in PRA.

assigned to STG_k, and 0.0 otherwise. This assignment is performed by a source-term analysis.

5. $P(CM \in I_l|STG_k)$: Conditional probability of consequence measure CM being in interval I_l, given occurrence of source-term group k. For a fixed source-term group, a consequence value is not uniquely determined because it depends on probabilistic factors such as a combination of wind direction and weather. Typically, 2500 weather trials were performed in NUREG-1150 for each STG_k to estimate the conditional probability. Denote by W_n a particular weather trial. The conditional probability is

$$P(CM \in I_l|STG_k) = \sum_n P(CM \in I_l|W_n, STG_k)P(W_n) \tag{3.7}$$

where $P(CM \in I_l|W_n, STG_k)$ is unity for a particular interval I_l because the source-term group and weather condition are both fixed. Figure 3.18 shows conditional probability $P(CM \in I_l|STG_k)$ reflecting latent cancer fatality variations due to weather conditions.

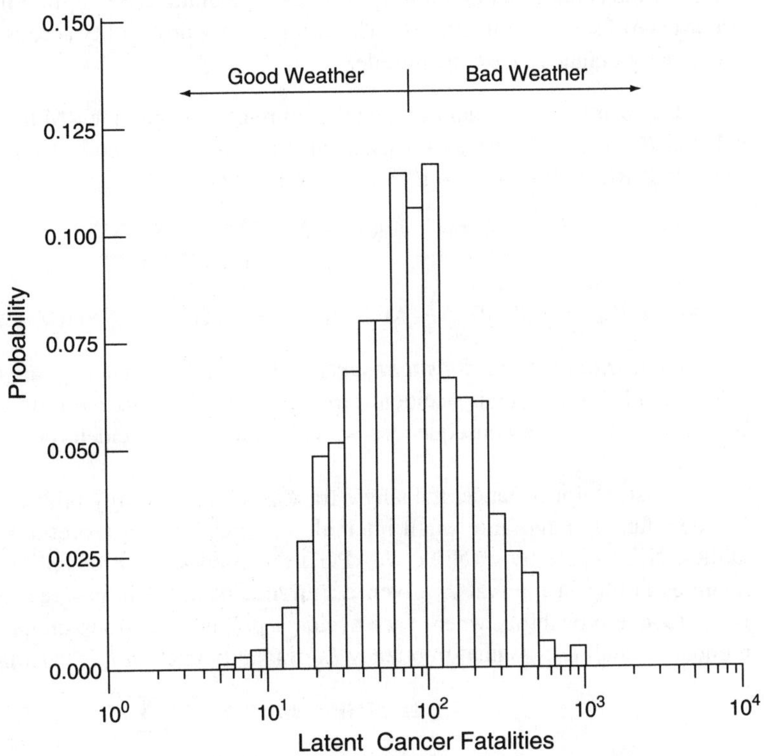

Figure 3.18. Variation of cancer fatalities by weather, given a source-term group.

Risk profile. Likelihood L_l (frequency per year) of consequence measure CM falling in interval I_l can be calculated by

$$L_l \equiv f(CM \in I_l) = \sum_h f(IE_h)P(CM \in I_l|IE_h) \tag{3.8}$$

$$= \sum_h \sum_i \sum_j \sum_k \tag{3.9}$$

$$f(IE_h)P(ASG_i|IE_h)P(APG_j|ASG_i)P(STG_k|ASG_j)P(CM \in I_l|STG_k) \tag{3.10}$$

A risk profile for consequence measure CM is obtained from pairs (L_l, I_l), $l = 1, \ldots, m$. A large number of risk profiles such as this are generated by uncertainty analysis.

Expected consequence. Denote by $E(\text{CM}|\text{STG}_k)$ a conditional expected value of consequence measure CM, given source-term group STG_k. This value was calculated by a (weighted) sample mean of 2500 weather trials. An unconditional expected value $E(\text{CM})$ of consequence measure CM can be calculated by

$$E(\text{CM}) = \sum_h \sum_i \sum_j \sum_k \tag{3.11}$$

$$f(\text{IE}_h)P(\text{ASG}_i|\text{IE}_h)P(\text{APG}_j|\text{ASG}_i)P(\text{STG}_k|\text{ASG}_j)E(\text{CM}|\text{STG}_k) \tag{3.12}$$

3.4.2 The Level 2 PRA Risk Profile

Release magnitude. Consider a level 2 PRA dealing with releases of a toxic material. Divide the release-magnitude range into small intervals I_l. Denote by $P(\text{RM} \in I_l|\text{STG}_k)$ the conditional probability of release magnitude RM falling in interval I_l, given occurrence of source-term group k. This is a zero–one probability because each source-term group has a unique release magnitude.

Risk profile. Annual frequency L_l of release magnitude RM falling in interval I_l is calculated in the same way as a consequence-measure likelihood. A risk profile for release magnitude RM is obtained from pairs (L_l, I_l).

$$L_l \equiv f(\text{RM} \in I_l) = \sum_h \sum_i \sum_j \sum_k \tag{3.13}$$

$$f(\text{IE}_h)P(\text{ASG}_i|\text{IE}_h)P(\text{APG}_j|\text{ASG}_i)P(\text{STG}_k|\text{ASG}_j)P(\text{RM} \in I_l|\text{STG}_k) \tag{3.14}$$

Plant without hazardous materials. If hazardous materials are not involved, then a level 2 PRA only yields accident-progression groups; source-term analyses need not be performed. Onsite consequences are calculated after accident-progression groups are identified.

Consider, for instance, the single track passenger railway problem in Section 3.1.2. Divide a fatality range into small intervals I_l. Each interval represents a subrange of fatalities, NF. Denote by $P(\text{NF} \in I_l|\text{APG}_j)$ the conditional probability of the number of fatalities falling in interval I_l, given occurrence of accident-progression group j. This is a zero–one probability where each accident-progression group uniquely determines the number of fatalities. Annual frequency L_l of fatality interval I_l is calculated as

$$L_l \equiv f(\text{NF} \in I_l) = \sum_h \sum_i \sum_j \tag{3.15}$$

$$f(\text{IE}_h)P(\text{ASG}_i|\text{IE}_h)P(\text{APG}_j|\text{ASG}_i)P(\text{NF} \in I_l|\text{APG}_j) \tag{3.16}$$

A risk profile for the number of fatalities NF is obtained from pairs (L_l, I_l).

3.4.3 The Level 1 PRA Risk Profile

A level 1 PRA deals mainly with accident frequencies; for instance, the annual frequency of railway collisions. Denote by $P(A|\text{ASG}_i)$ the conditional probability of accident A, given occurrence of accident-sequence group i. This is a zero–one probability. Annual frequency L of accident A is given by

$$L \equiv f(A) = \sum_{h} \sum_{i} f(\mathrm{IE}_h) P(\mathrm{ASG}_i|\mathrm{IE}_h) P(A|\mathrm{ASG}_i) \tag{3.17}$$

3.4.4 Uncertainty of Risk Profiles

Likelihood samples. The accident-frequency analyses, accident-progression analyses, and source-term analyses are performed several hundred times (200 in NUREG-1150) by sampling frequencies and probabilities from failure data distributions. This yields several hundred combinations of the three analyses. Each sample or observation uniquely determines initiating-event frequency $f(\mathrm{IE}_h)$, accident-sequence-group probability $P(\mathrm{ASG}_i|\mathrm{IE}_h)$, accident-progression-group probability $P(\mathrm{APG}_j|\mathrm{ASG}_i)$, source-term-group probability $P(\mathrm{STG}_k|\mathrm{ASG}_j)$, and consequence probability $P(\mathrm{CM} \in I_l|\mathrm{STG}_k)$.

Uncertainty as distributions. Each observation yields a unique risk profile for a consequence measure, and several hundred risk profiles are obtained by random sampling. Distribution patterns of these risk profiles indicate uncertainty in the risk profile. Figure 3.19 shows a 95% upper bound, 5% lower bound, mean, and median risk profiles on a log arithmetic scale.

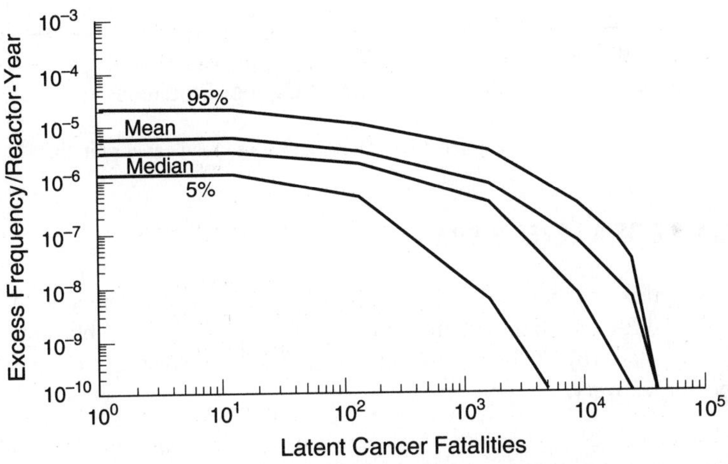

Figure 3.19. Distribution of latent cancer fatality risk profiles.

Samples of expected consequence $E(\mathrm{CM})$ of consequence measure CM are obtained in a similar way. If conditional expected values $E(\mathrm{CM}|\mathrm{STG}_k)$ obtained from weather trials are used for a fixed source-term group, repetition of time-consuming consequence calculations are avoided as long as an observation yields the source-term group. Variations of expected consequence $E(\mathrm{CM})$ are depicted in Figure 3.20, which includes 95% upper bound, 5% lower bound, median and mean values.

3.4.5 Summary

Risk profiles are calculated in three PRA levels by using conditional probabilities. Level 3 risk profiles refer to consequence measures, level 2 profiles to release magnitudes, and level 1 profiles to accident occurrence. Uncertainties in risk profiles are quantified in terms of profile distributions.

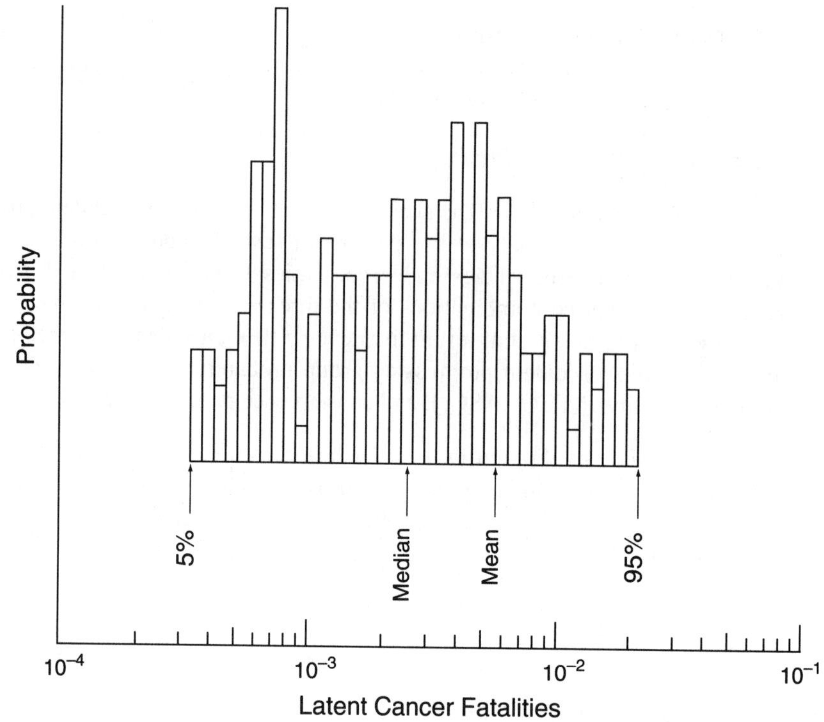

Figure 3.20. Distribution of mean cancer fatalities.

3.5 EXAMPLE OF A LEVEL 3 PRA

A schematic event tree for a LOCA is given in Figure 3.5. Appendix A.3 describes in detail a level 3 PRA starting with the initiating event, that is, station blackout (SBO) for a nuclear power plant [6]. This example also includes an interesting timing problem involving ac power recovery.

3.6 BENEFITS, DETRIMENTS, AND SUCCESSES OF PRA

Quantitative risk profiles are only one of the PRA products and indeed may be less important than others [24]. VonHerrmann and Wood interviewed ten U.S. nuclear power utilities that have undertaken significant PRA activities [1]. This section summarizes their results. Some benefits are tangible, others are intangible. Some utilities use PRAs only once while others use them routinely. The results obtained by vonHerrmann and Wood apply to PRAs for industries other than nuclear power, although nuclear reactor safety studies are usually considerably more elaborate.

3.6.1 Tangible Benefits in Design and Operation

Benefits in design. PRA has the following beneficial impacts on plant design.

1. Demonstration of a low risk level: Some utilities initiated PRA activities and submitted elaborate PRAs to the NRC based on the belief that demonstration

of a low level of risk from their plants would significantly speed their licensing process. (They were wrong. Regulatory malaise, public hearings, and lawsuits are the major delay factors in licensing.)

2. Identification of hitherto unrecognized deficiencies in design.
3. Identification of cost-beneficial design alternatives. Some utilities routinely use PRAs to evaluate the cost and safety impact of proposed plant modifications. PRAs can be useful in industry-regulatory agency jousts:
   - **(a)** To obtain exemption from an NRC proposed modification that would not improve safety in a cost-beneficial manner.
   - **(b)** Replacement of an NRC proposed modification with a significantly more cost-beneficial modification.

Benefits in operation. This includes improvements in procedures and control.

1. Improved procedures: Some utilities identified specific improvements in maintenance, testing, and emergency procedures that have a higher safety impact than hardware modifications. These utilities have successfully replaced an expensive NRC hardware requirement with more cost-effective procedure upgrades.
2. Improved control: One utility was able to demonstrate that additional water-level measuring would not enhance safety, and that the addition of another senior reactor operator in the control room had no safety benefit.

3.6.2 Intangible Benefits

Staff capabilities. PRA brings the following staff-capability benefits.

1. Improved plant knowledge: Engineering and operations personnel, when exposed to the integrated perspective of a PRA, are better able to understand overall plant design and operation, especially the interdependencies between and among systems.
2. Improved operator training: Incorporation of PRA models and results in operator training programs has significantly enhanced ability to diagnose and respond to incidents.

Benefits in NRC interaction. PRA yields the following benefits in interactions with the NRC.

1. Protection from NRC-sponsored studies: One utility performed their own study to convince the NRC not to make their plant the subject of an NRC study. The utility believes that:
   - **(a)** NRC-sponsored studies, because they are performed by outside personnel who may have insufficient understanding of the plant-specific features, might identify false issues or problems or provide the NRC with inaccurate information.
   - **(b)** The utility could much more effectively interact with the NRC in an intelligent manner concerning risk issues if they performed their own investigation.
   - **(c)** Even where valid issues were identified by NRC-sponsored studies, the recommended modifications to address these issues were perceived to be both ineffective and excessively costly.

2. Enhanced credibility with the NRC: Some utilities strongly believe that their PRA activities have allowed them to establish or enhance their reputation with the NRC, thus leading to a significantly improved regulatory process. The NRC now has a higher degree of faith that the utility is actively taking responsibility for safe operation of their plant.
3. Efficient response to the NRC: PRAs allow utilities to more efficiently and effectively respond to NRC questions and concerns.

3.6.3 PRA Negatives

Utilities cited potential negatives in the following areas. The first two can be resolved by PRAs, although the resources expended in clearing up the issues could be excessive.

1. Identification of problems of little safety importance: A few utilities cited the danger that, if PRAs were submitted to the NRC, NRC staff would inappropriately use the study to magnify minor safety problems. The utilities stated that PRA provided them with the means to identify effective resolutions to these problems but resources to clear up the issues were excessive and unwarranted.

   For example, in response to a PRA submittal that focused on a problem, the NRC initiated inquiries into the adequacy of a plant's auxiliary feedwater system (AFWS) reliability. The AFWS was modeled in a conservative manner in the submission. The NRC took the AFWS reliability estimate out of context and required the utility to divert resources to convince the NRC that no problems actually existed with the AFWS.
2. Familiarization with the study: The utilities must ensure that the individuals who interact with the NRC are familiar with the PRA study. Failure to do this can produce modest negative impacts on the utility-regulator relationship. The question of whether a utility should send lawyers and/or engineers to deal with the NRC is discussed in Chapter 12.

Although the major focus in Section 3.6 has been on the nuclear field, NRC-type procedures and policies are being adopted by the EPA, FDA, and state air and water quality agencies, whose budgets have more than quadrupled over the last twenty years (while manufacturing employment has dropped 15%).

3.6.4 Success Factors of PRA Program

3.6.4.1 Three PRA levels. The PRA successes can be defined in terms of the ability to complete the PRA, ability to derive significant benefits from a PRA after it is completed, and ability to produce additional analyses without dependence on outside contractor support.

The majority of level 3 PRAs were motivated by the belief that the nuclear reactor licensing process would be appreciably enhanced by submittal of a PRA that demonstrated a low level of risk. No utility performed a full level 2 PRA to evaluate source terms. This indicates that utilities believe that the logical end points of a PRA are either an assessment of core damage frequency (level 1) or public health consequences (level 3).

PRA programs, whose primary motivation is to prioritize plant modification activities, deal with level 1 PRAs. It is generally believed that a level 1 PRA provides an adequate basis for evaluating, comparing, and prioritizing proposed changes to plant design and operation.

3.6.4.2 Staffing requirements

In-house versus contractor staff. All of the utilities used considerable contract support in their initial studies and all indicated that this was important in getting their programs started in an efficient and successful manner. However, a strong corporate participation in the development process is a necessary condition for success.

Attributes of an in-house PRA team. Utilities that have assigned personnel with the following characteristics to their PRA team report benefits from their PRA expenditures.

1. Possess detailed knowledge of plant design and dynamic behavior. Experienced plant personnel have a more detailed knowledge of plant design and operation than contractors.
2. Be known and respected by managers and decision makers throughout the organization.
3. Have easy access to experienced personnel.
4. Possess the ability to communicate PRA insights and results in terms familiar to designers, operators, and licensing personnel.
5. Understand the PRA perspective and be inclined toward investigative studies.

On the other hand, utilities that have assigned personnel who are disconnected from other members of the utility staff in design, operations, and licensing and are unable to effectively or credibly interact with other groups have experienced the least benefits from their PRAs, regardless of the PRA training or skills of these individuals.

Roles of in-house staff. Successful programs have used either of the following two approaches.

1. Use of company personnel in a detailed technical review role. This takes advantage of their plant-specific knowledge and their access to knowledgeable engineers and operators. It also provides an effective mechanism for them to learn the details of the models and how they are consolidated into an overall risk model.
2. An evolutionary technology transfer process in which the utility personnel receive initial training, and then perform increasingly responsible roles as the tasks progress and as their demonstrated capabilities increase.

3.6.4.3 Technical tools and methods

Details of models. Detailed plant models were essential because

1. these models were required for identifying unrecognized deficiencies in design and operation, and for identifying effective alternatives
2. the models created confidence outside the PRA group

Computer software. Utilities interviewed developed large, detailed fault-tree models and used mainframe computer codes such as SETS or WAM to generate cut sets and quantify the accident sequences. Most utilities warned against overreliance on "intelligent" software; the computer software plus a fundamental understanding of the models by experienced engineers are necessary.

Methodology. There are methodological options such as large versus small event trees, fault trees versus block diagrams, or SETS or WAM. The PRA successes are less dependent on these methodological options.

Documentation. Clear documentation of the system models is essential. It is also important to provide PRA models, results, and insights written expressly for non-technical groups to present this information in familiar terms.

3.6.4.4 Visible senior management advocacy. This produces the following benefits.

1. Continued program funding
2. Availability of quality personnel
3. Evaluation of PRA potential in an unbiased manner by other groups
4. An increased morale and commitment of the PRA team to make the PRA produce the benefits expected by upper management
5. An increased commitment to modify the plant design and operation, even if the cost is significant, if the PRA analysis identifies such a need, and documents its cost-effectiveness

3.6.5 Summary

PRA provides tangible benefits in improved plant design and operation, and intangible benefits in strengthening staff capability and interaction with regulatory agencies. PRA also has some detriments. Factors for a successful PRA are presented from points of view of in-house versus contractor staff, attributes of in-house PRA teams, roles of in-house staff, depth of modeling detail, computer software, methodology and documentation, and senior management advocacy.

REFERENCES

[1] vonHerrmann, J. L., and P. J. Wood. "The practical application of PRA: An evaluation of utility experience and USNRC perspectives," *Reliability Engineering and System Safety*, vol. 24, no. 2, pp. 167–198, 1989.

[2] Papazoglou, I. A., O. Aneziris, M. Christou, and Z. Nivoliantou. "Probabilistic safety analysis of an ammonia storage plant." In *Probabilistic Safety Assessment and Management*, edited by G. Apostolakis, pp. 233–238. New York: Elsevier, 1991.

[3] USNRC. "Reactor safety study: An assessment of accident risk in U.S. commercial nuclear power plants." USNRC, WASH-1400, NUREG-75/014, 1975.

[4] IAEA. "Computer codes for level 1 probabilistic safety assessment." IAEA, IAEA-TECDOC-553, June 1990.

[5] Apostolakis, G. E., J. H. Bickel, and S. Kaplan. "Editorial: Probabilistic risk assessment in the nuclear power utility industry," *Reliability Engineering and System Safety*, vol. 24, no. 2, pp. 91–94, 1989.

[6] USNRC. "Severe accident risks: An assessment for five U.S. nuclear power plants." USNRC, NUREG-1150, vol. 2, 1990.

[7] USNRC. "PRA procedures guide: A guide to the performance of probabilistic risk assessments for nuclear power plants." USNRC, NUREG/CR-2300, 1983.

[8] Holloway, N. J. "A method for pilot risk studies." In *Implications of Probabilistic Risk Assessment*, edited by M. C. Cullingford, S. M. Shah, and J. H. Gittus, pp. 125–140. New York: Elsevier Applied Science, 1987.

[9] Lambert, H. E. "Fault tree in decision making in systems analysis." Lawrence Livermore Laboratory, UCRL-51829, 1975.

[10] Department of Defense. "Procedures for performing a failure mode, effects and criticality analysis." Department of Defense, MIL-STD-1629A.

[11] Taylor, R. RISϕ National Laboratory, Roskilde, Denmark. Private Communication.

[12] Villemeur, A. *Reliability, Availability, Maintainability and Safety Assessment*, vol. 1 and 2. New York: John Wiley & Sons, 1992.

[13] Mckinney, B. T. "FMECA, the right way." In *Proc. Annual Reliability and Maintainability Symposium*, pp. 253–259, 1991.

[14] Hammer, W. *Handbook of System and Product Safety*. Englewood Cliffs, NJ: Prentice-Hall, 1972.

[15] Lawley, H. G. "Operability studies and hazard analysis," *Chemical Engineering Progress*, vol. 70, no. 4, pp. 45–56, 1974.

[16] Roach, J. R., and F. P. Lees. "Some features of and activities in hazard and operability (Hazop) studies," *The Chemical Engineer*, pp. 456–462, October, 1981.

[17] Kletz, T. A. "Eliminating potential process hazards," *Chemical Engineering*, pp. 48–68, April 1, 1985.

[18] Suokas, J. "Hazard and operability study (HAZOP)." In *Quality Management of Safety and Risk Analysis*, edited by J. Suokas and V. Rouhiainen, pp. 84–91. New York: Elsevier, 1993.

[19] Venkatasubramanian, V., and R. Vaidhyanathan. "A knowledge-based framework for automating HAZOP analysis," *AIChE Journal*, vol. 40, no. 3, pp. 496–505, 1994.

[20] Russomanno, D. J., R. D. Bonnell, and J. B. Bowles. "Functional reasoning in a failure modes and effects analysis (FMEA) expert system." In *Proc. Annual Reliability and Maintainability Symposium*, pp. 339–347, 1993.

[21] Hake, T. M., and D. W. Whitehead. "Initiating event analysis for a BWR low power and shutdown accident frequency analysis." In *Probabilistic Safety Assessment and Management*, edited by G. Apostolakis, pp. 1251–1256. New York: Elsevier, 1991.

[22] Arrieta, L. A., and L. Lederman. "Angra I probabilistic safety study." In *Implications of Probabilistic Risk Assessment*, edited by M. C. Cullingford, S. M. Shah, and J. H. Gittus, pp. 45–63. New York: Elsevier Applied Science, 1987.

[23] Swain, A. D. "Accident sequence evaluation program: Human reliability analysis procedure." Sandia National Laboratories, NUREG/CR-4722, SAND86-1996, 1987.

[24] Konstantinov, L. V. "Probabilistic safety assessment in nuclear safety: International developments." In *Implications of Probabilistic Risk Assessment*, edited by M. C. Cullingford, S. M. Shah, and J. H. Gittus, pp. 3–25. New York: Elsevier Applied Science, 1987.

[25] Ericson, D. M., Jr., et al. "Analysis of core damage frequency: Internal events methodology." Sandia National Laboratories, NUREG/CR-4550, vol. 1, Rev. 1, SAND86-2084, 1990.

CHAPTER THREE APPENDICES

A.1 CONDITIONAL AND UNCONDITIONAL PROBABILITIES

A.1.1 Definition of Conditional Probabilities

Conditional probability $\Pr\{A|C\}$ is the probability of occurrence of event A, given that event C occurs. This probability is defined by

$$\Pr\{A|C\} = \text{proportion of the things resulting in event } A \text{ among the set of things yielding event } C\text{. This proportion is defined as zero when the set is empty.} \quad \text{(A.1)}$$

The conditional probability is different from unconditional probabilities $\Pr\{A\}$, $\Pr\{C\}$, or $\Pr\{A, C\}$:*

$$\Pr\{A\} = \text{proportion of the things resulting in event } A \text{ among the set of all things} \quad \text{(A.2)}$$

$$\Pr\{C\} = \text{proportion of the things resulting in event } C \text{ among the set of all things} \quad \text{(A.3)}$$

$$\Pr\{A, C\} = \text{proportion of the things resulting in the simultaneous occurrence of events } A \text{ and } C \text{ among the set of all things} \quad \text{(A.4)}$$

Example A—Unconditional and conditional probabilities. There are six balls that are small or medium or large; red or white or blue.

BALL 1	BALL 2	BALL 3	BALL 4	BALL 5	BALL 6
SMALL BLUE	SMALL RED	MEDIUM WHITE	LARGE WHITE	SMALL RED	MEDIUM RED

Obtain the following probabilities.

1. Pr{BLUE}
2. Pr{SMALL}
3. Pr{BLUE, SMALL}
4. Pr{BLUE|SMALL}

Solution: There are six balls. Among them, one is blue, three are small, and one is blue and small. Thus,

$$\begin{aligned} \Pr\{\text{BLUE}\} &= 1/6 \\ \Pr\{\text{SMALL}\} &= 3/6 = 1/2 \\ \Pr\{\text{BLUE, SMALL}\} &= 1/6 \end{aligned} \quad \text{(A.5)}$$

Among the three small balls, only one is blue. Thus,

$$\Pr\{\text{BLUE}|\text{SMALL}\} = 1/3 \quad \text{(A.6)}$$

■

Conditional probability $\Pr\{A|B, C\}$ is the probability of the occurrence of event A, given that both events B and C occur. This probability is defined by

---

*Joint probability $\Pr\{A, C\}$ is denoted by $\Pr\{A \cap C\}$ in some texts.

$$\Pr\{A|B, C\} = \text{proportion of the things yielding event } A \text{ among the set of things resulting in the simultaneous occurrence of events } B \text{ and } C \tag{A.7}$$

Example B—Conditional probability. Obtain

1. Pr{BALL 2}
2. Pr{SMALL, RED}
3. Pr{BALL 2, SMALL, RED}
4. Pr{BALL 2|SMALL, RED}
5. Pr{BALL 1|SMALL, RED}

Solution: Among the six balls, two are small and red, and one is at the same time ball 2, small and red. Thus,

$$\begin{aligned} \Pr\{\text{BALL } 2\} &= 1/6 \\ \Pr\{\text{SMALL, RED}\} &= 2/6 = 1/3 \\ \Pr\{\text{BALL } 2, \text{SMALL, RED}\} &= 1/6 \end{aligned} \tag{A.8}$$

Ball 2 is one of the two small red balls; therefore

$$\Pr\{\text{BALL } 2|\text{SMALL, RED}\} = 1/2 \tag{A.9}$$

Ball 1 does not belong to the set of the two small red balls. Thus

$$\Pr\{\text{BALL } 1|\text{SMALL, RED}\} = 0/2 = 0 \tag{A.10}$$

■

A.1.2 Chain Rule

The simultaneous existence of events A and C is equivalent to the existence of event C plus the existence of event A under the occurrence of event C. Symbolically,

$$(A, C) \Leftrightarrow C \text{ and } (A|C) \tag{A.11}$$

This equivalence can be extended to probabilities:

$$\Pr\{A, C\} = \Pr\{C\}\Pr\{A|C\} \tag{A.12}$$

More generally,

$$\Pr\{A_1, A_2, \ldots, A_n\} = \Pr\{A_1\}\Pr\{A_2|A_1\} \cdots \Pr\{A_n|A_1, A_2, \ldots, A_{n-1}\} \tag{A.13}$$

If we think of the world (the entire population) as having a certain property W, then equation (A.12) becomes:

$$\Pr\{A, C|W\} = \Pr\{C|W\}\Pr\{A|C, W\} \tag{A.14}$$

These equations are the chain rule relationships. They are useful for calculating simultaneous (unconditional) probabilities from conditional probabilities. Some conditional probabilities can be calculated more easily than unconditional probabilities, because conditions narrow the world under consideration.

Example C—Chain rule. Confirm the chain rules:

1. Pr{BLUE, SMALL} = Pr{SMALL}Pr{BLUE|SMALL}
2. Pr{BALL 2, SMALL|RED} = Pr{SMALL|RED}Pr{BALL 2|SMALL, RED}

Solution: From Example A

$$\begin{aligned} \Pr\{\text{BLUE, SMALL}\} &= 1/6 \\ \Pr\{\text{SMALL}\} &= 1/2 \\ \Pr\{\text{BLUE}|\text{SMALL}\} &= 1/3 \end{aligned} \tag{A.15}$$

The first chain rule is confirmed, because

$$1/6 = (1/2)(1/3) \tag{A.16}$$

Among the three red balls, two are small, and one is at the same time small and ball 2. Thus

$$\begin{aligned} \Pr\{\text{BALL 2, SMALL}|\text{RED}\} &= 1/3 \\ \Pr\{\text{SMALL}|\text{RED}\} &= 2/3 \end{aligned} \tag{A.17}$$

Only one ball is ball 2 among the two small red balls.

$$\Pr\{\text{BALL 2}|\text{SMALL, RED}\} = 1/2 \tag{A.18}$$

Thus the second chain rule is confirmed, because

$$\frac{1}{3} = (2/3)(1/2) \tag{A.19}$$

■

A.1.3 Alternative Expression of Conditional Probabilities

From the chain rule of equations (A.12) and (A.14), we have

$$\Pr\{A|C\} = \frac{\Pr\{A, C\}}{\Pr\{C\}} \tag{A.20}$$

$$\Pr\{A|C, W\} = \frac{\Pr\{A, C|W\}}{\Pr\{C|W\}} \tag{A.21}$$

We see that the conditional probability is the ratio of the unconditional simultaneous probability to the probability of condition C.

Example D—Conditional probability expression. Confirm:

1. Pr{BLUE|SMALL} = Pr{BLUE, SMALL}/Pr{SMALL}
2. Pr{BALL 2|SMALL, RED} = Pr{BALL 2, SMALL|RED}/Pr{SMALL|RED}

Solution: From Example C

$$\begin{aligned} 1/3 &= \frac{1/6}{1/2} = 1/3, \quad \text{for the first equation} \\ 1/2 &= \frac{1/3}{2/3} = 1/2, \quad \text{for the second equation} \end{aligned} \tag{A.22}$$

■

A.1.4 Independence

Event A is independent of event C if and only if

$$\Pr\{A|C\} = \Pr\{A\} \tag{A.23}$$

This means that the probability of event A is unchanged by the occurrence of event C. Equations (A.20) and (A.23) give

$$\Pr\{A, C\} = \Pr\{A\}\Pr\{C\} \tag{A.24}$$

This is another expression for independence. We see that if event A is independent of event C, then event C is also independent of event A.

Example E—Independent events. Is event "BLUE" independent of "SMALL"?

Solution: It is not independent because

$$\Pr\{\text{BLUE}\} = 1/6, \quad \text{Example A} \tag{A.25}$$

$$\Pr\{\text{BLUE}|\text{SMALL}\} = 1/3, \quad \text{Example B} \tag{A.26}$$

Event "BLUE" is more likely to occur when "SMALL" occurs. In other words, the possibility "BLUE" is increased by the observation, "SMALL." ■

A.1.5 Bridge Rule

To further clarify conditional probabilities, we introduce intermediate events, each of which acts as a bridge from event C to event A (see Figure A3.1).

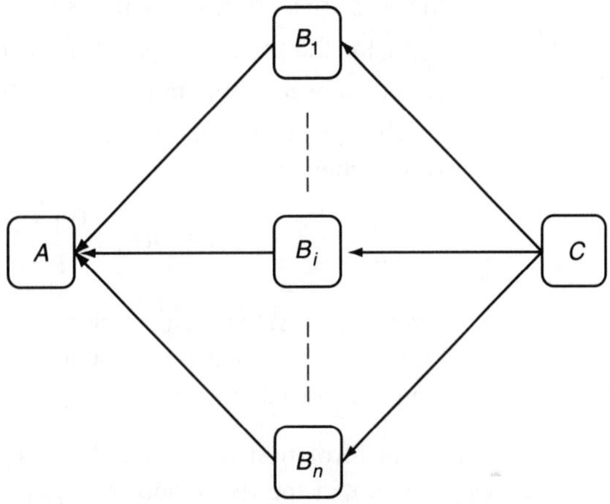

Figure A3.1. Bridges $B_1, \ldots, B_n$.

We assume that intermediate events $B_1, \ldots, B_n$ are mutually exclusive and cover all cases, i.e.,

$$\Pr\{B_i, B_j\} = 0, \quad \text{for } i \neq j \tag{A.27}$$

$$\Pr\{B_1 \text{ or } B_2 \text{ or} \cdots \text{or } B_n\} = 1 \tag{A.28}$$

Then the conditional probability $\Pr\{A|C\}$ can be written as

$$\Pr\{A|C\} = \sum_{i=1}^{n} \Pr\{B_i|C\}\Pr\{A|B_i, C\} \tag{A.29}$$

Event A can occur through any one of the n events $B_1, \ldots, B_n$: Intuitively speaking, $\Pr\{B_i|C\}$ is the probability of the choice of bridge B_i, and $\Pr\{A|B_i, C\}$ is the probability of the occurrence of event A when we have passed through bridge B_i.

Example F—Bridge rule. Calculate Pr{BLUE|SMALL} by letting B_i be "BALL i."

Solution: Equation (A.29) becomes

$$\begin{aligned}\Pr\{\text{BLUE}|\text{SMALL}\} &= \Pr\{\text{BLUE 1}|\text{SMALL}\}\Pr\{\text{BLUE}|\text{BALL 1, SMALL}\}\\ &\quad + \Pr\{\text{BLUE 2}|\text{SMALL}\}\Pr\{\text{BLUE}|\text{BALL 2, SMALL}\}\\ &\quad + \cdots + \Pr\{\text{BLUE 6}|\text{SMALL}\}\Pr\{\text{BLUE}|\text{BALL 6, SMALL}\} \qquad \text{(A.30)}\\ &= (1/3)(1) + (1/3)(0) + (0)(0) + (0)(0) + (1/3)(0) + (0)(0)\\ &= 1/3\end{aligned}$$

When there is no ball satisfying the condition, the corresponding conditional probability is zero. Thus

$$\Pr\{\text{BLUE}|\text{BALL 3, SMALL}\} = 0 \tag{A.31}$$

Equation (A.30) confirms the result of Example A. ■

A.1.6 Bayes Theorem for Discrete Variables

Bayes theorem, in a modified and useful form, may be stated as:

$$\text{Posterior probabilities} \propto \text{prior probabilities} \times \text{likelihoods} \tag{A.32}$$

where the symbol $\propto$ means "are proportional to." This relation may be formulated in a general form as follows: if

1. the A_i's are a set of mutually exclusive and exhaustive events, for $i = 1, \ldots, n$;
2. $\Pr\{A_i\}$ is the prior (or a priori) probability of A_i before observation;
3. B is the observation; and
4. $\Pr\{B|A_i\}$ is the likelihood, that is, the probability of the observation, given that A_i is true, then

$$\Pr\{A_i|B\} = \frac{\Pr\{A_i, B\}}{\Pr\{B\}} = \frac{\Pr\{A_i\}\Pr\{B|A_i\}}{\sum_i \Pr\{A_i\}\Pr\{B|A_i\}} \tag{A.33}$$

where $\Pr\{A_i|B\}$ is the posterior (or a posteriori) probability, meaning the probability of A_i now that B is known. Note that the denominator of equation (A.33) is simply a normalizing constant for $\Pr\{A_i|B\}$, ensuring $\sum \Pr\{A_i|B\} = 1$.

The transformation from $\Pr\{A_i\}$ to $\Pr\{A_i|B\}$ is called the Bayes's transform. It utilizes the fact that the likelihood of $\Pr\{B|A_i\}$ is more easily calculated than $\Pr\{A_i|B\}$. If we think of probability as a degree of belief, then our prior belief is changed, by the evidence observed, to a posterior degree of belief.

Example G—Bayes theorem. A randomly sampled ball turns out to be small. Use Bayes theorem to obtain the posterior probability that the ball is ball 1.

Solution: From Bayes theorem

$$\Pr\{\text{BALL 1}|\text{SMALL}\} = \frac{\Pr\{\text{SMALL}|\text{BALL 1}\}\Pr\{\text{BALL 1}\}}{\sum_{i=1}^{6} \Pr\{\text{SMALL}|\text{BALL } i\}\Pr\{\text{BALL } i\}} \tag{A.34}$$

Because the ball is sampled randomly, we have prior probabilities before the small ball observation:

$$\Pr\{\text{BALL } i\} = 1/6, \quad i = 1, \ldots, 6 \tag{A.35}$$

From the ball data of Example A, likelihoods of small ball observation are

$$\Pr\{\text{SMALL}|\text{BALL } i\} = \begin{cases} 1, & i = 1, 2, 5, \\ 0, & i = 3, 4, 6 \end{cases} \tag{A.36}$$

Thus the Bayes formula is calculated as

$$\Pr\{\text{BALL 1}|\text{SMALL}\} = \frac{1 \times (1/6)}{(1+1+0+0+1+0)(1/6)} = \frac{1}{3} \tag{A.37}$$

This is consistent with the fact that ball 1 and two other balls are small. ■

A.1.7 Bayes Theorem for Continuous Variables

Let

1. $x =$ the continuous valued parameter to be estimated;
2. $p\{x\} =$ the prior probability density of x before observation;*
3. $\mathbf{y} = (y_1, \ldots, y_N)$: N observations of an attribute of x;
4. $p\{\mathbf{y}|x\} =$ likelihood, that is, the probability density of the observations given that x is true; and
5. $p\{x|\mathbf{y}\} =$ the posterior probability density of x.

From the definition of conditional probabilities,

$$p\{x|\mathbf{y}\} = \frac{p\{x, \mathbf{y}\}}{p\{\mathbf{y}\}} = \frac{p\{x, \mathbf{y}\}}{\int [\text{numerator}]dx} \tag{A.38}$$

The numerator can be rewritten as

$$p\{x, \mathbf{y}\} = p\{x\}p\{\mathbf{y}|x\} \tag{A.39}$$

yielding Bayes theorem for the continuous valued parameter x.

$$p\{x|\mathbf{y}\} = \frac{p\{x\}p\{\mathbf{y}|x\}}{\int [\text{numerator}]dx} \tag{A.40}$$

Bayes theorem for continuous x and discrete B is

$$p\{x|B\} = \frac{p\{x\}\Pr\{B|x\}}{\int [\text{numerator}]dx} \tag{A.41}$$

For discrete A_i and continuous $\mathbf{y}$

$$\Pr\{A_i|\mathbf{y}\} = \frac{\Pr\{A_i\}p\{\mathbf{y}|A_i\}}{\sum_i [\text{numerator}]} \tag{A.42}$$

A.2 VENN DIAGRAMS AND BOOLEAN OPERATIONS

A.2.1 Introduction

In Venn diagrams the set of all possible causes is denoted by rectangles, and a rectangle becomes a universal set. Some causes in the rectangle result in an event but others do not. Because the event occurrence is equivalent to the occurrence of its causes, the event is represented by a closed region—that is, a subset—within the rectangle.

Example H—Venn diagram expression. Assume an experiment where we throw a dice and observe its outcome as a cause of events. Consider the events A, B, and C, which are defined as

$$\begin{aligned} A &= \{\text{outcome} = 3,\ 4,\ 6\} \\ B &= \{3 \le \text{outcome} \le 5\} \\ C &= \{3 \le \text{outcome} \le 4\} \end{aligned}$$

Represent these events by a Venn diagram.

---

*Denote by X a continuous random variable having probability density $p\{x\}$. Quantity $p\{x\}dx$ is the probability that random variable X has a value in a small interval $(x, x + dx)$.

Solution: The rectangle (universal set) consists of six possible outcomes 1, 2, 3, 4, 5, and 6. The event representation is shown in Figure A3.2. Event C forms an intersection of events A and B. ■

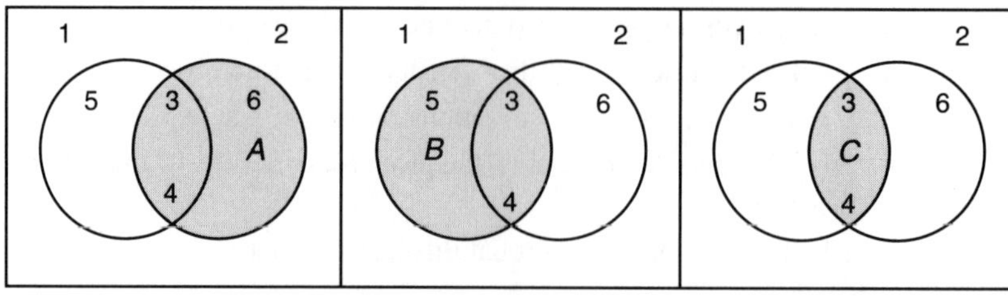

Figure A3.2. Venn diagram for Example H.

Venn diagrams yield a visual tool for handling events, Boolean variables, and event probabilities; their use is summarized in Table A3.1.

TABLE A3.1. Venn Diagram, Event, Boolean Variable, and Probability

Venn Diagram	Event	Boolean Variable	Probability $Pr\{\}$ [$S\{\}$: Area]
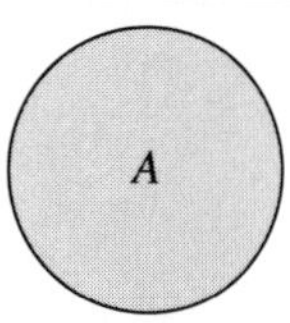	A	$Y_A = \begin{cases} 1, \text{ in } A \\ 0, \text{ otherwise} \end{cases}$	$Pr\{A\} = S\{A\}$
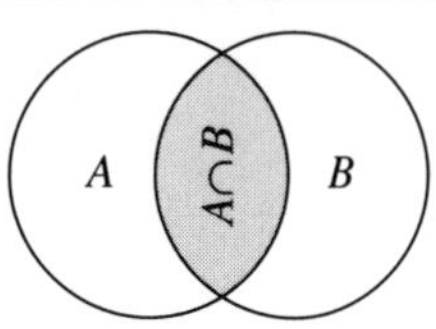	Intersection $A \cap B$	$Y_{A \cap B} = Y_A \wedge Y_B$ $= \begin{cases} 1, \text{ in } A \cap B \\ 0, \text{ otherwise} \end{cases}$ $= Y_A Y_B$	$\Pr\{A \cap B\} = S\{A \cap B\}$
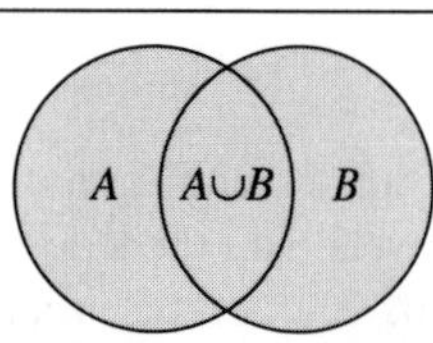	Union $A \cup B$	$Y_{A \cup B} = Y_A \vee Y_B$ $= \begin{cases} 1, \text{ in } A \cup B \\ 0, \text{ otherwise} \end{cases}$ $= 1 - [1 - Y_A][1 - Y_B]$	$\Pr\{A \cup B\} = S\{A \cup B\}$ $= S\{A\} + S\{B\} -$ $S\{A \cap B\}$ $= Pr\{A\} + Pr\{B\} -$ $Pr\{A \cap B\}$
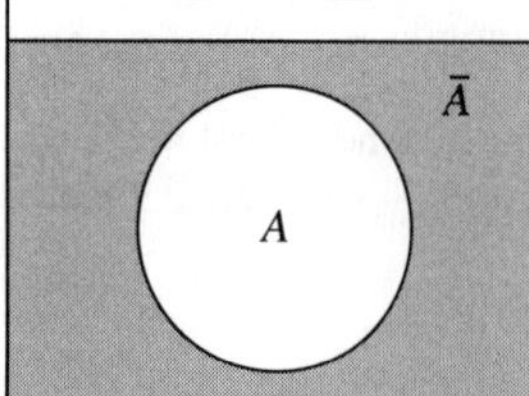	Complement $\bar{A}$	$Y_{\bar{A}} = \bar{Y}_A$ $= \begin{cases} 1, \text{ in } \bar{A} \\ 0, \text{ otherwise} \end{cases}$ $= 1 - Y_A$	$\Pr\{\bar{A}\} = S\{\bar{A}\}$ $= 1 - S\{A\}$ $= 1 - Pr\{A\}$

A.2.2 Event Manipulations via Venn Diagrams

The intersection $A \cap B$ of events A and B is the set of points that belong to both A and B (column 1, row 2 in Table A3.1). The intersection is itself an event, and the common causes of events A and B become the causes of event $A \cap B$. The union $A \cup B$ is the set of points belonging to either A or B (column 1, row 3). Either causes of event A or B can create event $A \cup B$. The complement $\overline{A}$ consists of points outside event A.

Example I—Distributive set operation. Prove

$$A \cap (B \cup C) = (A \cap B) \cup (A \cap C) \tag{A.43}$$

Solution: Both sides of the equation correspond to the shaded area of Figure A3.3. This proves equation (A.43). ■

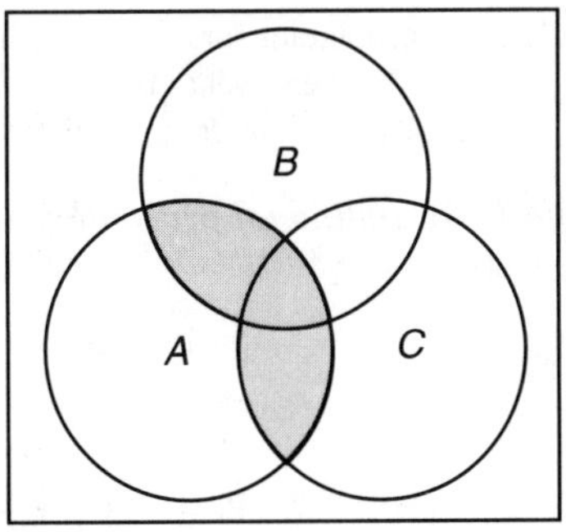

Figure A3.3. Venn diagram for $A \cap (B \cup C) = (A \cap B) \cup (A \cap C)$.

A.2.3 Probability and Venn Diagrams

Let the rectangle have an area of unity. Denote by $S(A)$ the area of event A. Then the probability of occurrence of event A is given by the area $S(A)$ (see column 4, row 1, Table A3.1):

$$\Pr\{A\} = S(A) \tag{A.44}$$

Other probabilities, $\Pr\{A \cap B\}, \Pr\{A \cup B\}, \Pr\{\overline{A}\}$ are defined by the areas $S(A \cap B)$, $S(A \cup B)$, and $S(\overline{A})$, respectively (column 4, Table A3.1). This definition of probabilities yields the relationship:

$$\begin{aligned} \Pr\{A \cup B\} &= \Pr\{A\} + \Pr\{B\} - \Pr\{A \cap B\} \\ \Pr\{\overline{A}\} &= 1 - \Pr\{A\} \end{aligned}$$

Example J—Complete dependence. Assume the occurrence of event A results in the occurrence of event B. Then prove that

$$\Pr\{A \cap B\} = \Pr\{A\} \tag{A.45}$$

Solution: Whenever event A occurs, event B must occur. This means that any cause of event A is also a cause of event B. Therefore, set A is included in set B as shown in Figure A3.4. Thus the area $S(A \cap B)$ is equal to $S(A)$, proving equation (A.45). ■

Conditional probability $\Pr\{A|C\}$ is defined by

$$\Pr\{A|C\} = \frac{S(A \cap C)}{S(C)} \tag{A.46}$$

In other words, the conditional probability is the proportion of event A in the set C as shown in Figure A3.5.

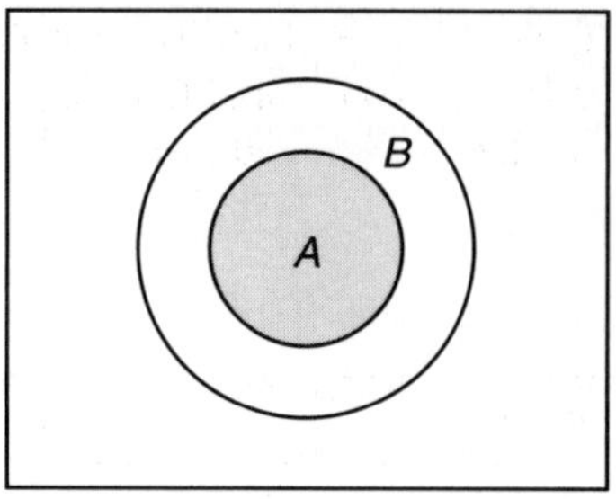

Figure A3.4. Venn diagram for $A \cap B$ when event A results in event B.

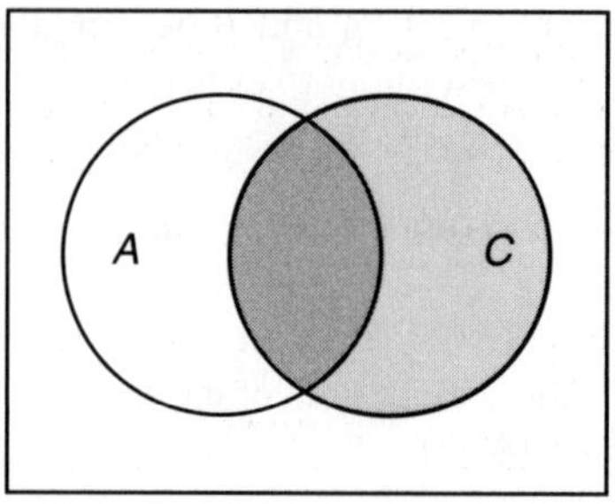

Figure A3.5. Venn diagram for conditional probability $\Pr\{A|C\}$.

Example K—Conditional probability simplification. Assume that event C results in event B. Prove that

$$\Pr\{A|B, C\} = \Pr\{A|C\} \tag{A.47}$$

Solution:

$$\Pr\{A|B, C\} = \frac{S(A \cap B \cap C)}{S(B \cap C)} \tag{A.48}$$

Because set C is included in set B, as shown in Figure A3.6, then

$$S(A \cap B \cap C) = S(A \cap C)$$
$$S(B \cap C) = S(C)$$

Thus

$$\Pr\{A|B, C\} = \frac{S(A \cap C)}{S(C)} = \Pr\{A|C\} \tag{A.49}$$

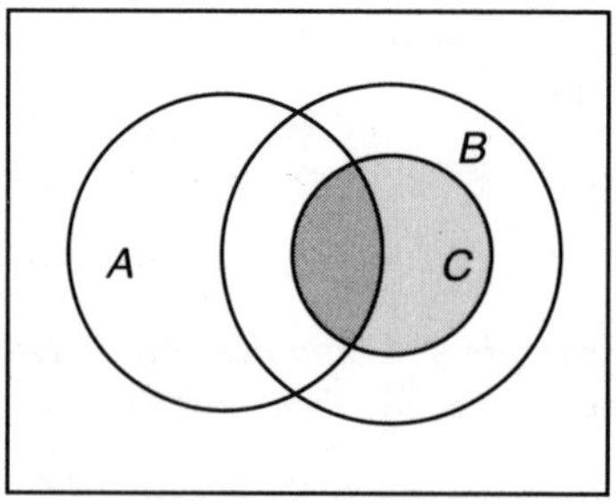

Figure A3.6. Venn diagram when event C results in event B.

This relation is intuitive, because the additional observation of B brings no new information as it was already known when event C happened. ■

A.2.4 Boolean Variables and Venn Diagrams

The Boolean variable Y_A is an indicator variable for set A, as shown in column 3, row 1 in Table A3.1. Other variables such as $Y_{A \cup B}$, $Y_{A \cap B}$, $Y_{\overline{A}}$ are defined similarly. The event unions and intersections, $\cup$ and $\cap$, used in the set expressions to express relationships between events, correspond to the Boolean operators $\vee$ (OR) and $\wedge$ (AND), and to the usual algebraic operations $-$ and $\times$ as shown in Table A3.2. Probability equivalences are also in Table A3.2; note that $\Pr\{B_i\} = E\{Y_i\}$; thus for zero–one variable Y_i, $E\{\}$ is an expected number, or probability. Variables $Y_{A\cup B}$, $Y_{A\cap B}$, and $Y_{\overline{A}}$ are equal to $Y_A \vee Y_B$, $Y_A \wedge Y_B$, and $\overline{Y}_A$, respectively.

TABLE A3.2. Event, Boolean, and Algebraic Operations

Event	Boolean	Algebraic	Note
B_i	$Y_i = 1$	$Y_i = 1$	Event i exists
$\overline{B_i}$	$Y_i = 0$	$Y_i = 0$	Event i does not exist
$B_i \cap B_j$	$Y_i \wedge Y_j = 1$	$Y_i Y_j = 1$	$\Pr\{B_i \cap B_j\} = E\{Y_i \wedge Y_j\}$
$B_i \cup B_j$	$Y_i \vee Y_j = 1$	$1 - [1 - Y_i][1 - Y_j] = 1$	$\Pr\{B_i \cup B_j\} = E\{Y_i \vee Y_j\}$
$B_1 \cap \cdots \cap B_n$	$Y_1 \wedge \cdots \wedge Y_n = 1$	$Y_1 \times \cdots \times Y_n = 1$	$\Pr\{B_1 \cap \cdots \cap B_n\}$ $= E\{Y_1 \wedge \cdots \wedge Y_n\}$
$B_1 \cup \cdots \cup B_n$	$Y_1 \vee \cdots \vee Y_n = 1$	$1 - \prod_{i=1}^{n} [1 - Y_i] = 1$	$\Pr\{B_1 \cup \cdots \cup B_n\}$ $= E\{Y_1 \vee \cdots \vee Y_n\}$

Addition (+) and product (·) symbols are often used as Boolean operation symbols $\vee$ and $\wedge$, respectively, when there is no confusion with ordinary algebraic operations; the Boolean product symbol is often omitted.

$$Y_A \vee Y_B = Y_A + Y_B \tag{A.50}$$

$$Y_A \wedge Y_B = Y_A \cdot Y_B = Y_A Y_B \tag{A.51}$$

Example L—De Morgan's law. Prove

$$\overline{Y_A \vee Y_B} = \overline{Y}_A \wedge \overline{Y}_B \tag{A.52}$$

Solution: By definition, $\overline{Y_A \vee Y_B}$ is the indicator for the set $\overline{A \cup B}$, whereas $\overline{Y}_A \wedge \overline{Y}_B$ is the indicator for the set $\overline{A} \cap \overline{B}$. Both sets are the shaded region in Figure A3.7 and de Morgan's law is proven. ■

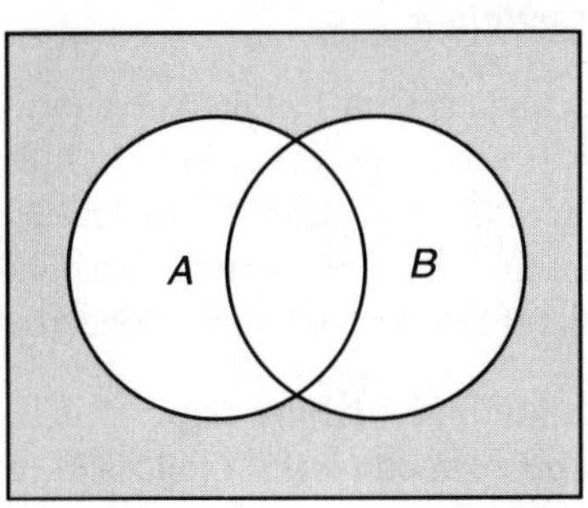

Figure A3.7. Venn diagram for de Morgan's law $\overline{A \cup B} = \overline{A} \cap \overline{B}$.

A.2.5 Rules for Boolean Manipulations

The operators $\vee$ and $\wedge$ can be manipulated in accordance with the rules of Boolean algebra. These rules and the corresponding algebraic interpretations are listed in Table A3.3.

TABLE A3.3. Rules for Boolean Manipulations

Laws	Algebraic Interpretation
Idempotent laws:	
$Y \vee Y = Y$	$1 - [1 - Y][1 - Y] = Y$
$Y \wedge Y = Y$	$YY = Y$
Commutative laws:	
$Y_1 \vee Y_2 = Y_2 \vee Y_1$	$1 - [1 - Y_1][1 - Y_2] = 1 - [1 - Y_2][1 - Y_1]$
$Y_1 \wedge Y_2 = Y_2 \wedge Y_1$	$Y_1 Y_2 = Y_2 Y_1$
Associative laws:	
$Y_1 \vee (Y_2 \vee Y_3) = (Y_1 \vee Y_2) \vee Y_3$	
$Y_1 \wedge (Y_2 \wedge Y_3) = (Y_1 \wedge Y_2) \wedge Y_3$	
Distributive laws:	
$Y_1 \wedge (Y_2 \vee Y_3) = (Y_1 \wedge Y_2) \vee (Y_1 \wedge Y_3)$	
$Y_1 \vee (Y_2 \wedge Y_3) = (Y_1 \vee Y_2) \wedge (Y_1 \vee Y_3)$	
Absorption laws:	
$Y_1 \wedge (Y_1 \wedge Y_2) = Y_1 \wedge Y_2$	$Y_1 Y_1 Y_2 = Y_1 Y_2$
$Y_1 \vee (Y_1 \wedge Y_2) = Y_1$	$1 - [1 - Y_1][1 - Y_1 Y_2] = Y_1$
Complementation:	
$Y \vee \overline{Y} = 1$	$1 - [1 - Y][1 - (1 - Y)] = 1$
$Y \wedge \overline{Y} = 0$	$Y[1 - Y] = 0$
Operations with 0 and 1:	
$Y \vee 0 = Y$	$1 - [1 - Y][1 - 0] = Y$
$Y \vee 1 = 1$	$1 - [1 - Y][1 - 1] = 1$
$Y \wedge 0 = 0$	$Y \cdot 0 = 0$
$Y \wedge 1 = Y$	$Y \cdot 1 = 1$
De Morgan's laws:	
$\overline{Y_1 \vee Y_2} = \overline{Y_1} \wedge \overline{Y_2}$	$1 - \{1 - [1 - Y_1][1 - Y_2]\} = [1 - Y_1][1 - Y_2]$
$\overline{Y_1 \wedge Y_2} = \overline{Y_1} \vee \overline{Y_2}$	$1 - Y_1 Y_2 = 1 - [1 - (1 - Y_1)][1 - (1 - Y_2)]$
$Y_1 \vee Y_2 = \overline{\overline{Y_1} \wedge \overline{Y_2}}$	$1 - [1 - Y_1][1 - Y_2] = 1 - \{[1 - Y_1][1 - Y_2]\}$

A.3 A LEVEL 3 PRA—STATION BLACKOUT

A.3.1 Plant Description

The target plant is Unit 1 of the Surry Power Station, which has two units. The station blackout occurs if offsite power is lost (LOSP: loss of offsite power) and the emergency ac power system fails. A glossary of nuclear power plant technical terms is listed in Table A3.4. Important time data are summarized in Table A3.5. Features of Unit 1 relevant to the station blackout initiator are summarized below:

C1: Reactor and turbine trip. It is assumed that the reactor and main steam turbine are tripped correctly when the loss of offsite power occurs.

C2: Diesel generators. Three emergency diesel generators, DG1, DG2, and DG3, are available. DG1 supplies power only to Unit 1, DG2 supplies power only to Unit 2, and DG3 supplies power to either unit with the priority Unit 2 first, then Unit 1. Thus the availability of the diesel generators is as shown in Table A3.6, which shows that the emergency ac power system (EACPS) for Unit 1 fails if both DG1 and DG2 fail, or both DG1 and DG3 fail.

TABLE A3.4. Glossary for Nuclear Power Plant PRA

Abbreviation	Description
ac	Alternating current
AFWS	Auxiliary feedwater system
APET	Accident progression event tree
BWS	Backup water supply
CCI	Core-concrete interaction
CM	Core melt
CST	Condensate storage tank
DG	Diesel generator
EACPS	Emergency ac power system
ECCS	Emergency core-cooling system
FO	Failure of operator
FS	Failure to start
FTO	Failure to operate
HPIS	High-pressure injection system
HPME	High-pressure melt ejection
LOCA	Loss of coolant accident
LOSP	Loss of offsite power
NREC-AC-30	Failure to restore ac power in 30 min
OP	Offsite power
PORV	Pressure-operated relief valve
PWR	Pressurized water reactor
RCI	Reactor coolant integrity
RCP	Reactor coolant pump
RCS	Reactor coolant system
SBO	Station blackout
SG	Steam generator
SGI	Steam generator integrity
SRV	Safety-relief valve (secondary loop)
TAF	Top of active fuel
UTAF	Uncovering of top of active fuel
VB	Vessel breach

TABLE A3.5. Time Data for Station Blackout PRA

Event	Time Span	Condition
Condensate storage tank (CST) depletion	1 hr	SRV sticks open
Uncovering of top of active fuel	1 hr	1. Steam-driven AFWS failure 2. Motor-driven AFWS failure
Start of core-coolant injection	30 min	After ac power recovery

C3: Secondary loop pressure relief. In a station blackout (SBO), a certain amount of the steam generated in the steam generators (SGs) is used to drive a steam-driven AFWS pump (see description of C5). The initiating LOSP causes isolation valves to close to prevent the excess steam from flowing to the main condenser. Pressure relief from the secondary system takes place through one or more of the secondary loop safety-relief valves (SRVs).

C4: AFWS heat removal. All systems capable of injecting water into the reactor coolant system (RCS) depend on pumps driven by ac motors. Thus if decay heat cannot be

TABLE A3.6. Emergency Power Availability for Units 1 and 2

DG1	DG2	DG3	Unit 1 Power	Unit 2 Power
UP	UP	UP	OK	OK
UP	UP	DOWN	OK	OK
UP	DOWN	UP	OK	OK
UP	DOWN	DOWN	OK	NOT OK
DOWN	UP	UP	OK	OK
DOWN	UP	DOWN	NOT OK	OK
DOWN	DOWN	UP	NOT OK	OK
DOWN	DOWN	DOWN	NOT OK	NOT OK

removed from the RCS, the pressure and temperature of the water in the RCS will increase to the point where it flows out through the pressure-operated relief valves (PORVs), and there will be no way to replace this lost water. The decay heat removal after shutdown is accomplished in the secondary loop via steam generators, that is, heat exchangers. However, if the secondary loop safety-relief valves repeatedly open and close, and the water is lost from the loop, then the decay heat is removed by the AFWS, which injects water into the secondary loop to remove heat from the steam generators.

C5: AFWS trains. The AFWS consists of three trains, two of which have ac-motor-driven pumps, and one train that has a steam-turbine-driven pump. With the loss of ac power (SBO), the motor-driven trains will not work. The steam-driven train is available as long as steam is generated in the steam generators (SGs), and dc battery power is available for control purposes.

C6: Manual valve operation. If one or more of the secondary loop SRVs fails, water is lost from the secondary loop at a significant rate. The AFWS draws water from the 90,000-gallon condensate storage tank (CST). If the SRV sticks open, the AFWS draws from the CST at 1500 gpm to replace the water lost through the SRV, thus depleting the CST in one hour. A 300,000-gallon backup water supply (BWS) is available, but the AFWS cannot draw from this tank unless a valve is opened manually. If the secondary loop SRV correctly operates, then the water loss is not significant.

C7: Core uncovering. With the failure of the steam-driven AFWS, and no ac power to run the motor-driven trains, the RCS heats up until the pressure forces steam through the PORVs. Water loss through the PORVs continues, with the PORVs opening and closing, until enough water has been lost to reduce the liquid water level below the top of active fuel (TAF). The uncovering of the top of active fuel (UTAF) occurs approximately 60 min after the three AFWS train failures. The onset of core degradation follows shortly after the UTAF.

C8: AC power recovery. A 30-min time delay is assumed from the time that ac power is restored to the time that core-coolant injection can start. Thus, ac power must be recovered within 30 min after the start of an AFWS failure to prevent core uncovering. There are two recovery options from the loss of ac power. One is the restoration of offsite power, and the other is recovery of a failed diesel generator (DG).

A.3.2 Event Tree for Station Blackout

Figure A3.8 shows a portion of an event tree for initiating event SBO at Unit 1.

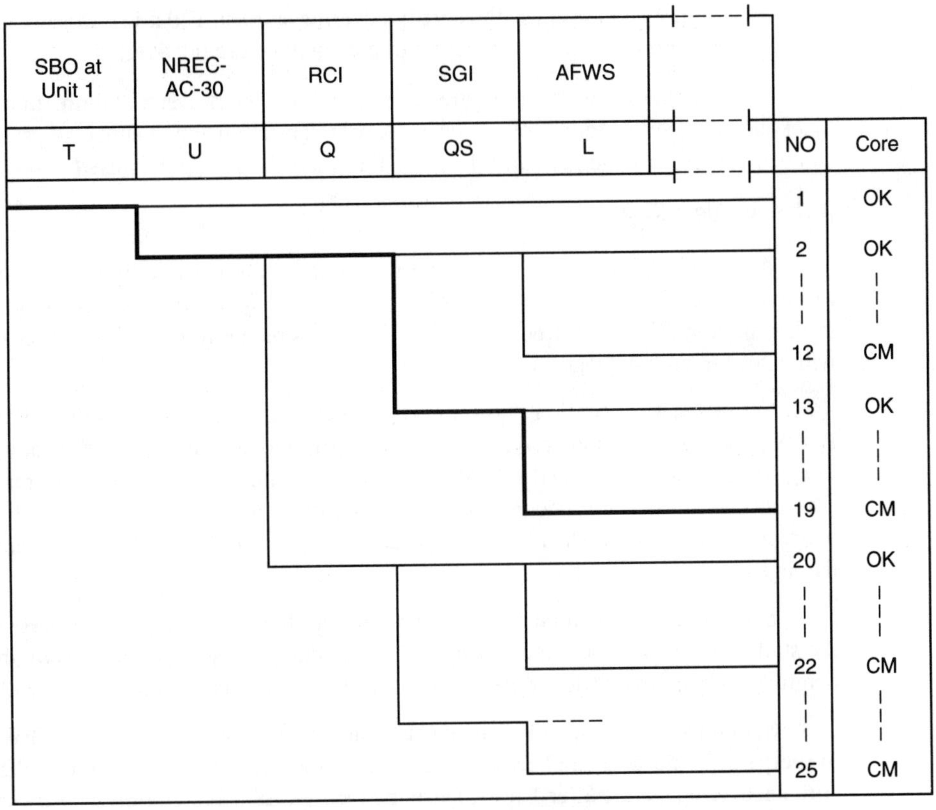

Figure A3.8. Station blackout event tree.

Event-tree headings. The event tree has the following headings and labels.

1. SBO at Unit 1 (T): This initiating event is defined by failure of offsite power, and failure of emergency diesel power supply to Unit 1.
2. NREC-AC-30 (U): This is a failure to recover ac power within 30 min, where symbols N, REC, and AC denote No, Recovery, and ac power, respectively.
3. RCI (Q): This is a failure of reactor-coolant integrity. The success of RCI means that the PORVs operate correctly and do not stick open.
4. SGI (QS): This denotes steam-generator integrity at the secondary loop side. If the secondary loop SRVs stick open, this failure occurs.
5. AFWS (L): This is an AFWS failure. Note that this failure can occur at different points in time. If the steam turbine pump fails to start, then the AFWS failure occurs at 0 min, that is, at the start of the initiating event. The description of C7 in Section A.3.1 indicates that the fuel uncovering occurs in approximately 60 min; C8 shows there is a 30-min time delay for re-establishing support systems; thus ac power must be recovered within 30 min after the start of the initiating event, which justifies the second heading NREC-AC-30. On the other hand, if the steam turbine pump starts correctly, the steam-driven AFWS runs until the CST is depleted in about 60 min under SRV failures. The AFWS fails at that time if the operators fail to switch the pump suction to the BWS. In this case, ac power must be recovered

within 90 min because the core uncovering starts in 120 min and there is a 30-min time delay for coolant injection to prevent the core uncovering.

Note that the event tree in Figure A3.8 includes support-system failure, that is, station blackout and recovery failure of ac power sources. The inclusion of support-system failures can be made more systematically if a large ET/small FT approach is used.

A.3.3 Accident Sequences

An accident sequence is an initiating event followed by failure of the systems to respond to the initiator. Sequences are defined by specifying what systems fail to respond to the initiator. The event tree of Figure A3.8 contains the following sequences, some of which lead to core damage.

Sequence 1. Station blackout occurs and there is a recovery within 30 min. The PORVs and SRVs operate correctly, hence reactor coolant integrity and steam generator integrity are both maintained. AFWS continuously removes heat from the reactor, thus core uncovering will not occur. One hour from the start of the accident, feed and bleed operations are re-established because the ac power is recovered within 30 min, thus core damage is avoided.

Sequence 2. Similar to sequence 1 except that ac power is recovered 1 hr from the start of accident. Core uncovering will not occur because heat removal by the AFWS continues. Core damage does not occur because feed and bleed operations start within 1.5 hr.

Sequence 12. Ac power is not re-established within 30 min. The AFWS fails at the very start of the accident because of a failure in the steam-turbine-driven AFWS train. A core uncovering occurs after 1 hr because the feed and bleed operation by primary coolant injection cannot be re-established within 1 hr.

Sequence 13. Ac power is not restored within 30 min. The reactor coolant integrity is maintained but steam generator integrity is not. However, AFWS continuously removes the decay heat, providing enough time to recover ac power. Core damage is avoided.

Sequence 19. Similar to sequence 12 except that AFWS fails after 1 hr because the operators did not open the manual valve to switch the AFWS suction to a BWS. This sequence contains an operator error. A core uncovering starts at 2 hr after the initiating event. Core damage occurs because feed and bleed operation cannot be re-established within 2 hr if the ac power is not re-established within 1.5 hr.

Sequence 20. Similar to sequence 13 except that RCI, instead of the SGI, fails. Core damage is avoided because the AFWS continuously removes heat, thus preventing the reactor coolant from overheating.

Sequence 22. Similar to sequence 19 except that RCI, instead of the SGI, fails. Failure of AFWS results in core damage if ac power is not re-established in time.

Sequence 25. This is a more severe accident sequence than 19 or 22 because the RCI and SGI both fail, in addition to the AFWS failure. Core damage occurs.

A.3.4 Fault Trees

In an accident-frequency analysis, fault trees, down to the hardware level of detail, are constructed for each event-tree heading. Failure rates for equipment such as pumps and valves are developed ideally from failure data specific to the plant being analyzed.

Initiating-event fault tree. Consider the event tree in Figure A3.8. The initiating event is a station blackout, which is a simultaneous failure of offsite ac power and emergency ac power. The unavailability of emergency ac power from DG1 is depicted by the fault tree shown in Figure A3.9. The emergency ac power system fails if DG1 and DG3 both fail, or if DG1 and DG2 both fail.

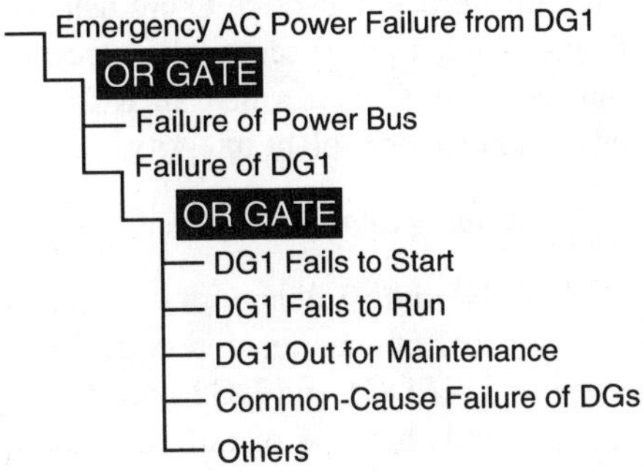

Figure A3.9. Fault tree for emergency power failure from diesel generator DG1.

AFWS-failure fault tree. A simplified fault tree for an AFWS failure is shown in Figure A3.10. Ac-motor-drive trains A and B have failed because of the SBO. Failure probabilities for these trains are unity ($P = 1$) in the fault tree.

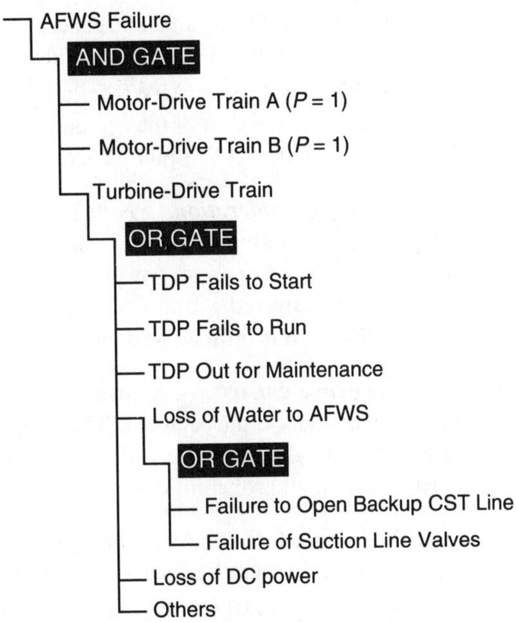

Figure A3.10. Fault tree for AFWS failure.

A.3.5 Accident-Sequence Cut Sets

Cut sets. Large event-tree and fault-tree models are analyzed by the computer programs that calculate accident-sequence cut sets, which are failure combinations that lead to the core damage. Each cut set consists of the initiating event and the specific hardware or operator failures that produce the accident. For example, in Figure 3.14 the water injection system fails because the pump fails to start or because the normally closed, motor-operated discharge valve fails to open.

Sequence expression. Consider accident sequence 19 in Figure A3.8. The logic expression for this sequence, according to the column headings, is

$$\text{Sequence } 19 = \text{T} \wedge \text{U} \wedge \overline{\text{Q}} \wedge \text{QS} \wedge \text{L}, \tag{A.53}$$

where $\overline{\text{Q}}$ indicates not-Q, or success and symbol $\wedge$ is a logic conjunction (a Boolean AND). System-success states like $\overline{\text{Q}}$ are usually omitted during quantification if the state results from a single event, because the success values are close to 1.0 in a well-designed system. Success state $\overline{\text{Q}}$ means that all RCS PORVs successfully operate during the SBO, thus ensuring reactor coolant integrity.

Heading analysis. Headings T, U, Q, QS, and L are now considered in more detail.

1. Heading T denotes a station blackout, which consists of offsite power failure and loss of emergency power. The emergency power fails if DG1 and DG3 both fail or if DG1 and DG2 both fail. The fault tree in Figure A3.9 indicates that DG1 fails because of failure to start, failure to run, out of service for maintenance, common-cause failure, or others. DG3 fails similarly.
2. Heading U is a failure to restore ac power within 30 min. This occurs when neither offsite nor emergency ac power is restored. Emergency ac power is restored when DG1 OR (DG2 AND DG3) are functional.
3. Heading Q is a reactor coolant integrity failure.
4. Heading QS is a steam generator integrity failure at the secondary side. This occurs if an SRV in the secondary system is stuck open.
5. Heading L is an AFWS failure. For accident sequence 19, this failure occurs 1 hr after the start of the accident when the operators fail to open a manual valve to switch the AFWS pump suction to backup condensate water storage tank, BWS.

Timing consideration. Note here that the AFWS time to failure is 1 hr for sequence 19. A core uncovering starts after 2 hr. Thirty minutes are required for re-establishing the support systems after an ac power recovery. Thus accident sequence 19 holds only if ac power is not recovered within 1.5 hr. This means that NREC-AC-30 should be rewritten as NREC-AC-90. It is difficult to do a PRA without making mistakes.

Sequence cut sets. A cut set for accident sequence 19 defines a combination of failures that leads to the accident. There are 216 of these cut sets. From the above section, "Heading Analysis," starting with T, a cut set C1 consisting of nine events is defined. The events—and their probabilities—are

1. LOSP (0.0994): An initiating-event element, that is, loss of offsite power, with an annual failure frequency of 0.0994.
2. FS-DG1 (0.0133): DG1 fails to start.
3. $\overline{\text{FTO-DG2}}$ (0.966): Success of DG2. Symbol FTO (fails to operate) includes a failure to start. The DG2 failure implies additional SBO for Unit 2, yielding a more serious situation.
4. FS-DG3 (0.0133): DG3 fails to start.
5. NREC-OP-90 (0.44): Failure to restore offsite electric power within 1.5 hr.
6. NREC-DG-90 (0.90): Failure to restore DG within 1.5 hr.
7. $\overline{\text{R-PORV}}$ (0.973): RCS PORVs successfully close during SBO.

8. R-SRV (0.0675): At least one SRV in the secondary loop fails to reclose after opening one or more times.
9. FO-AFW (0.0762): Failure of operator to open the manual valve in the AFWS pump suction to BWS.

Each fractional number in parentheses denotes an annual frequency or a probability. For this observation, the frequency of cut set C1 is 3.4×10^{-8}/year, the product of (1) to (9).

Cut set equation. There are 216 cut sets that produce accident sequence 19. The cut set equation for this sequence is

$$\text{Sequence 19} = C1 \vee \cdots \vee C216 \tag{A.54}$$

where symbol $\vee$ is a logic disjunction (a Boolean OR).

A.3.6 Accident-Sequence Quantification

Quantification of an accident sequence is achieved by quantifying the individual hardware or human failures that comprise the cut sets. This involves sampling from distribution of failure probability or frequency. Cut set C1 of accident sequence 19 of Figure A3.8 was quantified as follows.

1. Event LOSP (Loss of offsite power): This frequency distribution was modeled using historical data. Had historical data not been available, the entire offsite power system would have to be modeled first.
2. Event FS-DG1 (Failure of DG1): The distribution of this event probability was derived from the plant records of DG operation from 1980 to 1988. In this period, there were 484 attempts to start the DGs and 19 failures. Eight of these failures were ignored because they occurred during maintenance. The distribution of this probability was obtained by fitting the data to a log-normal distribution.*
3. Event $\overline{\text{FO-DG2}}$ (DG2 has started and is supplying power to Unit 2): The probability was sampled from a distribution.
4. Event FS-DG3 (Failure of DG3): The same distribution was used for both DG1 and DG3. Note that the sampling is fully correlated, that is, the same value (0.0133) is used for DG1 and DG3.
5. Event NREC-OP-90 (Failure to restore offsite electric power within 1.5 hr): A Bayesian model was developed for the time to recovery of the offsite power.† The probability used was sampled from a distribution derived from the model.
6. Event NREC-DG-90 (Failure to restore DG1 or DG3 to operation within 1.5 hr): The probability of this event was sampled from a distribution using the Accident-Sequence Evaluation Program (ASEP) database [25].
7. Event $\overline{\text{R-PORV}}$ (RCS PORVs successfully reclose during SBO): The probability was sampled from an ASEP distribution.
8. Event R-SRV (SRV in the secondary loop fails to reclose): The probability was sampled from an ASEP generic database distribution based on the number of times an SRV is expected to open.

---

*Log-normal distribution is discussed in Chapter 11.

†Bayesian models are described in Chapter 11.

9. FO-AFW (Failure of operator to open the manual valve from the AFWS pump suction to BWS): The probability was sampled from a distribution derived using a standard method for estimating human reliability. This event is a failure to successfully complete a step-by-step operation following well-designed emergency operating procedures under a moderate level of stress.*

A.3.7 Accident-Sequence Group

ASG. An accident-frequency analysis identifies significant accident sequences, which can be numerous. The accident-progression analysis, which is a complex and lengthy process, can be simplified if accident sequences that progress in a similar fashion are grouped together as ASGs. For example, sequences 12, 19, and 22 in Figure A3.8 can be grouped in the same ASG.

Cut sets and effects. A cut set consists of specific hardware faults and operator failures. Many cut sets on an accident sequence are essentially equivalent because the failure mode is irrelevant. Thus equivalent cut sets can be grouped together in an ASG. In theory, it is possible that the cut sets from a single accident sequence are separable into two (or more) different groups. However, this happens only rarely. Grouping into ASGs can usually be performed on an accident-sequence level.

For example, referring to Figure A3.9, it would make little difference whether there is no ac power because DG1 is out of service for maintenance or whether DG1 failed to start. The fault is different, and the possibilities for recovery may be different, but the result on a system level is the same. Exactly how DG1 failed must be known to determine the probability of failure and recovery, but it is less important in determining how the accident progresses after UTAF. Most hardware failures under an OR gate are equivalent in that they lead to the same top event.

A.3.8 Uncertainty Analysis

Because component-failure and human-error probabilities are sampled from distributions, the quantification process yields a distribution of occurrence probabilities for each accident sequence. Four measures are commonly used for the accident-sequence-probability distribution: mean, median, 5th percentile value, and 95th percentile value.

A.3.9 Accident-Progression Analysis

A.3.9.1 Accident-progression event tree. This analysis is based on an APET. Each event-tree heading on an APET corresponds to a question relating to an ASG. Branching operations are performed after each question. Branching ratios and parameter values are determined by expert panels or computer codes. Examples of parameters include containment pressure before vessel breach, containment pressure rise at vessel breach, and containment failure pressure. The following questions for sequence 19 or accident-sequence group ASG1 illustrate accident-progression analysis based on APET. Some questions are not listed for brevity. Each question is concerned with core recovery prior to vessel breach, in-vessel accident progression, ex-vessel accident progression, or containment building integrity.

1. **RCS integrity at UTAF?** Accident-sequence group ASG1 involves no RCS pressure boundary failure. A relevant branch, "PORVs do not stick open," is chosen.

---

*Human reliability analysis is described in Chapter 10.

2. **AC power status?** ASG1 indicates that ac power is available throughout the plant if offsite power is recovered after UTAF. Recovery of offsite power after the onset of core damage but before vessel failure is more likely than recovery of power from the diesel generators. Recovery of power would allow the high-pressure injection system (HPIS) and the containment sprays to operate and prevent vessel failure. One progression path thus assumes offsite ac power recovery before vessel failure; the other path does not.
3. **Heat removal from SGs?** The steam-turbine-driven AFWS must fail for accident-sequence group ASG1 to occur, but the electric-motor-driven AFWS is available when power is restored. A relevant branch is taken to reflect this availability.
4. **Cooling for RCP seals?** Accident-sequence group ASG1 implies no cooling water to the RCP seals, so there is a LOCA risk by seal failure unless ac power is available.
5. **Initial containment failure?** The containment is maintained below atmospheric pressure. Pre-existing leaks are negligible and the probability of a containment failure at the start of the accident is 0.0002. There are two possible branches. The more likely branch, no containment failure, is followed in this example.
6. **RCS pressure at UTAF?** The RCS must be at the setpoint pressure of the PORVs, about 2500 psi. The branch indicating a pressure of 2500 psi is followed.
7. **PORVs stick open?** These valves will need to operate at temperatures well in excess of design specifications in the event of an AFWS failure. They may fail. The PORVs reclose branch is taken.
8. **Temperature-induced RCP seal failure?** If a flow of relatively cool water through the seal is not available, the seal material eventually fails. In accident sequence 19, seal failure can only occur after UTAF, which starts at 2 hr. Whether the seals fail or not determines the RCS pressure when the vessel fails. The containment loads at VB (vessel breach) depend strongly on the RCS pressure at that time. There are two possibilities, and seal failure is chosen.
9. **Temperature-induced steam generator tube rupture?** If hot gases leaving the core region heat the steam generator tubes sufficiently, failure of the tubes occurs. The expert panel concluded that tube rupture is not possible because the failure of the RCP seals has reduced the RCS pressure below the setpoint of the PORVs.
10. **Temperature-induced hot leg failure?** There is no possibility of this failure because the RCS pressure is below the setpoint of the PORVs.
11. **AC power early?** The answer to this question determines whether offsite power is recovered in time to restore coolant injection to the core before vessel failure. A branch that proceeds to vessel breach is followed in this example.
12. **RCS pressure at VB?** It is equally likely that the RCS pressure at VB is in a high range, an intermediate range, or a low range. In this example, the intermediate range was selected.
13. **Containment pressure before VB?** The results of a detailed simulation indicated that the containment atmospheric pressure will be around 26 psi. Parameter P_1 is set at 26 psi.
14. **Water in reactor cavity at VB?** There is no electric power to operate the spray pumps in this blackout accident; the cavity is dry at VB in the path followed in this example.

15. **Alpha-mode failure?** This is a steam explosion (fuel-coolant interaction) in the vessel. The path selected for this example is "no alpha-mode failure."

16. **Type of vessel breach?** The possible failure modes are pressurized ejection, gravity pour, or gross bottom head failure. Pressurized ejection after vessel breach is selected.

17. **Size of hole in vessel?** The containment pressure rise depends on hole size. There are two possibilities: small hole and large hole. This example selects the large hole.

18. **Pressure rise at VB?** Pressure, $P_2 = 56.8$ psi, is selected.

19. **Ex-vessel steam explosion?** A significant steam explosion occurs when the hot core debris falls into water in the reactor cavity after vessel breach. In this example, the cavity is dry, so there is no steam explosion.

20. **Containment failure pressure?** This example selects a failure pressure of $P_3 =$ 163.1 psi.

21. **Containment failure?** From question 13, containment pressure before VB is $P_1 = 26$ psi. From question 18, pressure rise at VB is $P_2 = 56.8$ psi. Thus the load pressure, $P_1 + P_2 = 82.8$ psi, is less than the failure pressure $P_3 = 163.1$, so there is no containment failure at vessel breach.

22. **AC power late?** This question determines whether offsite power is recovered after vessel breach, and during the initial CCI (core-concrete interaction) period. The initial CCI period means that no appreciable amount of hydrogen has been generated by the CCI. This period is designated the "Late" period. Power recovery is selected.

23. **Late sprays?** Containment sprays now operate because the power has been restored.

24. **Late burn? Pressure rise?** The restoration of power means that ignition sources may be present. The sprays condense most of the steam in the containment and may convert the atmosphere from one that was inert because of the high steam concentration to one that is flammable. The pressure rise question asks "what is the total pressure that results from the ensuing deflagration?" For the current example, the total load pressure is $P_4 = 100.2$ psi.

25. **Containment failure and type of failure?** The failure pressure is $P_3 = 163.1$ psi. The load pressure is $P_4 = 100.2$ psi, so there is no late containment failure.

26. **Amount of core in CCI?** The path being followed has pressurized ejection at VB and a large fraction of the core ejected from the vessel. Pressurized ejection means that a substantial portion of the core material is widely distributed throughout the containment. For this case, it is estimated that between 30% and 70% of the core would participate in CCI.

27. **Does prompt CCI occur?** The reactor cavity is dry at VB because the sprays did not operate before VB, so CCI begins promptly. If the cavity is dry at VB, the debris will heat up and form a noncoolable configuration; even if water is provided at some later time, the debris will remain hot. Thus prompt CCI occurs.

28. **Very large ignition?** Because an ignition source has been present since the late burn, any hydrogen that accumulates after the burn will ignite whenever a flammable concentration is reached. Therefore, the ignition branch is not taken.

29. **Basemat melt-through?** It is judged that eventual penetration of the basemat by the CCI has only a 5% probability. However, the basemat melt-through branch is selected because the source-term analysis in Section A.3.9.3 and consequence analyses in Section A.3.9.4 are not of much interest if there is no failure of the containment.
30. **Final containment condition?** This summarizes the condition of the containment a day or more after the start of the accident. In the path followed through the APET, there were no aboveground failures, so basemat melt-through is selected.

A.3.9.2 Accident-progression groups. There are so many paths through the APET that they cannot all be considered individually in a source-term analysis. Therefore, these paths are condensed into APGs.

For accident sequence 19, 22 APGs having probabilities above 10^{-7} exist. For example, the alpha-mode steam explosion probability is so low that all the alpha-mode paths are truncated and there are no accident-progression groups with containment alpha-mode failures. The most probable group, with probability 0.55, has no VB and no containment failure. It results from offsite ac power recovery before the core degradation process had gone too far (see the second question in Section A.3.9.1).

An accident-progression group results from the path followed in the example in Section A.3.9.1. It is the most likely (0.017) group that has both VB and containment failures. Basemat melt-through occurs a day or more after the start of the accident. The group is characterized by:

1. containment failure in the final period
2. sprays only in the late and very late periods
3. prompt CCI, dry cavity
4. intermediate pressure in the RCS at VB
5. high-pressure melt ejection (HPME) occurred at VB
6. no steam-generator tube rupture
7. a large fraction of the core is available for CCI
8. a high fraction of the Zr is oxidized
9. high amount of core in HPME
10. basemat melt-through
11. one effective hole in the RCS after VB

A.3.9.3 Source-term analysis

Radionuclide classes. A nuclear power plant fuel meltdown can release 60 radionuclides. Some radionuclides behave similarly both chemically and physically, so they can be considered together in the consequence analysis. The 60 isotopes comprise nine radionuclide classes: inert gases, iodine, cesium, tellurium, strontium, ruthenium, lanthanum, cerium, and barium. There are two types of releases: an early release due to fission products that escape from the fuel while the core is still in the RCS, that is, before vessel breach; and a late release largely due to fission products that escape from the fuel after VB.

Early- and late-release fractions. The radionuclides in the reactor and their decay constant are known for each class at the start of the source-term analysis. For an accident-progression group, the source-term analysis yields the release fractions for each radionuclide class. These fractions are estimated for the early and late releases. Radionuclide inventory multiplied by an early-release fraction gives the amount released from the containment in the early period. A late release is calculated similarly.

Consider as an example the release fraction ST for an early release of iodine. This fraction consists of three subfractions and one factor that describes core, vessel, containment, and environment:

$$\text{ST} = [\text{FCOR} \times \text{FVES} \times \text{FCONV}/\text{DFE}] + \text{OTHERS} \tag{A.55}$$

where

1. FCOR: fraction of the core iodine released in the vessel before VB
2. FVES: fraction of the iodine released from the vessel
3. FCONV: fraction of the iodine released from the containment
4. DFE: decontamination factor (sprays, etc.)

These subfractions and the decontamination factor are established by an expert panel and reflect the results of computer codes that consider chemical and physical properties of fission products, and flow and temperature conditions in the reactor and the containment. For instance, sample data such as FCOR = 0.98, FVES = 0.86, FCONV = 10^{-6}, OTHERS = 0.0, and DFE = 34.0 result in ST = 2.5×10^{-8}. The release fraction ST is a very small fraction of the original iodine core inventory because, for this accident-progression group, the containment failure takes place many hours after VB and there is time for natural and engineered removal processes to operate.

Early- and late-release fractions are shown in Table A3.7 for a source-term group caused by an accident-progression group dominated by a late release.

TABLE A3.7. Early and Late Release Fractions for a Source Term

Fission Products	Early Release	Late Release	Total Release
Xe, Kr	0.0	1.0	1.0
I	0.0	4.4*E*-3	4.4*E*-3
Cs,Rb	0.0	8.6*E*-8	8.6*E*-8
Te, Sc, Sb	0.0	2.3*E*-7	2.3*E*-7
Ba	0.0	2.8*E*-7	2.8*E*-7
Sr	0.0	1.2*E*-9	1.2*E*-9
Ru, etc.	0.0	3.0*E*-8	3.0*E*-8
La, etc.	0.0	3.1*E*-8	3.1*E*-8
Ce, Np, Pu	0.0	2.0*E*-7	2.0*E*-7

Other characteristics of source terms. The source-term analysis calculates for early and late releases: start times, durations, height of release source, total energy. Each release involves nine isotope groups.

Partitioning into source-term groups. The accident-frequency analysis yields accident-sequence groups. Each accident-sequence group is associated with many accident-progression groups developed through APET. Each accident-progression group yields source terms. For instance, a NUREG-1150 study produced a total of 18,591 source terms from all progression groups. This is far too many, so a reduction step must be performed before a consequence analysis is feasible. This step is called a partitioning.

Source terms having similar adverse effects are grouped together. Two types of adverse effects are considered here: early fatality and chronic fatality. These adverse effects are caused by early and late fission product releases.

Early fatality weight. Each isotope class in a source term is converted into an equivalent amount of ^{131}I by considering the following factors for the early release and late release.

1. Isotope conversion factor
2. Inventory of the isotope class at the start of the accident
3. Release fraction
4. Decay constant for the isotope class
5. Start of release
6. Release duration

The early-fatality weight factor is proportional to the inventory and release fraction. Because a source term contains nine isotope classes, a total early fatality weight for the source term is determined as a sum of $9 \times 2 = 18$ weights for early and late releases.

Chronic fatality weight. This is calculated for each isotope class in a source term by considering the following.

1. Inventory of the isotope class at the start of the accident
2. Release fractions for early and late releases
3. Number of latent cancer fatalities due to early exposure from an isotope class, early exposure being defined as happening in the first seven days after the accident
4. Number of latent cancer fatalities due to late exposure from an isotope class, late exposure being defined as happening after the first seven days

Note that the early release, in theory, also contributes to the late exposure to a certain extent because of residual contamination.

The chronic-fatality weight factor is proportional to inventory, release fractions, and number of cancer fatalities. Each source term contains nine isotope classes, and thus has nine chronic fatality weights. A chronic fatality weight for the source terms is a sum of these nine weights.

Evacuation timing. Recall that each source term is associated with early release start time and late release start time. The early and late releases in a source term are classified into categories according to evacuation timings that depend on the start time of the release. (In reality everybody would run as fast and as soon as they could.)

1. Early evacuation: Evacuation can start at least 30 min before the release begins.
2. Synchronous evacuation: Evacuation starts between 30 min before and 1 hr after the release begins.
3. Late evacuation: Evacuation starts one or more hours after the release begins.

Stratified grouping. Each source term now has three attributes: early fatality weight, chronic fatality weight, and evacuation timing. The three-dimensional space is now divided into several regions. Source terms are grouped together if they are in the same region. A representative or mean source term for each group is identified. Table A3.8 shows a source-term group and evacuation characteristics.

TABLE A3.8. Source-Term Group with Early Evacuation Characteristics

Property	Minimum Value	Maximum Value	Frequency Weighted Mean
Release Height (m)	10	10	10
Warning Time (s)	2.2*E*+4	3.6*E*+4	2.5*E*+4
Start Early Release (s)	4.7*E*+4	5.1*E*+4	4.8*E*+4
Duration Early Release (s)	0.0	3.6*E*+3	3.3*E*+2
Energy Early Release (W)	0.0	7.0*E*+8	9.2*E*+5
ERF Xe, Kr	0.0	1.0*E*+0	1.4*E*-1
ERF I	0.0	1.5*E*-1	7.3*E*-3
ERF Cs, Rb	0.0	1.1*E*-1	5.4*E*-3
ERF Te, Sc, Sb	0.0	2.9*E*-2	1.2*E*-3
ERF Ba	0.0	1.4*E*-2	1.2*E*-4
ERF Sr	0.0	2.4*E*-3	2.3*E*-5
ERF Ru, etc.	0.0	1.1*E*-3	6.6*E*-6
ERF La, etc.	0.0	5.2*E*-3	2.8*E*-5
ERF Ce, Np, Pu	0.0	1.4*E*-2	1.4*E*-4
Start Late Release (s)	4.7*E*+4	1.3*E*+5	1.1*E*+5
Duration Late Release (s)	1.0*E*+1	2.2*E*+4	1.2*E*+4
Energy Late Release (W)	0.0	7.0*E*+8	9.2*E*+5
LRF Xe, Kr	0.0	1.0*E*+0	8.1*E*-1
LRF I	5.0*E*-6	1.3*E*-1	4.0*E*-2
LRF Cs, Rb	0.0	5.0*E*-2	3.9*E*-4
LRF Te, Sc, Sb	3.4*E*-11	9.6*E*-2	2.7*E*-4
LRF Ba	6.3*E*-14	1.7*E*-2	4.9*E*-5
LRF Sr	1.0*E*-18	1.4*E*-3	2.7*E*-6
LRF Ru, etc.	5.2*E*-18	1.6*E*-3	4.2*E*-6
LRF La, etc.	5.2*E*-18	1.7*E*-3	6.5*E*-6
LRF Ce, Np, Pu	1.6*E*-13	1.4*E*-2	4.2*E*-5

ERF: Early release fraction
LRF: Late release fraction

A.3.9.4 Consequence analysis. The inventory of fission products in the reactor at the time of the accident and the release fractions for each radionuclide class are used to calculate the amount released for each of the 60 isotopes. Then, for a large number of weather situations, the transport and dispersion of these radionuclides in the air downstream from the plant is calculated. The amount deposited on the ground is computed for each distance downwind. Doses are computed for a hypothetical human at each distance due to exposure to the contaminated air—from breathing the contaminated air, from the exposure due to radioactive material deposited on the ground, and from drinking water and eating food contaminated by radioactive particles.

For each of 16 wind directions, the consequence calculation is performed for about 130 different weather situations. The wind direction determines the population over which the plume from the accident passes. The atmospheric stability is also important because it determines the amount of dispersion in the plume downwind from the plant. Deposition is much more rapid when it is raining.

Table A3.9 shows a result of consequence analysis for a source-term group. These consequences assume that the source term has occurred. Different results are obtained for different weather assumptions. Figure 3.19 shows latent cancer fatality risk profiles. Each profile reflects uncertainty caused by weather conditions, given a source-term group; the 95%, 5%, mean, and median profiles represent uncertainty caused by variations of basic likelihoods.

TABLE A3.9. Result of Consequence Analysis for a Source-Term Group

Early Fatalities	0.0
Early Injuries	4.2*E*-6
Latent Cancer Fatalities	1.1*E*+2
Population Dose—50 mi	2.7*E*+5 person-rem
Population Dose—region	6.9*E*+5 person-rem
Economic Cost (dollars)	1.8*E*+8
Individual Early Fatality Risk—1 mi	0.0
Individual Latent Cancer Fatality Risk—10 mi	7.6*E*-5

A.3.10 Summary

A level 3 PRA for a station-blackout initiating event was developed. First, an event tree is constructed to enumerate potential accident sequences. Next, fault trees are constructed for the initiating event and mitigation system failures. Each sequence is characterized and quantified by accident sequence cut sets that include timing considerations. Accident-sequence groups are determined and an uncertainty analysis is performed for a level 1 PRA.

An accident-progression analysis is performed using an accident-progression event tree (APET), which is a question-answering technique to determine the accident-progression paths. The APET output is grouped in accident-progression groups and used as the input to a source-term analysis. This analysis considers early and late releases. The relatively small number of source-term groups relate to early fatality weight, chronic fatality weight, and evacuation timing. A consequence analysis is performed for each source-term group using different weather conditions. Risk profiles and their uncertainty are determined.

PROBLEMS

3.1. Give seven basic tasks for a reactor safety study (WASH-1400).

3.2. Give five tasks for WASH-1400 update, NUREG-1150. Identify three PRA levels.

3.3. Compare PRA applications to nuclear reactor, railway, oil tanker, and disease problems.

3.4. Enumerate seven major and three supporting activities for a level 1 PRA.

3.5. Briefly discuss benefits and detriments of PRA

3.6. Explain the following concepts: 1) hazardous energy sources, 2) hazardous process and events, 3) generic failure modes.

3.7. Give examples of guide words for HAZOPS.

3.8. Figure P3.8 is a diagram of a domestic hot-water system (Lambert, UCID-16328, May 1973). The gas valve is operated by the controller, which, in turn, is operated by the temperature measuring and comparing device. The gas valve operates the main burner in full-on/full-off modes. The check valve in the water inlet prevents reverse flow due to overpressure in the hot-water system, and the relief valve opens when the system pressure exceeds 100 psi.

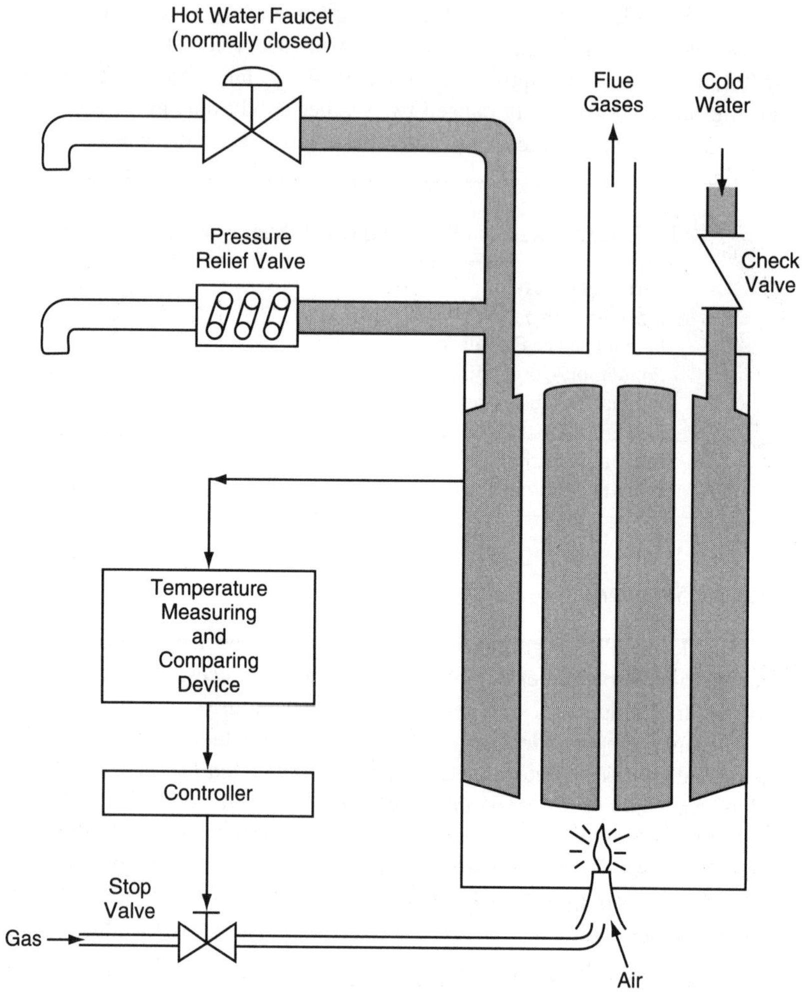

Figure P3.8. Schematic of domestic hot water system.

Control of the temperature is achieved by the controller opening and closing the main gas valve when the water temperature goes outside the preset limits (140°–180°F). The pilot light is always on.

(a) Formulate a list of undesired safety and reliability events.

(b) Do a preliminary hazard analysis on the system.

(c) Do a failure modes and effects analysis.

(d) Do a qualitative criticality ranking.

3.9. **(a)** Suppose we are presented with two indistinguishable urns. Urn 1 contains 30 red balls and 70 green ones, and Urn 2 contains 50 red balls and 50 green ones. One urn is selected at random and a ball withdrawn. What is the probability that the ball is red?

(b) Suppose the ball drawn was red. What is the probability of its being from Urn 1?

4

Fault-Tree Construction

4.1 INTRODUCTION

Accidents and losses. The primary goal of any reliability or safety analysis is to reduce the probability of accidents and the attending human, economic, and environmental losses. The human losses include death, injury, and sickness or disability and the economic losses include production or service shutdowns, off-specification products or services, loss of capital equipment, legal costs, and regulatory agency fines. Typical environmental losses are air and water pollution and other environmental degradations such as odor, vibration, and noise.

Basic failure events. Accidents occur when an initiating event is followed by safety-system failures. The three types of basic failure events most commonly encountered are (see Figure 2.8):

1. events related to human beings: operator error, design error, and maintenance error
2. events related to hardware: leakage of toxic fluid from a valve, loss of motor lubrication, and an incorrect sensor measurement
3. events related to the environment: earthquakes or ground subsidence; storm, flood, tornado, lightning; and outside ignition sources

Failure and propagation prevention. Accidents are frequently caused by a combination of failure events, that is, a hardware failure plus human error and/or environmental faults. Typical policies to minimize these accidents include

1. Equipment redundancies
2. Inspection and maintenance
3. Safety systems such as sprinklers, fire walls, and relief valves
4. Fail-safe and fail-soft design

Identification of causality. A primary PRA objective is to identify the causal relationships between human, hardware, and environmental events that result in accidents, and to find ways of ameliorating their impact by plant redesign and upgrades.

The causal relations can be developed by event and fault trees, which are analyzed both qualitatively and quantitatively. After the combination of the basic failure events that lead to accidents are identified, the plant can be improved and accidents reduced.

4.2 FAULT TREES

Fault-tree value. Fussell declares the value of a fault tree to be [1]:

1. directing the analysis to ferret out failures
2. pointing out the aspects of the system important to the system failure of interest
3. providing a graphic aid in giving visibility to those in systems management who are removed from plant design changes
4. providing options for qualitative and quantitative system-reliability analysis
5. allowing the analyst to concentrate on one particular system failure at a time
6. providing an insight into system behavior

To this, one might add that a fault tree, like any other engineering report, is a communication tool and, as such, must be a clear and demonstratable record.

Fault-tree structure. The tree structure is shown in Figure 4.1. An undesired system-failure event such as an initiating event or a safety-system failure appears as the top event, and this is linked to more basic failure events by event statements and logic gates. The central advantage of the fault tree vis-à-vis other techniques such as FMEA is that the analysis is restricted only to the identification of the system and component causes that lead to one particular top event.

Fault-tree construction. In large fault trees, mistakes are difficult to find, and the logic is difficult to follow or obscured. The construction of fault trees is perhaps as much of an art as a science. Fault-tree structures are not unique; no two analysts construct identical fault trees (although the trees should be equivalent in the sense that they yield the same cut set or combination of causes).

4.3 FAULT-TREE BUILDING BLOCKS

To find and visualize causal relations by fault trees, we require building blocks to classify and connect a large number of events. There are two types of building blocks: gate symbols and event symbols.

4.3.1 Gate Symbols

Gate symbols connect events according to their causal relations. The symbols for the gates are listed in Table 4.1. A gate may have one or more input events but only one output event.

AND and OR gates. The AND gate output event occurs if all input events occur simultaneously, and the OR gate output event happens if any one of the input events occurs.

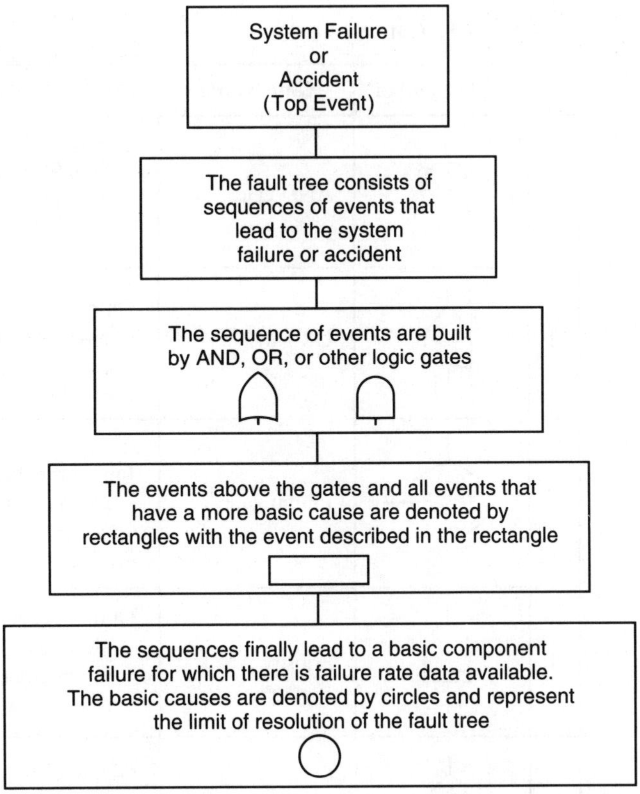

Figure 4.1. Fundamental fault-tree structure.

Examples of OR and AND gates are shown in Figure 4.2. The system event "fire breaks out" happens when two events, "leak of flammable fluid" and "ignition source is near the fluid," occur simultaneously. The latter event happens when either one of the two events, "spark exists" or "employee is smoking" occurs.* By showing these events as rectangles implies they are system states. If the event "flammable fluid leak," for example, were a basic cause it would be circled and become a basic hardware failure event.

The causal relation expressed by an AND gate or OR gate is deterministic because the occurrence of the output event is controlled by the input events. There are causal relations that are not deterministic. Consider the two events: "a person is struck by an automobile" and "a person dies." The causal relation here is probabilistic, not deterministic, because an accident does not always result in a death.

Inhibit gate. The hexagonal inhibit gate in row 3 of Table 4.1 is used to represent a probabilistic causal relation. The event at the bottom of the inhibit gate in Figure 4.3 is an input event, whereas the event to the side of the gate is a conditional event. The conditional event takes the form of an event conditioned by the input event. The output event occurs if both the input event and the conditional event occur. In other words, the input event causes the output event with the (usually constant, time-independent) probability of occurrence of the conditional event. In contrast to the probability of equipment failure, which is usually

*Events such as "spark exists" are frequently not shown because ignition sources are presumed to be always present.

TABLE 4.1. Gate Symbols

	Gate Symbol	Gate Name	Causal Relation
1		AND gate	Output event occurs if all input events occur simultaneously.
2		OR gate	Output event occurs if any one of the input events occurs.
3	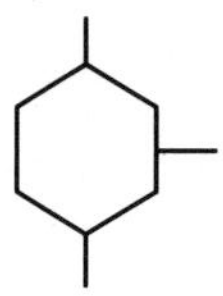	Inhibit gate	Input produces output when conditional event occurs.
4	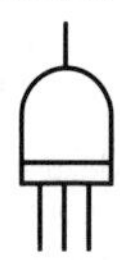	Priority AND gate	Output event occurs if all input events occur in the order from left to right.
5		Exclusive OR gate	Output event occurs if one, but not both, of the input events occur.
6	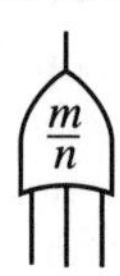 *n* inputs	*m*-out-of-*n* gate (voting or sample gate)	Output event occurs if *m*-out-of-*n* input events occur.

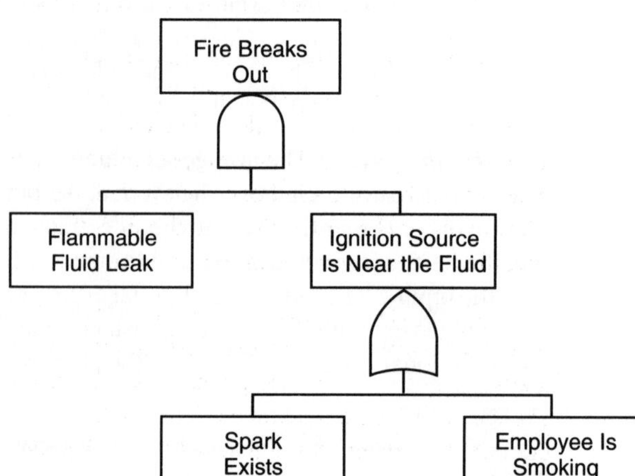

Figure 4.2. Example of AND gate and OR gate.

time dependent, the inhibit gate frequently appears when an event occurs with a probability according to a demand. It is used primarily for convenience and can be replaced by an AND gate, as shown in Figure 4.4.

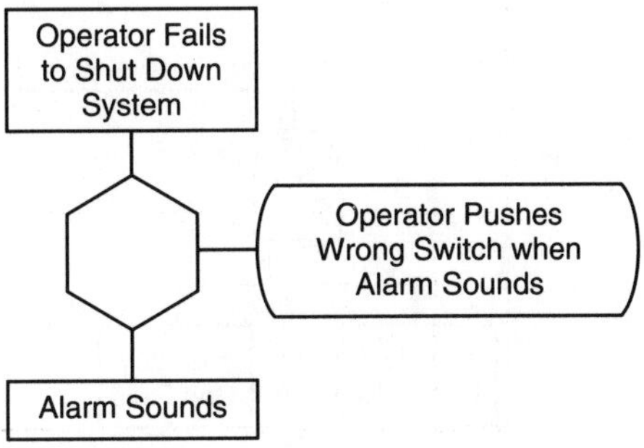

Figure 4.3. Example of inhibit gate.

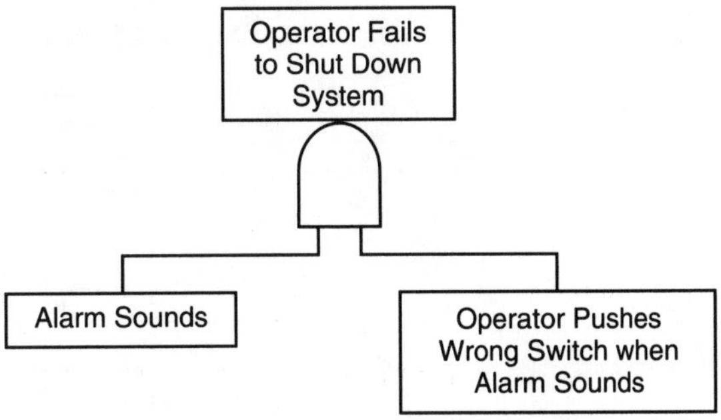

Figure 4.4. Expression equivalent to inhibit gate.

Priority AND gate. The priority AND gate in row 4 of Table 4.1 is logically equivalent to an AND gate, with the additional requirement that the input events occur in a specific order [2]. The output event occurs if the input events occur in the order that they appear from left to right. The occurrence of the input events in a different order does not cause the output event. Consider, for example, a system that has a principal power supply and a standby power supply. The standby power supply is switched into operation by an automatic switch when the principal power supply fails. Power is unavailable in the system if

1. the principal and standby units both fail, or
2. the switch controller fails first and then the principal unit fails

It is assumed that the failure of the switch controller after the failure of the principal unit does not yield a loss of power because the standby unit has been switched correctly when the principal unit failed. The causal relations in the system are shown in Figure 4.5. The priority AND gate can be represented by a combination of an AND gate and an inhibit gate, and it has already been shown that inhibit gates can be represented by AND gates. The conditional event to the inhibit gate is that the input events to the AND gate occur in the specified order. Representations equivalent to Figure 4.5 are shown in Figures 4.6 and 4.7.

Exclusive OR gate. Exclusive OR gates (Table 4.1, row 5) describe a situation where the output event occurs if either one, not both, of the two input events occur. Consider a system powered by two generators. A partial loss of power can be represented by the exclusive OR gate shown in Figure 4.8. The exclusive OR gate can be replaced by a combination of an AND gate and an OR gate, as illustrated in Figure 4.8. Usually, we avoid having success states such as "generator operating" appear in fault trees, because

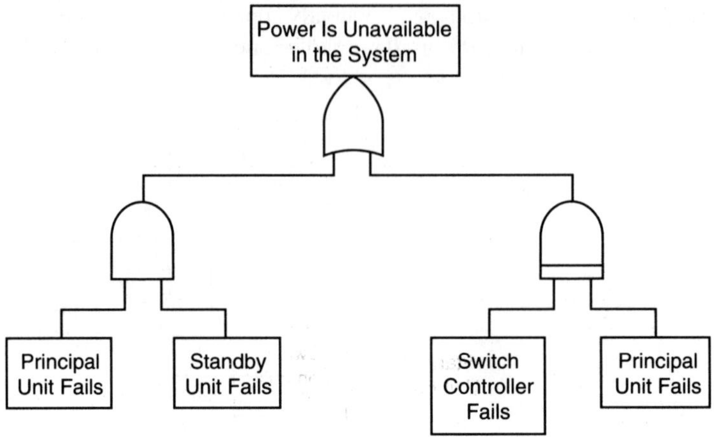

Figure 4.5. Example of priority AND gate.

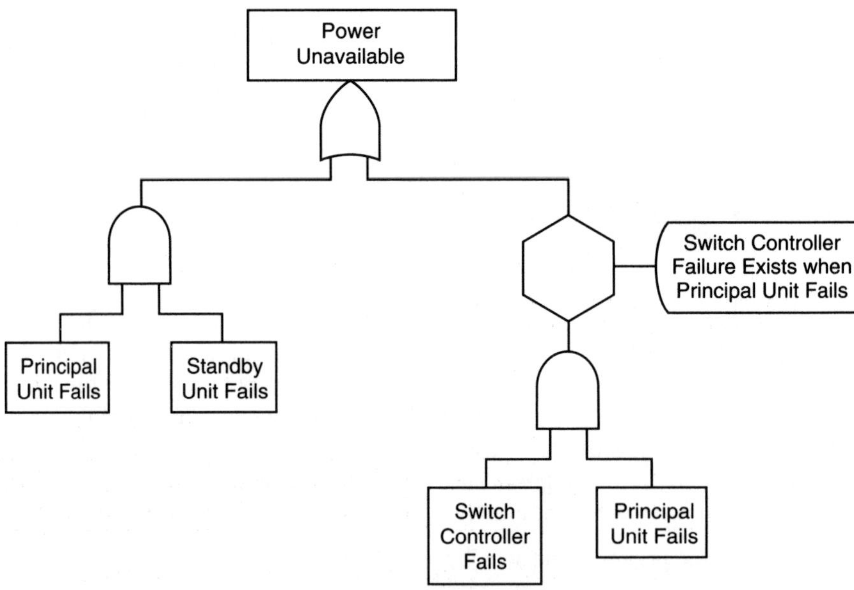

Figure 4.6. Expression equivalent to priority AND gate.

these greatly complicate the qualitative analysis. A prudent and conservative policy is to replace exclusive OR gates by OR gates.

Voting gate. An m-out-of-n voting gate (row 6, Table 4.1) has n input events, and the output event occurs if at least m-out-of-n input events occur. Consider a shutdown system consisting of three monitors. Assume that system shutdown occurs if and only if two or more monitors generate shutdown signals. Thus unnecessary shutdowns occur if two or more monitors create spurious signals while the system is in its normal state. This situation can be expressed by the two-out-of-three gate shown in Figure 4.9. The voting

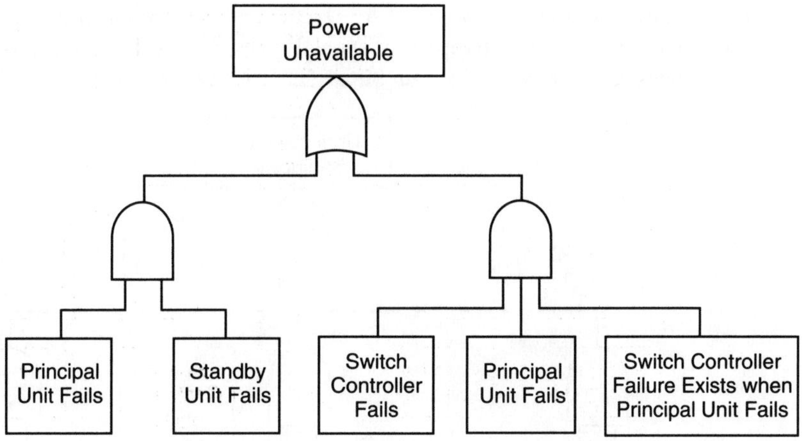

Figure 4.7. Equivalent expression to priority AND gate.

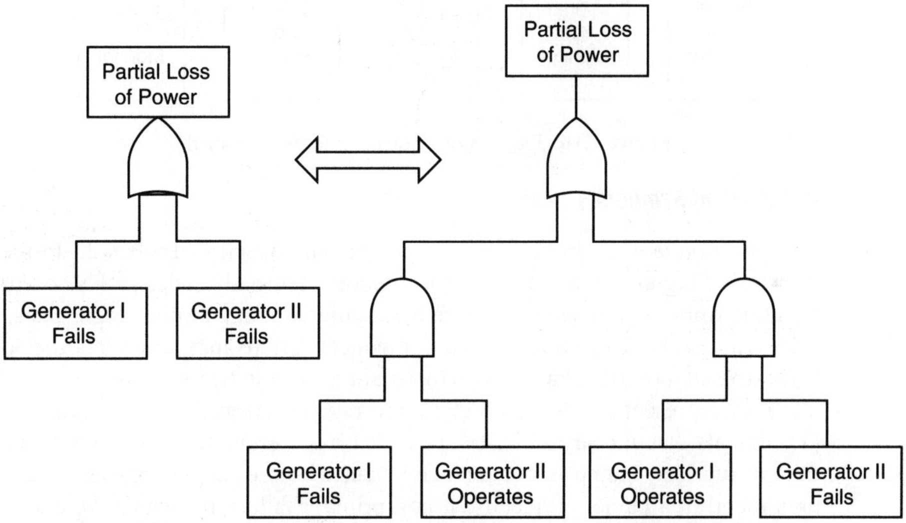

Figure 4.8. Example of exclusive OR gate and its equivalent expression.

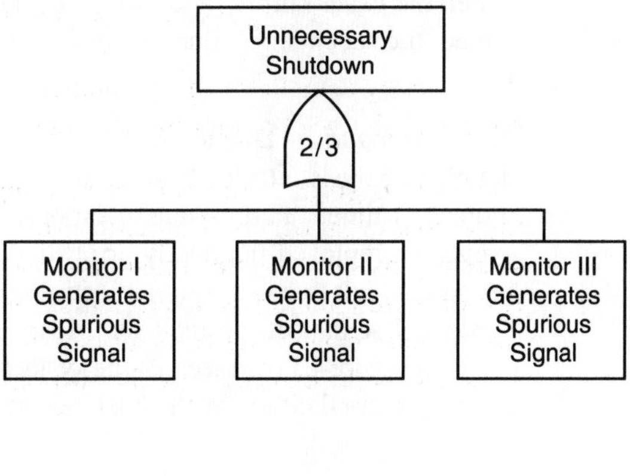

Figure 4.9. Example of two-out-of-three gate.

gate is equivalent to a combination of AND gates and OR gates as illustrated in Figure 4.10. New gates can be defined to represent special types of causal relations. We note that most special gates can be rewritten as combinations of AND and OR gates.

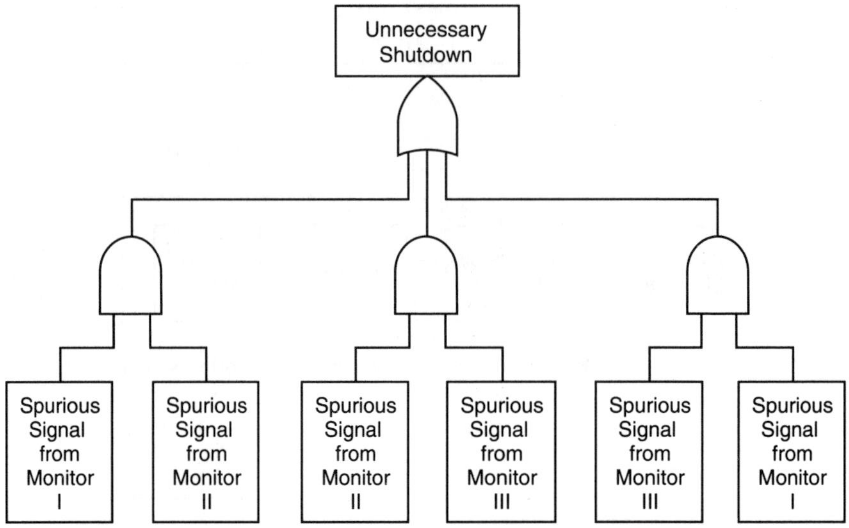

Figure 4.10. Expression equivalent to two-out-of-three voting gate.

4.3.2 Event Symbols

Rectangle and circle. Event symbols are shown in Table 4.2. In the schematic fault tree of Figure 4.1, a rectangular box denotes a (usually undesirable) system event state resulting from a combination of more basic failures acting through logic gates.

The circle designates a basic component failure that represents the lowest level, highest resolution of a fault tree. To obtain a quantitative solution for a fault tree, circles must represent events for which failure-rate (occurrence-likelihood) data are available [1]. Events that appear as circles are called basic events. "Pump fails to start," "pump fails to run," or "pump is out for maintenance" are examples of basic component failures found in a circle. Typically, it is a primary failure for which the component itself is responsible, and once it occurs the component must be repaired, replaced, recovered, or restored. See Section 2.2.3.1 for basic, primary, and secondary events or failures. When the exact failure mode for a secondary failure is identified and failure data are obtained, the secondary failure becomes a basic event and can be shown as circles in a fault tree.

Diamond. Diamonds are used to signify undeveloped events, in the sense that a detailed analysis into the basic failures is not carried out because of lack of information, money, or time. "Failure due to sabotage" is an example of an undeveloped event. Such events are removed frequently prior to a quantitative analysis. They are included initially because a fault tree is a communication tool, and their presence serves as a reminder of the depth and bounds of the analysis. Most secondary failures are diamond events.

In Figure 4.11 we see that the system failure, "excessive current in circuit," is analyzed as being caused either by the basic event, "shorted wire," or the undeveloped event, "line

TABLE 4.2. Event Symbols

	Event Symbol	Meaning of Symbol
1	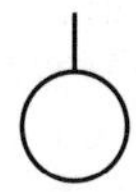 Circle	Basic component failure event with sufficient data
2	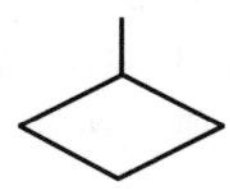 Diamond	Undeveloped event
3	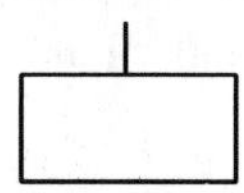 Rectangle	State of system or component event
4	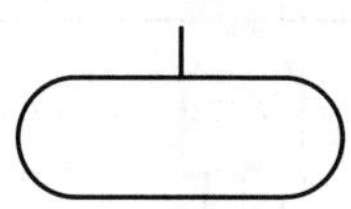 Oval	Conditional event with inhibit gate
5	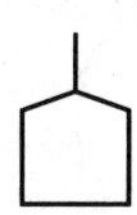 House	House event. Either occurring or not occurring
6	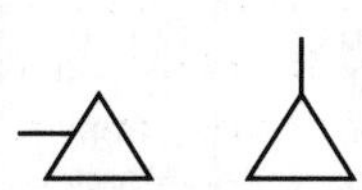 Triangles	Transfer symbol

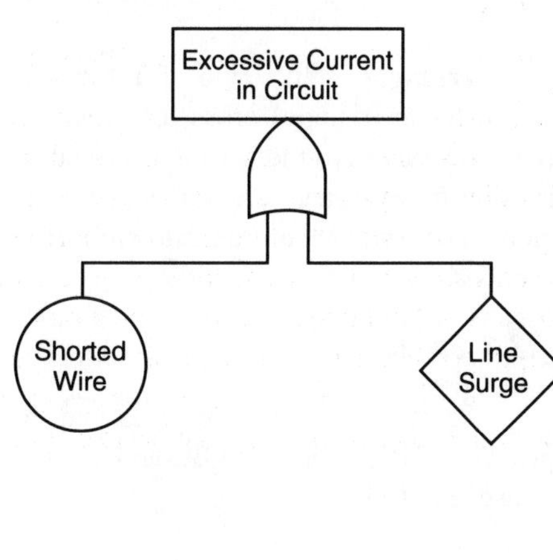

Figure 4.11. Example of event in diamond.

surge." Had we chosen to develop the event "line surge" more fully, a rectangle would have been used to show that this is developed to more basic events, and then the analysis would have to be carried further back, perhaps to a generator or another in-line hardware component.

House. Sometimes we wish to examine various special fault-tree cases by forcing some events to occur and other events not to occur. For this purpose, we could use the house event (row 5, Table 4.2). When we turn on the house event, the fault tree presumes the occurrence of the event and vice versa when we turn it off.

We can also delete causal relations below an AND gate by turning off a dummy house event introduced as an input to the gate; the output event from the AND gate can then never happen. Similarly, we can assume relations below an OR gate by turning on a house event to the gate.

The house event is illustrated in Figure 4.12. When we turn on the house event, monitor I is assumed to be generating a spurious signal. Thus we have a one-out-of-two gate, that is, a simple OR gate with two inputs, II and III. If we turn off the house event, a simple AND gate results.

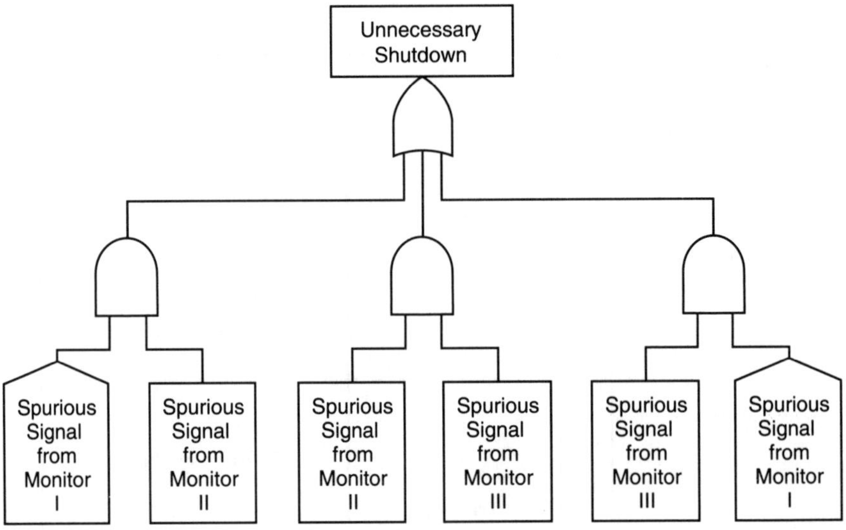

Figure 4.12. Example of house event.

Triangle. In row 6 of Table 4.2 the pair of triangles (a transfer-out triangle and a transfer-in triangle) cross references two identical parts of the causal relations. The two triangles have the same identification number. The transfer-out triangle has a line to its side from a gate, whereas the transfer-in triangle has a line from its apex to another gate. The triangles are used to simplify the representation of fault trees, as illustrated in Figure 4.13.

4.3.3 Summary

Fault trees consist of gates and events. Gate symbols include AND, OR, inhibit, priority AND, exclusive OR, and voting. Event symbols are rectangle, circle, diamond, house, and triangle.

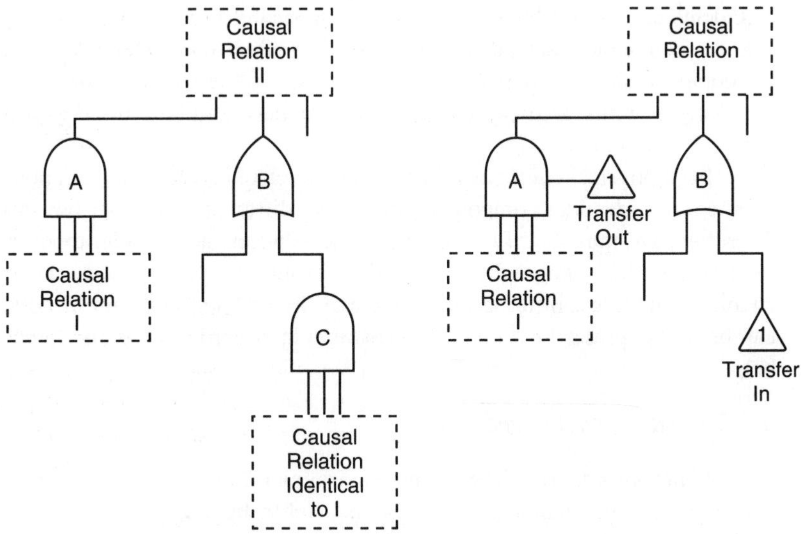

Figure 4.13. Use of transfer symbol.

4.4 FINDING TOP EVENTS

4.4.1 Forward and Backward Approaches

There are two approaches for analyzing causal relations. One is forward analysis, the other is backward analysis. A forward analysis starts with a set of failure events and proceeds forward, seeking possible effects resulting from the events. A backward analysis begins with a particular event and traces backward, searching for possible causes of the event. As was discussed in Chapter 3, the cooperative use of these two approaches is necessary to attain completeness in finding causal relations including enumeration of initiating events.

Backward approach. The backward analysis—that is, the fault-tree analysis—is used to identify the causal relations leading to events such as those described by event-tree headings. A particular top event may be only one of many possible events of interest; the fault-tree analysis itself does not identify possible top events in the plant. Large plants have many different top events, and thus fault trees.

Forward approach. Event tree, failure mode and effects analysis, criticality analysis, and preliminary hazards analysis use the forward approach (see Chapter 3). Guide words for HAZOPS are very helpful in a forward analysis.

The forward analysis, typically event-tree analysis (ETA), assumes sequences of events and writes a number of scenarios ending in plant accidents. Relevant FTA top events may be found by event-tree analysis. The information used to write good scenarios is component interrelations and system topography, plus accurate system specifications. These are also used for fault-tree construction.

4.4.2 Component Interrelations and System Topography

A plant consists of hardware, materials, and plant personnel, is surrounded by its physical and social environment, and suffers from aging (wearout or random failure).

Accidents are caused by one or a set of physical components generating failure events. The environment, plant personnel, and aging affect the system only through the physical components. Components are not necessarily the smallest constituents of the plant; they may be units or subsystems; a plant operator can be viewed as a physical component.

Each physical component in a system is related to the other components in a specific manner, and identical components may have different characteristics in different plants. Therefore, we must clarify component interrelations and system topography. The interrelations and the topography are found by examining plant piping, electrical wiring, mechanical couplings, information flows, and the physical location of components. These can be best expressed by a plant schematic; plant word models and logic flow charts also help.

4.4.3 Plant Boundary Conditions

Plant boundary. The system environment, in principle, includes the entire world outside the plant, so an appropriate boundary for the environment is necessary to prevent the initiating-event and event-tree analyses from diverging. Only major, highly probable, or critical events should be considered in the initial steps of the analysis. FMECA can be used to identify these events. We can include increasingly less probable or less serious events as the analysis proceeds, or choose to ignore them.

Initial conditions. System specification requires a careful delineation of component initial conditions. All components that have more than one operating state generate initial conditions. For example, if the initial quantity of fluid in a tank is unspecified, the event "tank is full" is one initial condition, while "tank is empty" is another. For the railway in Figure 3.1, the position of train B is an initial condition for the initiating event, "train A unscheduled departure." The time domain must also be specified; start-up or shutdown conditions, for example, can generate different accidents than a steady-state operation.

When enough information on the plant has been collected, we can write event-tree scenarios and define fault-tree top events. Causal relations leading to each top event are then found by fault-tree analysis. Combinations of failures (cut sets) leading to an accident sequence are determined from these causal relations.

4.4.4 Example of Preliminary Forward Analysis

System schematic. Consider the pumping system in Figure 4.14 [3,4]. This schematic gives the component relationships described by the following model:

Word model. In the start-up mode, to start the pumping, reset switch S1 is closed and then immediately opened. This allows current to flow in the control branch circuit, activating relay coils K1 and K2; relay K1 contacts are closed and latched, while K2 contacts close and start the pump motor.

In the shutdown mode, after approximately 20 s, the pressure switch contacts should open (since excess pressure should be detected by the pressure switch), deactivating the control circuit, de-energizing the K2 coil, opening the K2 contacts, and thereby shutting the motor off. If there is a pressure switch hang-up (emergency shutdown mode), the timer

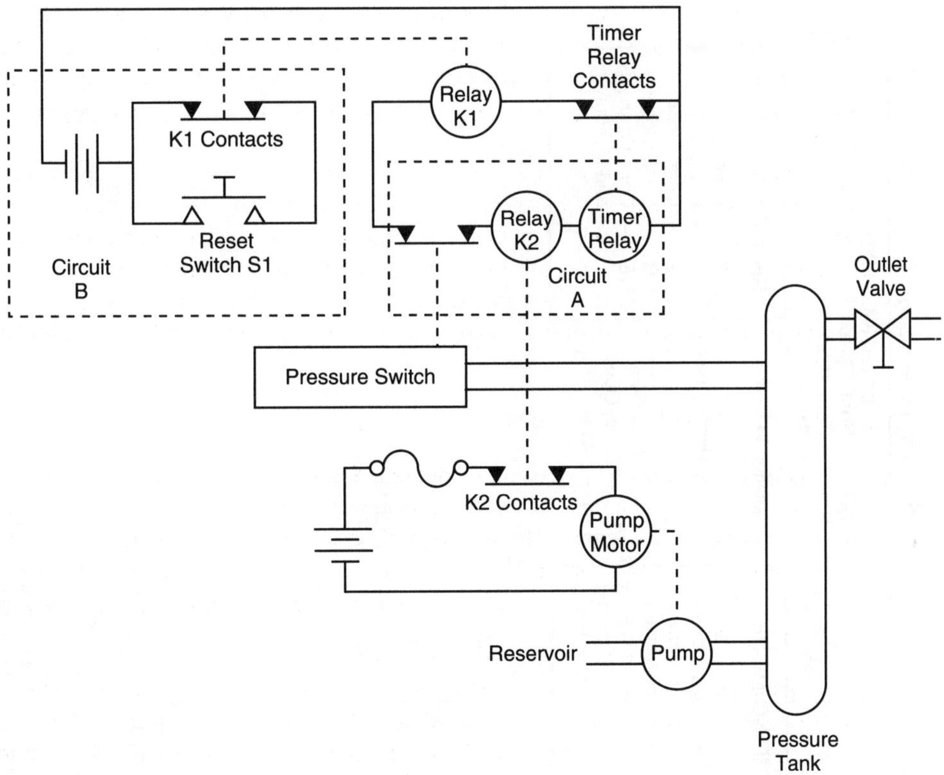

Figure 4.14. System schematic for a pumping system.

relay contacts should open after 60 s, de-energizing the K1 coil, which in turn de-energizes the K2 coil, shutting off the pump. We assume that the timer resets itself automatically after each trial, that the pump operates as specified, and that the tank is emptied of fluid after every run.

Sequence flow chart. We can also introduce the Figure 4.15 flow chart, showing the sequential functioning of each component in the system with respect to each operational mode.

Preliminary forward analysis. Forward analyses such as PHA and FMEA are carried out, and we detect sequences of component-failure events leading to the accidents. For the pumping system of Figure 4.14:

1. Pressure switch fails to open → timer fails to time-out → overpressure → rupture of tank
2. Reset switch fails to open → pressure switch fails to open → overpressure → rupture of tank
3. Reset switch fails to close → pump does not start → fluid from the tank becomes unavailable
4. Leak of flammable fluid from tank → relay sparks → fire

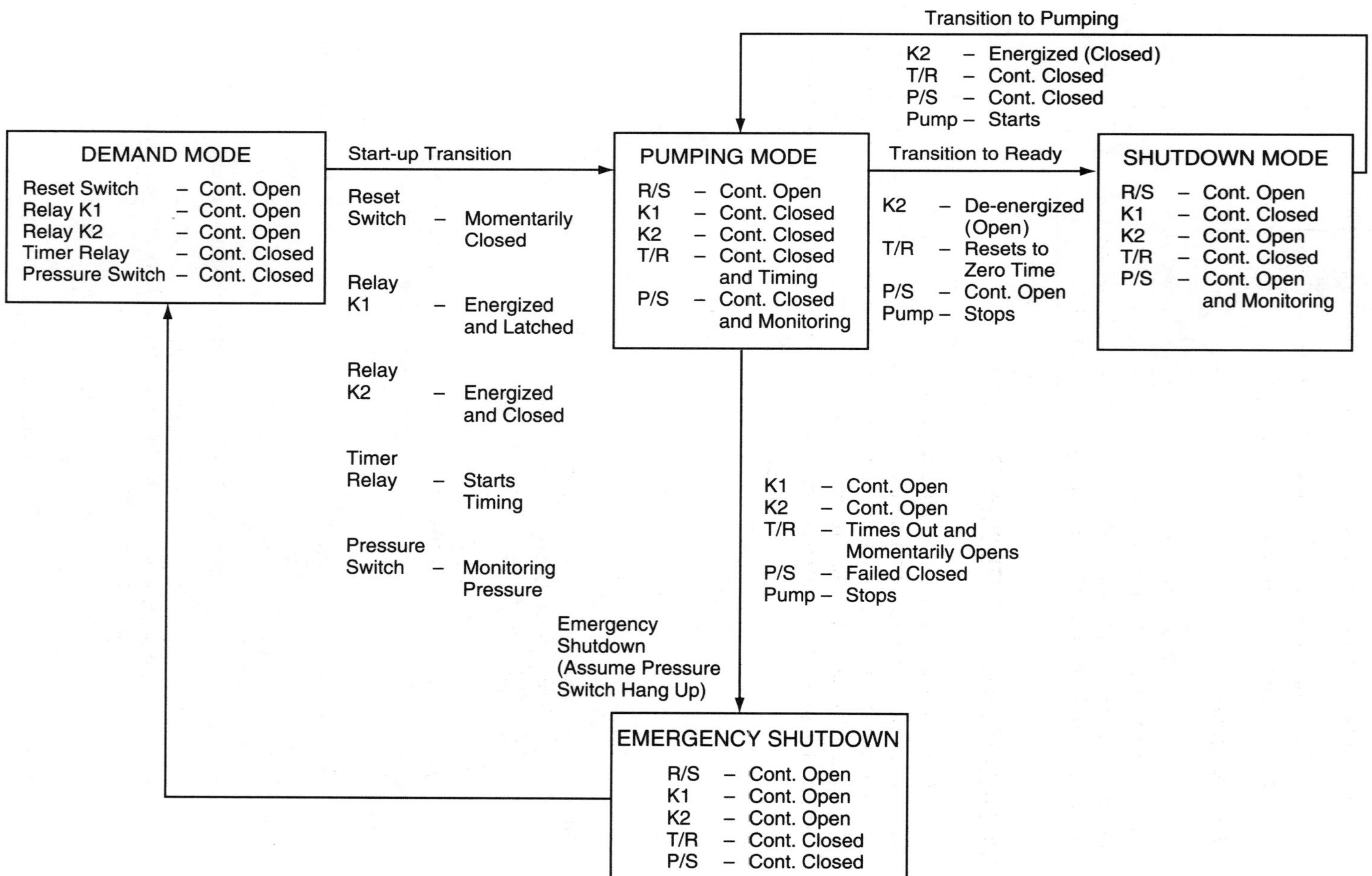

Figure 4.15. Pumping system flow chart.

By an appropriate choice of the environmental boundary, these system hazards can be traced forward in the system and into its environment. Examples are

1. Tank rupture: loss of capital equipment, death, injury, and loss of production
2. No fluid in tank: production loss, runaway reaction, and so on

4.4.5 Summary

A forward analysis typified by ETA is used to define top events for the backward analysis, FTA. Prior to the forward and backward analysis, component interrelations, system topography, and boundary conditions must be established. An example of a preliminary forward analysis for a simple pumping system is provided.

4.5 PROCEDURE FOR FAULT-TREE CONSTRUCTION

Primary, secondary, and command failure. Component failures are key elements in causal relation analyses. They are classified as either primary failures, secondary failures, or command failures (see Chapter 2). The first concentric circle about "component failure" in Figure 4.16 shows that failure can result from primary failure, secondary failure, or command failures. These categories have the possible causes shown in the outermost circle.

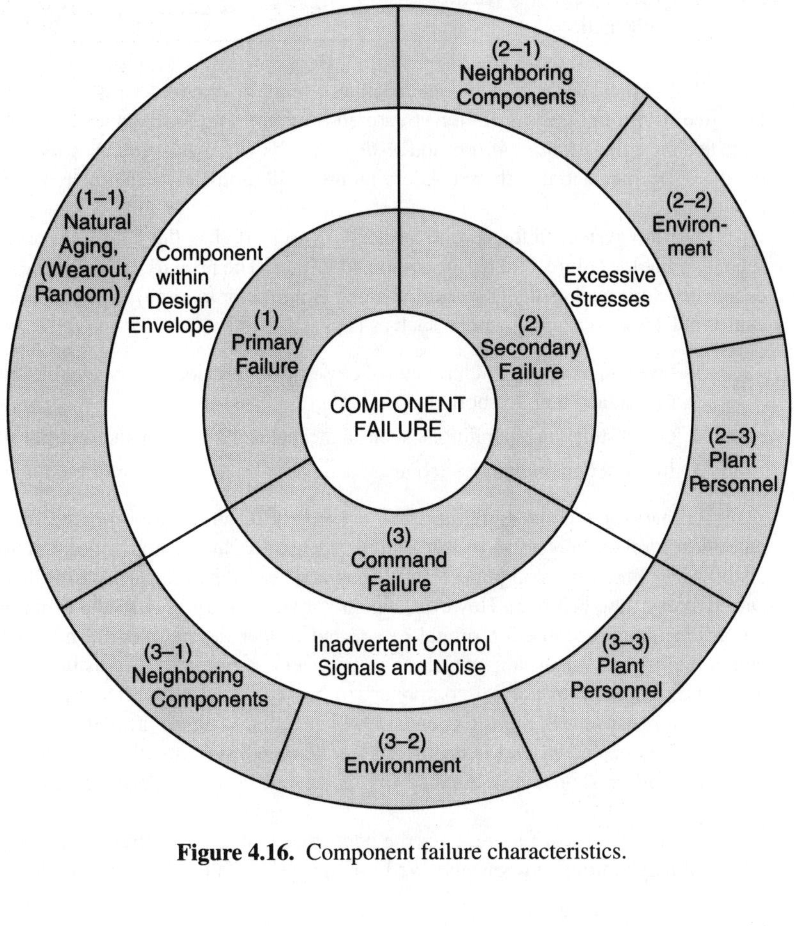

Figure 4.16. Component failure characteristics.

4.5.1 Fault-Tree Example

Structured-programming format. A fault tree is a graphic representation of causal relations obtained when a top event is traced backward to search for its possible causes. This representation can also be expressed as a structured programming format. This format is used in this book because it is more compact and modular, the first example being the format in Figure 1.27.

Example 1—Simple circuit with fuse. As an example of fault-tree construction, consider the top event, "motor fails to start," for the system of Figure 4.17. A clear definition of the top event is necessary even if the event is expressed in abbreviated form in the fault tree. In the present case, the complete top event is "motor fails to start when switch is closed at time t." Variable t can be expressed in terms other than time; for example, transport reliability information is usually expressed in terms of mileage. The variable sometimes means cycles of operation.

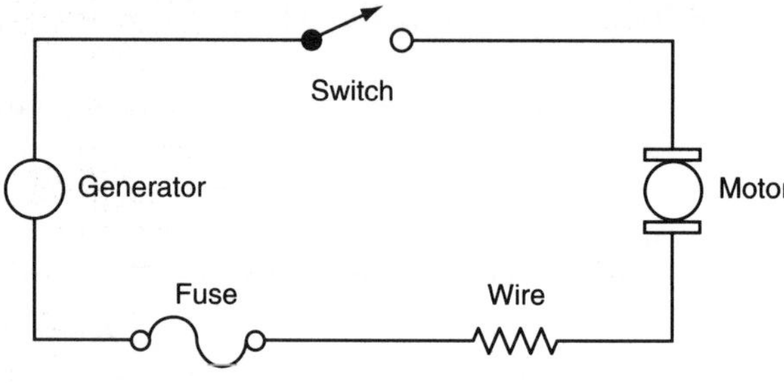

Figure 4.17. Electric circuit system schematic.

The classification of component-failure events in Figure 4.16 is useful for constructing the fault tree shown in Figure 4.18 in a structured-programming format and an ordinary representation. Note that the terms *primary failure* and *basic failure* become synonymous when the failure mode (and data) are specified and that the secondary failures will ultimately either be removed or become basic events.

The top system-failure event "motor fails to start" has three causes: primary motor failure, secondary motor failure, and motor command failure. The primary failure is the motor failure in the design envelope and results from natural aging (wearout or random). The secondary failure is due to causes outside the design envelope such as [1]:

1. Overrun, that is, switch remained closed from previous operation, causing motor windings to heat and then to short or open circuit.
2. Out-of-tolerance conditions such as mechanical vibration and thermal stress.
3. Improper maintenance such as inadequate lubrication of motor bearings.

Primary or secondary failures are caused by disturbances from the sources shown in the outermost circle of Figure 4.16. A component can be in the nonworking state at time t if past disturbances broke the component and it has not been repaired. The disturbance could have occurred at any time before t. However, we do not go back in time, so the primary or the secondary failures at time t become a terminal event, and further development is not carried out. In other words, fault trees are instant snapshots of a system at time t. The disturbances are factors controlling transition from normal component to broken component. The primary event is enclosed by a circle because it is a basic event for which failure data are available. The secondary failure is an undeveloped event and is enclosed by a diamond. Quantitative failure characteristics of the secondary failure should be estimated by appropriate methods, in which case it becomes a basic event.

As was shown in Figure 4.16, the command failure "no current to motor" is created by the failure of neighboring components. We have the system-failure event "wire does not carry current"

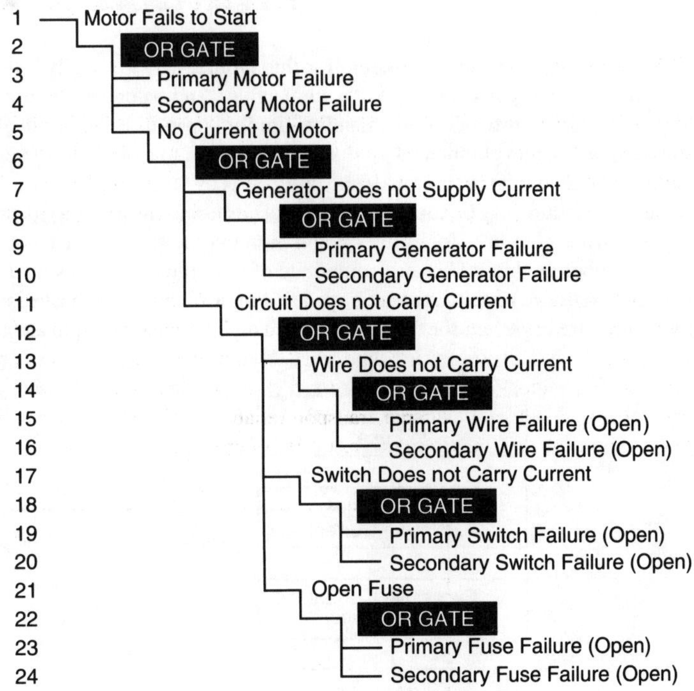

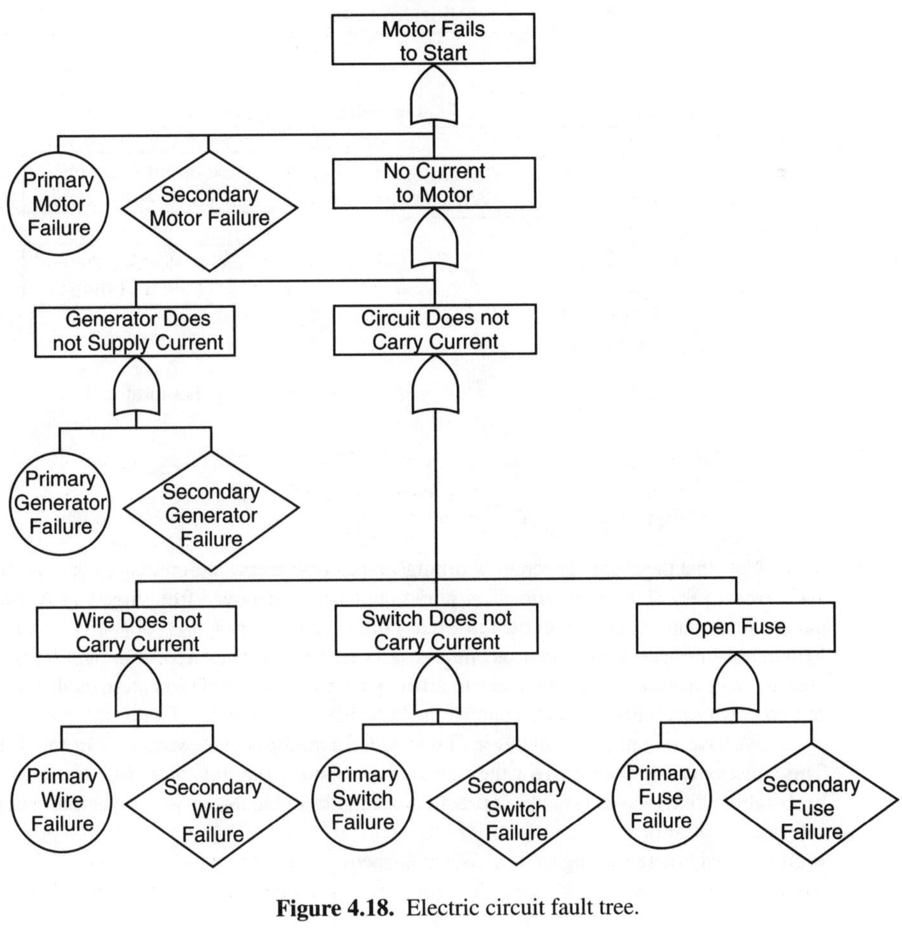

Figure 4.18. Electric circuit fault tree.

in Figure 4.18. A similar development is possible for this failure, and we finally reach the event "open fuse." We have the primary fuse failure by "natural aging," and secondary failure possibly by "excessive current." We might introduce a command failure for "open fuse" as in category (3-1) of Figure 4.16. However, there is no component commanding the fuse to open. Thus, we can neglect this command failure, and the fault tree is complete.

The secondary fuse failure may be caused by present or past excessive current from neighboring components. Any excessive current before time t could burn out the fuse. We cannot develop the event "excessive current before time t" because an infinite of past times are involved. However, we can develop the event "excessive current exists at a specified time t^*" by the fault tree in Figure 4.19 where secondary failures are neglected for convenience, and an inhibit gate is equivalent to an AND gate.

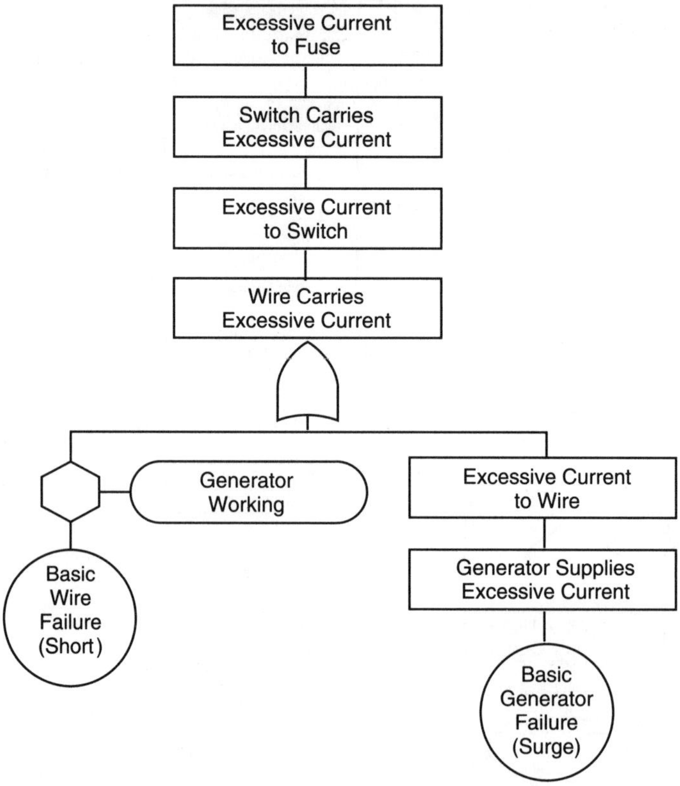

Figure 4.19. Fault tree with the top event "excessive current to fuse."

Note that the event "generator working" exists with a very high probability, say 0.999. We call such events *very high probability events*, and they can be removed from inputs to AND (or inhibit) gates without major changes in the top-event probabilities. Very high probability events are typified by component success states that, as emphasized earlier, should not appear in fault trees. Failure rate data are not generally accurate enough to justify such subtleties. Simplification methods for very high or very low probability events are shown in Table 4.3.

We have a simplified fault tree in Figure 4.20 for the top event "excessive current" in Figure 4.19. This fault tree can be quantified (by the methods described in a later chapter) to determine an occurrence probability of excessive current as a function of time from the last inspection and maintenance. This information, in turn, is used to quantify the secondary fuse failure and finally, the probability of the occurrence of "motor failing to start" is established. ■

TABLE 4.3. Simplifications for Very High or Very Low Probability Events

<table>
<tr><th></th><th>Original Causal Relation</th><th>Simplified Causal Relation</th></tr>
<tr><td>Simplification by very high probability event (AND gate with two inputs)</td><td>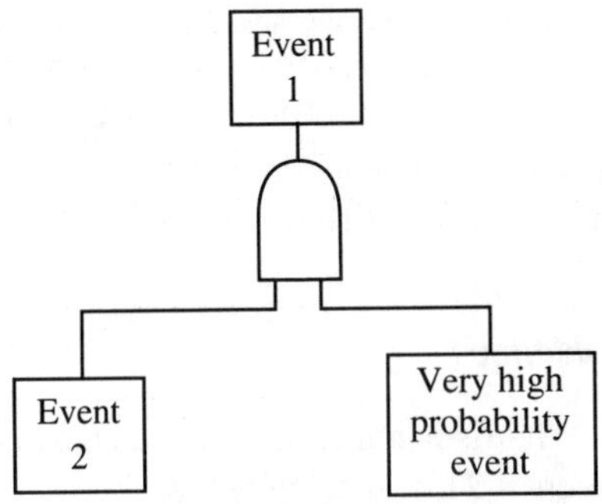
</td><td>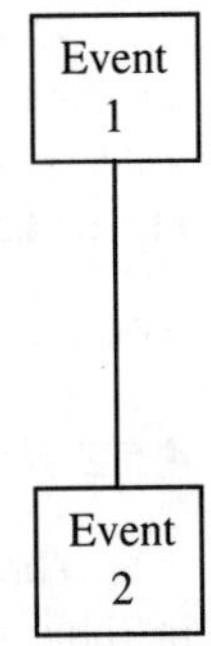
</td></tr>
<tr><td>Simplification by very high probability event (AND gate with three or more inputs)</td><td>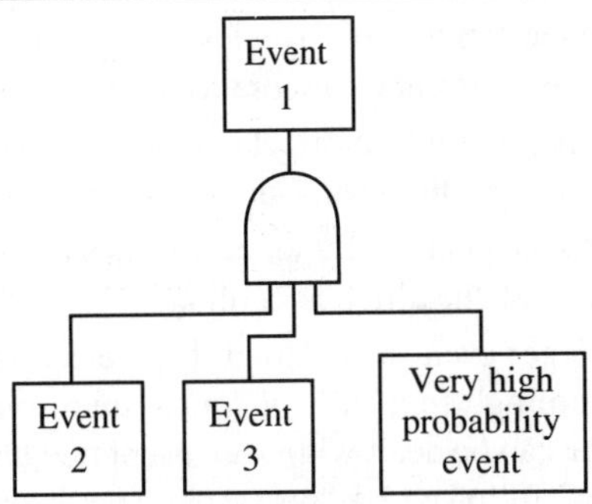
</td><td>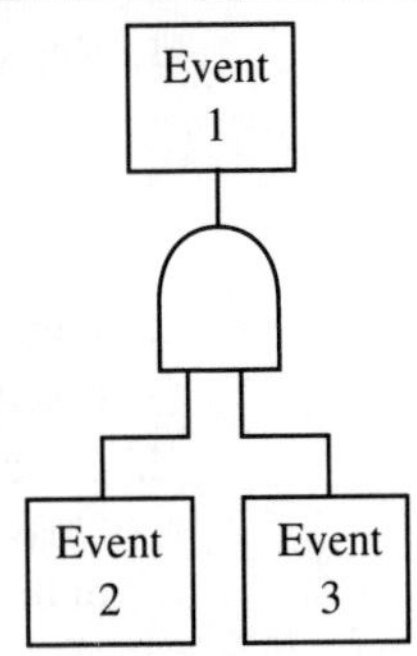
</td></tr>
<tr><td>Simplification by very low probability event (OR gate with two inputs)</td><td>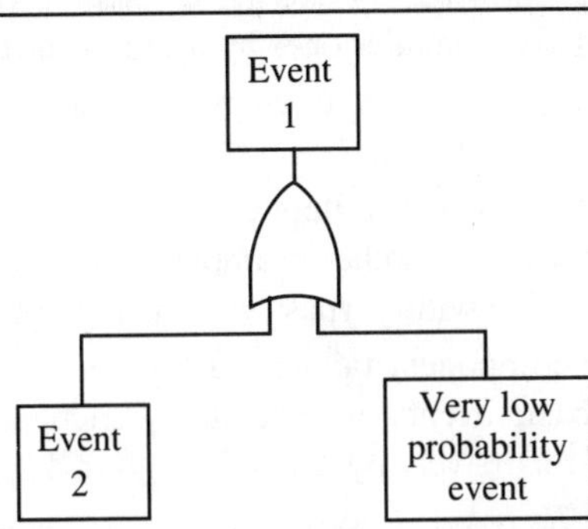
</td><td>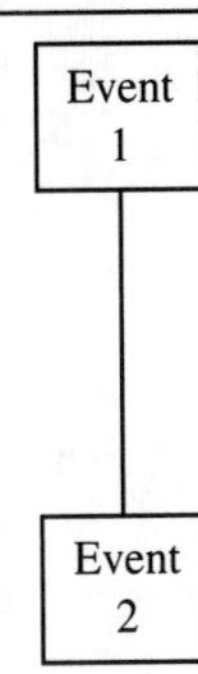
</td></tr>
<tr><td>Simplification by very low probability event (OR gate with three or more inputs)</td><td>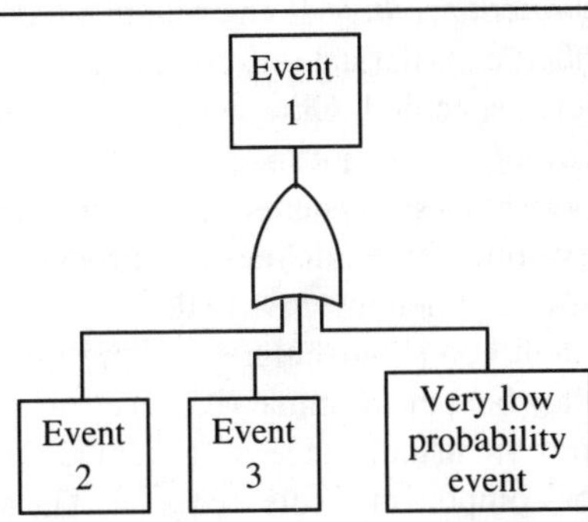
</td><td>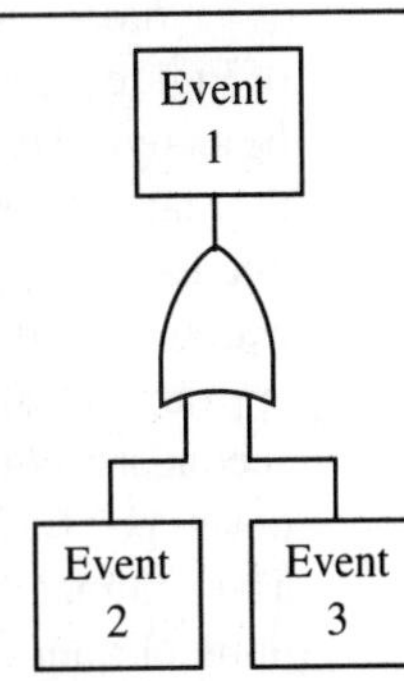
</td></tr>
</table>

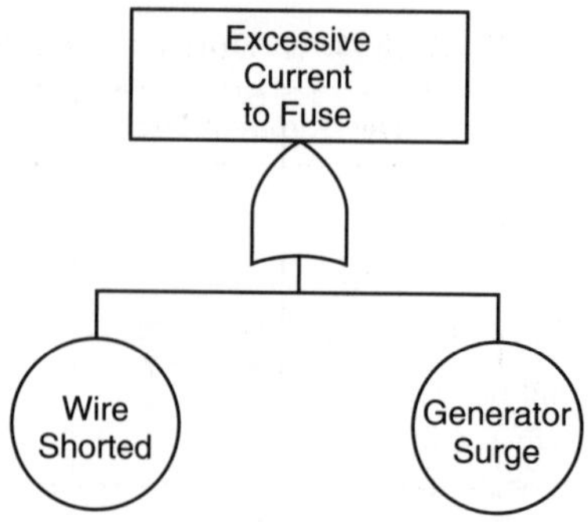

Figure 4.20. Fault tree obtained by neglecting generator not dead event.

4.5.2 Heuristic Guidelines

Guidelines. Heuristic guidelines for the construction of fault trees are summarized in Table 4.4 and Figure 4.21, and given below.

1. Replace an abstract event by a less abstract event. Example: "motor operates too long" versus "current to motor too long."
2. Classify an event into more elementary events. Example: "tank rupture" versus "rupture by overfilling" or "rupture due to runaway reaction."
3. Identify distinct causes for an event. Example: "runaway reaction" versus "large exotherm" and "insufficient cooling."
4. Couple trigger event with "no protective action." Example: "overheating" versus "loss of cooling" coupled with "no system shutdown." Note that causal relations of this type can be dealt with in an event tree that assumes an initiating event "loss of cooling" followed by "no system shutdown"; a single large fault tree can be divided into two smaller ones by using event-tree headings.
5. Find cooperative causes for an event. Example: "fire" versus "leak of flammable fluid" and "relay sparks."
6. Pinpoint a component-failure event. Example: "no current to motor" versus "no current in wire." Another example is "no cooling water" versus "main valve is closed" coupled with "bypass valve is not opened."
7. Develop a component failure via Figure 4.21. As we trace backward to search for more basic events, we eventually encounter component failures that can be developed recursively by using the Figure 4.21 structure.

State-of-component event. If an event in a rectangle can be developed in the form of Figure 4.21, Lambert calls it a state-of-component event [3]. In this case, a component to be analyzed is explicitly specified. Otherwise, an event is called a state-of-system event. For the state-of-system event, we cannot specify a particular component to analyze. More than one hardware component or subsystems are responsible for a state-of-system event. Such events should be developed by guidelines (1) through (6) until state-of-component events appear. The state-of-component events are developed further in terms of primary failures, secondary failures, and command failures. If the primary or secondary failures are not developed further, they become terminal (basic) events in the fault tree under construction. The command failures are usually state-of-system failure events that are developed further until relevant state-of-component events are found. The resulting state-of-component events are again developed via Figure 4.21. The procedure is repeated, and the development is eventually terminated when there is no possibility of command failures.

TABLE 4.4. Heuristic Guidelines for Fault-Tree Construction

	Development Policy	**Corresponding Part of Fault Tree**
1	Equivalent but less abstract event *F*	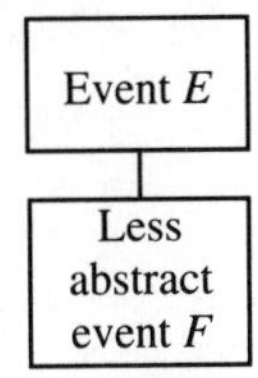
2	Classification of event *E*	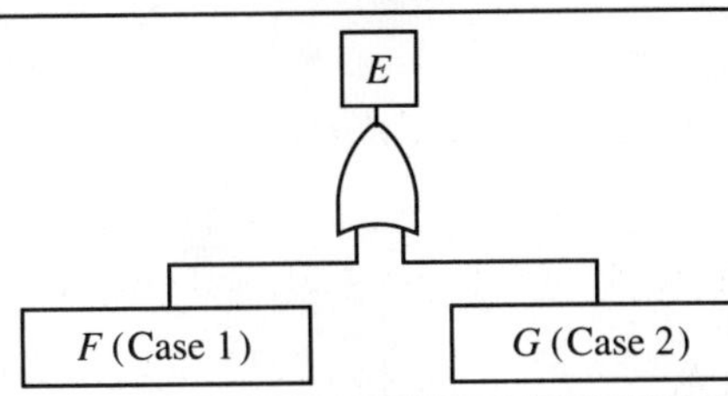
3	Distinct causes for event *E*	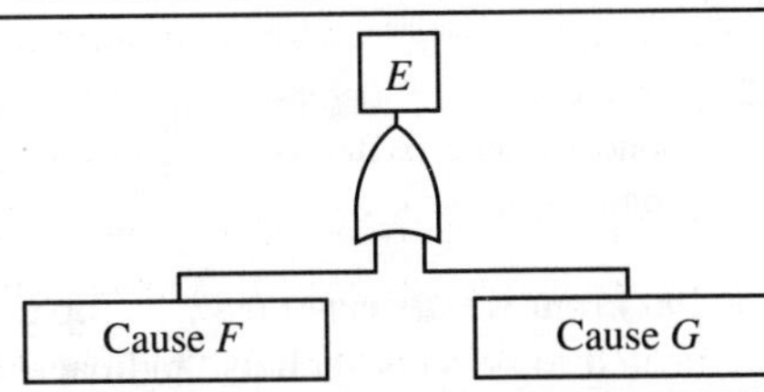
4	Trigger versus no protective event	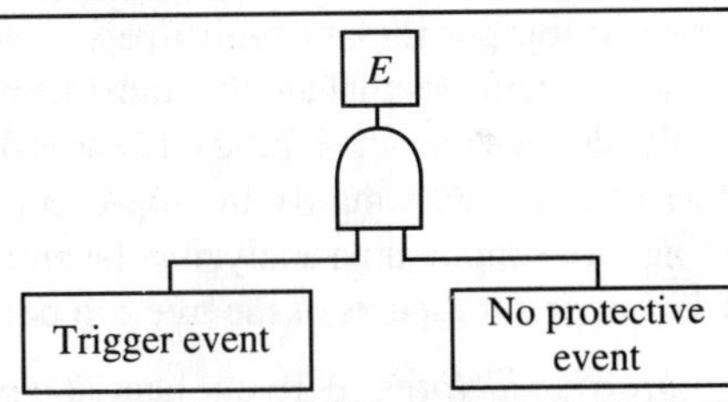
5	Cooperative cause	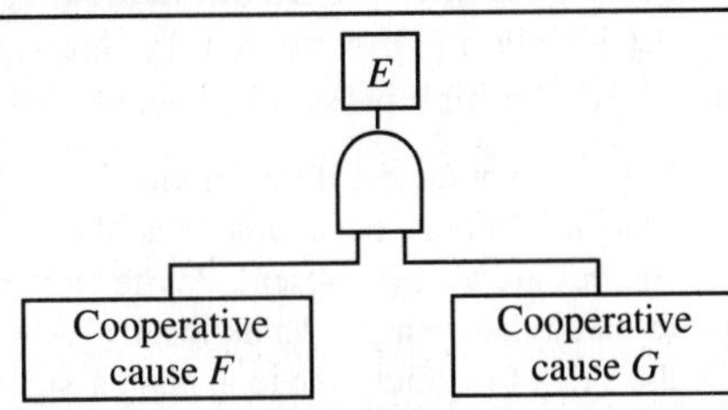
6	Pinpoint a component failure event	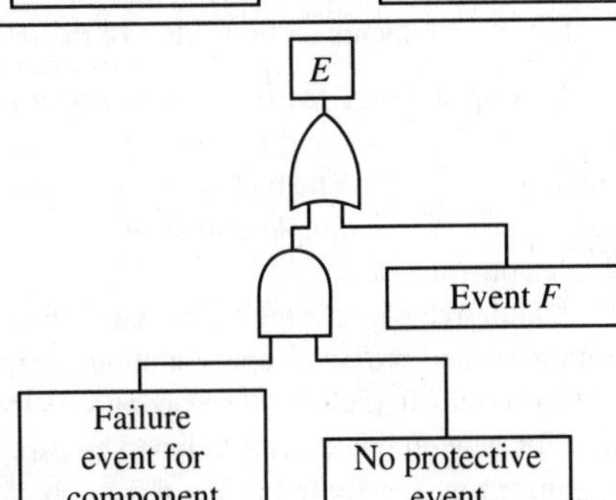

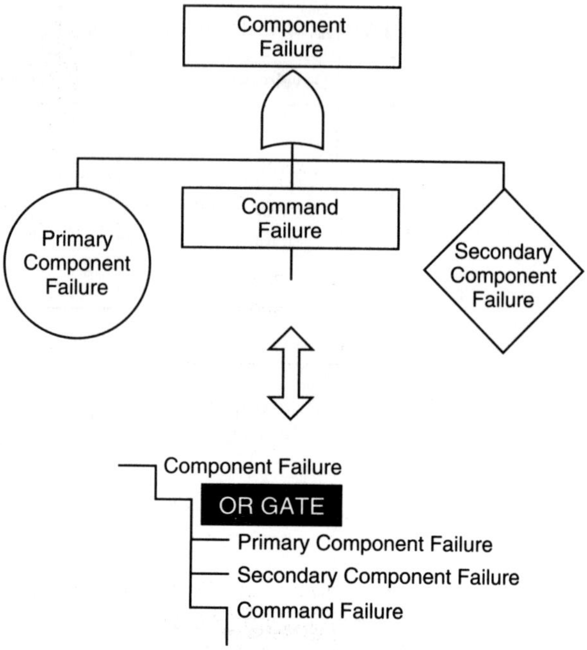

Figure 4.21. Development of a component failure (state-of-component event).

Top event versus event tree. Top events are usually state-of-system failure events. Complicated top events such as "radioactivity release" and "containment failure" are developed in top portions of fault trees. The top portion includes undesirable events and hazardous conditions that are the immediate causes of the top event. The top event must be carefully defined and all significant causes of the top event identified. The marriage of fault and event trees can simplify the top-event development because top events as event-tree headings are simpler than analyzing the entire accident by a large, single fault tree. In other words, important aspects of the tree-top portions can be included in an event tree.

More guidelines. To our heuristic guidelines, we can add a few practical considerations by Lambert [3]. Note that the description about normal function is equivalent to the removal of very high probability events from the fault tree (see Table 4.3).

> Expect no miracles; if the "normal" functioning of a component helps to propagate a failure sequence, it must be assumed that the component functions "normally": assume that ignition sources are always present. Write complete, detailed failure statements. Avoid direct gate-to-gate relationships. Think locally. Always complete the inputs to a gate. Include notes on the side of the fault tree to explain assumptions not explicit in the failure statements. Repeat failure statements on both sides of the transfer symbols.

Example 2—A fault tree without an event tree. This example shows how the heuristic guidelines of Table 4.4 and Figure 4.21 can be used to construct a fault tree for the pressure tank system in Figure 4.22. The fault tree is not based on an event tree and is thus larger in size than those in Figure 1.10. This example also shows that the marriage of fault and event trees greatly simplifies fault-tree construction.

A fault tree with the top event "tank rupture" is shown in Figures 4.23 and 4.24 in a structured-programming and ordinary representations, respectively. This tree shows which guidelines are used to develop events in the tree. The operator in this example can be regarded as a system component, and the OR gate on line 23 is developed by using the guidelines of Figure 4.21 conveniently denoted as imaginary row 7 of Table 4.4. A primary operator failure means that the operator functioning within

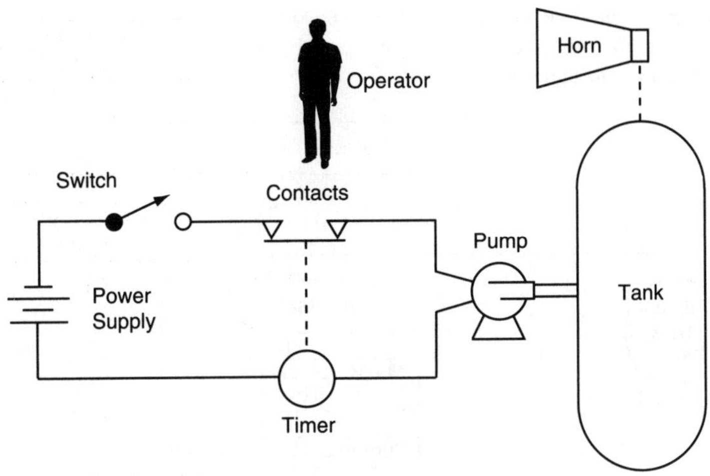

Figure 4.22. Schematic diagram for a pumping system.

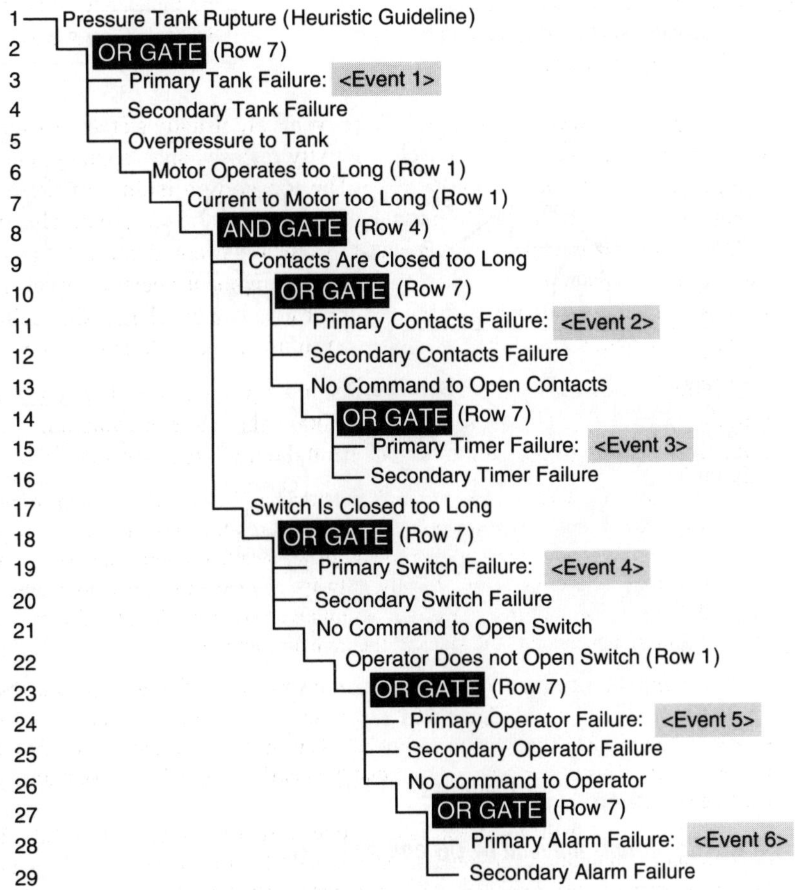

Figure 4.23. Fault tree for pumping system.

the design envelope fails to push the panic button when the alarm sounds. A secondary operator failure is, for example, "operator was dead when the alarm sounded." The command failure for the operator is "no alarm sounds." ■

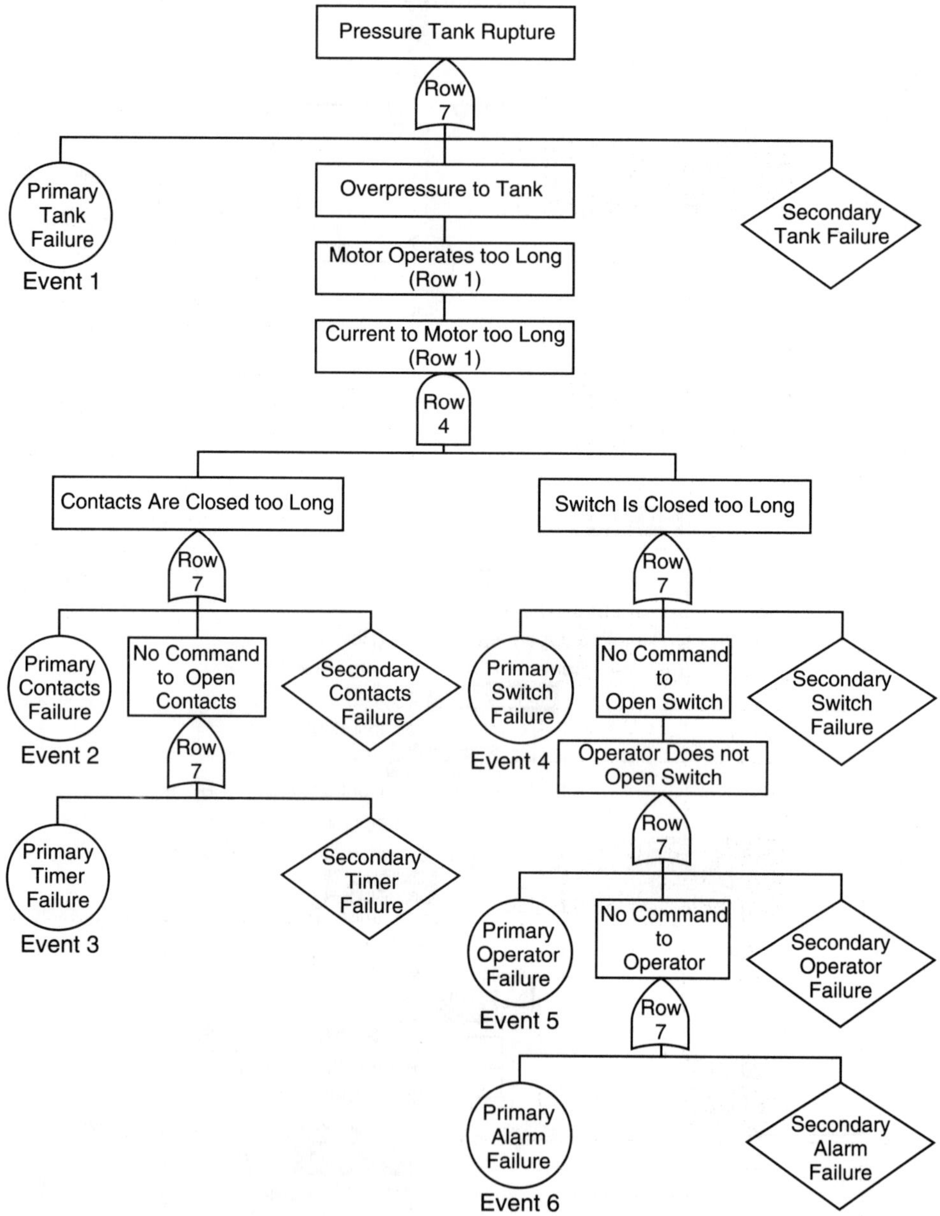

Figure 4.24. Fault tree for pumping system.

4.5.3 Conditions Induced by OR and AND Gates

We have three applications for OR gates. These are shown in rows 1 through 3 of Table 4.5. Row 1 has two events, A and B, and these two will overlap as shown in the figure by the corresponding Venn diagram.

TABLE 4.5. Conditions Induced by OR and AND Gates

	Venn Diagram	Fault Tree	Remark
1	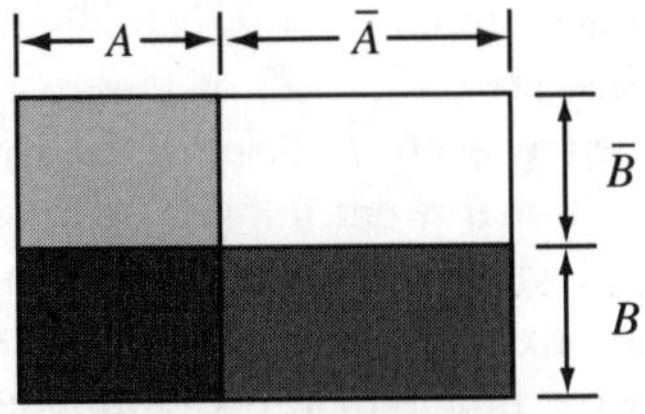	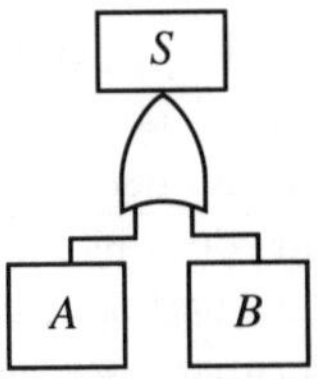	
2	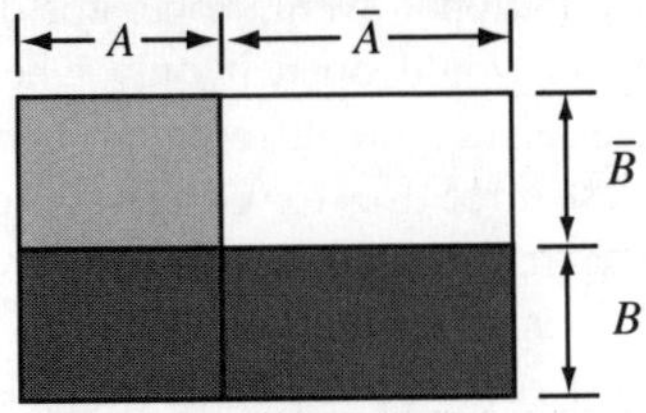	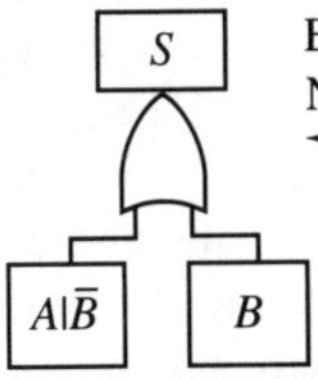	Normal Event $\bar{B}$ is Neglected 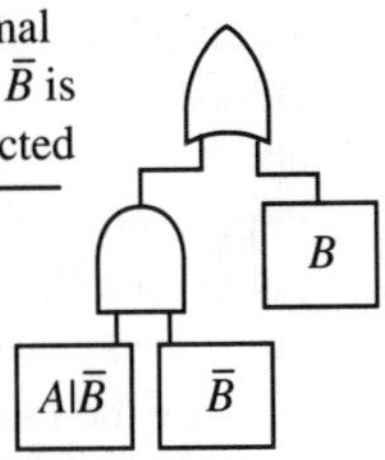
3	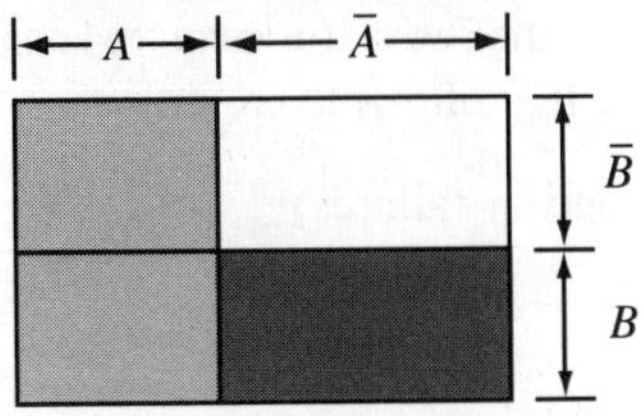	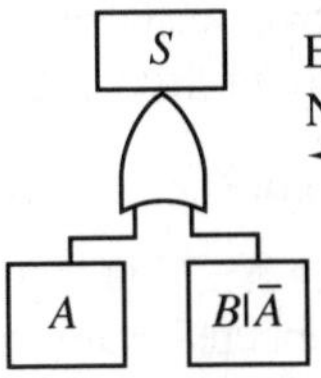	Normal Event $\bar{A}$ is Neglected 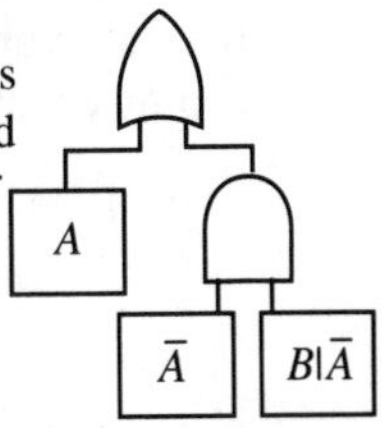
4	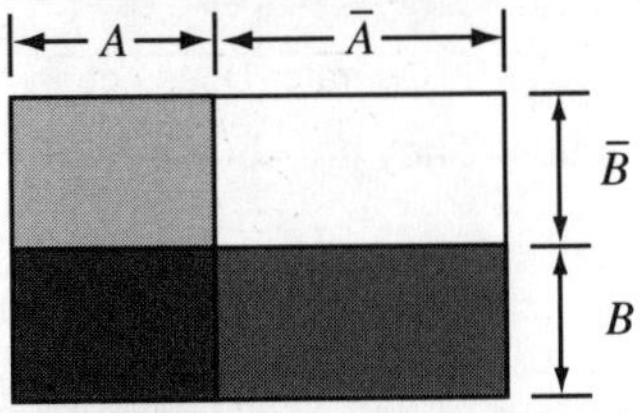	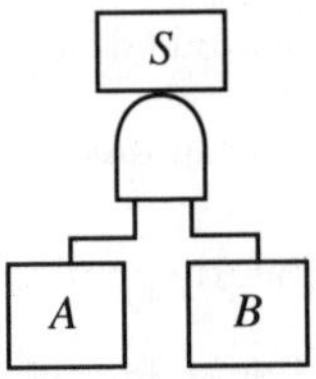	
5	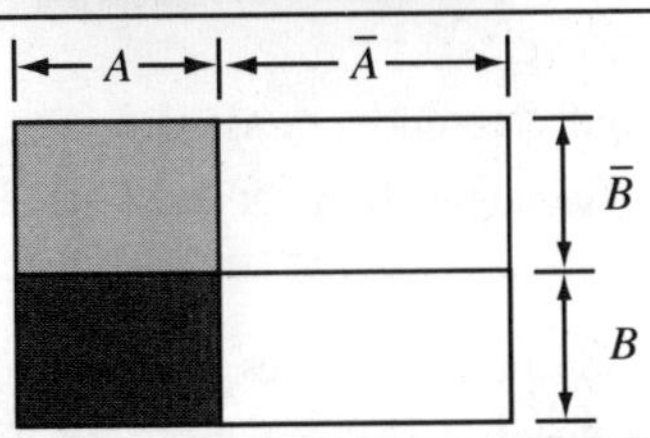	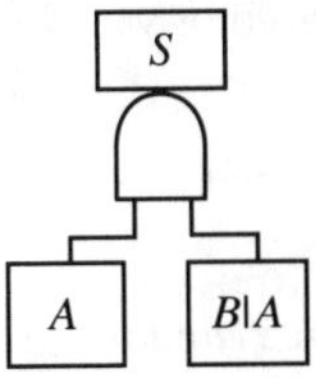	
6	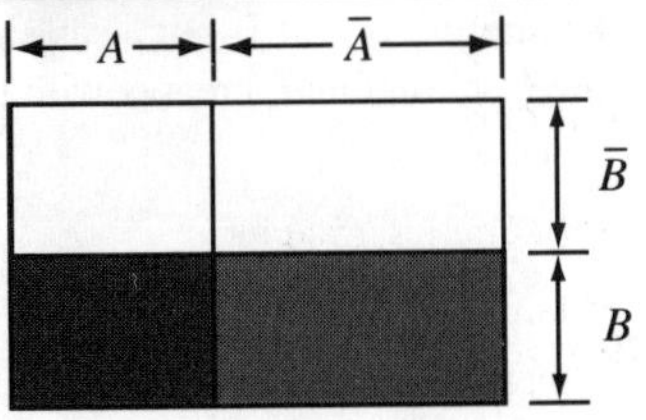	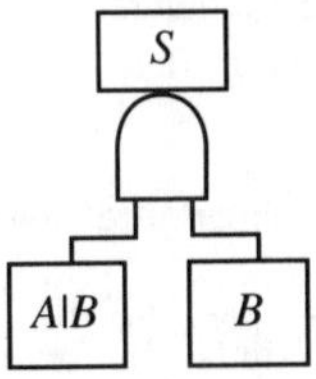	

Note: $A\,|\,\bar{B}$ and $A\,|\,B$ are often written simply as A in the development of fault trees. Similarly, $B\,|\,\bar{A}$ and $B\,|\,A$ are abbreviated as B.

Row 2 subdivides the Venn diagram into two parts: event B plus complement $\overline{B}$ AND A. The latter part is equivalent to the conditional event $A|\overline{B}$ coupled with $\overline{B}$ (see the tree in the last column). Conditional event $A|\overline{B}$ means that event A is observed when event $\overline{B}$ is true, that is, when event B is not occurring. Because $\overline{B}$ is usually a very high probability event, it can be removed from the AND gate and the tree in row 2, column 2 is obtained.

An example of this type of OR gate is the gate on line 23 of Figure 4.23. Event 5, "primary operator failure," is an event conditioned by event $\overline{B}$ meaning "alarm to operator." (event B is "no alarm to operator"). This conditional event implies that the operator (in a normal environment) does not open the switch when there is an alarm. In other words, the operator is careless and neglects the alarm or opens the wrong switch. Considering condition $\overline{B}$ for the primary operator failure, we estimate that this failure has a relatively small probability. On the other hand, the unconditional event, "operator does not open switch," has a very high probability, because he would open it only when the tank is about to explode and the alarm horn sounds. These are quite different probabilities, which depend on whether the event is conditioned. These three uses for OR gates provide a useful background for quantifying primary or secondary failure in fault trees.

Rows 2 and 3 of Table 4.5 introduce conditions for fault-tree branching. They account for why the fault tree of Figure 4.18 in Example 1 could be terminated by the primary and secondary fuse failures. All OR gates in the tree are used in the sense of row 3. We might have been able to introduce a command failure for the fuse. However, the command failure cannot occur, because at this final stage we have the following conditions.

1. Normal motor (i.e., no primary or secondary failures)
2. Generator is working (same as above)
3. Wire is connected (same as above)
4. Switch is closed (same as above)
5. Fuse is connected (same as above)

Three different situations exist for AND gates. They are shown by rows 4 through 6 in Table 4.5.

Table 4.5, if properly applied:

1. clarifies and quantifies events
2. finds very high or very low probability events
3. terminates further development of a fault tree under construction
4. provides a clear background and useful suggestions at each stage of fault-tree construction

Example 3—A reaction system. The temperature increases with the feed rate of flow-controlled stream D in the reaction system in Figure 4.25 [5]. Heat is removed by water circulation through a water-cooled exchanger. Normal reactor temperature is 200°F, but a catastrophic runaway will start if this temperature reaches 300°F because the reaction rate increases with temperature. In view of this situation:

1. The reactor temperature is monitored.
2. Rising temperature is alarmed at 225°F (see horn).
3. An interlock shuts off stream D at 250°F, stopping the reaction (see temperature sensor, solenoid, and valve A).
4. The operator can initiate the interlock by punching the panic switch.

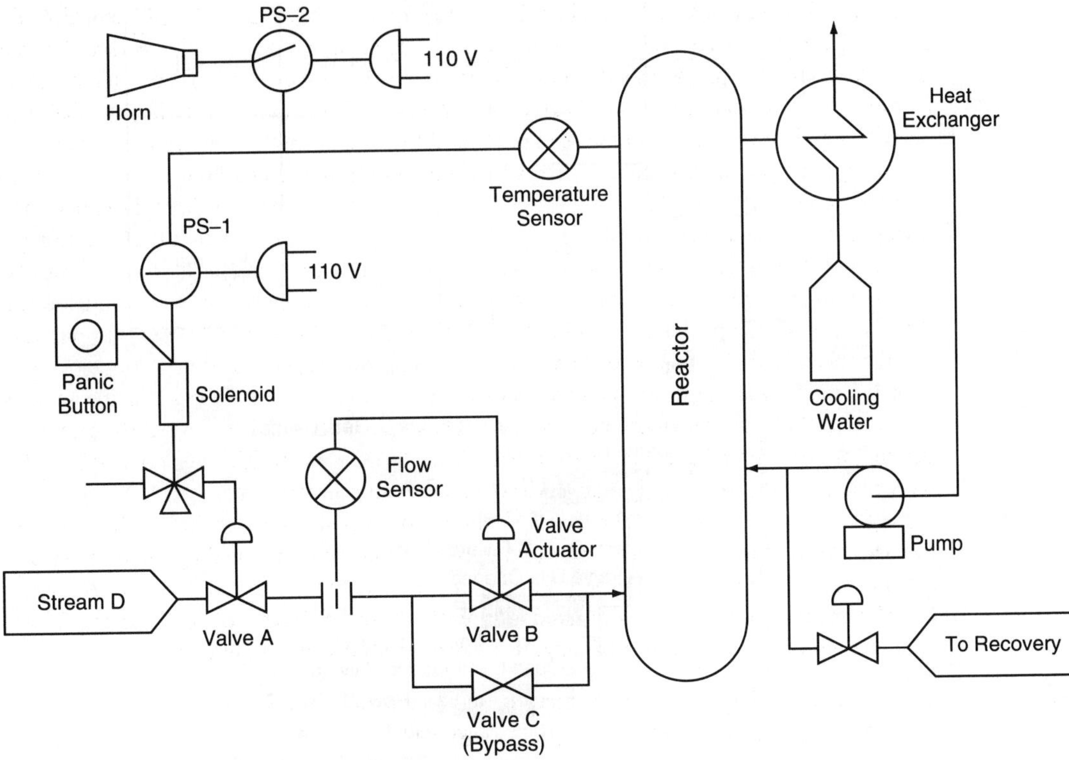

Figure 4.25. Schematic diagram for reactor.

Two safety systems are observed; one is an automatic shutdown of stream D, and the other is a manual shutdown. The initiating event is a large increase in feed. A system event tree is shown in Figure 4.26. Construct fault trees for the initiating event, automatic shutdown system failure, and manual shutdown system failure. Also construct a fault tree for the simultaneous failure of the automatic and manual shutdown systems when the two safety systems are aggregated into one system in the function event tree in Figure 4.27.

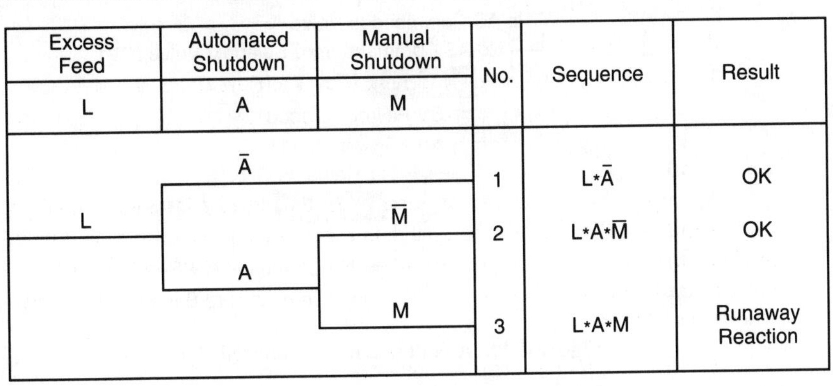

Figure 4.26. A reactor plant system event tree.

Solution: Fault trees for the event tree of Figure 4.26 are shown in Figures 4.28, 4.29, and 4.30, while the event tree of Figure 4.27 results in the fault trees in Figure 4.28 and Figure 4.31. Secondary

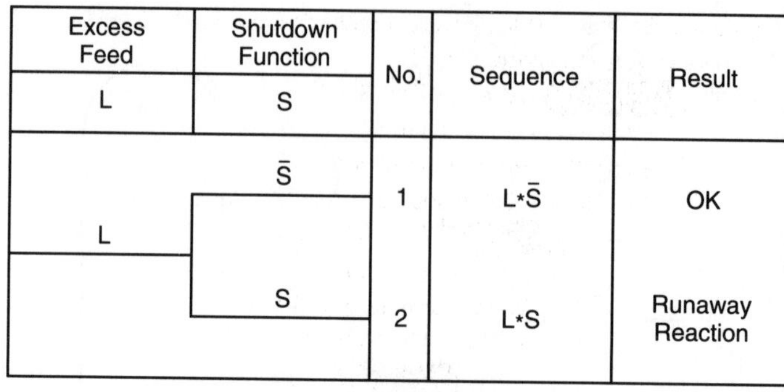

Figure 4.27. A reactor plant function event tree.

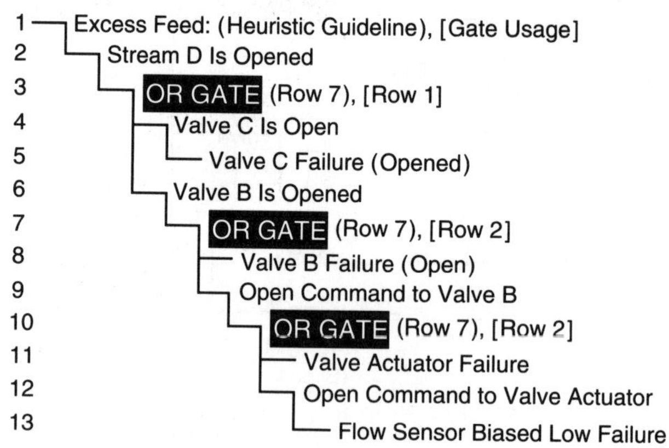

Figure 4.28. A fault tree with top event "excess feed."

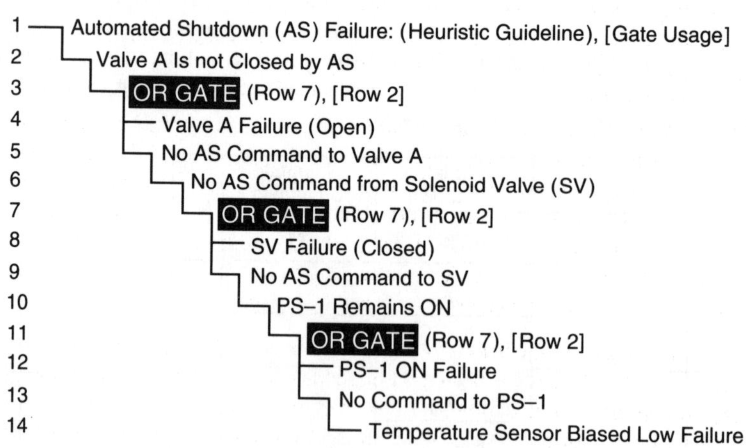

Figure 4.29. A fault tree for "automated shutdown failure."

failures are neglected. It is further assumed that the alarm signal always reaches the operator whenever the horn sounds, that is, the alarm has a sufficiently large signal-to-noise ratio. Heuristic guidelines and gate usages are indicated in the fault trees. Note that row 7 of the heuristic guidelines refers to Figure 4.21. It is recommended that the reader trace them.

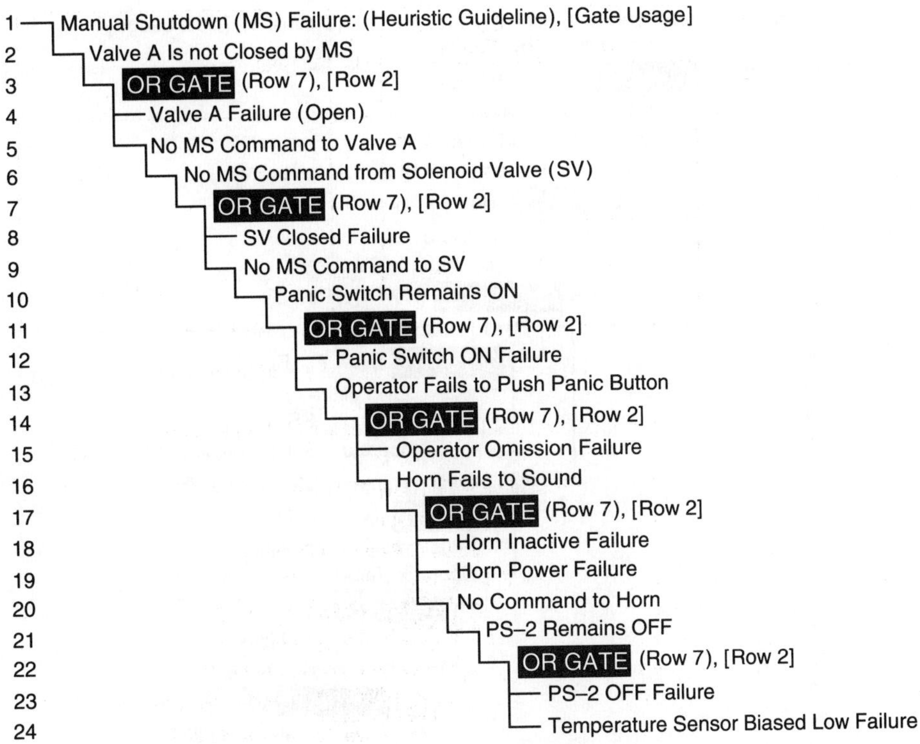

Figure 4.30. A fault tree for "manual shutdown failure."

One might think that event "valve A is open" on line 4 of Figure 4.29 is a very high probability event because the valve is open if the system is in normal operation. This is not true, because this open valve is conditioned by the initiating event of the event tree in Figure 4.26. Under this circumstance, the shutdown system will operate, and "valve A is open" has a small probability of occurrence. This event can be regarded as an input to an AND gate in accident sequence L*A*M in Figure 4.26, and should not be neglected.

We note that a single large fault tree without an event tree is given in our previous text [6,7]. In this fault tree, AND gates appear to show that the plant is designed so as to protect it from a single failure event, that is, an initiating event in this case. The fault trees in Figures 4.28 to 4.30 have no AND gate because protection features have been included in headings of the system event tree. The fault tree in Figure 4.31 has an AND gate because this represents simultaneous failures of automatic and manual shutdown features. The reaction system may have another initiating event, "loss of coolant," for which event trees and fault trees should be constructed in a similar way. ■

Example 4—A pressure tank system. Consider the pressure tank system shown in Figure 4.14. This system has been a bit of a straw-man since it was first published by Vesely in 1971 [8]. It appears also in Barlow and Proschan [9]. A single large fault tree is given in our previous text [6,7] and shown as Figure 4.32. It is identical to that given by Lambert [3] except for some minor modifications. The fault tree can be constructed by the heuristic guidelines of Table 4.4. It demonstrates the gate usages of Table 4.5.

We now show other fault trees for this system constructed by starting with event trees. The plant in Figure 4.14 is similar to the plant in Figure 4.22. A marriage of event and fault trees considers as an initiating event, "pump overrun." Because the plant of Figure 4.14 has neither an operator nor a relief valve as safety systems, a relatively large fault tree for the initiating event would be constructed,

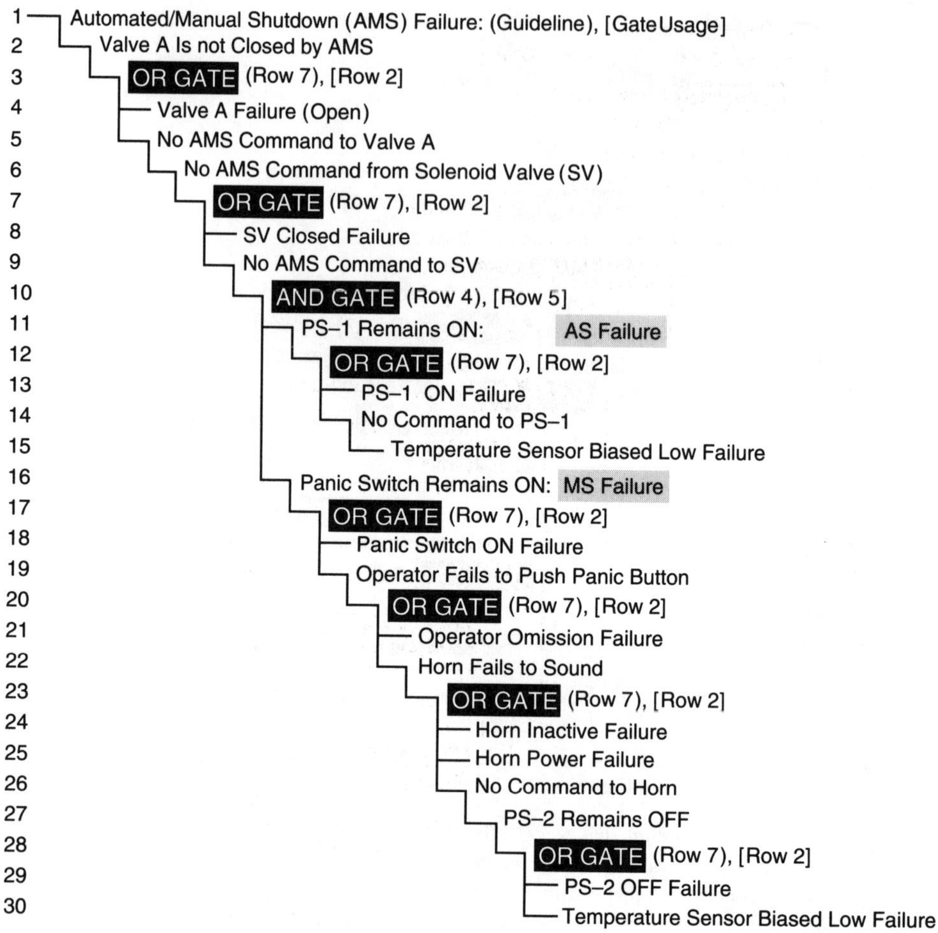

Figure 4.31. A fault tree for "automated/manual shutdown failure."

and this is the fault tree constructed in other texts and shown as Figure 4.32. If an initiating event is defined as "pump overrun before timer relay de-activation," then the timer relay becomes a safety system and the event tree in Figure 4.33 is obtained. Fault trees are constructed for the initiating event and the safety system, respectively, as shown in Figures 4.34 and 4.35. These small fault trees can be more easily constructed than the single large fault tree shown in Figure 4.32. These fault trees do not include a tank failure as a cause of tank rupture; the failure should be treated as another initiating event without any mitigation features. ■

4.5.4 Summary

Component failures are classified as primary failures, secondary failures, and command failures. A simple fault-tree-construction example based on this classification is given. Then more general heuristic guidelines are presented, and a fault tree is constructed for a tank rupture. Conditions induced by OR and AND gates are given, and fault trees are constructed for a reaction system and a pressure tank system with and without recourse to event trees.

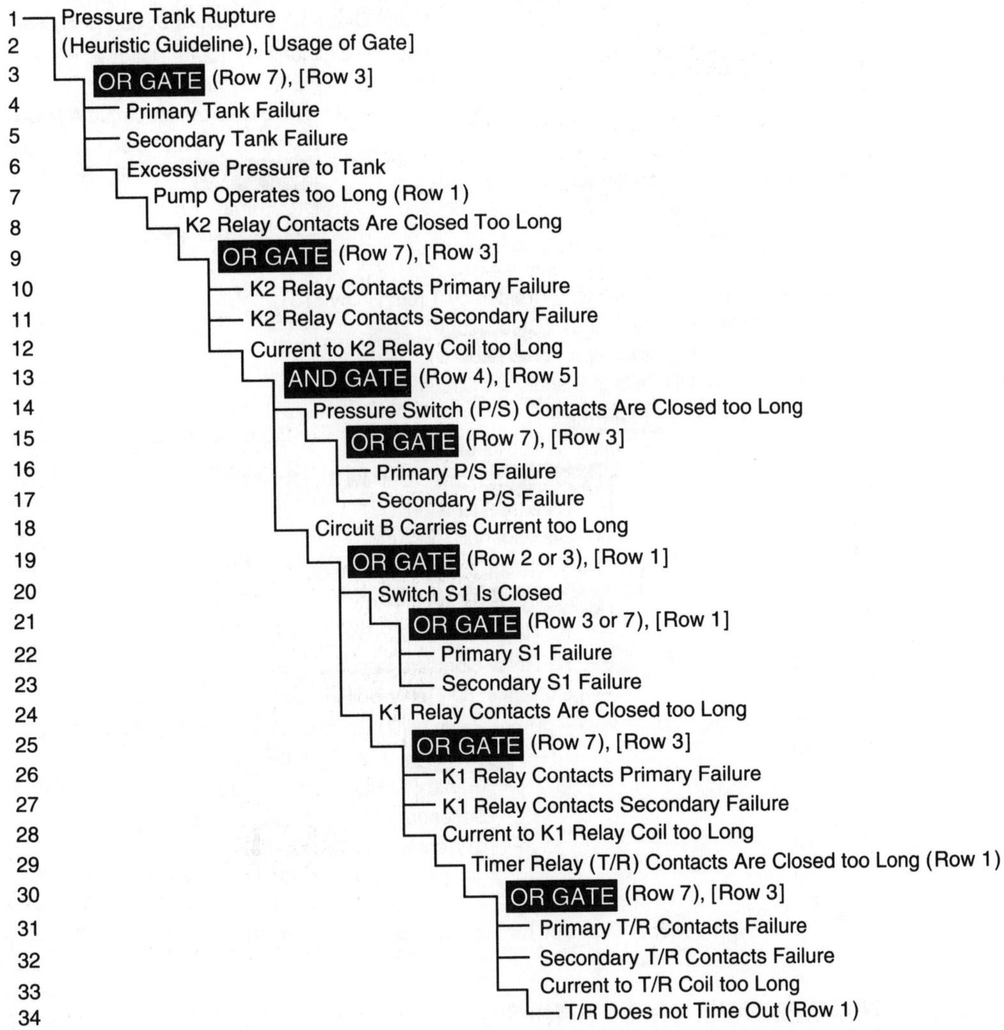

Figure 4.32. A single, large fault tree for pressure tank system.

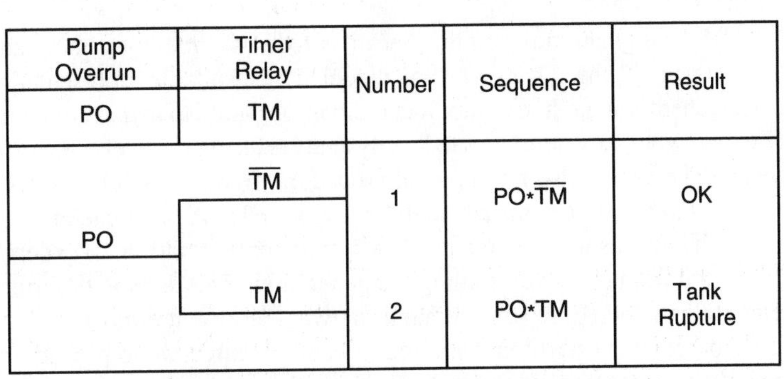

Figure 4.33. Event tree for pressure tank system.

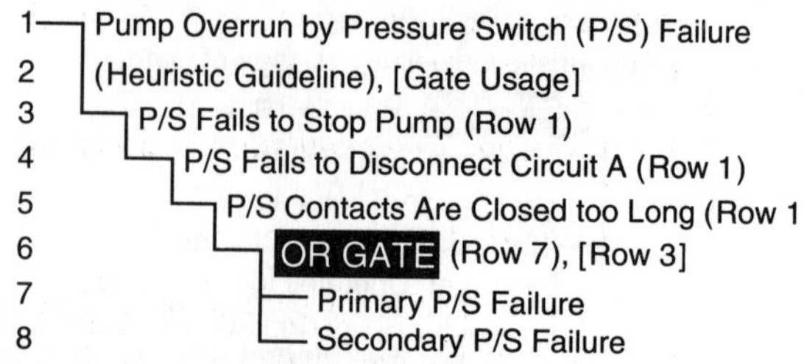

Figure 4.34. Fault tree for "pump overrun due to pressure switch failure."

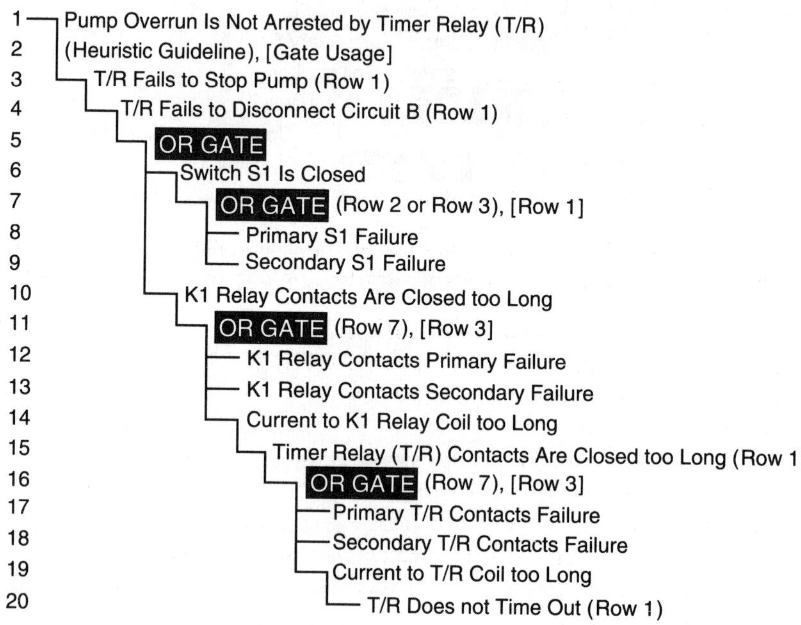

Figure 4.35. Fault tree for "pump overrun is not arrested by timer relay."

4.6 AUTOMATED FAULT-TREE SYNTHESIS

4.6.1 Introduction

Manual generation of fault trees is a tedious, time-consuming and error-prone task. To create an FT, the system must be modeled by a suitable representation method, because no FT-generation method can extract more information than that contained in the model. An FT expert would use heuristics to locally analyze an upper-level event in terms of lower-level events. The expert also has a global procedural framework for a systematic application of heuristics to generate, truncate, and decompose FTs. A practical, automated FT-generation approach requires three elements: 1) a system representation, 2) expert heuristics, and 3) a procedural framework for guiding the generation. This section describes a new automated generation method based on a semantic network representation of the system to be analyzed, a rule-based event development, and a recursive three-value procedure with normal- and impossible-event truncations and modular FT decompositions.

Automated FT-generation methods have been proposed and reviewed in Andrews and Brennan [10], Chang et al. [11,12] and in a series of papers by Kelly and Lees [13], Mullhi et al. [14], and Hunt et al. [15]. Some of the earliest works include Fussell [16],

Salem, Apostolakis, and Okrent [17], and Henley and Kumamoto [18]. None of the methods proposed to date is in general use.

4.6.2 System Representation by Semantic Networks

4.6.2.1 Flows.

Flow and event propagation. A flow is defined as any material, information, energy, activity, or phenomenon that can move or propagate through the system. A system can be viewed as a pipeline structure of flows and pieces of equipment along flow paths. A variety of flows travel the flow paths and cause events specific to the system. Typical flows are

1. material flow; liquid, gas, steam
2. information flow; signal, data, command, alarm
3. energy flow; light, heat, sound, vibration
4. activity and phenomenon; manual operation, fire, spark, high pressure

Light as a flow is generated when an electric flow is supplied to a bulb. Activities and phenomena are regarded as flows because they propagate through the system to cause events.

Flow rate, generation rate, and aperture. We focus mainly on the three attributes of a flow: flow rate, generation rate, and aperture. The aperture and generation rate are determined by plant equipment in the flow path. The flow rate is determined from aperture and generation rate.

The flow aperture is defined similarly to a valve; an open valve corresponds to an on switch, whereas a closed valve corresponds to an off switch. The flow aperture is closed if, for instance, one or more valve apertures in series are closed, or at least one switch in series is off. The generation rate is a potential. The potential causes the positive flow rate when the aperture is open. The positive flow rate implies existence of a flow, and a zero flow rate implies a nonexistence.

Flow rate, generation rate, and aperture values. Aperture attribute values are Fully_Closed (F_Cl), Increase (Inc), Constant (Cons), Decrease (Dec), Fully_Open (F_Op), Open, and Not_Fully_Open (Not_F_Op). The values Inc, Cons, and Dec, respectively, mean that the aperture increases, remains constant, and decreases between F_Cl (excluded) and F_Op (excluded), as shown in Figure 4.36. In a digital representation, only two attribute values are considered, that is, F_Cl and F_Op.

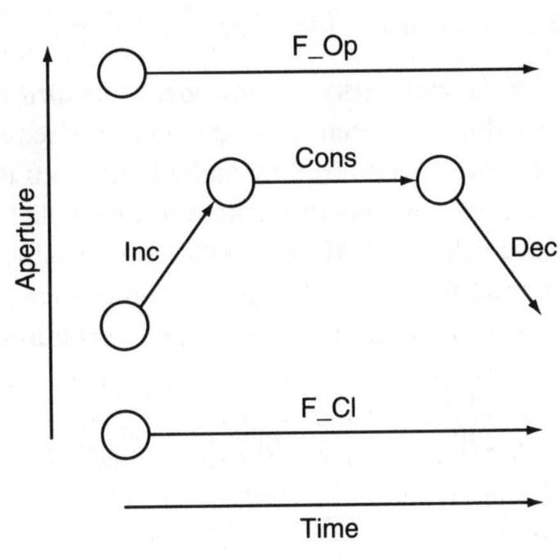

Figure 4.36. Five aperture values.

In Table 4.6 aperture values are shown in column A. Attribute values Open and N_F_Op are composite, while values F_Cl, Inc, Cons, Dec, and F_Op are basic.

TABLE 4.6. Flow Rate as a Function of Aperture and Generation Rate

Flow Aperture ↓				Positive			
		↓ A →	Zero	Inc	Cons	Dec	Max
	Not_F_Op	F_CL	Zero	Zero	Zero	Zero	Zero
Open	Not_F_Op	Inc	Zero	Inc	Inc	Inc, Dec	Inc
Open	Not_F_Op	Cons	Zero	Inc	Cons	Dec	Cons
Open	Not_F_Op	Dec	Zero	Inc, Dec	Dec	Dec	Dec
Open		F_Op	Zero	Inc	Cons	Dec	Max
			Not_Max				

Generation Rate →

As shown in row A of Table 4.6, the generation rate has attribute values Zero, Inc, Cons, Dec, Max, Positive, and Not_Max. The first five values are basic, while the last two are composite. The flow rate has the same set of attribute values as the generation rate. See Table 4.6 where each cell denotes a flow rate value.

Relations between aperture, generation rate, and flow rate. The three attributes are not independent of each other. The flow rate of a flow becomes zero if its aperture is closed or its generation rate is zero. For instance, the flow rate of electricity through a bulb is zero if the bulb has a filament failure or the battery is dead.

The flow rate is determined when the aperture and the generation rate are specified. Table 4.6 shows the relationship. Each row has a fixed aperture value, which is denoted in column A, and each column has a fixed generation rate value denoted in row A. Each cell is a flow rate value. The flow rate is Zero when the aperture is F_Cl or the generation rate is Zero. The flow rate is not uniquely determined when the aperture is Inc and the generation rate is Dec. A similar case occurs for the Dec aperture and the Inc generation rate. In these two cases, the flow rate is either Inc or Dec; we exclude the rare chance of the flow rate becoming Cons. The two opposing combinations of aperture and generation rate in Table 4.6 become causes of the flow rate being Inc (or Dec).

Relations between flow apertures and equipment apertures. Table 4.7 shows the relationships between flow apertures and equipment apertures, when equipment 1 and 2 are in series along the flow path. Each column has the fixed aperture value of equipment 1, and each row has the fixed aperture value of equipment 2. Each cell denotes a flow-aperture value. The flow aperture is either Inc or Dec when one equipment aperture is Inc and the other is Dec. Tables 4.6 and 4.7 will be used in Section 4.6.3.3 to derive a set of event-development rules that search for causes of events related to the flow rate.

Flow triple event. A flow triple is defined as a particular combination (flow, attribute, value). For example, (electricity, flow rate, Zero) means that electricity does not exist.

TABLE 4.7. Flow Aperture as Function of Equipment Apertures in Series

Aperture 2 ↓		A →	Open				
			F_Cl	**Inc**	**Cons**	**Dec**	**F_Op**
	Not_F_Op	**F_Cl**	F_Cl	F_Cl	F_Cl	F_Cl	F_Cl
	Not_F_Op	**Inc**	F_Cl	Inc	Inc	Inc, Dec	Inc	Open
	Not_F_Op	**Cons**	F_Cl	Inc	Cons	Dec	Cons	Open
	Not_F_Op	**Dec**	F_Cl	Inc, Dec	Dec	Dec	Dec	Open
		F_Op	F_Cl	Inc	Cons	Dec	F_Op	Open
			Not_F_Op	Not_F_Op	Not_F_Op	Not_F_Op	

Aperture 1 →

4.6.2.2 Basic equipment library. Equipment that controls an aperture or generation rate is catalogued in Figures 4.37 and 4.38 where a fragment of a semantic network is associated with each piece (second column). Examples are given in the third column. A circle represents a flow node, while a box, hexagon, or gate is an equipment node. A labeled arrow between flow and equipment node represents a relationship between the flow and the equipment. The effect to cause (backward) direction essential to fault-tree construction is represented by the arrow.

(A) Aperture controller. Two types of equipment, those with and those without command modes, are used for aperture control. Equipment 1 and 3 in Figure 4.37 are devices without command. Flow F_2 to equipment 2, 4, 5, and 6 is the command. Equipment 1 through 5 are digital devices with only two aperture values, F_Cl or F_Op, while equipment 6 is an analog device.

Aperture Controller without Command

1. **Normally Closed Equipment (NCE):** This is digital equipment that is normally closed (F_Cl). It has no command mode and its F_Op state is caused by failure of the NCE itself. Examples include normally closed valve, normally off switch, plug, insulator, and oil barrier.

   In the NCE semantic network, symbol F_1 denotes a flow that is stopped by the NCE. The vertical black stripe in the NCE box indicates a normally closed state. The arrow labeled NCE points to the equipment that closes the F_1 aperture. Suppose that the F_1 flow aperture is Open. This can be traced back to an Open failure of the NCE box.

2. **Normally Open Equipment (NOE):** This is digital equipment that is normally open (F_Op), a dual of NCE. Examples include normally open valve, normally on switch, pipe, and electric wire.

Aperture Controller with Command. Some types of equipment can be commanded to undergo an aperture change.

1. **Closed to Open Equipment (COE):** Normally this equipment is in an F_Cl state. When a transition from an F_Cl to an F_Op state occurs because of a command,

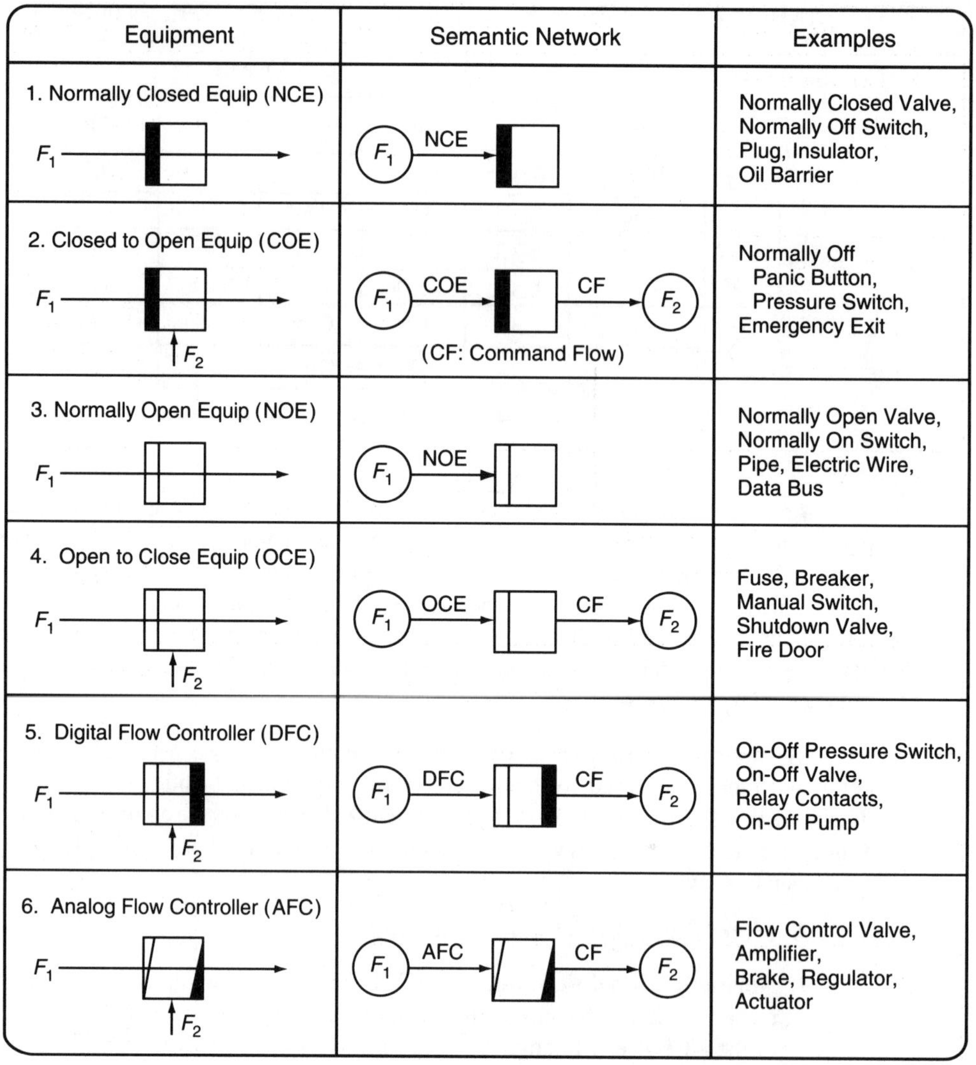

Figure 4.37. Aperture controllers and semantic networks.

we treat the command like a flow triple: (command, flow rate, Positive). This transition also occurs when the equipment spuriously changes its state when no command occurs. The reverse transition occurs by the failure of the COE, possibly after the command changes the equipment aperture to F_Op.

An emergency button normally in an off state is an example of a COE. An oil barrier can be regarded as a COE and a human action removing the barrier is a command to the COE. Symbol F_1 for the COE in Figure 4.37 denotes an aperture-controlled flow. Symbol F_2 represents the command flow. The arrow labeled COE points to the COE itself, while the arrow labeled CF points to the command flow.

Two types of COE exist: a positive gain and a negative gain. Note that in the following definitions the positive gain, in general, means that equipment aperture is a monotonically increasing function of the flow rate of command flow F_2.

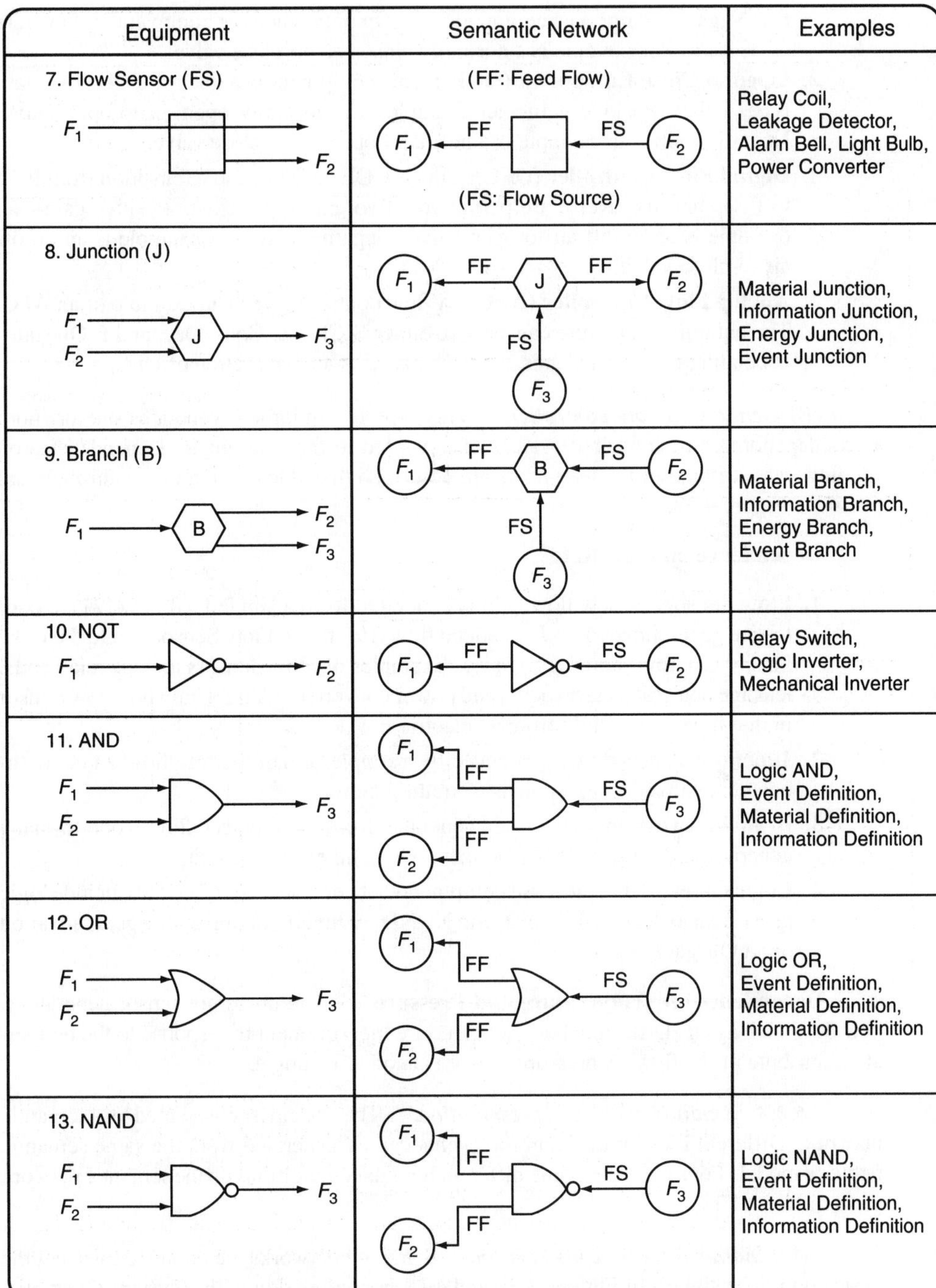

Figure 4.38. Generation rate controllers and semantic networks.

(1) Positive gain: The equipment is F_Op only when the command F_2 flow rate is Positive. An example is a normally closed air-to-open valve that is opened by command event (air, flow rate, Positive).

(2) **Negative gain:** The equipment is F_Op only when the command F_2 flow rate is Zero. An example is a normally closed air-to-close valve.

2. **Open to Close Equipment (OCE):** This equipment is a dual of COE. Two gain types exist: Positive gain—an example is a normally open air-to-open valve; Negative gain—an example is a normally open air-to-close valve.
3. **Digital Flow Controller (DFC):** This is COE or OCE, and a transition from F_Cl to F_Op and its reverse are permitted. Two gain types exist: Positive gain—an example is an on-off air-to-open valve; Negative gain—an example is an on-off air-to-close valve.
4. **Analog Flow Controller (AFC):** A flow control valve is an example of an AFC. The equipment aperture can assume either F_Cl, Inc, Cons, Dec, and F_Op states depending on the AFC gain type. The AFC is an elaboration of DFC.

(B) Generation rate controller. This type of equipment generates one or more flows depending on the attribute values of flows fed to the equipment. Dependencies on the flow-rate attribute of the feed flows are described first. Generation rate controllers are shown in Figure 4.38.

Dependence on Flow Rate

1. **Flow Sensor:** A new flow (F_2) is generated from a single feed flow (F_1), a one-to-one generation. Flow F_1 is a feed flow (FF) to the Flow Sensor, while the Flow Sensor is a flow source (FS) of F_2. Examples of Flow Sensors include relay coils, leakage detectors, alarm bells, and power converters. A light bulb is a Flow Sensor in that it generates light from an electric flow.
2. **Junction:** A new flow is generated by a simple sum of the feed flows, a many-to-one generation. An example is a circuit junction.
3. **Branch:** Two or more flows are generated from a single feed flow, a one-to-many generation. An example is a branch node in an electric circuit.
4. **Logic Gates:** Other pieces of equipment that control generation rates include logic gates such as NOT, OR, AND, and NAND. A Junction is an analog generalization of an OR gate.

Dependence on Temperature and Pressure. A temperature sensor generates a new flow such as an alarm signal or a temperature measurement in response to the temperature attribute of the flow. A pressure sensor is another example.

4.6.2.3 Semantic network representation. The system is represented by a semantic network. Different FTs for different top events can be generated from the same semantic network model. For a fixed top event, different boundary conditions on the semantic network yield different FTs.

(A) Semantic network construction. Semantic networks are obtained by using the basic equipment library in Figures 4.37 and 4.38 in conjunction with a system schematic. First, a correspondence between the basic equipment library and the system components is established. Then, semantic networks representing the pieces of equipment are integrated to yield a system semantic network.

Consider the schematic of Figure 4.39. This is a simplified portion of an ECCS (emergency core-cooling system) of a nuclear reactor. Lines A and AA are electric wires with a dc voltage difference. PS1 is a pressure switch; S1 and S2 are manual switches;

R2 is a relay contact. PS1 is on when a drywell pressure is high. As a result, dc current D1 flows through relay coil R2_COIL as current D3 if S1 is on. This, in turn, energizes the R2_COIL. As a result, relay contact R2 is turned on by an EMG (electromagnetic) command from R2_COIL, and dc current D2 flows if S2 is on. Currents D1 and D2 are joined at Junction J1, and D3 flows through R2_COIL even if current D1 stops flowing for some reason, such as PS1 (incorrectly) going off. In a real ECCS, the EMG signal energized by R2_COIL is used as a signal to activate an emergency cooling pump. A semantic network is shown in Figure 4.40. Switches (PS1, S1, S2) and relay contact (R2) are modeled as DFCs. Relay coil (R2_COIL) is represented as a Flow Sensor. Flows are dc currents (D1, D2, D3), EMG command (R2_CM), manual operations (OP1, OP2), and drywell pressure-high phenomenon (DWPH). The semantic network contains a loop consisting of R2_CM, R2_COIL, D3, J1, D2, R2, and R2_CM. This loop represents the locking capability of the relay circuit in Figure 4.39.

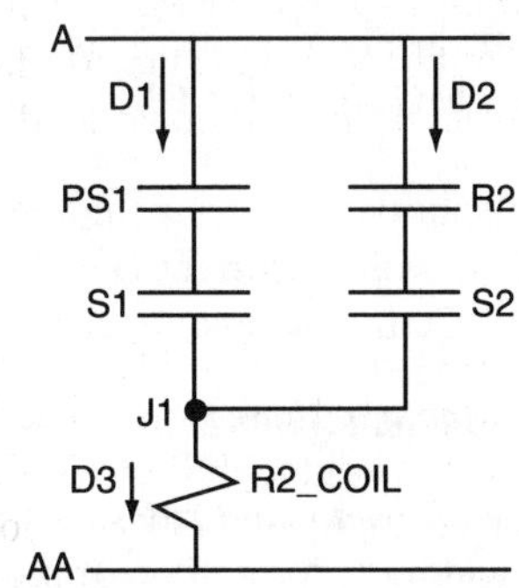

Figure 4.39. A simple relay circuit.

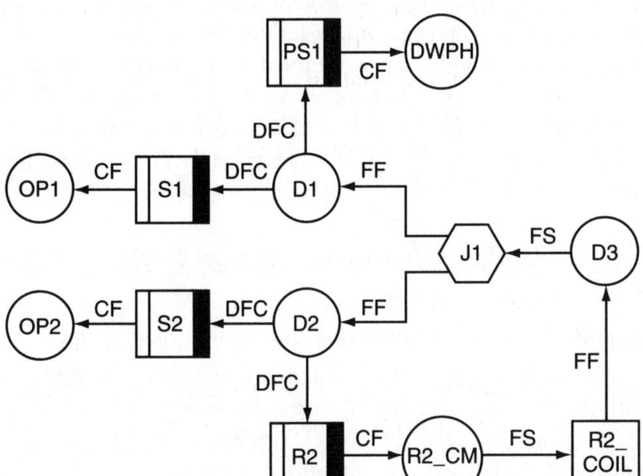

Label	Description
CF DFC FF FS	Command Flow Digital Flow Controller Feed Flow Flow Source
S1,S2 R2 R2_COIL J1	Manual Switches Relay Contact Relay Coil Junction
D1,D2,D3 R2_CM OP1,OP2 DWPH	DC Currents EMG Command to R2 S1,S2 Manual Operations Drywell Pressure High

Figure 4.40. A relay circuit semantic network representation.

(B) Boundary conditions. Fixed and/or free boundary conditions can be specified explicitly for flow or equipment nodes in a semantic network.

Conditions at Flow Nodes. A boundary condition at a flow node is described by a flow triple. Consider again the relay system and network in Figures 4.39 and 4.40. It is assumed that power lines A and AA are intact, and have a voltage difference. Thus, the generation rates (or flow potentials) of D1 and D2 are always positive. This fixed boundary condition is expressed as (D1, generation rate, Positive) and (D2, generation rate, Positive). The drywell pressure-high phenomenon may or may not occur. It can be represented as (DWPH, flow rate, ?) where the symbol ? denotes a free value. Similarly, (OP1, flow rate, ?) and (OP2, flow rate, ?) hold. Fixed or free flow rate boundary conditions are required for terminal flow nodes such as DWPH, OP1, and OP2. Generation rate conditions are required for intermediate flow nodes (D1, D2) without generation rate controllers pointed to by FS arrows.

Conditions at Equipment Nodes. Some equipment-failure boundary conditions are obvious from equipment definitions. For instance, consider developing the F_1 flow-rate Zero event for NCE in Figure 4.37. The NCE being closed is a cause. This is a normal event by definition of the NCE. Possibilities such as this normal closure propagating upward toward the top event via a three-value logic interrogation are described shortly.

Equipment failure modes are explicitly stated for the semantic network. Consider the relay coil R2_COIL in Figure 4.40. This is modeled as a Flow Sensor because the relay coil generates the EMG signal R2_CM when dc current D3 is applied. In general, a Flow Sensor may generate a spurious flow in spite of a Zero feed-flow rate. However, for the relay coil, such a spurious failure is improbable. Thus the relay-coil failure—R2_COIL remaining energized without current D3—is prohibited. This is registered as a boundary condition at the R2_COIL equipment node.

4.6.3 Event Development Rules

4.6.3.1 Type of events and rules. Figure 4.41 shows (in round boxes) two more types of events in addition to the flow triple events about flow rate, generation rate, and aperture (shown in rectangles). These are equipment_suspected (generation-rate-controller suspected and aperture-controller suspected) and equipment-failure events (generation-rate-controller failure and aperture-controller failure). The equipment_suspected event indicates that a piece of equipment is suspected as being the cause of an event. This event is developed as an equipment failure, that is, a failure of the equipment itself, a command-flow failure, or a feed-flow failure. The latter two failures are flow triple events such as (command, flow rate, Zero) and (feed, flow rate, Zero). An equipment failure usually becomes a basic FT event.

The three types of events are related to each other through event development rules, shown by arrows in Figure 4.41.

1. **Flow triple to flow triple:** Consider, for instance, the flow triple (D1, flow rate, Zero) in the semantic network of Figure 4.40. There are two DFC aperture controllers PS1 and S1 around flow D1. The flow triple event can be developed into an OR combination of (D1, generation rate, Zero) or (D1, aperture, F_Cl); the second event is included because of the existence of aperture controllers around D1. The D1 flow-rate event is developed into the generation rate and aperture event at the same flow; this is a self-loop development. The triple (D1, generation rate, Zero) thus developed turns out to be impossible because of the boundary condition at node D1, (D1, generation rate, Positive).
2. **Flow triple to equipment_suspected:** Consider again the triple (D1, aperture, F_Cl) in Figure 4.40. All aperture controllers around flow D1 are suspected, thus yielding an OR combination of two equipment_suspected events: PS1 is suspected of being F_Cl or S1 is suspected of being F_Cl. The aperture event at D1 is developed into events at adjacent equipment nodes, PS1 and S1.

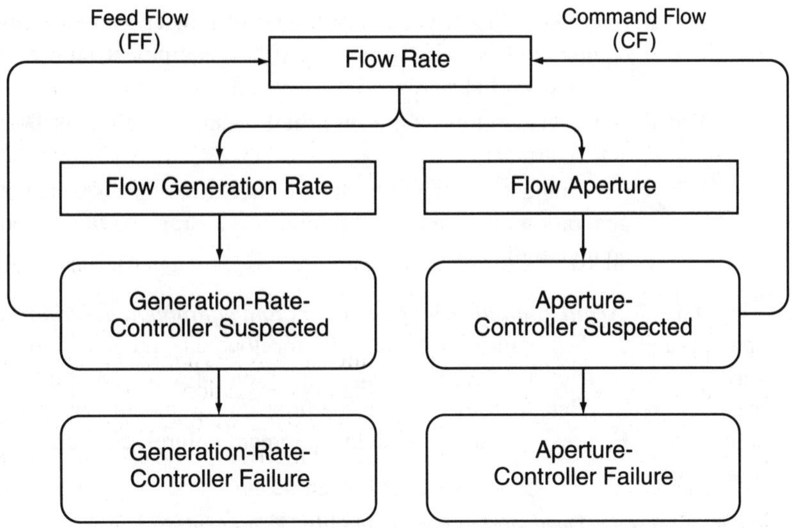

Figure 4.41. Flow rate event development.

3. **Equipment_suspected to flow triple:** Consider the equipment_suspected event that PS1 is F_Cl. PS1 is a DFC with a positive gain, and has command DWPH, as shown in Figure 4.40. Thus an event development rule for DFC yields a triple (DWPH, flow rate, Zero) for the command flow. The equipment_suspected event at PS1 is developed into an event at adjacent flow node DWPH.

   Consider next an equipment_suspected event about Junction J1. This Junction was suspected as a cause of (D3, generation rate, Zero). Thus, the equipment suspected is developed into an AND combination of the two feed-flow (FF) triples: (D1, flow rate, Zero) and (D2, flow rate, Zero).

4. **Equipment_suspected to equipment failure:** Consider the equipment_suspected event that PS1 is F_Cl. This is developed into the equipment failure, that is, pressure switch is inadvertently stuck in an off state.

   A flow node event is eventually developed into events at adjacent equipment nodes via a self-loop. An equipment-node event is analyzed into adjacent-flow-node event and equipment-failure events. This process is repeated. Event development rules determine local directions to be followed on semantic network paths.

4.6.3.2 Examples of rules.

R1: if ((flow, flow rate, Zero) **and** (there exists an equipment-controlling aperture for the flow)) **then** ((flow, aperture, F_Cl) **or** (flow, generation rate, Zero)).

R2: if ((flow, flow rate, Zero) **and** (no equipment exists to control the flow aperture)) **then** (flow, generation rate, Zero).

R3: if (flow, aperture, F_Cl) **then** ((suspect flow-aperture controllers as OR causes for the F_Cl aperture).

R4: if ((equipment is suspected as a cause of flow aperture being F_Cl) **and** (the equipment is OCE, positive gain)) **then** (command flow rate to the equipment is Zero) **or** (F_Cl failure of the equipment).

R5: if ((equipment is suspected as a cause of flow aperture's being F_Cl) **and** (the equipment is NCE)) **then** ((the equipment-failure mode F_Cl is surely_occurring).

R6: if (flow, generation rate, Zero) **then** (suspect equipment pointed to by flow-source arrow).

R7: if ((equipment pointed to by flow-source arrow is suspected of causing a Zero generation rate) **and** (the equipment is a Branch)) **then** (feed-flow rate to the equipment is Zero).

4.6.3.3 Acquisition of rules from tables and equipment definitions. Event development rules can be obtained systematically for flow rate and generation rate and aperture attributes. Flow rates are developed into generation rates and apertures by Table 4.6. Table 4.7 is used to relate flow apertures to apertures for equipment along the flow. Equipment definitions in Figures 4.37 and 4.38 yield equipment failures, command failures, and feed-flow failures.

4.6.4 Recursive Three-Value Procedure for FT Generation

4.6.4.1 Procedural schematic and FT truncation. A top event is represented as a flow triple for a flow node. This node is called a top-event node. The FT generation process is illustrated in Figure 4.42 where the event, case, and rule layers appear in sequence. If two or more rules apply to an event, an OR gate is included in the case layer to represent the rule applications. A rule yielding an AND or OR combination of causes becomes an AND or OR gate in the rule layer. New causes are added to the event layer by executing the rule.

Consider as an example event 3 in Figure 4.42. Rules $R4$ and $R5$ are applicable to event 3, so OR gate C2 is introduced to reflect the two possible cases for event development. Rule $R4$ is triggered, yielding an AND combination of events 5 and 6. In a similar way, event 5 is developed using rules $R7$ and $R8$, yielding events $B6$ and $B7$, respectively; event 6 is developed by rule $R9$, yielding event $B8$.

As event development proceeds, we eventually encounter an event where one of three logic values, surely_occurring (*yes*), surely_not_occurring (*no*), and uncertain (*unknown*), can be assigned. The value assignment takes place in one of the following cases, and downward development is terminated: flow-node recurrence (see Section 4.6.4.2), a boundary condition, and an equipment failure. An example of a *yes* event is NCE being F_Cl. An example of a *no* event is that the generation rate of D1 in Figure 4.40 is Zero, which contradicts the Positive rate boundary condition. On the other hand, (OP1, flow rate, Zero) is an *unknown* value event because flow OP1 has a free boundary condition (OP1, flow rate, ?).

From upward propagation of these values, each event or gate is assigned a logic value. The three-value logic in Table 4.8 is used to propagate the values toward the tree top via intermediate events and gates. *Yes* and *no* events and gates are excluded from the FT because they represent FT boundary conditions. Only *unknown* events and gates are retained in the finished FT because they have small to medium probabilities.

A branch denoted by the solid line in Figure 4.42 consists of a continuous series of *unknown* values. Events $B6$, $B7$, and $B8$ have truth values *no*, *yes*, and *unknown*, respectively. These values are propagated upward, resulting in an *unknown* branch from $B8$ to the output of AND gate $R4$. Rule $R5$ yields event $B3$ with truth value *unknown*. This value is propagated upward, resulting in an *unknown* branch from $B3$ to the output of OR gate $R5$. The two branches are combined, yielding a subtree that develops event 3.

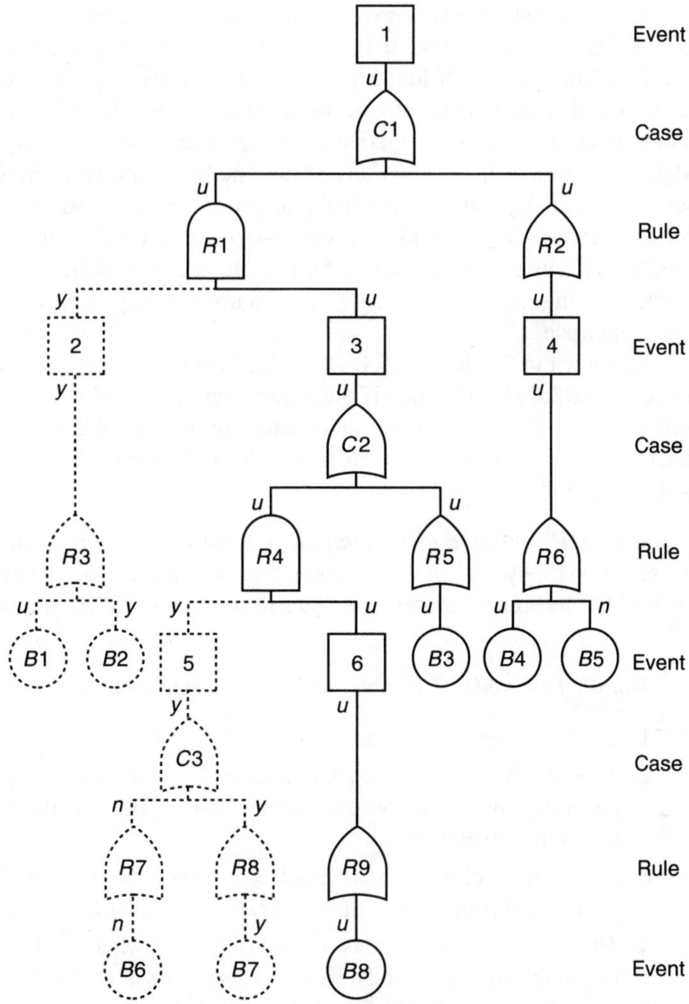

Figure 4.42. Downward event development and upward truth propagation.

TABLE 4.8. Three-Value Logic for Upward Truth Value Propagation

A	***B***	***A* AND *B***	***A* OR *B***
yes	*yes*	*yes*	*yes*
yes	*no*	*no*	*yes*
yes	*unknown*	*unknown*	*yes*
no	*yes*	*no*	*yes*
no	*no*	*no*	*no*
no	*unknown*	*no*	*unknown*
unknown	*yes*	*unknown*	*yes*
unknown	*no*	*no*	*unknown*
unknown	*unknown*	*unknown*	*unknown*

The general process illustrated in Figure 4.42 can be programmed into a recursive procedure that is a three-value generalization of a well-known backtracking algorithm [19].

4.6.4.2 Flow-node recurrence as house event. Consider the event, the flow rate of R2_CM is Zero, in the network in Figure 4.40. A cause is a Zero-generation-rate event at the same flow. This type of self-loop is required for a step-by-step event development. However, because the flow node is in a loop, the same flow node, R2_CM, will be encountered for reasons other than the self-loop, that is, the recurrence occurs via other equipment or flow nodes. To prevent infinite iterations of flow node, a truth value must be returned when a flow-node recurrence other than a self-loop type is encountered. The generation procedure returns *unknown*. This means that a one-step-earlier event at the recurring flow node is included as a house event in the FT. As a result, one-step-earlier time series conditions are specified for all recurrent flow nodes. The recurrence may occur for a flow node other than a top-event node.

As shown in Section 4.6.5.1, (R2_CM, flow rate, Zero) is included as a house event for the Zero R2_CM fault tree. If the house event is turned on, this indicates that the top event continues to exist. On the other hand, turning off the house event means that the R2_CM flow rate changes from Positive to Zero. Different FTs are obtained by assigning on-off values to house events.

4.6.4.3 FT module identification. Fault-tree modules considerably simplify FT representations, physical interpretations, and minimal cut set generations [20,21].* The proposed FT generation approach enables us to identify FT modules and their hierarchical structure.

Module flow node. Define the following symbols.

1. T: A top-event flow node.
2. $N \neq T$: A flow node reachable from T. This ensures a possibility that the FT generation procedure may encounter node N because the top-event development traces the labeled arrows.
3. $U(N)$: A set of flow nodes appearing in one or more paths from T to N. Node N is excluded from the definition of $U(N)$. Symbol U stands for upstream.
4. $D(N)$: A set of flow nodes reachable from N where each reachability check path is terminated immediately after it visits a node in $U(N)$. Node N is removed from the definition of $D(N)$. Symbol D stands for downstream.
5. $R(N) = U(N) \cap D(N)$: A set of flow nodes commonly included in $U(N)$ and $D(N)$. This is a set of nodes in $U(N)$ that may recur in $D(N)$. Symbol R stands for recurrence.

Consider, for instance, the semantic network in Figure 4.40. For top-event node $T = \text{R2\_CM}$ we observe:

$$U(\text{D1}) = \{\text{R2\_CM, D3}\}, \quad D(\text{D1}) = \{\text{OP1, DWPH}\}, \quad R(\text{D1}) = \phi \tag{4.1}$$

$$U(\text{D2}) = \{\text{R2\_CM, D3}\}, \quad D(\text{D2}) = \{\text{OP2, R2\_CM}\}, \quad R(\text{D2}) = \{\text{R2\_CM}\} \tag{4.2}$$

Flow node N is called a module node when either condition C1 or C2 holds. Module node N is displayed in Figure 4.43.

C1: Sets $U(N)$ and $D(N)$ are mutually exclusive, that is, $R(N) = \phi$.

C2: Each path from T to N has every node in $R(N)$.

---

*Minimal cut sets are defined in Chapter 5.

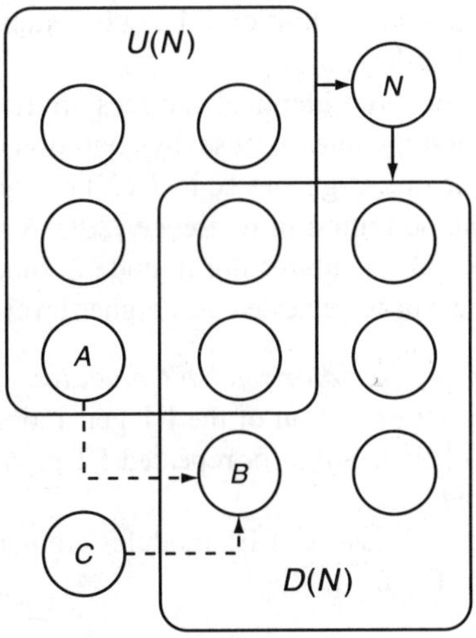

Figure 4.43. Module flow node N.

Nodes D1 and D2 satisfy conditions C1 and C2, respectively. Thus these are module flow nodes. The downstream development of a flow triple at node N remains identical for each access path through $U(N)$ because neither node in $U(N)$ recurs in $D(N)$ when condition C1 holds, and $R(N)$ nodes recur in $D(N)$ in the same way for each access path from T to N when condition C2 holds. One or more identical subtrees may be generated at node N, hence the name module flow node.

Repeated module node. Module node N is called a repeated module node when condition C3 holds.

C3: Node N is reachable from T by two or more access paths. Neither node D1 nor D2 satisfies this condition.

Suppose that the FT generation procedure creates the same flow triple at node N by the two or more access paths. This requirement is checked on-line, while conditions C1 to C3 can be examined off-line by the semantic network before execution of FT generation procedure. Two or more identical subtrees are generated for the same flow triple at node N.

Another set of access paths may create a different flow triple. However, the unique flow triple is likely to occur because node N in a coherent system has a unique role in causing the top event. The repeated structure simplifies FT representation and Boolean manipulations, although the structure cannot be replaced by a higher level basic event because a subtree at node B of Figure 4.43 may appear both in node N subtree and node A subtree. The repeated subtree is not a module in the sense of reference [20].

Solid-module node. Module node N is called a solid-module node when condition C4 holds.

C4: Each node in $D(N)$ is reachable from T only through N. In this case broken-line arrows do not exist in Figure 4.43. Nodes D1 and D2 are examples of solid-module nodes.

Suppose that the FT generation procedure creates a unique flow triple every time solid-module node N is visited through nodes in $U(N)$. The uniqueness is likely to occur for a coherent system. Condition C4 can be examined off-line, while the flow triple uniqueness is checked on-line.

One or more identical subtrees are now generated at node N. This subtree can be called a solid module because, by condition C4, the subtree provides a unique place where all the basic events generated in $D(N)$ can appear. The solid FT module is consistent with the module definition in reference [20]. A subtree at node B of Figure 4.43 may appear neither in node A subtree nor in node C subtree when condition C4 is satisfied. The solid FT module can be regarded as a higher level basic event.

Repeated- and/or solid-FT modules. Solid- or repeated-module nodes can be registered before execution of the FT generation procedure because conditions C1 to C4 are checked off-line. Solid- or repeated-FT modules are generated when relevant on-line conditions hold.

The two classes of FT modules are not necessarily exclusive, as shown by the Venn diagram of Figure 4.44:

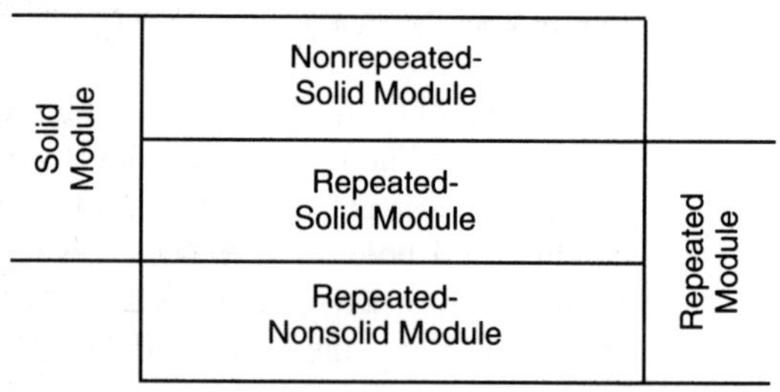

Figure 4.44. Venn diagram of solid and repeated modules.

1. A nonrepeated-solid module is obtained when solid-module node N does not satisfy condition C3. The single-occurrence solid module has a practical value because it is an isolated subtree that can be replaced by a higher level basic event. This class of FT modules is generated in Section 4.6.5.1 for node D1 and D2.
2. A repeated-solid module, which is qualitatively more valuable, is obtained when solid-module node N satisfies condition C3 or when repeated-module node N satisfies condition C4. The module corresponds to a repeated higher level basic event. Examples are given in Sections 4.6.5.2 and 4.6.5.3.
3. A repeated-nonsolid module is obtained when repeated-module node N does not satisfy condition C4. Such FT modules are generated in Section 4.6.5.2.

Hierarchical structure of FT modules. Suppose that node B in $D(N)$ of Figure 4.43 is also a solid- or repeated-module node. FT modules at node N now include an FT module at node B when a relevant on-line condition holds at node B. For a repeated-nonsolid-FT module at node N, the FT module at node B may appear not only in the module at node N but also in other upstream subtrees such as for nodes A or C of Figure 4.43. For a solid-FT module at node N, the FT module at node B only appears below this solid module. In each of these cases, a module hierarchy is generated. An example is given in Section 4.6.5.2.

4.6.5 Examples

4.6.5.1 A relay circuit. Consider the relay circuit shown in Figures 4.39 and 4.40. The top event is "Flow rate of drywell pressure high signal, R2_CM, is Zero" under the boundary conditions in Section 4.6.2.3. The fault tree generated is shown as Figure 4.45. Nodes D1 and D2 are solid-module nodes. The FT generation procedure generates a unique flow triple at each of these nodes. The SM1 subtree (line 5) and SM2 subtree (line 15) are identified as two nonrepeated-solid-FT modules.

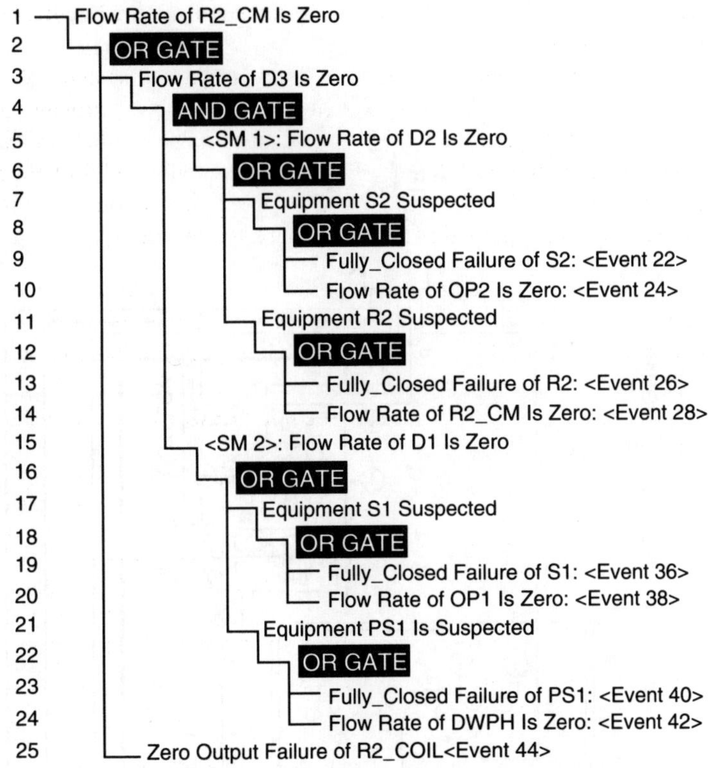

Figure 4.45. Relay-circuit fault tree.

A flow-node recurrence was encountered at Event 28 (line 14) dealing with the same flow-attribute pair as the top event, flow rate of R2_CM; the value *unknown* was returned.

Event 28 at the recurrent-flow node is a house event, and two cases exist:

1. If Event 28 is true, then the top event T becomes

$$T = 36 + 38 + 40 + 42 + 44 \tag{4.3}$$

This corresponds to the case where drywell pressure high signal, R2_CM, continues to remain off, thus causing the top event to occur. One event cut set {38} implies that the drywell pressure high signal remains off because manual switch S1 is left off.

2. If Event 28 is false, the top event is

$$T = (22 + 24 + 26)(36 + 38 + 40 + 42) + 44 \tag{4.4}$$

This corresponds to a case where the high pressure signal ceases to be on after its activation. Two-event cut set {22, 36} implies that both manual switches S1 and S2 are off, thus causing the deactivation.

The semantic network of Figure 4.40 can be used to generate an FT with the different top event "Flow rate of drywell pressure high signal R2_CM is Positive" under the boundary condition that the DWPH phenomenon does not exist. Such an FT shows possible causes of relay-circuit spurious activation. An FT similar to Figure 4.45 has been successfully generated for a large ECCS model. ■

4.6.5.2 A hypothetical swimming pool reactor. Consider the hypothetical swimming pool reactor in Figure 4.46 [22]. System components, flows, and a system-semantic network are shown in Figure 4.47.

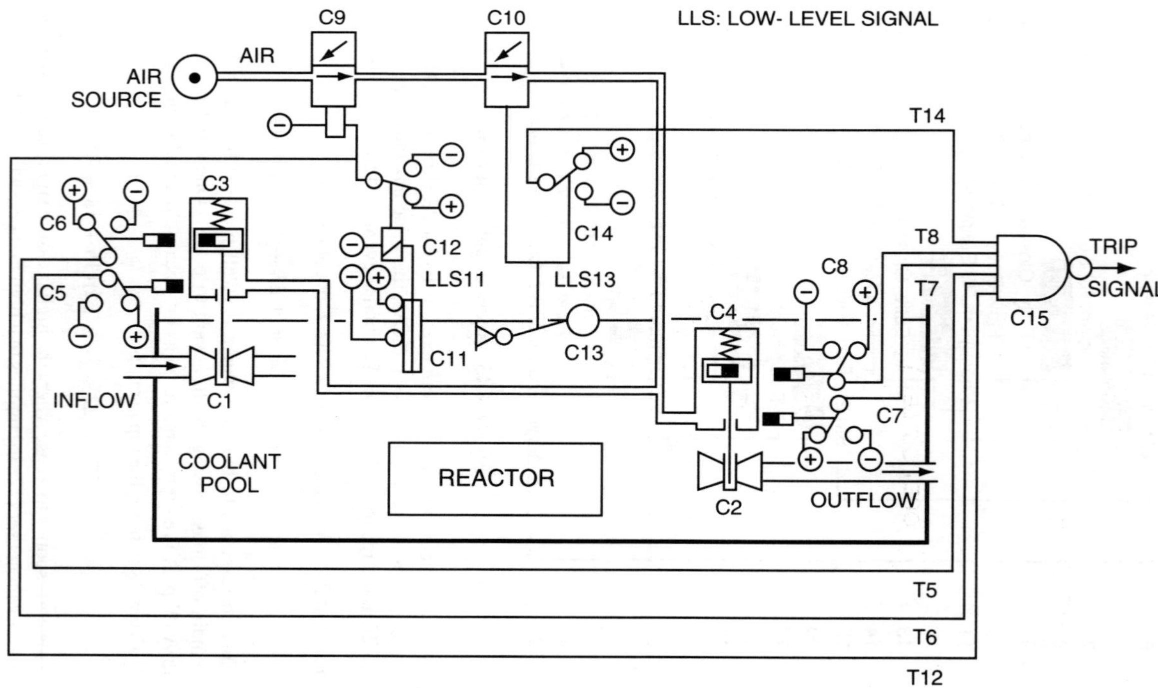

Figure 4.46 Hypothetical swimming pool reactor.

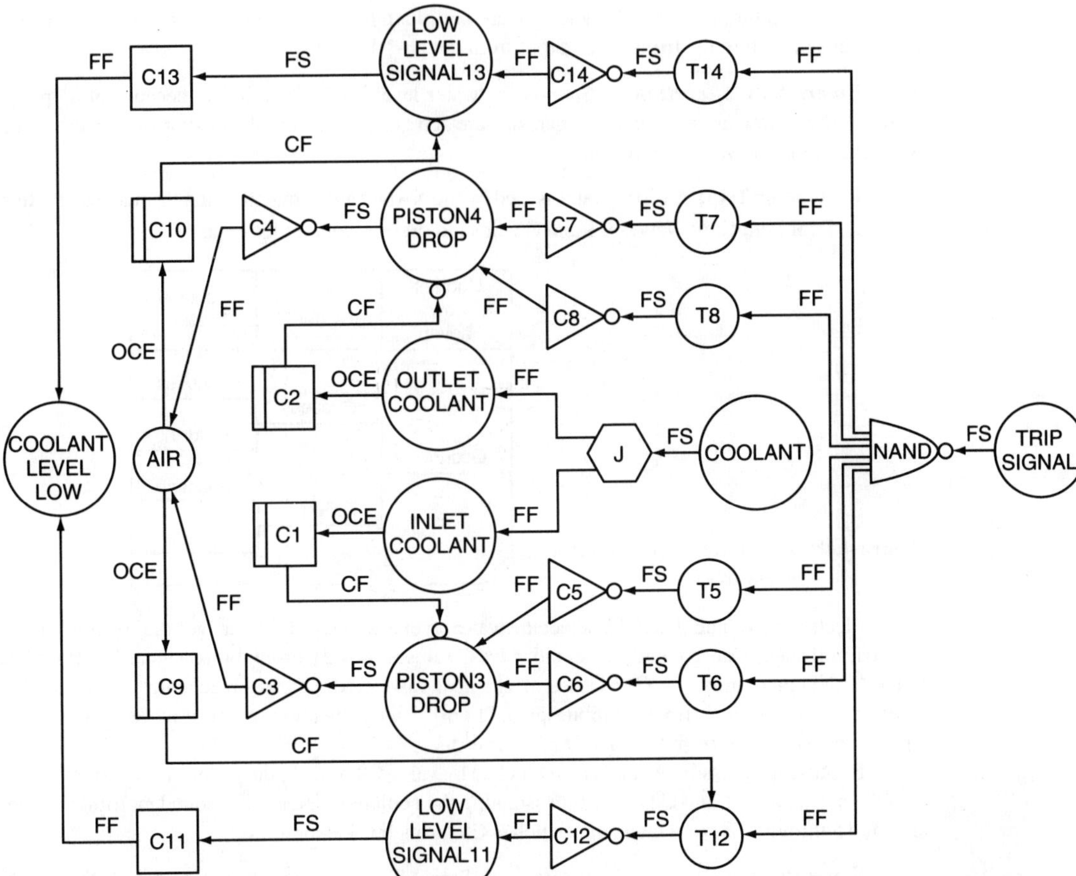

Equip.	Description	Library	Flow	Description
C1	Inlet valve	OCE	AIR	Actuator air
C2	Outlet valve	OCE	COOLANT	Coolant flow
C3	Inlet actuator	NOT	INLET COOLANT	Inlet coolant
C4	Outlet actuator	NOT	OUTLET COOLANT	Outlet coolant
C5	Magnet switch 5	NOT	COOLANT LEVEL LOW	Coolant level low phenomenon
C6	Magnet switch 6	NOT		
C7	Magnet switch 7	NOT	LOW LEVEL SIGNAL 11	Low level signal from electrode
C8	Magnet switch 8	NOT		
C9	Solenoid valve	OCE	LOW LEVEL SIGNAL 13	Low level signal from float
C10	Mechanical valve	OCE		
C11	Electrode bar	Flow Sensor	PISTON 3 DROP	C3 drop phenomenon
C12	Solenoid switch	NOT	PISTON 4 DROP	C4 drop phenomenon
C13	Float	Flow Sensor	Ti	Trip inhibition signal from Ci
C14	Mechanical switch	NOT		
NAND	NAND gate	NAND	TRIP SIGNAL	Trip signal from NAND gate
J	Junction node	Junction		

Figure 4.47. Swimming pool reactor semantic network representation.

Normal operation. Pressurized air (AIR) flows through solenoid valve C9 and mechanical valve C10 in series. Inlet and outlet actuators C3 and C4 respectively cause inlet and outlet valves C1 and C2 to open. The coolant enters the pool via inlet valve C1, and exits the pool via outlet valve

C2. Switches C5 through C8, C12, and C14 are on (plus), hence all the input signals to NAND gate are on, thus inhibiting the trip-signal output from the NAND gate.

Emergency operation. Suppose a "water level low" event occurs because of a "piping failure." The following protective mechanisms are activated to prevent the reactor from overheating. An event tree is shown in Figure 4.48.

1. **Reactor Trip:** A trip signal is issued by the NAND gate, thus stopping the nuclear reaction.
2. **Pool Isolation:** Valves C1 and C2 close to prevent coolant leakage.

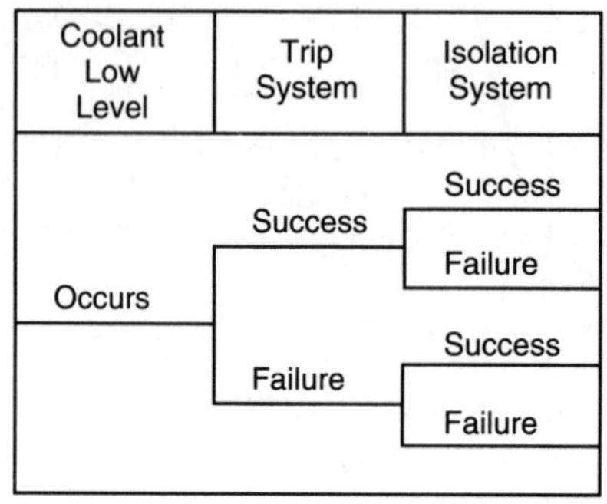

Figure 4.48. A swimming-pool reactor event tree.

Electrode C11 and float C13 detect the water level low event. C11 changes the solenoid switch C12 to its off state. Consequently, solenoid valve C9 closes, while trip-inhibition signal T12 from C12 to the NAND gate turns off. C13 closes mechanical valve C10, changes mechanical switch C14 to its off state, thus turning trip-inhibition signal T14 off. By nullification of one or more trip-inhibition signals, the trip signal from the NAND gate turns on.

Because the pressurized air is now blocked by valve C9 or C10, the pistons in actuators C3 and C4 fall, and valves C1 and C2 close, thus isolating the coolant in the pool. Redundant trip-inhibition signals T5 through T8 from magnetic switches C5 through C8 also turn off.

Semantic network representation. Signal T14 in Figure 4.46 goes to off, that is, the T14 flow rate becomes Zero when the flow rate of LOW LEVEL SIGNAL 13 from float is Positive. Therefore, mechanical switch C14 is modeled as a NOT. Switches C5, C6, C7, C8, and C12 are also modeled as NOTs.

The aperture controllers are C1, C2, C9, and C10. Mechanical valve C10 is changed from an open to a closed state by a LOW LEVEL SIGNAL 13 command, hence C10 is modeled as an OCE. The OCE gain is negative because the valve closes when the command signal exists. The negative gain is denoted by a small circle at the head of the arrow labeled CF from C10 to LOW LEVEL SIGNAL 13. Mechanical valve C10 controls the AIR aperture. The aperture is also controlled by solenoid valve C9, which is modeled as an OCE with command flow T12. The OCE gain is positive because C9 closes when T12 turns off. Two OCEs are observed around AIR in Figure 4.47.

The outlet coolant aperture is controlled by valve C2 as an OCE with command flow as the phenomenon "PISTON 4 DROP." The aperture of the inlet coolant is controlled by valve C1, an OCE. Flow COOLANT denotes either the inflowing or the outflowing movement of the coolant, and has Junction J as its generation-rate controller with feed flows of INLET COOLANT and OUTLET COOLANT. The COOLANT flow rate is Zero when the flow rates of INLET COOLANT and OUTLET COOLANT are both Zero. This indicates a successful pool isolation.

Boundary conditions. Assume the following boundary conditions for FT generation.

1. The COOLANT LEVEL LOW flow rate is a positive constant (Cons), causing the occurrence of a low level coolant phenomenon.

2. Generation rates of AIR, OUTLET COOLANT, and INLET COOLANT are positive and constant (Cons). This implies that the pool isolation occurs if and only if C1 and C2 apertures become F_Cl.

Trip-failure FT. Consider "Trip signal flow rate is Zero" as a top event. The fault tree of Figure 4.49 is obtained. The generation procedure traces the semantic network in the following order: 1) NAND gate as a flow source (FS) of the trip signal, 2) trip-inhibition signal T14 as a feed flow (FF) to the NAND gate, 3) mechanical switch C14 as a flow source for T14, 4) LOW LEVEL SIGNAL 13 as a feed flow to switch C14, 5) float C13 as a flow source of LOW LEVEL SIGNAL 13, 6) COOLANT LEVEL LOW as a feed flow to float C13, and so on.

FT modules. Despite the various monitor/control functions, the semantic-network model turns out to have no loops. Thus condition C1 in Section 4.6.4.3 is always satisfied. Condition C3 in Section 4.6.4.3 is satisfied for the following flow nodes: PISTON 3 DROP, PISTON 4 DROP, AIR, T12, LOW LEVEL SIGNAL 13, and COOLANT LEVEL LOW. These nodes are registered as repeated-module nodes (Table 4.9). At each of these nodes, a unique flow triple event is revisited, and repeated-FT modules are generated: RM92 for PISTON 3 DROP (lines 18, 22), RM34 for PISTON 4 DROP (lines 10, 14), RM40 for AIR (lines 28, 32), RSM54 for T12 (lines 24, 42), and RSM18 for LOW LEVEL SIGNAL 13 (lines 6, 38). COOLANT LEVEL LOW is a repeated-module node but the FT module is reduced to a surely_occurring event because of the boundary condition. LOW LEVEL SIGNAL 13 and T12 are also solid-module nodes satisfying condition C4 in Section 4.6.4.3, and RSM18 and RSM54 become repeated-solid-FT modules. RSM18 can be replaced by a repeated basic event, while RSM54 can be replaced by a repeated, higher level basic event. The module FTs form the hierarchical structure shown in Figure 4.50.

TABLE 4.9. List of repeated module nodes

Repeated Module Node
PISTON 3 DROP
PISTON 4 DROP
AIR
T12
LOW LEVEL SIGNAL 13
COOLANT LEVEL LOW

A fault tree for the pool isolation failure is shown in Figure 4.51. This corresponds to the third column heading in Figure 4.48. Fault trees for the two event-tree headings are generated using the same semantic network. ■

4.6.5.3 A chemical reactor.

Normal operation. Consider the chemical reactor shown in Figure 4.52. This plant is similar to the one in reference [5] and in Figure 4.25. Flow sensor FL-S1 monitors the feed-flow rate; the actuator air (A1) aperture is controlled by actuator ACT1; the flow-control valve FCV (air-to-open) aperture is controlled by the A1 flow rate; the flow rate of feed flow M1 is regulated by the feedback control. Bypass valve BV is normally closed.

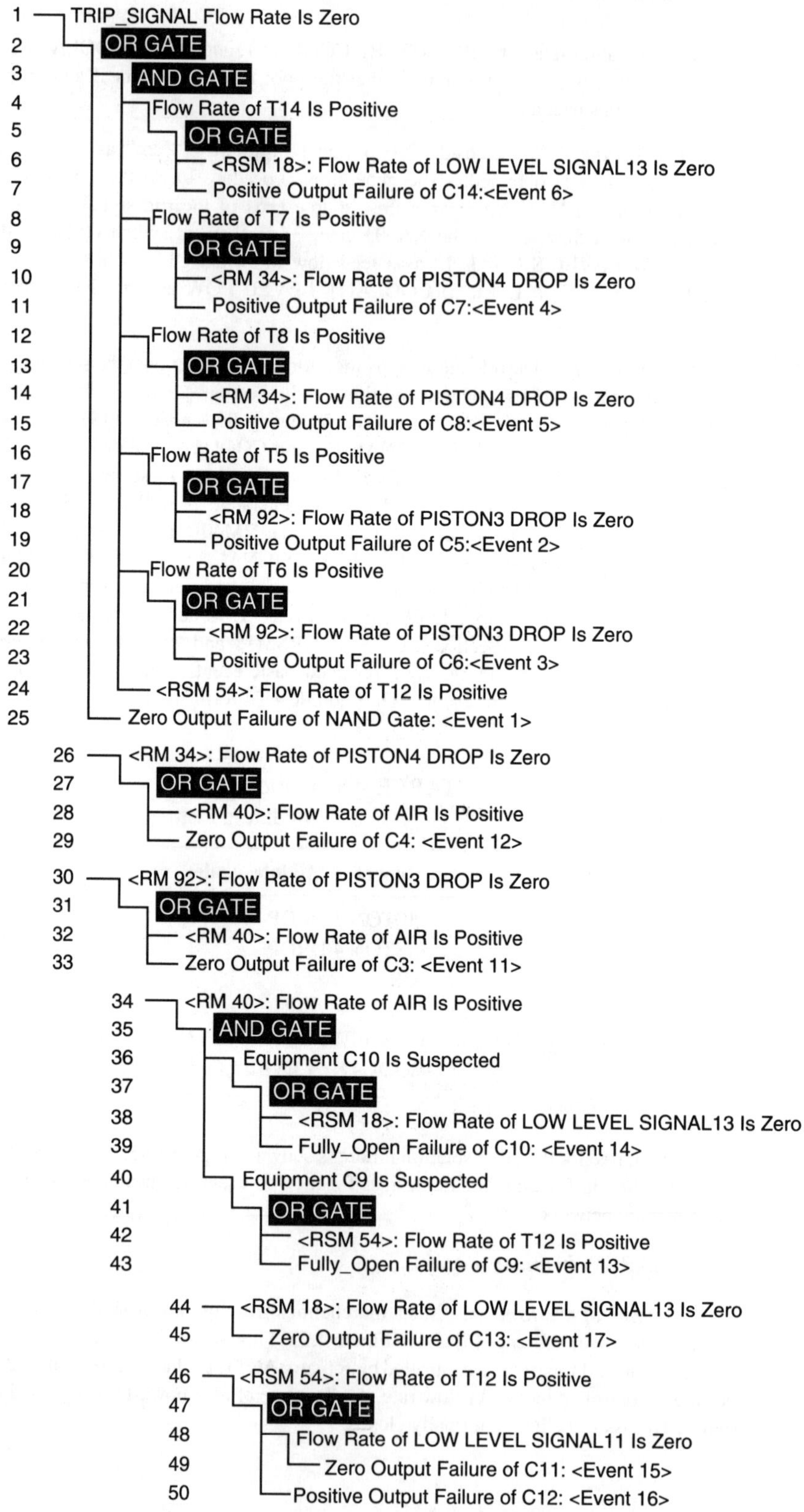

Figure 4.49. Swimming-pool-reactor fault tree for trip failure.

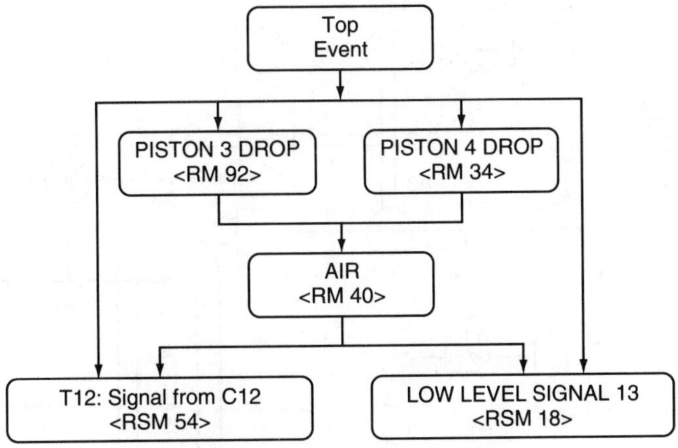

Figure 4.50. Module hierarchy.

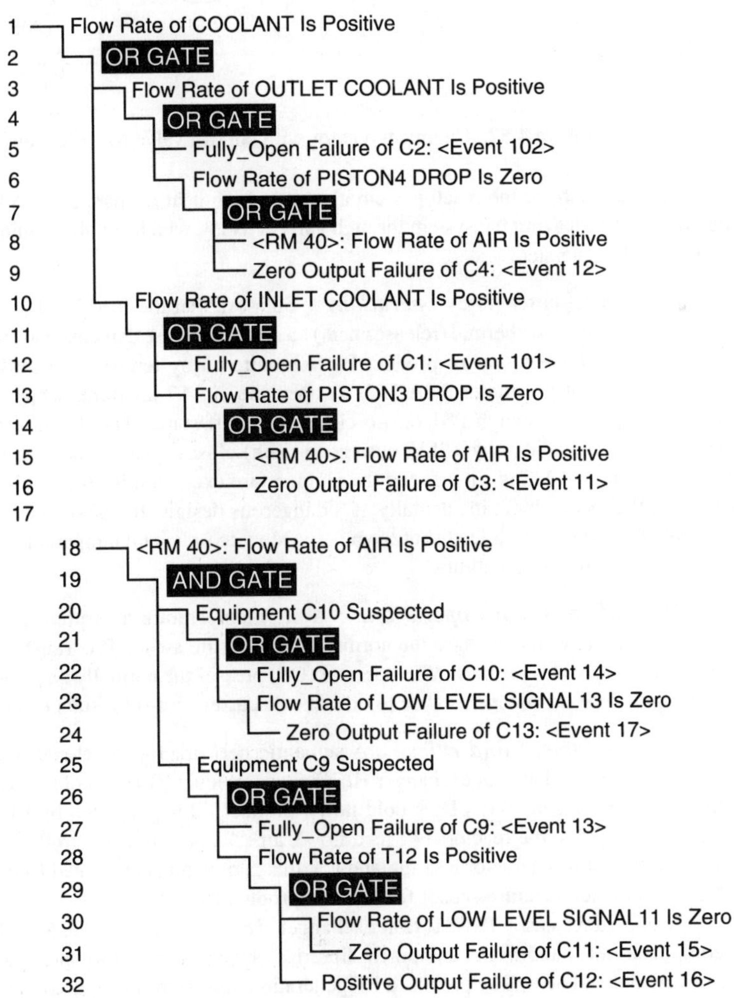

Figure 4.51. Pool-isolation-failure fault tree.

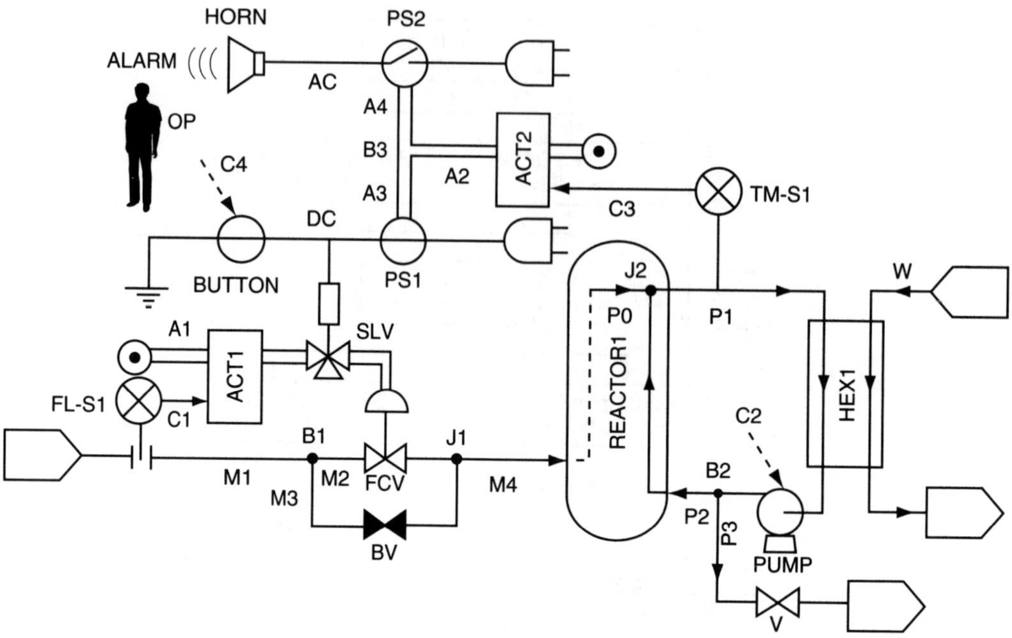

Figure 4.52. Chemical reactor with control valve for feed shutdown.

Product P1 from the reactor is circulated through heat exchanger HEX1 by pump (PUMP). The product flow leaving the system through valve V is P3, which equals P1 minus P2; flow P0 is the product newly generated.

Automated emergency operation. Suppose that the feed M4 flow rate increases. The chemical reaction is exothermic (releases heat) so a flow increase can create a dangerous temperature excursion. The temperature of product P1 is monitored by temperature sensor TM-S1. A high temperature activates actuator 2 (ACT2) to open the air A2 aperture, which in turn changes the normally on pressure switch PS1 (air-to-close) to its off state. The dc current is cut off, and the normally open solenoid valve (SLV; current-to-open) closes. Air A1 is cut off, flow-control valve FCV is closed, feed M2 is cut off, and the temperature excursion is prevented. The FCV is used to shut down the feed, which, incidentally, is a dangerous design. It is assumed for simplicity that the response of the system to a feed shutdown is too slow to prevent a temperature excursion by loss of heat exchanger cooling capability.

Manual emergency operation. A high-temperature measurement results in an air A4 flow rate increase, which changes the normally off pressure switch PS2 (air-to-open) to an on state. The ac current activates the horn. The operator (OP) presses the normally on panic button (BUTTON; operation-to-close) to change its state to off. The dc current cut-off results in a feed shutdown.

New equipment and rules. A semantic network for the chemical reactor is shown in Figure 4.53. We see that heat exchanger HEX1 cools product P1 (CS: cold source), the coolant flow to the heat exchange is W (CLD_F: cold flow), product P0 is generated by REACTOR1 (FS: flow source), M4 is fed to the reactor (FF: feed flow), air A2 aperture is controlled by actuator ACT2, a command flow of this actuator is command C3, this command is generated from temperature sensor TM-S1, and the temperature-sensor feed flow is product P1.

Temperature sensor TM-S1, heat exchanger HEX1, and reactor REACTOR1 are three pieces of equipment not found in the equipment libraries. New event development rules specific to these devices are defined here. The proposed FT-generation approach can be used for a variety of systems with only the addition of new types of equipment and rules.

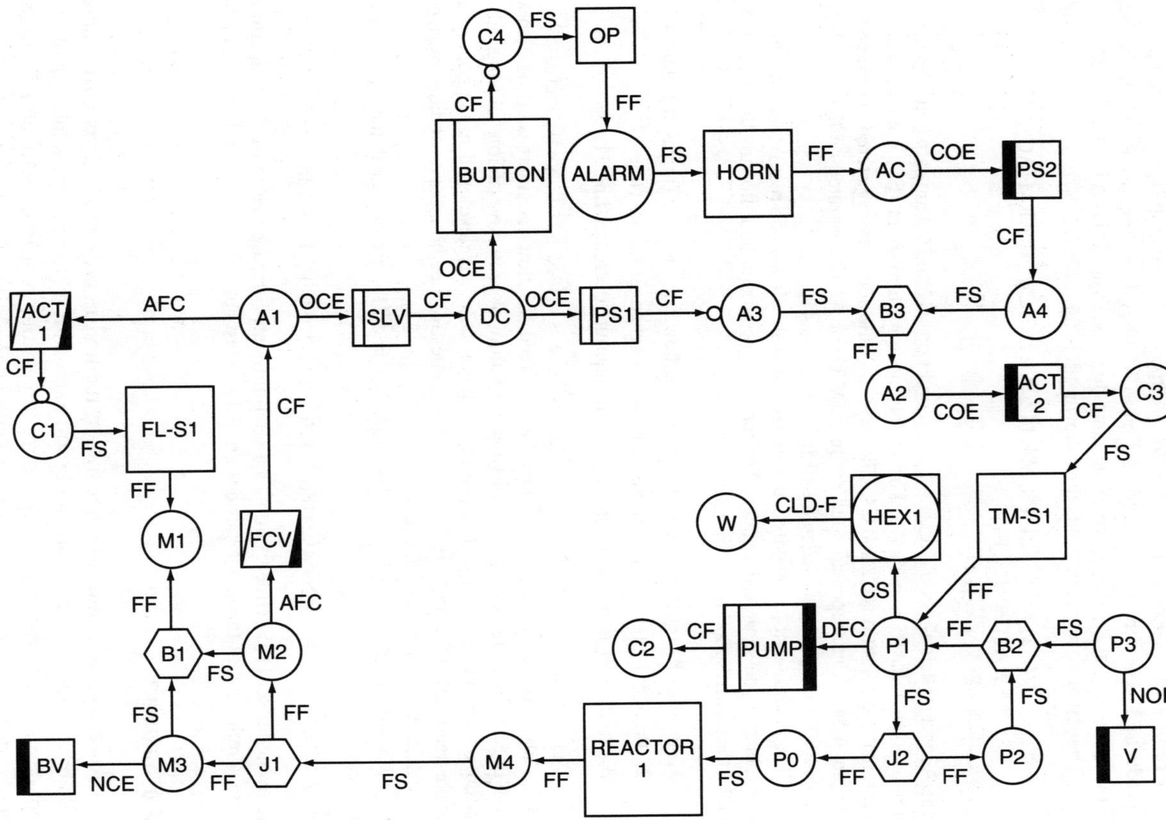

Figure 4.53. Chemical-reactor semantic-network representation.

Boundary conditions.

1. Flow rates of coolant W and command C2 are subject to free boundary conditions.
2. Generation rates of M1, A1, A2, DC, and AC are positive constants (Cons).

Temperature-excursion FT with modules. Consider the top event, temperature increase of product P2. The semantic network of Figure 4.53 has three loops: one is loop P2-B2-P1-J2-P2; the other two start at P1 and return to the same flow node via J2, J1, A1, DC, and B3.

The semantic network yields the following sets for node A2:

$$U(\text{A2}) = \{\text{P2, P1, P0, M4, M2, A1, DC, C4, ALARM, AC, A4, A3}\}$$
$$D(\text{A2}) = \{\text{C3, P1}\}$$
$$R(\text{A2}) = \{\text{P1}\}$$

Node A2 is a repeated-module node because conditions C2 and C3 are satisfied. We have long paths from top-event node P2 to node A2. Fortunately, node A1 turns out to be a nonrepeated-solid-module node satisfying conditions C2 and C4. These two module nodes are registered. The fault tree is shown in Figure 4.54. A nonrepeated-solid module SM65 for A1 is generated on line 16. Repeated-solid module RSM119 appears twice in the SM65 tree (lines 41, 48).

The *unknown* house-event values generated at the flow-node recurrence are changed to *no*'s, thus excluding one-step-earlier states. The top event occurs in the following three cases. The second and the third correspond to cooling system failures.

1. Product P1 temperature increase by feed-flow rate increase (line 3 of Figure 4.54)
2. Product P2 temperature increase by heat-exchanger failure (line 17)
3. Product P1 temperature increase by its aperture decrease (line 21)

The first case is divided into two causes: one is a feed M3 flow-rate increase because of a bypass-valve failure (line 5), while the other is a feed M2 flow-rate increase (line 7) described by an AND gate (line 11), which has as its input a failure of protective action "closing valve FCV by shutting off air A1" (line 16). The protective-action failure is developed in the nonrepeated-solid-module tree labeled SM65 (line 25). Flow-rate values for free boundary-condition variables W and C2 are determined at event 200 (line 19) and 214 (line 24).

When cooling-system causes (200, 202, 212, and 214) are excluded, the top-event expression becomes

$$T = 49 + 165 + (182 + 192)\,[80 + 126 + 136 + (90 + 111 + 138 + 140) \cdot 142)] \tag{4.5}$$

One-event cut set {165} (line 9) implies a feed-flow-rate increase due to the FCV aperture increase failure, a reflection of the dangerous design. The largest cut set size is three; there are eight such cut sets. ■

4.6.6 Summary

An automated fault-tree-generation method is presented. It is based on the flow, attribute, and value; an equipment library; a semantic-network representation of the system; event development rules; and a recursive three-value procedure with an FT truncation and modular-decomposition capability. Boundary conditions for the network can be specified at flow and equipment nodes. Event development rules are obtained systematically from tables and equipment definitions. The three-value logic is used to truncate FTs according to boundary conditions. Only *unknown* events or gates remain in the FT. Repeated- and/or solid-FT modules and their hierarchies can be identified. From the same semantic-network-system model, different FTs are generated for different top events and boundary conditions.

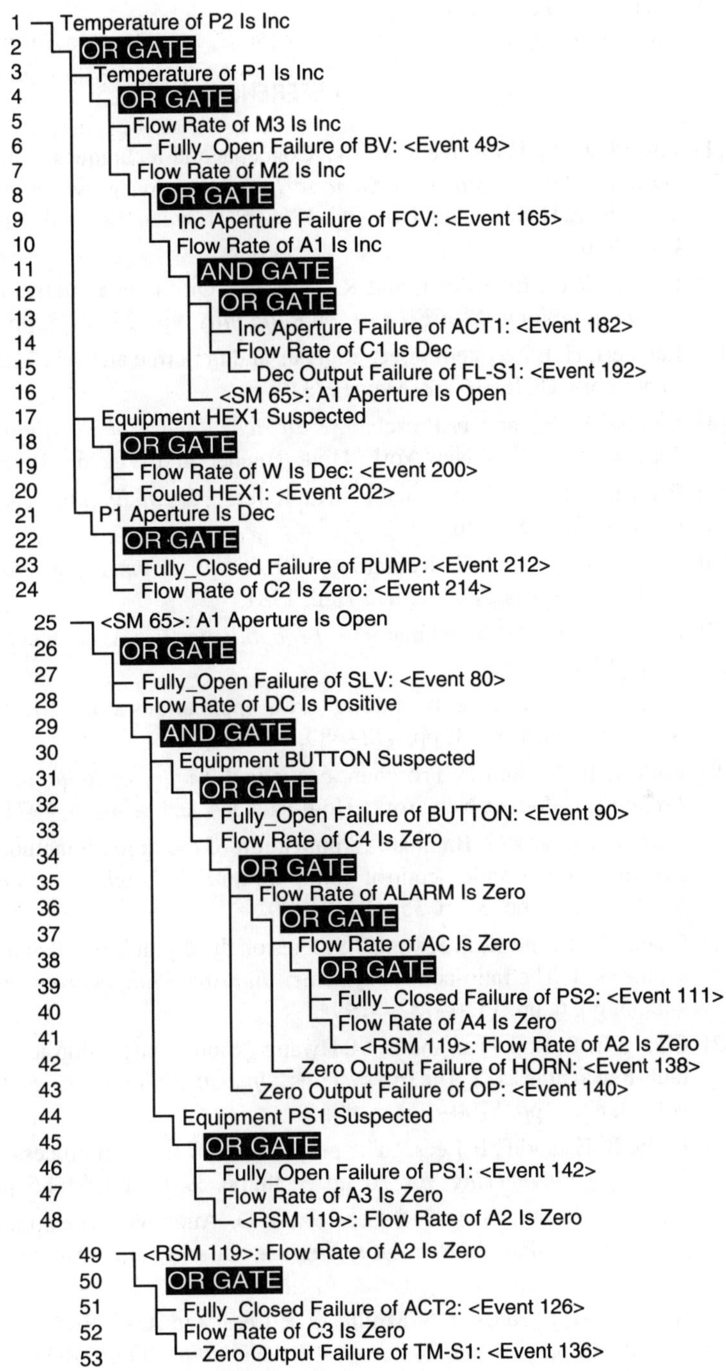

Figure 4.54. Fault tree for product temperature increase.

The generation method is demonstrated for a relay system, a hypothetical swimming-pool reactor, and a chemical reactor.

REFERENCES

[1] Fussell, J. B. "Fault tree analysis: Concepts and techniques." In *Proc. of the NATO Advanced Study Institute on Generic Techniques in Systems Reliability Assessment*, edited by E. Henley and J. Lynn, pp. 133–162. Leyden, Holland: Noordhoff Publishing Co., 1976.

[2] Fussell, J. B., E. F. Aber, and R. G. Rahl. "On the quantitative analysis of priority AND failure logic," *IEEE Trans. on Reliability*, vol. 25, no. 5, pp. 324–326, 1976.

[3] Lambert, H. E. "System safety analysis and fault tree analysis." Lawrence Livermore Laboratory, UCID-16238, May 1973.

[4] Barlow, R. E., and F. Proschan. *Statistical Theory of Reliability and Life Testing Probability Models*. New York: Holt, Rinehart and Winston, 1975.

[5] Browning, R. L. "Human factors in fault trees," *Chem. Engingeering Progress*, vol. 72, no. 6, pp. 72–75, 1976.

[6] Henley, E. J., and H. Kumamoto. *Reliability Engineering and Risk Assessment*. Englewood Cliffs, NJ: Prentice-Hall, 1981.

[7] Henley, E. J., and H. Kumamoto. *Probabilistic Risk Assessment*. New York: IEEE Press, 1992.

[8] Vesely, W. E. "Reliability and fault tress applications at the NRTS," *IEEE Trans. on Nucl. Sci.*, vol. 1, no. 1, pp. 472–480, 1971.

[9] Barlow, R. E., and E. Proschan. *Statistical Theory of Reliability and Life Testing Probability Models*. New York: Holt, Rinehart and Winston, 1975.

[10] Andrews, J., and G. Brennan. "Application of the digraph method of fault tree construction to a complex control configuration," *Reliability Engineering and System Safety*, vol. 28, no. 3, pp. 357–384, 1990.

[11] Chang, C. T., and K. S. Hwang. "Studies on the digraph-based approach for fault-tree synthesis. 1. The ratio-control systems," *Industrial Engineering Chemistry Research*, vol. 33, no. 6, pp. 1520–1529, 1994.

[12] Chang, C. T., D. S. Hsu, and D. M. Hwang. "Studies on the digraph-based approach for fault-tree synthesis. 2. The trip systems," *Industrial Engineering Chemistry Research*, vol. 33, no. 7, pp. 1700–1707, 1994.

[13] Kelly, B. E., and F. P. Lees. "The propagation of faults in process plants, Parts 1–4," *Reliability Engineering*, vol. 16, pp. 3–38, pp. 39–62, pp. 63–86, pp. 87–108, 1986.

[14] Mullhi, J. S., M. L. Ang, F. P. Lees, and J. D. Andrews. "The propagation of faults in process plants, Part 5," *Reliability Engineering and System Safety*, vol. 23, pp. 31–49, 1988.

[15] Hunt, A., B. E. Kelly, J. S. Mullhi, F. P. Lees, and A. G. Rushton. "The propagation of faults in process plants, Parts 6–10," *Reliability Engineering and System Safety*, vol. 39, pp. 173–194, pp. 195–209, pp. 211–227, pp. 229–241, pp. 243–250, 1993.

[16] Fussell, J. B. "A formal methodology for fault tree construction," *Nuclear Science Engineering*, vol. 52, pp. 421–432, 1973.

[17] Salem, S. L., G. E. Apostolakis, and D. Okrent. "A new methodology for the computer-aided construction of fault trees," *Annals of Nuclear Energy*, vol. 4, pp. 417–433, 1977.

[18] Henley, E. J., and H. Kumamoto. *Designing for Reliability and Safety Control.* Englewood Cliffs, NJ: Prentice-Hall, 1985.

[19] Nilsson, N. J. *Principles of Artificial Intelligence.* New York: McGraw-Hill, 1971.

[20] Rosental, A. "Decomposition methods for fault tree analysis," *IEEE Trans. on Reliability*, vol. 29, no. 2, pp. 136–138, 1980.

[21] Kohda, T., E. J. Henley, and K. Inoue. "Finding modules in fault trees," *IEEE Trans. on Reliability*, vol. 38, no. 2, pp. 165–176, 1989.

[22] Nicolescu, T., and R. Weber. "Reliability of systems with various functions," *Reliability Engineering*, vol. 2, pp. 147–157, 1981.

PROBLEMS

4.1. There are four way stations (Figure P4.1) on the route of the Deadeye Stages from Hangman's Hill to Placer Gulch. (Problem courtesy of J. Fussell.) The distances involved are:

Hangman's Hill–Station 1:	20 miles
Station 1–Station 2:	30 miles
Station 2–Station 3:	50 miles
Station 3–Station 4:	40 miles
Station 4–Placer Gulch:	40 miles

The maximum distance the stage can travel without a change of horses, which can only be accomplished at the way stations, is 85 miles. The stages change horses at every opportunity; however, the stations are raided frequently, and their stock driven off by marauding desperadoes.

Draw a fault tree for the system of stations.

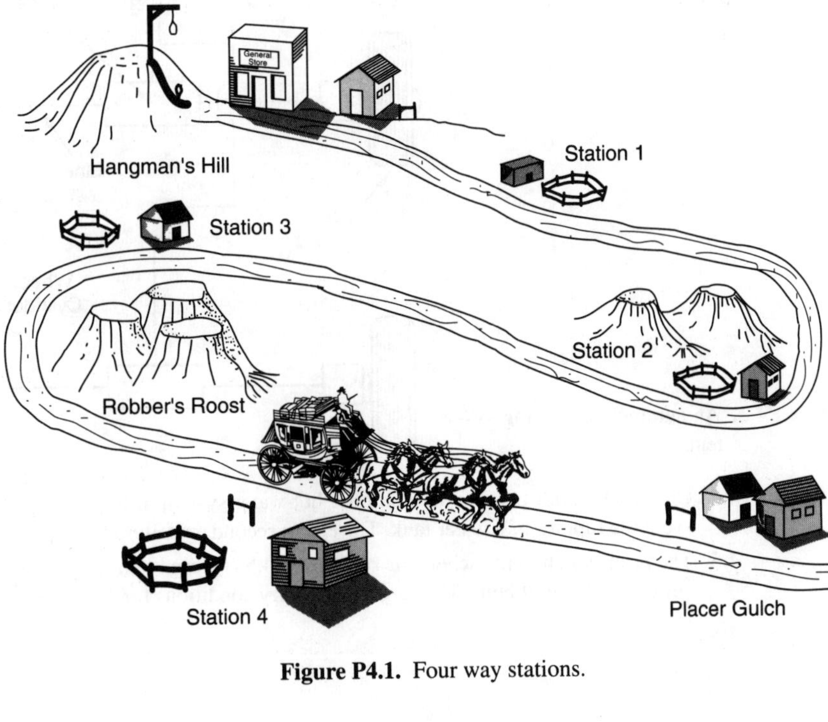

Figure P4.1. Four way stations.

4.2. Construct a fault tree for the circuit in Figure P4.2, with the top event "no light from bulb" and the boundary conditions.

Initial condition:	Switch is closed
Not-allowed events:	Failures external to the system
Existing events:	None

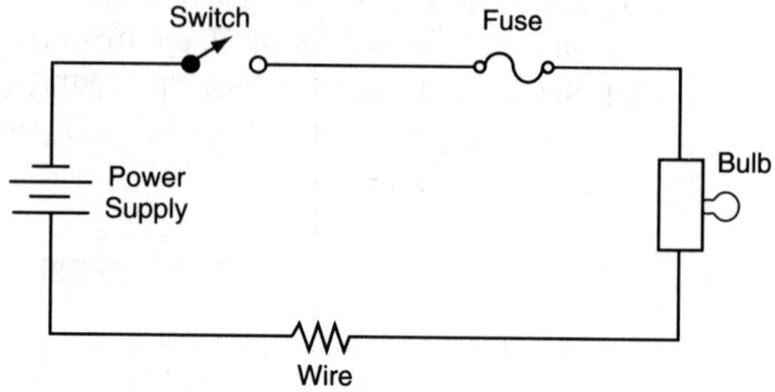

Figure P4.2. A simple electric circuit.

4.3. Construct a fault tree for the dual, hydraulic, automobile braking system shown in Figure P4.3.

System bounds:	Master cylinder assembly, front and rear brake lines, wheel cylinder, and brake shoe assembly
Top event:	Loss of all braking capacity
Initial condition:	Brakes released
Not-allowed events:	Failures external to system bounds
Existing events:	Parking brake inoperable

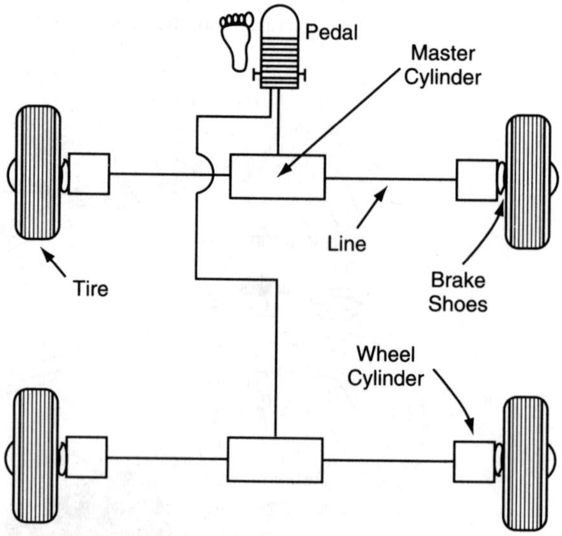

Figure P4.3. An automobile braking system.

4.4. Construct a fault tree for the domestic hot-water system in Problem 3.8. Take as a top event the rupture of a water tank. Develop a secondary failure listing.

4.5. The reset switch in the schematic of Figure P4.5 is closed to latch the circuit and provide current to the light bulb. The system boundary conditions for fault tree construction are:

Top event:	No current in circuit 1
Initial conditions:	Switch closed. Reset switch is closed momentarily and then opened
Not-allowed events:	Wiring failures, operator failures, switch failure
Existing events:	Reset switch open

Draw the fault tree, clarifying how it is terminated. (From Fussell, J.B., "Particularities of fault tree analysis," Aerojet Nuclear Co., Idaho National Lab., September 1974.)

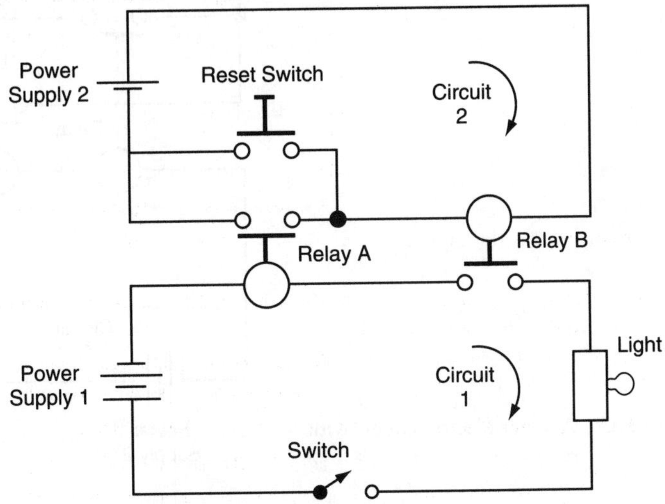

Figure P4.5. An electric circuit with relays.

4.6. A system (Figure P4.6) has two electric heaters that can fail by short circuiting to ground. Each heater has a switch connecting it to the power supply. If either heater fails with its switch closed, then the resulting short circuit will cause the power supply to short circuit, and the total system fails. If one switch fails open or is opened in error before its heater fails, then only that side of the system fails, and we can operate at half power.

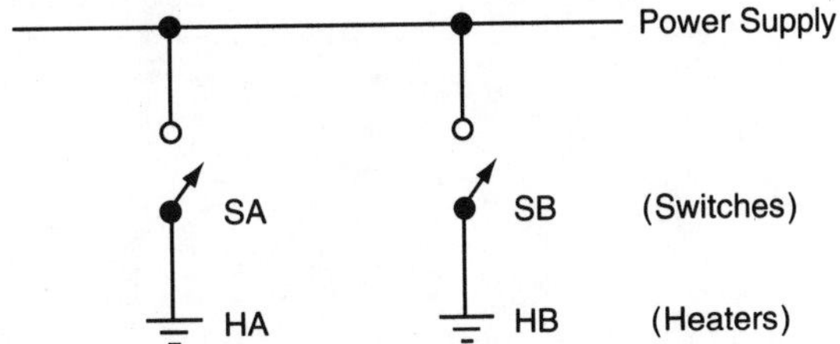

Figure P4.6. A heater system.

Draw the fault tree, and identify events that are mutually exclusive.

4.7. The purpose of the system of Figure P4.7 is to provide light from the bulb. When the switch is closed, the relay contacts close and the contacts of the circuit breaker, defined here as a normally closed relay, open. Should the relay contacts transfer open, the light will go out and the operator will immediately open the switch, which, in turn, causes the circuit breaker contacts to close and restore the light.

Draw the fault tree, and identify dependent basic events. The system boundary conditions are:

Top event:	No light
Initial conditions:	Switch closed
Not-allowed events:	Operator failures, wiring failures, secondary failures

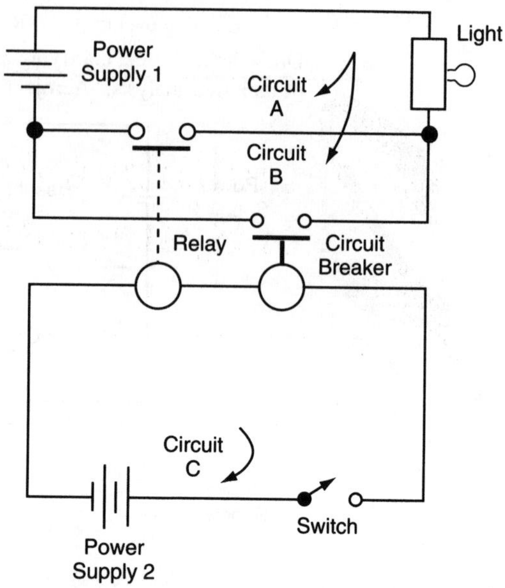

Figure P4.7. Another electric circuit with relays.

4.8. Construct semantic network models for the following circuits: 1) Figure P4.2, 2) Figure P4.5, 3) Figure P4.6, and 4) Figure P4.7.

5

Qualitative Aspects of System Analysis

5.1 INTRODUCTION

System failures occur in many ways. Each unique way is a system-failure mode, involving single- or multiple-component failures. To reduce the chance of a system failure, we must first identify the failure modes and then eliminate the most frequently occurring and/or highly probable. The fault-tree methods discussed in the previous chapter facilitate the discovery of failure modes; the analytical methods described in this chapter are predicated on the existence of fault trees.

5.2 CUT SETS AND PATH SETS

5.2.1 Cut Sets

For a given fault tree, a system-failure mode is clearly defined by a *cut set*, which is a collection of basic events; if all basic events occur, the top event is guaranteed to occur. Consider, for example, the fault tree of Figure 5.1, which is a simplified version of Figure 4.24 after removal of secondary failures. If events 2 and 4 occur simultaneously, the top event occurs, that is, if "contacts failure (stuck closed)" and "switch failure (stuck closed)" coexist, the top event, "pressure tank rupture," happens. Thus set {2,4} is a cut set. Also, {1} and {3,5} are cut sets.

Figure 5.2 is a reliability block-diagram representation equivalent to Figure 5.1. We observe that each cut set disconnects left and right terminal nodes denoted by circles.

5.2.2 Path Sets (Tie Sets)

A *path set* is the dual concept of a cut set. It is a collection of basic events, and if none of the events in the set occur, the non-occurrence of the top event is guaranteed. When

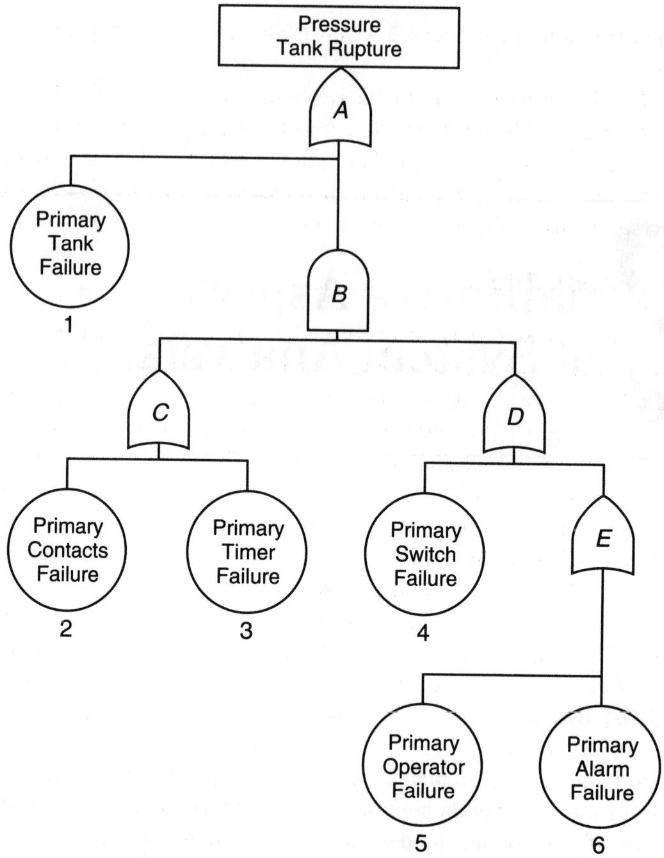

Figure 5.1. A pressure-tank-rupture fault tree.

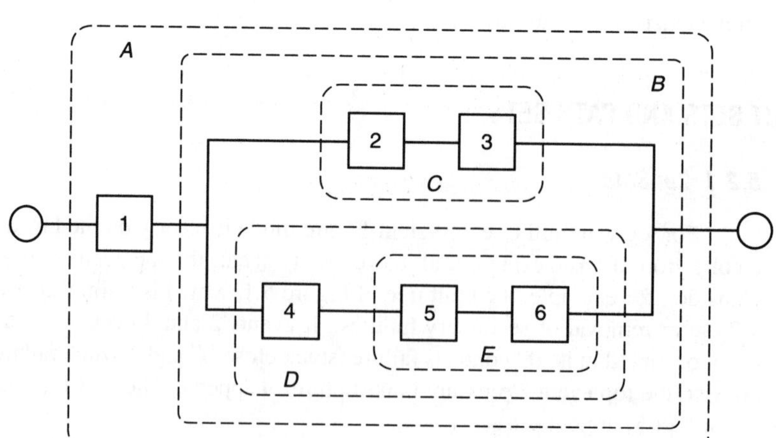

Figure 5.2. A pressure-tank-rupture reliability block diagram.

the system has only one top event, the non-occurrence of the basic failure events in a path set ensures successful system operation. The non-occurrence does not guarantee system success when more than one top event is specified. In such cases, a path set only ensures the non-occurrence of a particular top event. A path set is sometimes called a *tie set.*

For the fault tree of Figure 5.1, if failure events 1, 2, and 3 do not occur, the top event cannot happen. Hence if the tank, contacts, and timer are normal, the tank will not rupture. Thus {1,2,3} is a path set. Another path set is {1,4,5,6}, that is, the tank will not rupture if these failure events do not happen. In terms of the reliability block diagram of Figure 5.2, a path set connects the left and right terminal nodes.

5.2.3 Minimal Cut Sets

A large system has an enormous number of failure modes; hundreds of thousands of cut sets are possible for systems having between 40 and 90 components. If there are hundreds of components, billions of cut sets may exist. To simplify the analysis, it is necessary to reduce the number of failure modes. We require only those failure modes that are general, in the sense that one or more of them must happen for a system failure to occur. Nothing is lost by this restriction. If it were possible to improve the system in such a way as to eliminate all general failure modes, that would automatically result in the elimination of all system-failure modes.

A *minimal cut set* clearly defines a general failure mode. A minimal cut set is such that, if any basic event is removed from the set, the remaining events collectively are no longer a cut set. A cut set that includes some other sets is not a minimal cut set. The minimal-cut-set concept enables us to reduce the number of cut sets and the number of basic events involved in each cut set. This simplifies the analysis.

The fault tree of Figure 5.1 has seven minimal cut sets {1}, {2,4}, {2,5}, {2,6}, {3,4}, {3,5}, {3,6}. Cut set {1,2,4} is not minimal because it includes {1} or {2,4}. Both failure modes {1} and {2,4} must occur for mode {1,2,4} to occur. All failure modes are prevented from occurring when the modes defined by the minimal cut sets are eliminated.

5.2.4 Minimal Path Sets

A *minimal path set* is a path set such that, if any basic event is removed from the set, the remaining events collectively are no longer a path set. The fault tree of Figure 5.1 has two minimal path sets, {1,2,3} and {1,4,5,6}. If either {1,2,3} or {1,4,5,6} do not fail, the tank operates.

5.2.5 Minimal Cut Generation (Top-Down)

The MOCUS (method of obtaining cut sets) computer code can be used to generate minimal cut sets [1]. It is based on the observation that OR gates increase the number of cut sets, whereas AND gates enlarge the size of the cut sets. The MOCUS algorithm can be stated as follows.

1. Alphabetize each gate.
2. Number each basic event.
3. Locate the uppermost gate in the first row of a matrix.
4. Iterate either of the fundamental permutations a or b below in a top-down fashion. (When intermediate events are encountered, replace them by equivalent gates or basic events.)
   - **(a)** Replace an OR gate by a vertical arrangement of the input to the gate, and increase the number of cut sets.

(b) Replace an AND gate by a horizontal arrangement of the input to the gate, and enlarge the size of the cut sets.

5. When all gates are replaced by basic events, obtain the minimal cut sets by removing supersets. A *superset* is a cut set that includes other cut sets.

Example 1—Top-down generation. As an example, consider the fault tree of Figure 5.1 without intermediate events. The gates and the basic events have been labeled. The uppermost gate A is located in the first row:

$$A$$

This is an OR gate, and it is replaced by a vertical arrangement of the input to the gate:

$$\begin{array}{c} 1 \\ B \end{array}$$

Because B is an AND gate, it is permuted by a horizontal arrangement of its input to the gate:

$$\begin{array}{c} 1 \\ \hline C,D \end{array}$$

OR gate C is transformed into a vertical arrangement of its input:

$$\begin{array}{c} 1 \\ \hline 2,D \\ 3,D \end{array}$$

OR gate D is replaced by a vertical arrangement of its input:

$$\begin{array}{c} 1 \\ \hline 2,4 \\ 2,E \\ \hline 3,4 \\ 3,E \end{array}$$

Finally, OR gate E is permuted by a vertical arrangement of the input:

$$\begin{array}{c} 1 \\ \hline 2,4 \\ \hline 2,5 \\ 2,6 \\ \hline 3,4 \\ \hline 3,5 \\ 3,6 \end{array}$$

We have seven cut sets, {1},{2,4},{2,5},{2,6},{3,4},{3,5}, and {3,6}. All seven are minimal, because there are no supersets.

When supersets are uncovered, they are removed in the process of replacing the gates. Assume the following result at one stage of the replacement.

$$\begin{array}{c}1,2,G\\1,2,3,G\\1,2,K\end{array}$$

A cut set derived from $\{1,2,3,G\}$ always includes a set from $\{1,2,G\}$. However, the cut set from $\{1,2,3,G\}$ may not include any sets from $\{1,2,K\}$ because the development of K may differ from that of G. We have the following simplified result:

$$\begin{array}{c}1,2,G\\1,2,K\end{array}$$

When an event appears more than two times in a horizontal arrangement, it is aggregated into a single event. For example, the arrangement $\{1,2,3,2,H\}$ should be changed to $\{1,2,3,H\}$. This corresponds to the idempotence rule of Boolean algebra: 2 AND 2 = 2.* ■

Example 2—Boolean top-down generation. The fault tree of Figure 5.1 can be represented by a set of Boolean expressions:

$$\begin{array}{ll}A = 1 + B, \quad B = C \cdot D, & C = 2 + 3\\ D = 4 + E, \quad E = 5 + 6 & \end{array} \tag{5.1}$$

The top-down algorithm corresponds to a top-down expansion of the top gate A.

$$A = 1 + B = 1 + C \cdot D \tag{5.2}$$
$$= 1 + (2 + 3) \cdot D = 1 + 2 \cdot D + 3 \cdot D \tag{5.3}$$
$$= 1 + 2 \cdot (4 + E) + 3 \cdot (4 + E) = 1 + 2 \cdot 4 + 2 \cdot E + 3 \cdot 4 + 3 \cdot E \tag{5.4}$$
$$= 1 + 2 \cdot 4 + 2 \cdot (5 + 6) + 3 \cdot 4 + 3 \cdot (5 + 6) \tag{5.5}$$
$$= 1 + 2 \cdot 4 + 2 \cdot 5 + 2 \cdot 6 + 3 \cdot 4 + 3 \cdot 5 + 3 \cdot 6 \tag{5.6}$$

where a centered dot $(\cdot)$ and a plus sign $(+)$ stand for AND and OR operations, respectively. The dot symbol is frequently omitted when there is no confusion.

The above expansion can be expressed in matrix form:

$$A = \left|\begin{array}{c}1\\B\end{array}\right| = \left|\begin{array}{c}1\\C\cdot D\end{array}\right| = \left|\begin{array}{c|c}\multicolumn{2}{c}{1}\\2 & D\\3 & \end{array}\right| = \left|\begin{array}{c|c}\multicolumn{2}{c}{1}\\2 & 4\\3 & E\end{array}\right| = \left|\begin{array}{c|c}\multicolumn{2}{c}{1}\\2 & 4\\3 & 5\\ & 6\end{array}\right| = \left|\begin{array}{c}1\\2\cdot 4\\2\cdot 5\\2\cdot 6\\3\cdot 4\\3\cdot 5\\3\cdot 6\end{array}\right| \tag{5.7}$$

■

5.2.6 Minimal Cut Generation (Bottom-Up)

MOCUS is based on a top-down algorithm. MICSUP (minimal cut sets, upward) [2] is a bottom-up algorithm. In the bottom-up algorithm, minimal cut sets of an upper-level gate are obtained by substituting minimal cut sets of lower-level gates. The algorithm starts with gates containing only basic events, and minimal cut sets for these gates are obtained first.

Example 3—Boolean bottom-up generation. Consider again the fault tree of Figure 5.1. The minimal cut sets of the lowest gates, C and E, are:

$$C = 2 + 3 \tag{5.8}$$
$$E = 5 + 6 \tag{5.9}$$

*See appendix to Chapter 3 for Boolean operations and laws.

Gate E has parent gate D. Minimal cut sets for this parent gate are obtained:

$$C = 2 + 3 \tag{5.10}$$

$$D = 4 + E = 4 + 5 + 6 \tag{5.11}$$

Gate B is a parent of gates C and D:

$$B = C \cdot D = (2 + 3)(4 + 5 + 6) \tag{5.12}$$

Finally, top-event gate A is a parent of gate B:

$$A = 1 + B = 1 + (2 + 3)(4 + 5 + 6) \tag{5.13}$$

An expansion of this expression yields the seven minimal cut sets.

$$A = 1 + 2 \cdot 4 + 2 \cdot 5 + 2 \cdot 6 + 3 \cdot 4 + 3 \cdot 5 + 3 \cdot 6 \tag{5.14}$$

■

5.2.7 Minimal Path Generation (Top-Down)

The MOCUS top-down algorithm for the generation of minimal path sets makes use of the fact that AND gates increase the path sets, whereas OR gates enlarge the size of the path sets. The algorithm proceeds in the following way.

1. Alphabetize each gate.
2. Number each basic event.
3. Locate the uppermost gate in the first row of a matrix.
4. Iterate either of the fundamental permutations a or b below in a top-down fashion. (When intermediate events are encountered, replace them by equivalent gates or basic events.)
   - **(a)** Replace an OR gate by a horizontal arrangement of the input to the gate, and enlarge the size of the path sets.
   - **(b)** Replace an AND gate by a vertical arrangement of the input to the gate, and increase the number of path sets.
5. When all gates are replaced by basic events, obtain the minimal path sets by removing supersets.

Example 4—Top-down generation. As an example, consider again the fault tree of Figure 5.1. The MOCUS algorithm generates the minimal path sets in the following way.

A

replacement of A

1,B

replacement of B

1,C

1,D

replacement of C

1,2,3

– – – – –

1,D

replacement of D

1,2,3

$$\begin{array}{c} - - - - - \\ 1,4,E \\ \text{replacement of } E \\ \hline 1,2,3 \\ - - - - - \\ \\ 1,4,5,6 \end{array}$$

We have two path sets: {1,2,3} and {1,4,5,6}. These two are minimal because there are no supersets. ■

A dual fault tree is created by replacing OR and AND gates in the original fault tree by AND and OR gates, respectively. A minimal path set of the original fault tree is a minimal cut set of the dual fault tree, and vice versa.

Example 5—Boolean top-down generation. A dual representation of equation (5.1) is given by:

$$\begin{array}{lll} A = 1 \cdot B, & B = C + D, & C = 2 \cdot 3 \\ D = 4 \cdot E, & E = 5 \cdot 6 & \end{array} \tag{5.15}$$

The minimal path sets are obtained from the dual representation in the following way:

$$A = \begin{vmatrix} 1 & B \end{vmatrix} = \begin{vmatrix} 1 & \begin{matrix} C \\ D \end{matrix} \end{vmatrix} = \begin{vmatrix} 1 & \begin{matrix} 2 \cdot 3 \\ D \end{matrix} \end{vmatrix} \tag{5.16}$$

$$= \begin{vmatrix} 1 & \begin{matrix} 2 \cdot 3 \\ 4 \cdot E \end{matrix} \end{vmatrix} = \begin{vmatrix} 1 & \begin{matrix} 2 \cdot 3 \\ 4 \cdot 5 \cdot 6 \end{matrix} \end{vmatrix} = \begin{vmatrix} 1 \cdot 2 \cdot 3 \\ 1 \cdot 4 \cdot 5 \cdot 6 \end{vmatrix} \tag{5.17}$$

■

5.2.8 Minimal Path Generation (Bottom-Up)

Minimal path sets of an upper-level gate are obtained by substituting minimal path sets of lower-level gates. The algorithm starts with gates containing only basic events.

Example 6—Boolean bottom-up generation. Consider the fault tree of Figure 5.1. Minimal path sets of the lowermost gates C and E are obtained first:

$$\begin{array}{l} C = 2 \cdot 3 \\ E = 5 \cdot 6 \end{array}$$

Parent gate D of gate E is developed:

$$\begin{array}{l} C = 2 \cdot 3 \\ D = 4 \cdot E = 4 \cdot 5 \cdot 6 \end{array}$$

Gate B is a parent of gates C and D:

$$B = C + D = 2 \cdot 3 + 4 \cdot 5 \cdot 6$$

Finally, top-event gate A is developed:

$$A = 1 \cdot B = 1 \cdot (2 \cdot 3 + 4 \cdot 5 \cdot 6)$$

An expansion of the gate A expression yields the two minimal path sets.

$$A = 1 \cdot 2 \cdot 3 + 1 \cdot 4 \cdot 5 \cdot 6 \tag{5.18}$$

■

5.2.9 Coping with Large Fault Trees

5.2.9.1 Limitations of cut-set enumeration. The greatest problem with cut-set enumeration for evaluating fault trees is that the number of possible cut sets grows exponentially with the size of the fault tree. Thus [3]:

1. It is impossible to enumerate the cut sets of very large trees.
2. When there are tens of thousands or more cut sets, it is difficult for a human analyst to identify an important cut set.
3. High memory requirements rule out running safety software on-line on small in-plant computers.

5.2.9.2 Fault-tree modules

Simple module. If a large fault tree is divided into subtrees called modules, then these subtrees can be analyzed independently and the above difficulties are alleviated. The definition of a fault-tree module is a gate that has only single-occurrence basic events that do not appear in any other place of the fault tree. Figure 5.3 shows two simple modules; this tree can be simplified into the one in Figure 5.4. A simple module can be identified in the following way [4]:

1. Find the single-occurrence basic events in the fault tree.
2. If a gate is composed of all single-occurrence events, the gate is replaced by a module.
3. If a gate has single-occurrence and multi-occurrence events, only single-occurrence events are replaced with a module.
4. Arrange the fault tree.
5. Repeat the above procedures until no more modularization can be performed.

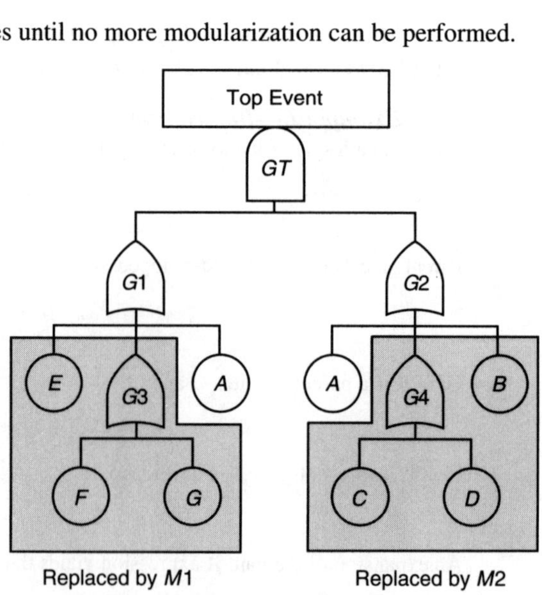

Figure 5.3. Examples of simple modules.

Sophisticated module. A more sophisticated module is a subtree having two or more basic events; the basic events (single-occurrence or repeated) only appear in the subtree;

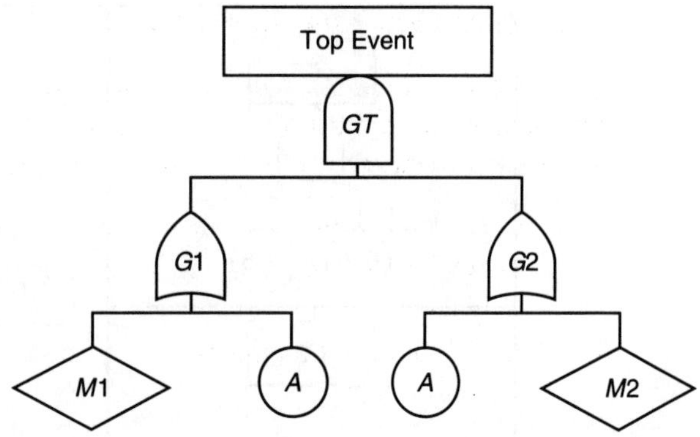

Figure 5.4. Fault-tree representation in terms of modules.

the subtree has no input except for these basic events; the subtree top gate is the only output port from the subtree [5]. The original fault tree itself always satisfies the above conditions, but it is excluded from the module. Note that the module subtree can contain repeated basic events. Furthermore, the output from a module can appear in different places of the original fault tree. A typical algorithm for finding this type of module is given in reference [5].

Because a module is a subtree, it can be identified by its top gate. Consider, as an example, the fault tree in Figure 5.5. This has two modules, $G11$ and $G2$. Module $G11$ has basic events $B15$ and $B16$, and module $G2$ has events $B5$, $B6$, and $B7$. The output from module $G11$ appears in two places in the original fault tree. Each of the two modules has no input except for the relevant basic events. The fault tree is represented in terms of modules as shown in Figure 5.6.

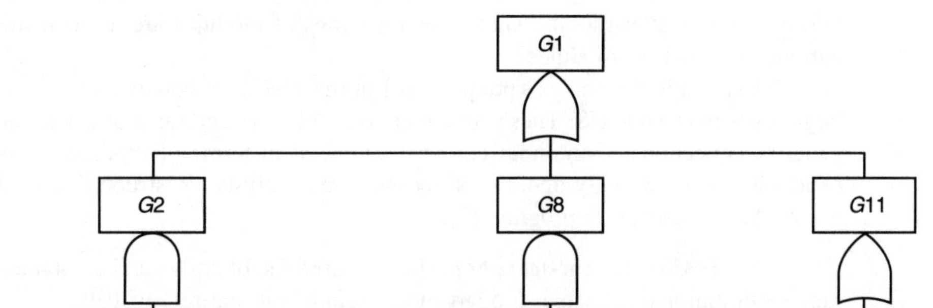

Figure 5.5. Fault-tree example.

Note that module $G11$ is not a module in the simple sense because it contains repeated events $B15$ and $B16$. Subtree $G8$ is not a module in a nonsimple nor the simple sense because basic event $B15$ also appears in subtree $G11$. Subtree $G8$ may be a larger module

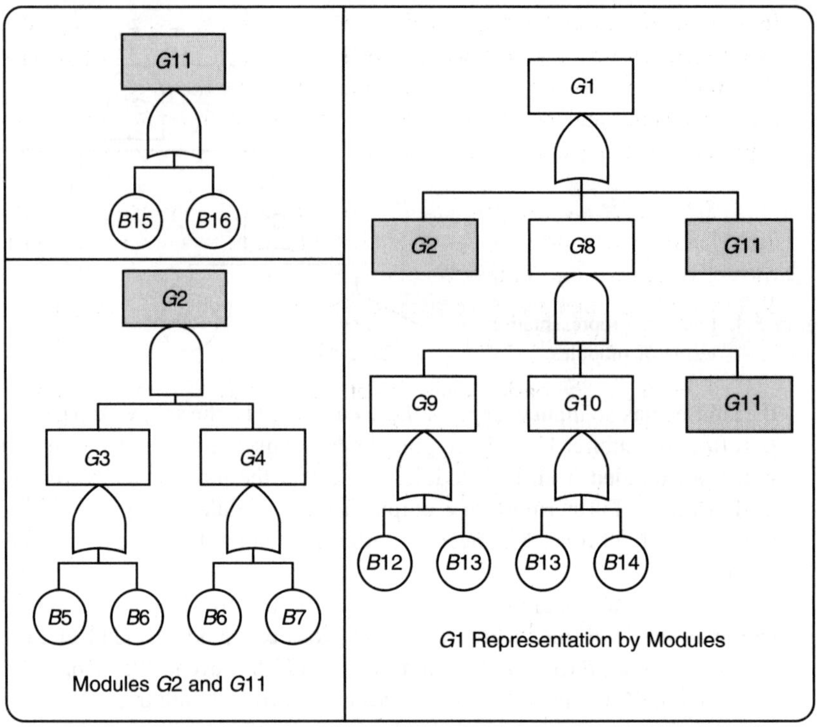

Figure 5.6. Fault-tree representation in terms of modules.

that includes smaller module $G11$. Such nestings of modules are not considered in the current definitions of modules.

FTAP (fault-tree analysis program) [6] and SETS [7] are said to be capable of handling larger trees than MOCUS. These computer codes identify certain subtrees as modules and generate collections of minimal cut sets expressed in terms of modules. This type of expression is more easily understood by fault-tree analysts. Restructuring is also part of the WAMCUT computer program [8].*

5.2.9.3 Minimal-cut-set subfamily. A useful subfamily can be obtained when the number of minimal cut sets is too large to be found in its entirety [6,10]:

1. The subfamily may consist only of sets not containing more than some fixed number of elements, or only of sets of interest.
2. The analyst can modify the original fault tree by declaring house event state variables.
3. The analyst can discard low-probability cut sets.

Assume that a minimal-cut-set subfamily is being generated and there is a size or probability cut-off criterion. A bottom-up rather than a top-down approach now has appreciable computational advantage [11]. This is because, during the cut-set evaluation procedure, exact probabilistic values can be assigned to the basic events, and not gates. Similarly, only basic events, and not gates, can contribute to the order of a term in the Boolean expression.

*See IAEA-TECDOC-553 [9] for other computer codes.

In the case of the top-down approach, at an intermediate stage of computation, the Boolean expression for the top gate contains mostly gates and so very few terms can be discarded. The Boolean expression can contain a prohibitive number of terms before the basic events are even reached and the cut-off procedure applied. In the bottom-up approach, the Boolean expression contains only basic events and the cut-off can be applied immediately.

5.2.9.4 MOCUS improvement. The MOCUS algorithm can be improved by gate development procedures such as FATRAM (fault-tree reduction algorithm) [12]. OR gates with only basic-event inputs are called *basic-event OR gates.* These gates are treated differently from other gates. Repeated events and nonrepeated events in the basic-event OR gates are processed differently:

1. Rule 1: The basic-event OR gates are not developed until all OR gates with one or more gate inputs and all AND gates with any inputs are resolved.
2. Rule 2: Remove any supersets before developing the basic-event OR gates.
3. Rule 3: First process repeated basic events remaining in the basic-event OR gates. For each repeated event do the following:
   (a) Replace the relevant basic-event OR gates by the repeated event, creating additional sets.
   (b) Remove the repeated event from the input list of the relevant basic-event OR gates.
   (c) Remove supersets.
4. Rule 4: Develop the remaining basic-event OR gates without any repeated events.

All sets become minimal cut sets without any superset examinations.

FATRAM can be modified to cope with a situation where only minimal cut sets up to a certain order are required [12].

Example 7—FATRAM. Consider the fault tree in Figure 5.7. The top event is an AND gate. The fault tree contains two repeated events, B and C. The top gate is an AND gate, and we obtain by MOCUS:

$$G1, G2$$

Gate $G1$ is an AND gate. Thus by Rule 1, it can be resolved to yield:

$$A, G3, G2$$

Both $G3$ and $G2$ are OR gates, but $G3$ is a basic-event OR gate. Therefore, $G2$ is developed next (Rule 1) to yield:

$$A, G3, B$$
$$A, G3, E$$
$$A, G3, G4$$

$G4$ is an AND gate and is the next gate to be developed (Rule 1):

$$A, G3, B$$
$$A, G3, E$$

\- - - - - - - - - -

$$A, G3, D, G5$$

The gates that remain, $G3$ and $G5$, are both basic-event OR gates. No supersets exist (Rule 2), so repeated events (Rule 3) are handled next.

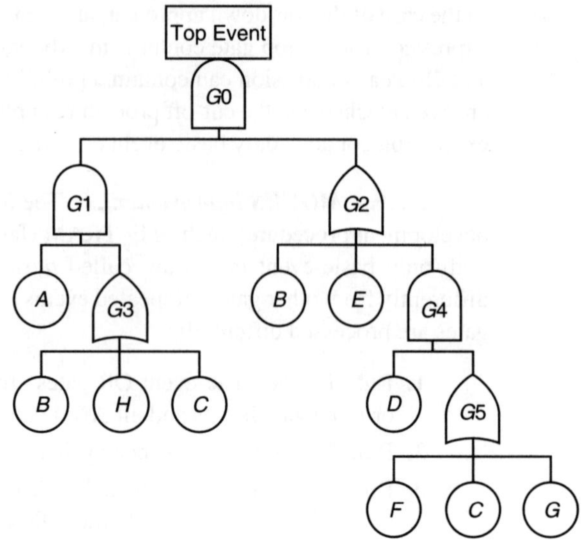

Figure 5.7. Example fault tree for MOCUS improvement.

Consider basic event B, which is input to gates $G2$ and $G3$. $G2$ has already been resolved but $G3$ has not. Everywhere $G3$ occurs in the sets it is replaced by B, thus creating additional sets:

$$A, G3, B$$
$$A, B, B \rightarrow A, B$$

- - - - - - - - - - -

$$A, G3, E$$
$$A, B, E$$

- - - - - - - - - - -

$$A, G3, D, G5$$
$$A, B, D, G5$$

Gate $G3$ (Rule 3-b) is altered by removing B as an input. Hence, $G3$ is now an OR gate with two basic-event inputs, C and H. Supersets are deleted (Rule 3-c):

$$A, B$$

- - - - - - - - - - -

$$A, G3, E$$

- - - - - - - - - - -

$$A, G3, D, G5$$

Basic event C is also a repeated event; it is an input to $G3$ and $G5$. By Rule 3-a replace $G3$ and $G5$ by C, thus creating additional sets:

$$A, B$$

- - - - - - - - - - -

$$A, G3, E$$
$$A, C, E$$

- - - - - - - - - - -

$$A, G3, D, G5$$
$$A, C, D, C \rightarrow A, C, D$$

Gate $G3$ now has only input H, and $G5$ has inputs F and G. Supersets are removed at this point (Rule 3-c) but none exist and all repeated events have been handled. We proceed to Rule 4, to obtain all minimal cut sets:

A,B

- - - - - - - - - - -

A,H,E
A,C,E

- - - - - - - - - - -

A,H,D,F
A,H,D,G
A,C,D

■

Example 8—Boolean explanation of FATRAM. The above procedure for developing gates can be written in matrix form.

$$\left| T \right| = \left| G1 \mid G2 \right| = \left| A \mid G3 \mid G2 \right| = \left| A \mid G3 \;\middle|\; \begin{array}{c} B \\ E \\ G4 \end{array} \right| = \left| A \mid G3 \;\middle|\; \begin{array}{l} B \\ E \\ D \mid G5 \end{array} \right| \tag{5.19}$$

Denote by X a Boolean expression. The following identities hold:

$$X \cdot A = (X|A = \text{true}) \cdot A \tag{5.20}$$

$$X \cdot \overline{A} = (X|A = \text{false}) \cdot \overline{A} \tag{5.21}$$

When expression X has no complement variables, then for Boolean variables A and B

$$A \cdot X + B \cdot X = A \cdot (X|A = \text{true}) + B \cdot (X|A = \text{false}) \tag{5.22}$$

Applying (5.22) to (5.19) with repeated event B as a condition,

$$T = \left| A \;\middle|\; \begin{array}{c} B \\ G3 \end{array} \;\middle|\; \begin{array}{l} B \\ E \\ D \mid G5 \end{array} \right| = \left| A \;\middle|\; \begin{array}{l} B \\ G3 \;\middle|\; \begin{array}{l} E \\ D \mid G5 \end{array} \end{array} \right| \tag{5.23}$$

Applying (5.22) with repeated event C as a condition,

$$T = \left| A \;\middle|\; \begin{array}{c} B \\ C \\ G3 \end{array} \;\middle|\; \begin{array}{l} E \\ D \;\middle|\; \begin{array}{c} C \\ G5 \end{array} \end{array} \right| = \left| A \;\middle|\; \begin{array}{l} B \\ C \;\middle|\; \begin{array}{l} E \\ D \end{array} \\ \\ G3 \;\middle|\; \begin{array}{l} E \\ D \mid G5 \end{array} \end{array} \right| \tag{5.24}$$

Replace $G3$ by H and $G5$ by F and G to obtain all minimal cut sets:

$$T = \left| A \;\middle|\; \begin{array}{l} B \\ C \;\middle|\; \begin{array}{l} E \\ D \end{array} \\ \\ H \;\middle|\; \begin{array}{l} E \\ D \;\middle|\; \begin{array}{c} F \\ G \end{array} \end{array} \end{array} \right| \tag{5.25}$$

■

5.2.9.5 Set comparison improvement. It can be proven that neither superset removal by absorption $x + xy = x$ nor simplification by idempotence $xx = x$ is required when a fault tree does not contain repeated events [13]. The minimal cut sets are those obtained by a simple development using MOCUS. When repeated events appear in fault trees, the number of set comparisons for superset removal can be reduced if cut sets are divided into two categories [13]:

1. K1: cut sets containing repeated events
2. K2: cut sets containing no repeated events

It can be shown that the cut sets in $K2$ are minimal. Thus superset removal can only be performed for the $K1$ cut sets. This approach can be combined with the FATRAM algorithm described in the previous section [13].

Example 9—Cut-set categories. Suppose that MOCUS yields the following minimal cut-set candidates.

$$K = \{1,\ 2,\ 3,\ 6,\ 8,\ 4 \cdot 6,\ 4 \cdot 7,\ 5 \cdot 7,\ 5 \cdot 6\} \tag{5.26}$$

Assume that only event 6 is a repeated event. Then

$$K1 = \{6,\ 4 \cdot 6,\ 5 \cdot 6\} \tag{5.27}$$

$$K2 = \{1,\ 2,\ 3,\ 8,\ 4 \cdot 7,\ 5 \cdot 7\} \tag{5.28}$$

The reduction is performed on three cut sets, the maximal number of comparisons being three, thus yielding the minimal cut set {6} from family $K1$. This minimal cut is added to family $K2$ to obtain all minimal cut sets:

$$\{1,\ 2,\ 3,\ 6,\ 8,\ 4 \cdot 7,\ 5 \cdot 7\} \tag{5.29}$$

When there is a large number of terms in repeated-event cut-set family $K1$, the set comparisons are time-consuming. A cut set, however, can be declared minimal without comparisons because a cut set is not minimal if and only if it remains a cut set when an element is removed from the set. Consider cut set C and element x in C. This cut set is not minimal when the top event still occurs when elements in set $C - \{x\}$ all occur and when other elements do not occur. This criterion can be calculated by simulating the fault tree. ■

5.3 COMMON-CAUSE FAILURE ANALYSIS

5.3.1 Common-Cause Cut Sets

Consider a system consisting of normally open valves A and B in two parallel, redundant, coolant water supply lines. Full blockage of the coolant supply system is the top event. The fault tree has as a minimal cut set:

{valve A closed failure, valve B closed failure}

This valve system will be far more reliable than a system with a single valve, if one valve incorrectly closes independently of the other. Coexistence of two closed-valve failures is almost a miracle. However, if one valve fails under the same conditions as the other, the double-valve system is only slightly more reliable than the single-valve system.

Two valves will be closed simultaneously, for example, if maintenance personnel inadvertently leave the two valves closed. Under these conditions, two are only as reliable as one. Therefore, there is no significant difference in reliability between one- and two-line systems. A condition or event that causes multiple basic events is called a *common cause*. An example of a common cause is a flood that causes all supposedly redundant components to fail simultaneously.

The minimal-cut-generation methods discussed in the previous sections give minimal cuts of various sizes. A cut set consisting of n basic events is called an n-*event cut set*. One-event cut sets are significant contributors to the top event unless their probability of occurrence is very small. Generally, hardware failures occur with low frequencies; hence, two-or-more-event cut sets can often be neglected if one-event sets are present because co-occurrence of rare events have extremely low probabilities. However, when a common cause is involved, it may cause multiple basic-event failures, so we cannot always neglect higher order cut sets because some two-or-more-event cut sets may behave like one-event cut sets.

A cut set is called a *common-cause cut set* when a common cause results in the co-occurrence of all events in the cut set. Taylor reported on the frequency of common causes in the U.S. power reactor industry [14]: "Of 379 component failures or groups of failures arising from independent causes, 78 involved common causes." In system-failure-mode analysis, it is therefore very important to identify all common-cause cut sets.

5.3.2 Common Causes and Basic Events

As shown in Figure 4.16, causes creating component failures come from one or more of the following four sources: aging, plant personnel, system environment, and system components (or subsystems).

There are a large number of common causes in each source category, and these can be further classified into subcategories. For example, the causes "water hammer" and "pipe whip" in a piping subsystem can be put into the category "impact." Some categories and examples are listed in Table 5.1 [15].

For each common cause, the basic events affected must be identified. To do this, a domain for each common cause, as well as the physical location of the basic event and component must be identified. Some common causes have only limited domains of influence, and the basic events located outside the domain are not affected by the causes. A liquid spill may be confined to one room, so electric components will not be damaged by the spill if they are in another room and no conduit exists between the two rooms. Basic events caused by a common cause are common-cause events of the cause.

Consider the fault tree of Figure 5.8. The floor plan is shown in Figure 5.9. This figure also includes the location of the basic events. We consider 20 common causes. Each common cause has the set of common-cause events shown in Table 5.2. This table also shows the domain of each common cause.

Only two basic events, 6 and 3, are caused by impact I1, whereas basic events 1,2,7,8 are caused by impact I2. This difference arises because each impact has its own domain of influence, and each basic event has its own location of occurrence. Neither event 4 nor event 12 are caused by impact I1 although they are located in domain 104 of I1. This is because these events occur independently of the impact, although they share the same physical location as event 3; in other words, neither event 4 nor 12 are susceptible to impact I1.

TABLE 5.1. Categories and Examples of Common Causes

Source	Symbol	Category	Examples
Environment, System, Components, Subsystems	I	Impact	Pipe whip, water hammer, missiles, earthquake, structural failure
	V	Vibration	Machinery in motion, earthquake
	P	Pressure	Explosion, out-of-tolerance system changes (pump overspeed, flow blockage)
	G	Grit	Airborne dust, metal fragments generated by moving parts with inadequate tolerances
	S	Stress	Thermal stress at welds of dissimilar metals, thermal stresses and bending moments caused by high conductivity and density
	T	Temperature	Fire, lightning, weld equipment, cooling-system fault, electrical short circuits
	E	Loss of energy source	Common drive shaft, same power supply
	C	Calibration	Misprinted calibration instruction
	F	Manufacturer	Repeated fabrication error, such as neglect to properly coat relay contacts. Poor workmanship. Damage during transportation
Plant Personnel	IN	Installation contractor	Same subcontractor or crew
	M	Maintenance	Incorrect procedure, inadequately trained personnel
	O	Operation	Operator disabled or overstressed, faulty operating procedures
	TS	Test	Fault test procedures that may affect all components normally tested together
Aging	A	Aging	Components of same materials

5.3.3 Obtaining Common-Cause Cut Sets

Assume a list of common causes, common-cause events, and basic events. Common-cause cut sets are readily obtained if all the minimal cut sets of a given fault tree are known. Large fault trees, however, may have an astronomically large number of minimal cut sets, and it is time-consuming to obtain them. For such fault trees, the generation methods discussed in the previous sections are frequently truncated to give, for instance, only two-or-less-event cut sets. However, this truncation should not be used when there is a possibility of common-cause failures because three-or-more-event cut sets may behave like one-event cut sets and hence should not be neglected.

One approach, due to Wagner et al. [15] is based on dissection of fault trees. An alternative method using a simplified fault tree is developed here.

A basic event is called a neutral event vis-à-vis a common cause if it is independent of the cause. For a given common cause, a basic event is thus either a neutral event or a common-cause event. The present approach assumes a probable situation for each common

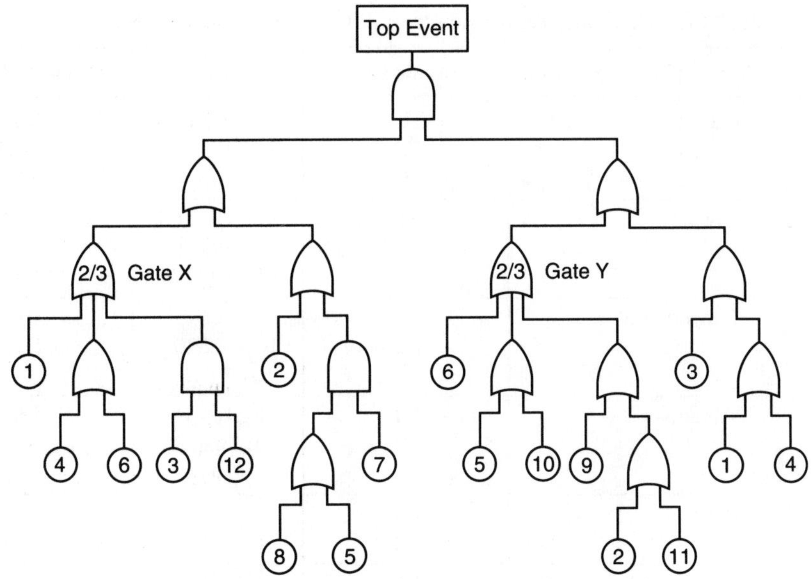

Figure 5.8. Fault tree for the example problem.

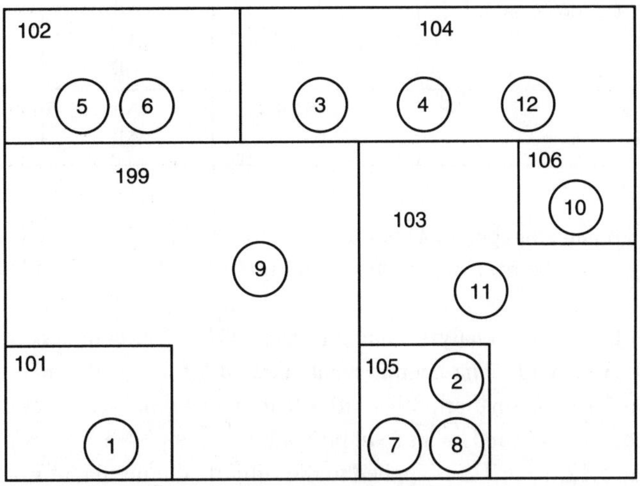

Figure 5.9. Example floor plan and location of basic events.

cause. This situation is defined by the statement: "Assume a common cause. Because most neutral events have far smaller possibilities of occurrence than common-cause events, these neutral events are assumed not to occur in the given fault tree." Other situations violating the above requirement can be neglected because they imply the occurrence of one or more neutral events.

The probable-situation simplifies the fault tree. It uses the fundamental simplification of Figure 5.10 in a bottom-up fashion. For the simplified fault tree, we can easily obtain the minimal cut sets. These minimal cut sets automatically become the common-cause cut sets.

TABLE 5.2. Common Causes, Domains, and Common-Cause Events

Category	Common Cause	Domain	Common-Cause Events
Impact	I1	102,104	6,3
	I2	101,103,105	1,2,7,8
	I3	106	10
Stress	S1	103,105,106	11,2,7,10
	S2	199	9
	S3	101,102,104	1,4
Temperature	T1	106	10
	T2	101,102,103, 104,105,199	5,11,8,12,3,4
Vibration	V1	102,104,106	5,6,10
	V2	101,103,105, 199	7,8
Operation	O1	All	1,3,12
	O2	All	5,7,10
Energy Source	E1	All	2,9
	E2	All	1,12
Manufacturer	F1	All	2,11
Installation Contractor	IN1	All	1,12
	IN2	All	6,7,10
	IN3	All	3,4,5,8,9,11
Test	TS1	All	2,11
	TS2	All	4,8

As an example, consider the fault tree of Figure 5.8. Note that the two-out-of-three gate, X, can be rewritten as shown in Figure 5.11. Gate Y can be represented in a similar way.

Let us first analyze common cause O1. The common-cause events of the cause are 1, 3, and 12. The neutral events are 2,4,5,6,7,8,9,10, and 11. Assume these neutral events have far smaller probabilities than the common-cause events when common cause O1 occurs. The fundamental simplification of Figure 5.10 yields the simplified fault tree of Figure 5.12. MOCUS is applied to the simplified fault tree of Figure 5.12 in the following way:

A
B, C
$1,3,12,C$
$1,3,12,3 \rightarrow 1,3,12$
$1,3,12,1 \rightarrow 1,3,12$

We have one common-cause cut set {1,3,12} for the common cause O1. Next, consider common cause I3 in Table 5.2. The neutral basic events are 1,2,3,4,5,6,7,8,9,11, and 12.

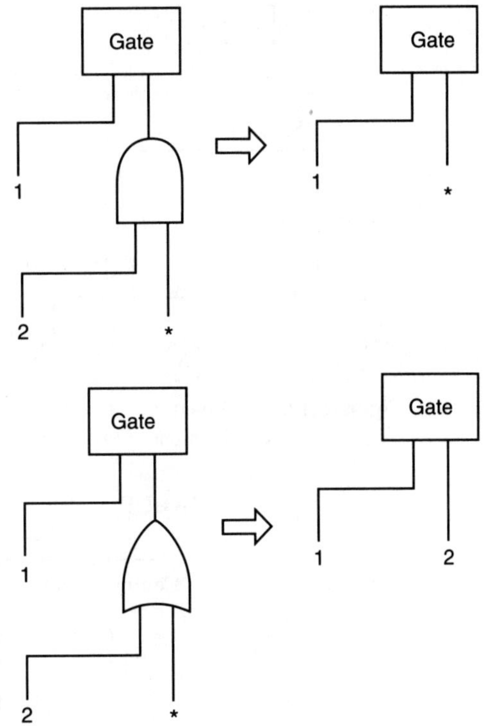

Figure 5.10. Fundamental simplification by zero-possibility branch (*).

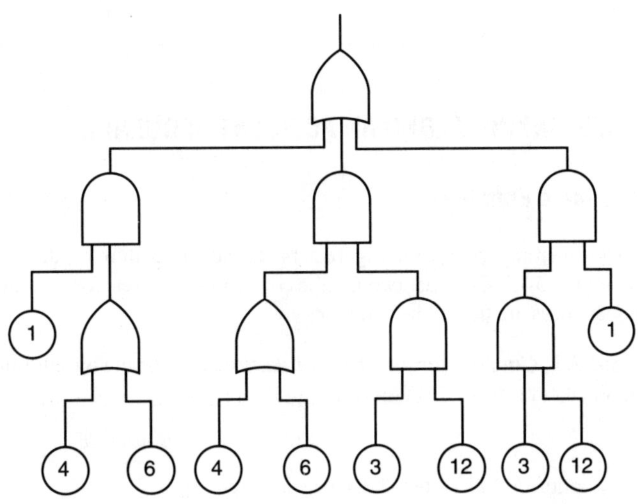

Figure 5.11. Equivalent expression for two-out-of-three gate X.

The fundamental simplifications yield the reduced fault tree of Figure 5.13. There are no common-cause cut sets for common cause I3.

The procedure is repeated for all other common causes to obtain the common-cause cut sets listed in Table 5.3.

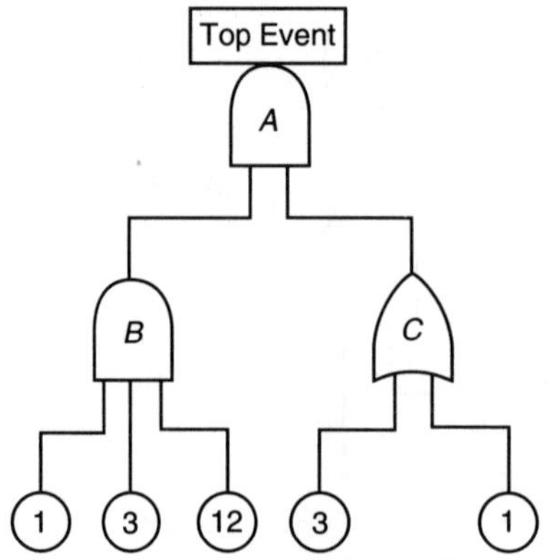

Figure 5.12. Simplified fault tree for common cause O1.

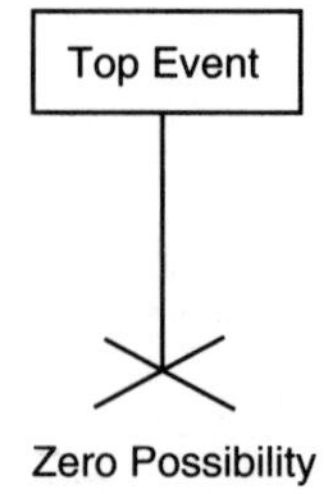

Figure 5.13. Simplified fault tree for common cause I3.

TABLE 5.3. Common Causes and Common-Cause Cut Sets

Common Cause	Common-Cause Cut Set
I2	{1,2}
I2	{1,7,8}
S3	{1,4}
S1	{2,10,11}
T2	{3,4,12}
O1	{1,3,12}

5.4 FAULT-TREE LINKING ALONG AN ACCIDENT SEQUENCE

5.4.1 Simple Example

Consider an event tree in Figure 5.14. Event-tree-failure headings are represented by the fault trees in Figure 5.15. Consider two families of minimal cut sets for accident sequence $S2$ and $S4$ [16]. Other sequences are treated in a similar way.

5.4.1.1 Cut sets for event-tree headings. Denote by $F1$ failure of system 1 (Fig. 5.15). The minimal cut sets for this failure are:

$$F1 = C + F + A \cdot B + D \cdot E \tag{5.30}$$

Similarly, failure $F2$ of system 2 can be expressed as:

$$F2 = A + F + G \tag{5.31}$$

■

5.4.1.2 Cut sets for sequence 2. In the second sequence $S2$, system 1 functions while system 2 is failed. Thus this sequence can be represented as:

$$S2 = \overline{F1} \cdot F2 \tag{5.32}$$

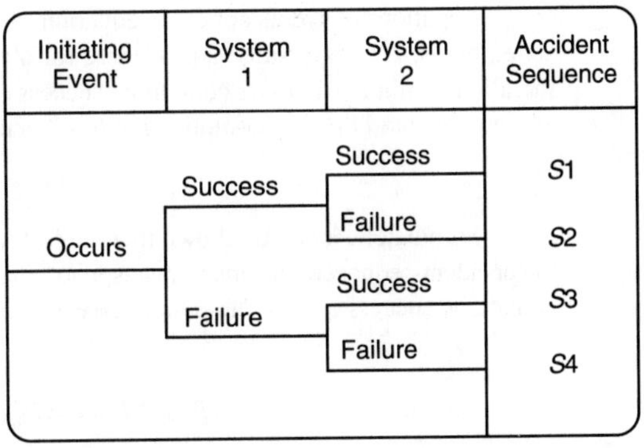

Figure 5.14. Simple event tree for demonstrating fault-tree linking.

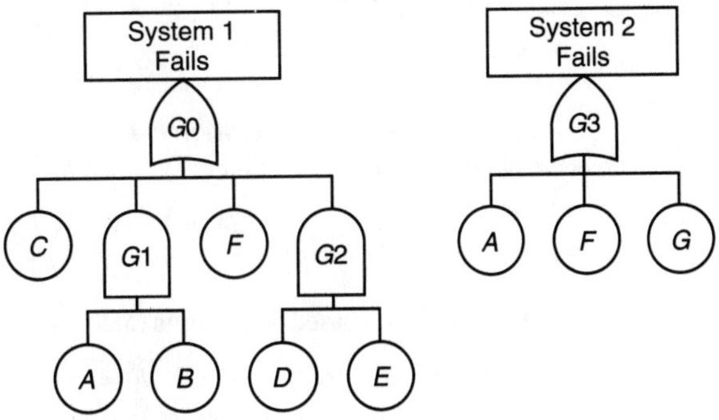

Figure 5.15. Simple fault trees for demonstrating fault-tree linking.

where symbol $\overline{F1}$ denotes success of system 1, that is, a negation of system 1 failure $F1$. By the de Morgan theorem (Appendix A.2, Chapter 3), this success can be expressed as:

$$\overline{F1} = \overline{C} \cdot \overline{F} \cdot (\overline{A} + \overline{B})(\overline{D} + \overline{E}) \tag{5.33}$$

This expression can be developed into an expression in terms of path sets:

$$\overline{F1} = \overline{A} \cdot \overline{C} \cdot \overline{D} \cdot \overline{F} + \overline{B} \cdot \overline{C} \cdot \overline{D} \cdot \overline{F} + \overline{A} \cdot \overline{C} \cdot \overline{E} \cdot \overline{F} + \overline{B} \cdot \overline{C} \cdot \overline{E} \cdot \overline{F} \tag{5.34}$$

The second sequence is:

$$S2 = \overline{F1} \cdot F2 = \overline{F1} \cdot A + \overline{F1} \cdot F + \overline{F1} \cdot G \tag{5.35}$$

Deletion of product terms containing a variable and its complement (for instance, A and $\overline{A}$), yields a sum of product expression for $S2$.

$$\begin{aligned} S2 = A \cdot \overline{B} \cdot \overline{C} \cdot \overline{D} \cdot \overline{F} + A \cdot \overline{B} \cdot \overline{C} \cdot \overline{E} \cdot \overline{F} + G \cdot \overline{A} \cdot \overline{C} \cdot \overline{D} \cdot \overline{F} \\ + G \cdot \overline{B} \cdot \overline{C} \cdot \overline{D} \cdot \overline{F} + G \cdot \overline{A} \cdot \overline{C} \cdot \overline{E} \cdot \overline{F} + G \cdot \overline{B} \cdot \overline{C} \cdot \overline{E} \cdot \overline{F} \end{aligned} \tag{5.36}$$

Assume that success states of basic events such as $\overline{A}$ are certain to occur. Then, the above expression on a sequence level simplifies to:

$$S2 = A + G \tag{5.37}$$

Note that erroneous cut set F appears if success states on a system level are assumed to be certain. In other words, if we assume $\overline{F1}$ to be true, then sequence $S2$ becomes:

$$S2 = F2 = A + F + G \tag{5.38}$$

Negations of events appear in equation (5.36) because sequence 2 contains the system success state, that is, $\overline{F1}$. Generally, a procedure for obtaining prime implicants must be followed for enumeration of minimal cut sets containing success events. Simplifications typified by the following rule are required, and this is a complication (see Section 5.5).

$$AB + A\overline{B} = A \tag{5.39}$$

Fortunately, it can be shown that the following simplification rules are sufficient for obtaining the accident-sequence minimal cut sets involving component success states if the original fault trees contain no success events. Note that success events are not included in fault trees $F1$ or $F2$:

$$\begin{aligned}
A^2 &= A, \quad \text{(Idempotent)} & (5.40)\\
AB + AB &= AB, \quad \text{(Idempotent)} & (5.41)\\
A + AB &= A, \quad \text{(Absorption)} & (5.42)\\
A \cdot \overline{A} &= \text{false}, \quad \text{(Complementation)} & (5.43)
\end{aligned}$$

■

5.4.1.3 Cut sets for sequence 4. In sequence $S4$, both systems fail and the sequence cut sets are obtained by a conjunction of system 1 and 2 cut sets.

$$\begin{aligned}
S4 &= F1 \cdot F2 = F1 \cdot (A + F + G)\\
&= F1 \cdot A + F1 \cdot F + F1 \cdot G
\end{aligned} \tag{5.44}$$

A manipulation based on equation (5.20) is simpler than the direct expansion of equation (5.44):

$$\begin{aligned}
S4 &= (F1|A = \text{true}) \cdot A + (F1|F = \text{true}) \cdot F + (F1|G = \text{true}) \cdot G\\
&= (C + F + B + D \cdot E) \cdot A + (\text{true}) \cdot F + (C + F + A \cdot B + D \cdot E) \cdot G\\
&= F + (C + F + B + D \cdot E) \cdot A + (C + F + A \cdot B + D \cdot E) \cdot G
\end{aligned} \tag{5.45}$$

Minimal cut F consists of only one variable. It is obvious that all cut sets of the form $F \cdot P$ where P is a product of Boolean variables can be deleted from the second and the third expressions of equation (5.45).

$$S4 = F + (C + B + D \cdot E) \cdot A + (C + A \cdot B + D \cdot E) \cdot G \tag{5.46}$$

This expression is now expanded:

$$S4 = F + A \cdot C + A \cdot B + A \cdot D \cdot E + C \cdot G + A \cdot B \cdot G + D \cdot E \cdot G \tag{5.47}$$

Cut set $A \cdot B \cdot G$ is a superset of $A \cdot B$, thus the family of minimal cut sets for sequence $S4$ is:

$$S4 = F + A \cdot C + A \cdot B + A \cdot D \cdot E + C \cdot G + D \cdot E \cdot G \tag{5.48}$$

■

5.4.2 A More Realistic Example

For the swimming pool reactor of Figure 4.46 and its event tree of Figure 4.48, consider the minimal cut sets for sequence $S3$ consisting of a trip system failure and an isolation system success. The two event headings are represented by the fault trees in Figures 4.49 and 4.51, and Table 5.4 lists their basic events. Events 1 through 6 appear only in the trip-system-failure fault tree, as indicated by symbol "Yes" in the fourth column; events 101 and 102 appear only in the isolation-system-failure fault tree; events 11 through 17 appear in both fault trees. Since the two fault trees have common events, the minimal cut sets of accident sequence $S3$ must be enumerated accordingly. Table 5.4 also shows event labels in the second column where symbols P, Z, and FO denote "Positive output failure," "Zero output failure," and "Fully_Open failure," respectively. Characters following each of

TABLE 5.4. Basic Events of the Two Fault Trees Along an Accident Sequence

Event	Label	Description	Trip	Isolation
1	ZNAND	Zero output failure of NAND gate	Yes	No
2	PC5	Positive output failure of C5	Yes	No
3	PC6	Positive output failure of C6	Yes	No
4	PC7	Positive output failure of C7	Yes	No
5	PC8	Positive output failure of C8	Yes	No
6	PC14	Positive output failure of C14	Yes	No
11	ZC3	Zero output failure of C3	Yes	Yes
12	ZC4	Zero output failure of C4	Yes	Yes
13	FOC9	Fully_Open failure of C9	Yes	Yes
14	FOC10	Fully_Open failure of C10	Yes	Yes
15	ZC11	Zero output failure of C11	Yes	Yes
16	PC12	Positive output failure of C12	Yes	Yes
17	ZC13	Zero output failure of C13	Yes	Yes
101	FOC1	Fully_Open failure of C1	No	Yes
102	FOC2	Fully_Open failure of C2	No	Yes

these symbols denote a relevant component; for instance, ZC11 for event 15 implies that component C11 has a "Zero output failure." ■

5.4.2.1 Trip system failure. The trip system failure is represented by the fault tree in Figure 4.49, which has four nested modules, RSM54, RSM18, RM40, RM92, and RM34. Inclusion relations are shown in Figure 4.50. Modules RSM54 and RSM18 are the most elementary; module RM40 includes modules RSM54 and RSM18; modules RM92 and RM34 contain module RM40.

Denote by T the top event of the fault tree, which can be represented as:

$$T = (M18 + 6)(M34 + 4)(M34 + 5)(M92 + 2)(M92 + 3)M54 + 1 \tag{5.49}$$

where symbol $M18$, for example, represents a top event for module RSM18.

The following identity is used to expand the above expression.

$$(A + X)(A + Y) = A + XY \tag{5.50}$$

where A, X, and Y are any Boolean expressions. In equation (5.49), $M34$ and $M92$ correspond to common expression A. Top event T can be written as:

$$T = (M18 + 6)(M34 + 4 \cdot 5)(M92 + 2 \cdot 3)M54 + 1 \tag{5.51}$$

Modules 34 and 92 are expressed in terms of module 40:

$$T = (M18 + 6)(M40 + 12 + 4 \cdot 5)(M40 + 11 + 2 \cdot 3)M54 + 1 \tag{5.52}$$

Applying equation (5.50) for $A \equiv M40$:

$$T = (M18 + 6)[M40 + (12 + 4 \cdot 5)(11 + 2 \cdot 3)]M54 + 1 \tag{5.53}$$

Module 40 is expressed in terms of modules 18 and 54:

$$T = (M18 + 6)[(M18 + 14)(M54 + 13) + (12 + 4 \cdot 5)(11 + 2 \cdot 3)]M54 + 1 \tag{5.54}$$

Applying equation (5.20) for $A \equiv M54$:

$$T = (M18 + 6)[M18 + 14 + (12 + 4 \cdot 5)(11 + 2 \cdot 3)]M54 + 1 \tag{5.55}$$

The equation (5.50) identity for $A = M18$ yields:

$$T = \{M18 + 6[14 + (12 + 4 \cdot 5)(11 + 2 \cdot 3)]\}M54 + 1 \tag{5.56}$$

Modules 18 and 54 are now replaced by basic events:

$$T = \{17 + 6[14 + (12 + 4 \cdot 5)(11 + 2 \cdot 3)]\}(15 + 16) + 1 \tag{5.57}$$

In matrix form:

$$T = \left| \begin{array}{l} 1 \\ \begin{array}{l|l} 15 & 17 \\ 16 & \begin{array}{l|l} 6 & \begin{array}{l} 14 \\ \begin{array}{l|l} \begin{array}{l} 12 \\ 4 \mid 5 \end{array} & \begin{array}{l} 11 \\ 2 \mid 3 \end{array} \end{array} \end{array} \end{array} \end{array} \end{array} \right| \tag{5.58}$$

An expansion of the above equation yields 13 minimal cut sets:

$$\begin{array}{l} 1, \\ 15 \cdot 17,\ 16 \cdot 17, \\ 6 \cdot 14 \cdot 15,\ 6 \cdot 14 \cdot 16, \\ 6 \cdot 11 \cdot 12 \cdot 15,\ 6 \cdot 11 \cdot 12 \cdot 16, \\ 6 \cdot 2 \cdot 3 \cdot 12 \cdot 15,\ 6 \cdot 2 \cdot 3 \cdot 12 \cdot 16, \\ 6 \cdot 4 \cdot 5 \cdot 11 \cdot 15,\ 6 \cdot 4 \cdot 5 \cdot 11 \cdot 16, \\ 6 \cdot 2 \cdot 3 \cdot 4 \cdot 5 \cdot 15,\ 6 \cdot 2 \cdot 3 \cdot 4 \cdot 5 \cdot 16 \end{array} \tag{5.59}$$

The fourth cut set $6 \cdot 14 \cdot 15$, in terms of components, is PC14 · FOC10 · ZC11. With reference to Figure 4.46 this means that switch C14 is sending a trip inhibition signal to the NAND gate (PC14), switches C7 and C8 stay at the inhibition side because valve C10 is fully open (FOC10), and switches C5, C6, and C12 remain in the inhibition mode because electrode C11 has zero output failure ZC11.

Equation (5.58) in terms of event labels is:

$$T = \left| \begin{array}{l} \text{ZNAND} \\ \begin{array}{l|l} \text{ZC11} & \text{ZC13} \\ \text{PC12} & \begin{array}{l|l} \text{PC14} & \begin{array}{l} \text{FOC10} \\ \begin{array}{l|l} \begin{array}{l} \text{ZC4} \\ \text{PC7} \mid \text{PC8} \end{array} & \begin{array}{l} \text{ZC3} \\ \text{PC5} \mid \text{PC6} \end{array} \end{array} \end{array} \end{array} \end{array} \end{array} \right| \tag{5.60}$$

This is a Boolean expression for the fault tree of Figure 4.49:

$$\begin{aligned} T &= G2 \cdot G1 + \text{ZNAND}, \\ G1 &= \text{ZC11} + \text{PC12}, \\ G2 &= \text{ZC13} + G3 \\ G3 &= \text{PC14}[\text{FOC10} + (\text{ZC4} + \text{PC7} \cdot \text{PC8})(\text{ZC3} + \text{PC5} \cdot \text{PC6})] \end{aligned} \tag{5.61}$$

Gate $G1$ implies that either electrode C11 with zero output failure or solenoid switch C12 failed at trip inhibition, thus forcing the electrode line trip system to become inactive. Gate $G2$ shows a trip system failure along the float line. Gate $G3$ is a float line failure when the float is functioning. ■

5.4.2.2 Isolation system failure. Denote by I an isolation system failure. From the fault tree in Figure 4.51, this failure can be expressed as:

$$I = 11 + 12 + 101 + 102 + M40, \quad M40 = (14 + 17)(13 + 15 + 16) \tag{5.62}$$

Ten minimal cut sets are obtained:

$$\begin{array}{l} 11,\ 12,\ 101,\ 102 \\ 13 \cdot 14,\ 14 \cdot 15,\ 14 \cdot 16 \\ 13 \cdot 17,\ 15 \cdot 17,\ 16 \cdot 17 \end{array} \tag{5.63}$$

■

5.4.2.3 Minimal cut sets for sequence 3. Rather than starting with expressions (5.59) and (5.63), which would involve time-consuming manipulations, consider (5.62), whereby the isolation system success $\overline{I}$ can be written as:

$$\overline{I} = \overline{11} \cdot \overline{12} \cdot \overline{101} \cdot \overline{102} \cdot \overline{M40}, \quad \overline{M40} = \overline{14} \cdot \overline{17} + \overline{13} \cdot \overline{15} \cdot \overline{16} \tag{5.64}$$

Take the Boolean AND of equations (5.57) and (5.64), and apply equation (5.21) by setting $\overline{A} = \overline{11} \cdot \overline{12}$, $\overline{A} \equiv \overline{14} \cdot \overline{17}$, and $\overline{A} = \overline{13} \cdot \overline{15} \cdot \overline{16}$. False of $A = 11 + 12$ implies that both 11 and 12 are false. A total of four minimal cut sets are obtained for accident sequence 3:

$$\begin{aligned} &1 \cdot \overline{11} \cdot \overline{12} \cdot \overline{14} \cdot \overline{17} \cdot \overline{101} \cdot \overline{102} \\ &2 \cdot 3 \cdot 4 \cdot 5 \cdot 6 \cdot 15 \cdot \overline{11} \cdot \overline{12} \cdot \overline{14} \cdot \overline{17} \cdot \overline{101} \cdot \overline{102} \\ &2 \cdot 3 \cdot 4 \cdot 5 \cdot 6 \cdot 16 \cdot \overline{11} \cdot \overline{12} \cdot \overline{14} \cdot \overline{17} \cdot \overline{101} \cdot \overline{102} \\ &1 \cdot \overline{11} \cdot \overline{12} \cdot \overline{13} \cdot \overline{15} \cdot \overline{16} \cdot \overline{101} \cdot \overline{102} \end{aligned} \tag{5.65}$$

Removing high-probability events by assigning a value of unity, the following minimal cut sets are identified.

$$\begin{aligned} &1 \\ &2 \cdot 3 \cdot 4 \cdot 5 \cdot 6 \cdot 15 \\ &2 \cdot 3 \cdot 4 \cdot 5 \cdot 6 \cdot 16 \end{aligned} \tag{5.66}$$

■

5.5 NONCOHERENT FAULT TREES

5.5.1 Introduction

5.5.1.1 Mutual exclusivity. A fault tree may have mutually exclusive basic events. Consider a heat exchanger that has two input streams, cooling water, and a hot acid stream. The acid-flow rate is assumed constant and its temperature is either normal or high. Outflow-acid high temperature is caused by zero cooling water flow rate due to coolant pump failure, OR an inflow acid temperature increase with the coolant pump operating normally. A fault tree is shown in Figure 5.16. This fault tree has two mutually exclusive events, "pump normal" and "pump stops."

Fault trees that contain EOR gates, working states, and so on, are termed *noncoherent* and their unique failure modes are called *prime implicants*. More rigorous definitions of coherency will be given in Chapter 8; in this section it is shown how prime implicants are obtained for noncoherent trees using Nelson's method and Quine's consensus method.

The Boolean simplification rules given by equations (5.40) to (5.43) do not guarantee a complete set of prime implicants, particularly if multistate components or success states exist.

The simplest approach to noncoherence is to assume occurrences of success states, because their effect on top-event probability is small, particularly in large systems and systems having highly reliable components.

5.5.1.2 Multistate components. When constructing a fault tree, mutual exclusivity should be ignored if at all possible; however, this is not always possible if the system hardware is multistate, that is, it has plural failure modes [17,18]. For example, a generator may have the mutually exclusive failure events, "generator stops" and "generator surge";

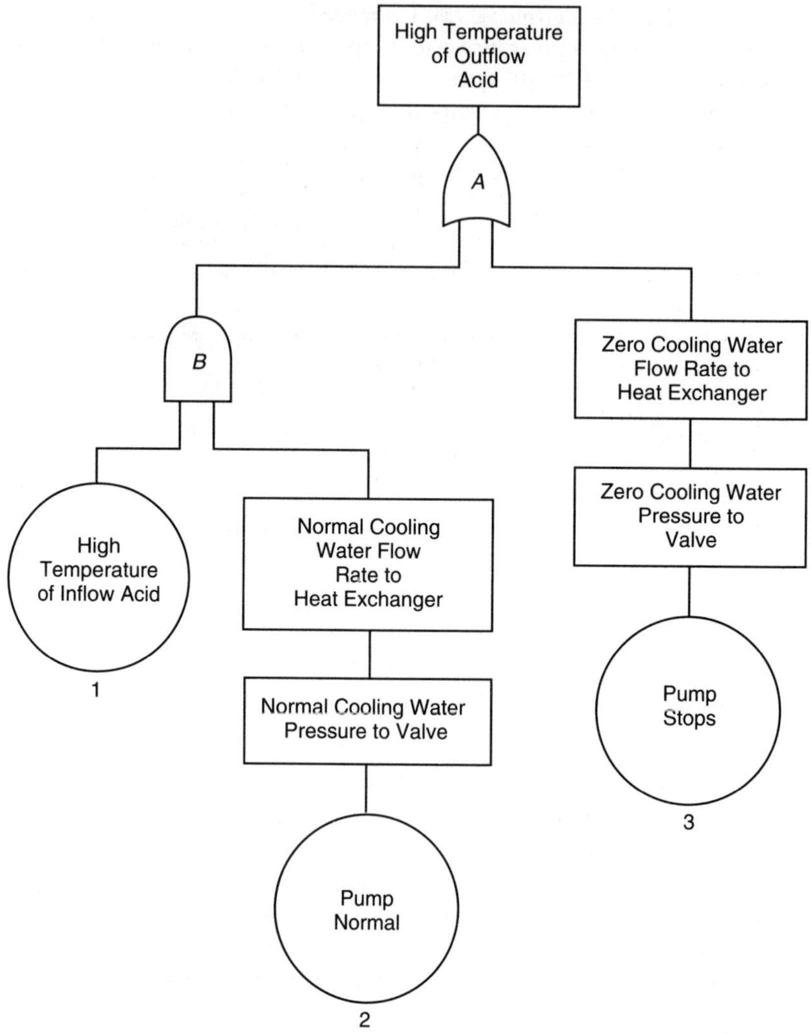

Figure 5.16. Fault tree for heat exchanger.

a relay may be "shorted" or remain "stuck open," and a pump may, at times, be a four-state component: state 1—no flow; state 2—flow equal to one third of full capacity; state 3—flow at least equal to two thirds of, but less than, full capacity; state 4—pump fully operational.

5.5.2 Minimal Cut Sets for a Binary Fault Tree

When a fault tree contains mutually exclusive binary events, the MOCUS algorithm does not always produce the correct minimal cut sets. MOCUS, when applied to the tree of Figure 5.16, for example, yields the cut sets {1,2} and {3}. Thus minimal cut set {1} cannot be obtained by MOCUS, although it would be apparent to an engineer, and numerically, the probability of {1} and {1,2} is the same for all practical purposes.

5.5.2.1 Nelson algorithm. A method of obtaining cut sets that can be applied to the case of binary exclusive events is a procedure consisting of first using MOCUS to obtain path sets, which represent system success by a Boolean function. The next step is to take a complement of this success function to obtain minimal cut sets for the original fault tree through expansion of the complement.

MOCUS is modified in such a way as to remove inconsistent path sets from the outputs, inconsistent path sets being sets with mutually exclusive events. An example is {generator normal, pump normal, pump stops} when the pump has only two states, "pump normal" and "pump stops." For this binary-state pump path set, one of the primary pump events always occurs, so it is not possible to achieve non-occurrence of all basic events in the path set, a sufficient condition of system success. The inconsistent set does not satisfy the path set definition and should be removed.

Example 10—A simple case. Consider the fault tree of Figure 5.16. Note that events 2 and 3 are mutually exclusive; event 2 is a pump success state, while event 3 is a pump failure. Denote by $\overline{3}$ the normal pump event. MOCUS generates path sets in the following way:

A
B,3
1,3
$\overline{3}$,3

Set {$\overline{3}$,3} is inconsistent; thus only path set {1,3} is a modified MOCUS output. Top event non-occurrence $\overline{T}$ is expressed as:

$$\overline{T} = \overline{1} \cdot \overline{3} \tag{5.67}$$

Note here that events $\overline{1}$ and $\overline{3}$ are "normal temperature of inflow acid" and "pump normal," respectively.

The above expression for $\overline{T}$ can also be obtained by a Boolean manipulation without MOCUS. The fault tree of Figure 5.16 shows that the top event T is:

$$T = 1 \cdot \overline{3} + 3 \tag{5.68}$$

The system success $\overline{T}$ is:

$$\overline{T} = \overline{1 \cdot \overline{3} + 3} = (\overline{1} + \overline{\overline{3}}) \cdot \overline{3} = (\overline{1} + 3) \cdot \overline{3} \tag{5.69}$$

An expansion of the above equation yields the same expression as (5.67):

$$\overline{T} = \overline{1} \cdot \overline{3} \tag{5.70}$$

The Nelson algorithm takes a complement of $\overline{T}$ to obtain two minimal cut sets {1} and {3} for top event T:

$$\overline{\overline{T}} = T = \overline{\overline{1} \cdot \overline{3}} = \overline{\overline{1}} + \overline{\overline{3}} = 1 + 3 \tag{5.71}$$

If MOCUS or a Boolean manipulation identifies three consistent path sets, $\overline{1} \cdot 2 \cdot 3$, $1 \cdot \overline{2} \cdot 3$, and $1 \cdot 2 \cdot \overline{3}$, by products of Boolean variables, top-event non-occurrence is represented by the following equation:

$$\overline{T} = \overline{1} \cdot 2 \cdot 3 + 1 \cdot \overline{2} \cdot 3 + 1 \cdot 2 \cdot \overline{3} \tag{5.72}$$

Minimal cut sets are obtained by taking the complement of this equation to obtain:

$$\overline{\overline{T}} = (1 + \overline{2} + \overline{3})(\overline{1} + 2 + \overline{3})(\overline{1} + \overline{2} + 3) \tag{5.73}$$

An expansion of this equation results in minimal cut sets for the top event:

$$\overline{\overline{T}} = T = \overline{1} \cdot \overline{3} + \overline{1} \cdot \overline{2} + \overline{2} \cdot \overline{3} + 1 \cdot 2 \cdot 3 \tag{5.74}$$

■

5.5.2.2 Generalized consensus. A method originally proposed by Quine [19,20] and extended by Tison [21] can be used to obtain all the prime implicants. The method is a consensus operation, because it creates a new term by mixing terms that already exist.

Example 11—Merging. Consider top event T expressed as:

$$T = A\overline{B} + AB \tag{5.75}$$

The following procedure is applied.

Step	Initial Set S	Biform Variable	Residues		New Consensi	Final Set
1	¶$A\overline{B}$ ¶AB	B	A	A	A	A

The initial set consists of product terms in the sum-of-products expression for the top event. We begin by searching for a two-event "biform" variable X such that each of the X and $\overline{X}$ appears in at least one term in the initial set. It is seen that variable B is biform because $\overline{B}$ is in the first term and B in the second.

The residue with respect to two-event variable B is the term obtained by removing B or $\overline{B}$ from a term containing it. Thus residues A and A are obtained. The residues are classified into two groups according to which event is removed from the terms.

The new consensi are all products of residues from different groups. In the current case, each group has only one residue, and a single consensus $AA = A$ is obtained. If a consensus has mutually exclusive events, it is removed from the list of the new consensi. As soon as a consensus is found, it is compared to the other consensi and to the terms in the initial set, and the longer products are removed from the table. We see that the terms $A\overline{B}$ and AB can be removed from the table because of consensus A. The terms thus removed are identified by the symbol ¶.

The final set of terms from step 1 is the union of the initial set and the set of new consensi. The final set is $\{A\}$. Because there is no biform variable in this initial set, the procedure is terminated. Otherwise, the final set would become the initial set for step 2. Event A is identified as the prime implicant.

$$T = A \tag{5.76}$$

This simplification is called merging, and can be expressed as:

$$T = A\overline{B} + AB = A \tag{5.77}$$

If two terms are the same except for exactly one variable with opposite truth values, the two terms can be merged. ■

Example 12—Reduction. Consider top event T expressed as:

$$T = ABC + A\overline{B} \tag{5.78}$$

The consensus procedure is:

Step	Initial Set S	Biform Variable	Residues		New Consensi	Final Set
1	¶ABC $A\overline{B}$	B	AC	A	AC	$A\overline{B}$ AC

The top event is simplified:

$$T = ABC + A\overline{B} = A\overline{B} + AC \tag{5.79}$$

This relation is called reduction; if two terms are comparable except for exactly one variable with opposite truth values, the larger of the two terms can be reduced by that variable. ■

The simplification operations (absorption, merging, reduction) are applied to the top-event expressions in cycles, until none of them is applicable. The resultant expression is then no longer reducible when this occurs.

Example 13—Two-step consensus operation. Consider top event T:

$$T = ABC + A\overline{B}C + AB\overline{C} + A\overline{B}\,\overline{C} \tag{5.80}$$

The two-step consensus operation is:

Step	Initial Set S	Biform Variable	Residues		New Consensi	Final Set
1	¶ABC ¶$A\overline{B}C$ ¶$AB\overline{C}$ ¶$A\overline{B}\,\overline{C}$	B	AC $A\overline{C}$	AC $A\overline{C}$	AC $A\overline{C}$	AC $A\overline{C}$
2	¶AC ¶$A\overline{C}$	C	A	A	A	A

Thus, the top event is:

$$T = A \tag{5.81}$$

■

5.5.2.3 *Modularization.* Because large trees lead to a large number of product-of-variables terms that must be examined during prime-implicant generation, computational times become prohibitive when all terms are investigated. Two approaches can be used [22].

Removal of singletons. Assume that a Boolean variable A is a cut set of top event T represented by a sum of products of basic events. Such a variable is called a *singleton.* The following operations to simplify T can be performed.

1. All terms of the form AP, where P is a product of basic events other than A itself, are deleted by absorption, that is, $A + AP = A$.
2. All terms of the form $\overline{A}P$ are replaced by P, that is, $A + \overline{A}P = A + P$.

Example 14—Simplification by singletons. Consider, as an example, top event T [22]:

$$\begin{aligned}
T = {} & x_8 + x_{18} + x_{21} + x_3x_{10} + x_6x_{10} + x_{10}x_{13} + x_3x_{14} + x_6x_{14} \\
& + x_{13}x_{14} + x_1x_2x_{10} + x_2x_{10}x_{24} + x_1x_2x_{14} \\
& + x_2x_{14}x_{24} + x_1x_5x_{10} + x_1x_{10}x_{25} + x_5x_{10}x_{24} \\
& + x_{10}x_{24}x_{25} + x_1x_5x_{14} + x_1x_{14}x_{25} + x_5x_{14}x_{24} + x_{14}x_{24}x_{25} \\
& + \bar{x}_9\bar{x}_{12}\bar{x}_{16}\bar{x}_{19}\bar{x}_{22}\bar{x}_{23} + \bar{x}_8\bar{x}_{12}\bar{x}_{16}\bar{x}_{18}\bar{x}_{20}\bar{x}_{21} + \bar{x}_9\bar{x}_{11}\bar{x}_{15}\bar{x}_{19}\bar{x}_{22}\bar{x}_{23} \\
& + \bar{x}_8\bar{x}_{11}\bar{x}_{15}\bar{x}_{18}\bar{x}_{20}\bar{x}_{21} + \bar{x}_9\bar{x}_{10}\bar{x}_{14}\bar{x}_{19}\bar{x}_{20}\bar{x}_{22}\bar{x}_{23} + \bar{x}_2\bar{x}_4\bar{x}_7\bar{x}_9\bar{x}_{17}\bar{x}_{19}\bar{x}_{22}\bar{x}_{23}\bar{x}_{25} \\
& + \bar{x}_2\bar{x}_4\bar{x}_7\bar{x}_8\bar{x}_{17}\bar{x}_{18}\bar{x}_{20}\bar{x}_{21}\bar{x}_{25} + \bar{x}_1\bar{x}_4\bar{x}_5\bar{x}_7\bar{x}_9\bar{x}_{17}\bar{x}_{19}\bar{x}_{22}\bar{x}_{23}\bar{x}_{24} \\
& + \bar{x}_1\bar{x}_4\bar{x}_5\bar{x}_7\bar{x}_8\bar{x}_{17}\bar{x}_{18}\bar{x}_{20}\bar{x}_{21}\bar{x}_{24} \\
& + \bar{x}_1\bar{x}_3\bar{x}_6\bar{x}_9\bar{x}_{13}\bar{x}_{19}\bar{x}_{20}\bar{x}_{22}\bar{x}_{23}\bar{x}_{24} + \bar{x}_2\bar{x}_3\bar{x}_5\bar{x}_6\bar{x}_9\bar{x}_{13}\bar{x}_{19}\bar{x}_{20}\bar{x}_{22}\bar{x}_{23}\bar{x}_{25}
\end{aligned} \tag{5.82}$$

Because x_8, x_{18}, and x_{21} are singletons, the above equation becomes:

$$\begin{aligned}
T = {} & x_8 + x_{18} + x_{21} + x_3x_{10} + x_6x_{10} + x_{10}x_{13} + x_3x_{14} + x_6x_{14} \\
& + x_{13}x_{14} + x_1x_2x_{10} + x_2x_{10}x_{24} + x_1x_2x_{14} \\
& + x_2x_{14}x_{24} + x_1x_5x_{10} + x_1x_{10}x_{25} + x_5x_{10}x_{24} \\
& + x_{10}x_{24}x_{25} + x_1x_5x_{14} + x_1x_{14}x_{25} + x_5x_{14}x_{24} + x_{14}x_{24}x_{25} \\
& + \bar{x}_9\bar{x}_{12}\bar{x}_{16}\bar{x}_{19}\bar{x}_{22}\bar{x}_{23} + \bar{x}_{12}\bar{x}_{16}\bar{x}_{20} + \bar{x}_9\bar{x}_{11}\bar{x}_{15}\bar{x}_{19}\bar{x}_{22}\bar{x}_{23} \\
& + \bar{x}_{11}\bar{x}_{15}\bar{x}_{20} + \bar{x}_9\bar{x}_{10}\bar{x}_{14}\bar{x}_{19}\bar{x}_{20}\bar{x}_{22}\bar{x}_{23} + \bar{x}_2\bar{x}_4\bar{x}_7\bar{x}_9\bar{x}_{17}\bar{x}_{19}\bar{x}_{22}\bar{x}_{23}\bar{x}_{25} \\
& + \bar{x}_2\bar{x}_4\bar{x}_7\bar{x}_{17}\bar{x}_{20}\bar{x}_{25} + \bar{x}_1\bar{x}_4\bar{x}_5\bar{x}_7\bar{x}_9\bar{x}_{17}\bar{x}_{19}\bar{x}_{22}\bar{x}_{23}\bar{x}_{24} + \bar{x}_1\bar{x}_4\bar{x}_5\bar{x}_7\bar{x}_{17}\bar{x}_{20}\bar{x}_{24} \\
& + \bar{x}_1\bar{x}_3\bar{x}_6\bar{x}_9\bar{x}_{13}\bar{x}_{19}\bar{x}_{20}\bar{x}_{22}\bar{x}_{23}\bar{x}_{24} + \bar{x}_2\bar{x}_3\bar{x}_5\bar{x}_6\bar{x}_9\bar{x}_{13}\bar{x}_{19}\bar{x}_{20}\bar{x}_{22}\bar{x}_{23}\bar{x}_{25}
\end{aligned} \tag{5.83}$$

■

Modularization. Let A and B be two basic events for which:

1. All terms that include A also include B
2. Neither term includes $\overline{A}\,\overline{B}$
3. For each term of the form $\overline{A}P$, there also exists a term of the form $\overline{B}P$

Then AB can be replaced by $Y \equiv (AB)$ or $\overline{Z} \equiv (AB)$ in each term that includes AB, the term $\overline{A}P$ is replaced by $\overline{Y}P$ or ZP, and term $\overline{B}P$ is deleted. A or B can be unnegated or negated variables and so modularization involves consideration of each of the pairs AB, $A\overline{B}$, $\overline{A}B$, or $\overline{A}\,\overline{B}$.

$$\begin{aligned}
ABX + \overline{A}P + \overline{B}P &= (AB)X + \overline{(AB)}P = YX + \overline{Y}P = \overline{Z}X + ZP \\
A\overline{B}X + \overline{A}P + BP &= (A\overline{B})X + \overline{(A\overline{B})}P = YX + \overline{Y}P = \overline{Z}X + ZP \\
\overline{A}BX + AP + \overline{B}P &= (\overline{A}B)X + \overline{(\overline{A}B)}P = YX + \overline{Y}P = \overline{Z}X + ZP \\
\overline{A}\,\overline{B}X + AP + BP &= (\overline{A}\,\overline{B})X + \overline{(\overline{A}\,\overline{B})}P = YX + \overline{Y}P = \overline{Z}X + ZP
\end{aligned} \tag{5.84}$$

Modularization replaces two basic events by one, and can be repeated for all possible parings of basic events, so that modularizing a group such as $A_1B_1A_2B_2$ is possible.

Example 15—A modularization process. Consider equation (5.83). All terms that include $\bar{x}_1$ also include $\bar{x}_{24}$, and for each term of the form x_1P, there also exists a term of the form

$x_{24}P$. Thus $\overline{x}_1\overline{x}_{24}$ can be replaced by $\overline{z}_1$ in each term that includes $\overline{x}_1\overline{x}_{24}$, the term $x_1 P$ is replaced by $y_1 P$, and the term $x_{24}P$ is deleted. Similar situations occur for pairs $(\overline{x}_2, \overline{x}_{25})$, $(\overline{x}_3, \overline{x}_6)$, $(\overline{x}_4, \overline{x}_7)$, $(\overline{x}_9, \overline{x}_{19})$, and so on:

$$\begin{aligned} T = {} & x_8 + x_{18} + x_{21} + u_3 z_6 + z_6 x_{13} \\ & + z_1 z_2 z_6 \\ & + z_1 x_5 z_6 \\ & + \overline{u}_5\overline{z}_8\overline{v}_5 + \overline{z}_8\overline{x}_{20} + \overline{u}_5\overline{z}_7\overline{v}_5 \\ & + \overline{z}_7\overline{x}_{20} + \overline{u}_5\overline{z}_6\overline{x}_{20}\overline{v}_5 + \overline{z}_2\overline{u}_4\overline{u}_5\overline{x}_{17}\overline{v}_5 \\ & + \overline{z}_2\overline{u}_4\overline{x}_{17}\overline{x}_{20} + \overline{z}_1\overline{u}_4\overline{x}_5\overline{u}_5\overline{x}_{17}\overline{v}_5 + \overline{z}_1\overline{u}_4\overline{x}_5\overline{x}_{17}\overline{x}_{20} \\ & + \overline{z}_1\overline{u}_3\overline{u}_5\overline{x}_{13}\overline{x}_{20}\overline{v}_5 + \overline{z}_2\overline{u}_3\overline{x}_5\overline{u}_5\overline{x}_{13}\overline{x}_{20}\overline{v}_5 \end{aligned} \tag{5.85}$$

where

$$\begin{aligned} &\overline{z}_1 = \overline{x}_1\overline{x}_{24}, \quad \overline{z}_2 = \overline{x}_2\overline{x}_{25}, \quad \overline{u}_3 = \overline{x}_3\overline{x}_6 \\ &\overline{u}_4 = \overline{x}_4\overline{x}_7, \quad \overline{u}_5 = \overline{x}_9\overline{x}_{19}, \quad \overline{v}_5 = \overline{x}_{22}\overline{x}_{23} \\ &\overline{z}_6 = \overline{x}_{10}\overline{x}_{14}, \quad \overline{z}_7 = \overline{x}_{11}\overline{x}_{15}, \quad \overline{z}_8 = \overline{x}_{12}\overline{x}_{16} \end{aligned} \tag{5.86}$$

Relevant pairs are observed in equation (5.85):

$$\begin{aligned} T = {} & x_8 + x_{18} + x_{21} + z_3 z_6 \\ & + z_1 z_2 z_6 \\ & + z_1 x_5 z_6 \\ & + \overline{z}_5\overline{z}_8 + \overline{z}_8\overline{x}_{20} + \overline{z}_5\overline{z}_7 \\ & + \overline{z}_7\overline{x}_{20} + \overline{z}_5\overline{z}_6\overline{x}_{20} + \overline{z}_2\overline{z}_4\overline{z}_5 \\ & + \overline{z}_2\overline{z}_4\overline{x}_{20} + \overline{z}_1\overline{z}_4\overline{x}_5\overline{z}_5 + \overline{z}_1\overline{z}_4\overline{x}_5\overline{x}_{20} \\ & + \overline{z}_1\overline{z}_3\overline{z}_5\overline{x}_{20} + \overline{z}_2\overline{z}_3\overline{x}_5\overline{z}_5\overline{x}_{20} \end{aligned} \tag{5.87}$$

where

$$\overline{z}_3 = \overline{u}_3\overline{x}_{13}, \quad \overline{z}_4 = \overline{u}_4\overline{x}_{17}, \quad \overline{z}_5 = \overline{u}_5\overline{v}_5 \tag{5.88}$$

Expression (5.87) is considerably easier to handle than (5.82). Furthermore, the sum of singletons $\overline{x}_8 + \overline{x}_{18} + \overline{x}_{21}$ can be treated as a module. ■

Module fault trees. Modules of noncoherent fault trees can be identified similarly to the coherent cases in Section 5.2.9.2 [5].

5.5.3 Minimal Cut Sets for a Multistate Fault Tree

Example 16—Nelson algorithm. Consider a top-event expression [18]:

$$T = X^{12}Z^{13} + X^2 Z^{123} + X^1 Y^2 Z^2 \tag{5.89}$$

Basic variables X and Y take values in set $\{0, 1, 2\}$ and variable Z in $\{0, 1, 2, 3\}$. Variable X^{12} becomes true when variable X is either 1 or 2. Other superfixed variables can be interpreted similarly. The top event occurs, for instance, when variables X and Z take the value 1.

By negation, there ensues:

$$\overline{T} = (X^0 + Z^{02})(X^{01} + Z^0)(X^{02} + Y^{01} + Z^{013}) \tag{5.90}$$

Then after development of the conjunctive form into the disjunctive form and simplifying,

$$\begin{aligned} \overline{T} &= (X^0 + X^0 Z^0 + X^{01} Z^{02} + Z^0)(X^{02} + Y^{01} + Z^{013}) && (5.91) \\ &= (X^0 + X^{01} Z^{02} + Z^0)(X^{02} + Y^{01} + Z^{013}) && (5.92) \\ &= X^0 + Z^0 + X^{01} Y^{01} Z^{02} && (5.93) \end{aligned}$$

Negation of this equation results in:

$$\bar{\bar{T}} = T = X^{12}Z^{123}(X^2 + Y^2 + Z^{13}) \tag{5.94}$$

Development of this conjunctive form and simplification lead to the top events expressed in terms of the disjunction of prime implicants:

$$T = X^{12}Z^{13} + X^2Z^{123} + X^{12}Y^2Z^{123} \tag{5.95}$$

Term $X^{12}Y^2Z^{123}$ covers a larger area than $X^1Y^2Z^2$ in (5.89). ■

Generalized consensus. The generalized consensus for binary variables can be extended to cases of multistate variables; however, the iterative process is time-consuming and tedious. The interested reader can consult reference [18].

REFERENCES

[1] Fussell, J. B., E. B. Henry, and N. H. Marshall. "MOCUS: A computer program to obtain minimal cut sets from fault trees." Aerojet Nuclear Company, ANCR-1156, 1974.

[2] Pande, P. K., M. E. Spector, and P. Chatterjee. "Computerized fault tree analysis: TREEL and MICSUP." Operation Research Center, University of California, Berkeley, ORC 75-3, 1975.

[3] Rosenthal, A. "Decomposition methods for fault tree analysis," *IEEE Trans. on Reliability*, vol. 26, no. 2, pp. 136–138, 1980.

[4] Han, S. H., T. W. Kim, and K. J. Yoo. "Development of an integrated fault tree analysis computer code MODULE by modularization technique," *Reliability Engineering and System Safety*, vol. 21, pp. 145–154, 1988.

[5] Kohda, T., E. J. Henley, and K. Inoue. "Finding modules in fault trees," *IEEE Trans. on Reliability*, vol. 38, no. 2, pp. 165–176, 1989.

[6] Barlow, R. E. "FTAP: Fault tree analysis program," *IEEE Trans. on Reliability*, vol. 30, no. 2, p. 116, 1981.

[7] Worrell, R. B. "SETS reference manual." Sandia National Laboratories, SAND 83-2675, 1984.

[8] Putney, B., H. R. Kirch, and J. M. Koren. "WAMCUT II: A fault tree evaluation program." Electric Power Research Institute, NP-2421, 1982.

[9] IAEA. "Computer codes for level 1 probabilistic safety assessment." IAEA, IAEA-TECDOC-553, June, 1990.

[10] Sabek, M., M. Gaafar, and A. Poucet. "Use of computer codes for system reliability analysis," *Reliability Engineering and System Safety*, vol. 26, pp. 369–383, 1989.

[11] Pullen, R. A. "AFTAP fault tree analysis program," *IEEE Trans. on Reliability*, vol. 33, no. 2, p. 171, 1984.

[12] Rasmuson, D. M., and N. H. Marshall. "FATRAM—A core efficient cut-set algorithm," *IEEE Trans. on Reliability*, vol. 27, no. 4, pp. 250–253, 1978.

[13] Limnios, N., and R. Ziani. "An algorithm for reducing cut sets in fault-tree analysis," *IEEE Trans. on Reliability*, vol. 35, no. 5, pp. 559–562, 1986.

[14] Taylor, J. R. RISϕ National Laboratory, Roskild, Denmark. Private Communication.

[15] Wagner, D. P., C. L. Cate, and J. B. Fussell. "Common cause failure analysis for complex systems." In *Nuclear Systems Reliability Engineering and Risk Assessment*, edited by J. Fussell and G. Burdick, pp. 289–313. Philadelphia: Society for Industrial and Applied Mathematics, 1977.

[16] USNRC. "PRA procedures guide: A guide to the performance of probabilistic risk assessments for nuclear power plants." USNRC, NUREG/CR-2300, 1983.

[17] Fardis, M., and C. A. Cornell. "Analysis of coherent multistate systems," *IEEE Trans. on Reliability*, vol. 30, no. 2, pp. 117–122, 1981.

[18] Garribba, S., E. Guagnini, and P. Mussio. "Multiple-valued logic trees: Meaning and prime implicants," *IEEE Trans. on Reliability*, vol. 34, no. 5, pp. 463–472, 1985.

[19] Quine, W. V. "The problem of simplifying truth functions," *American Mathematical Monthly*, vol. 59, pp. 521–531, 1952.

[20] Quine, W. V. "A way to simplify truth functions," *American Mathematical Monthly*, vol. 62, pp. 627–631, 1955.

[21] Tison, P. "Generalization of consensus theory and application to the minimization of Boolean functions," *IEEE Trans. on Electronic Computers*, vol. 16, no. 4, pp. 446–456, 1967.

[22] Wilson, J. M. "Modularizing and minimizing fault trees," *IEEE Trans. on Reliability*, vol. 34, no. 4, pp. 320–322, 1985.

PROBLEMS

5.1. Figure P5.1 shows a simplified fault tree for a domestic hot-water system in Problem 3.8. 1) Find the minimal cut sets. 2) Find the minimal path sets.

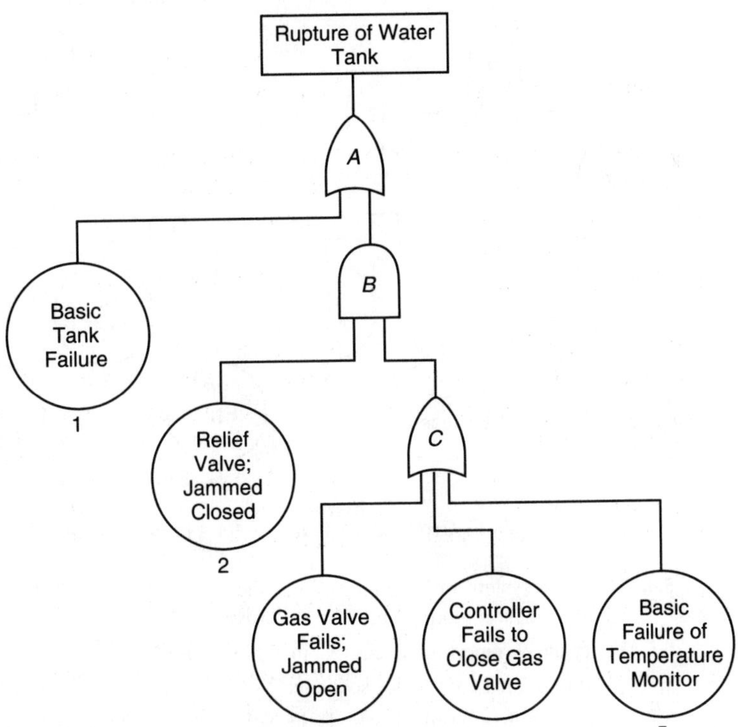

Figure P5.1. A simplified fault tree for a domestic hot-water system.

5.2. Figure P5.2 shows a simplified flow diagram for a chemical plant. Construct a fault tree, and find minimal path sets and cut sets for the event "plant failure."

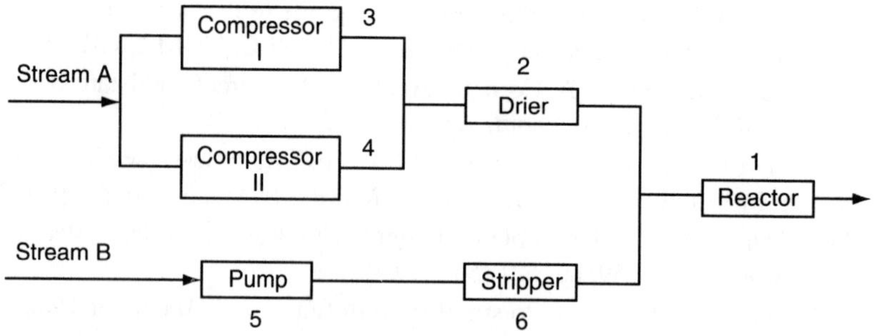

Figure P5.2. A simplified flow diagram for a chemical reactor.

5.3. Figure P5.3 shows a fault tree for the heater system of Problem 4.6. Obtain the minimal cut sets, noting the exclusive events.

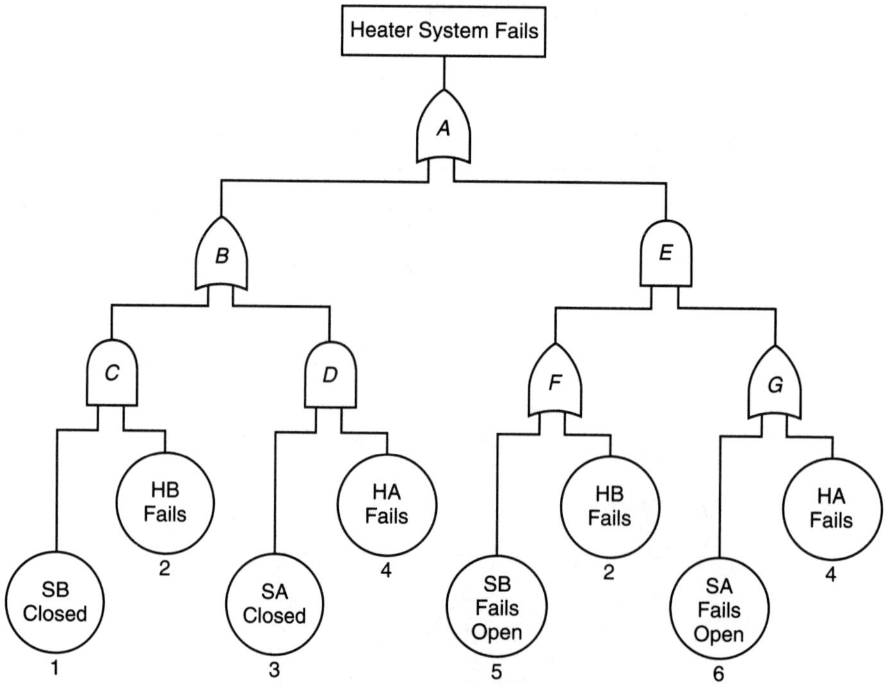

Figure P5.3. A fault tree for a heater system.

5.4. The relay system of Problem 4.7 has the fault tree shown in Figure P5.4. Obtain the minimal cut sets, noting mutually exclusive events.

5.5. Verify the common-mode cut sets in Table 5.3 for causes S3, S1, and T2.

5.6. Obtain minimal cut sets for sequence 3 of the Figure 5.14 event tree.

5.7. Prove the following equality by 1) the Nelson algorithm and 2) the generalized consensus.

$$\overline{A}B\overline{C} + \overline{A}BC + AB\overline{C} + ABC + A\overline{BC} + A\overline{B}C = A + B$$

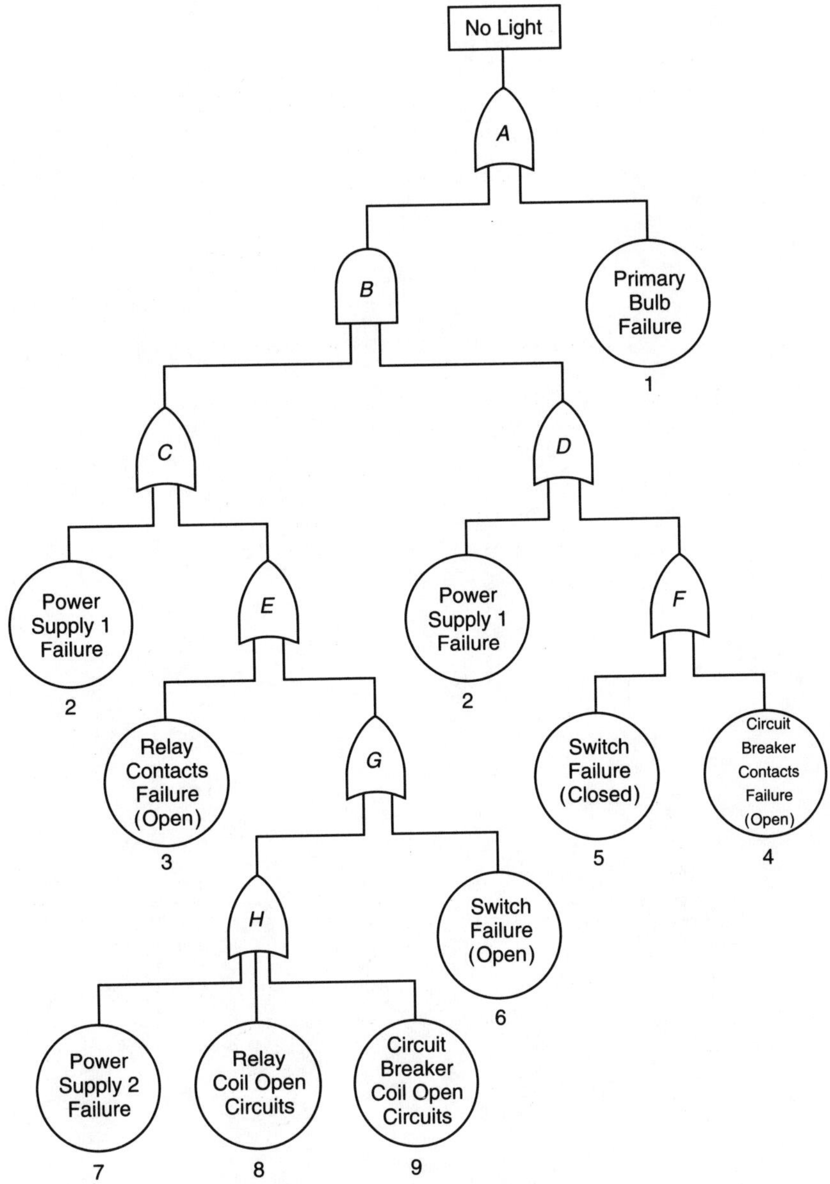

Figure P5.4. A fault tree for a relay system.

6

Quantification of Basic Events

6.1 INTRODUCTION

All systems eventually fail; nothing is perfectly reliable, nothing endures forever. A reliability engineer must assume that a system will fail and, therefore, concentrate on decreasing the frequency of failure to an economically and socially acceptable level. That is a more realistic and tenable approach than are political slogans such as "zero pollution," "no risk," and "accident-free."

Probabilistic statements are not unfamiliar to the public. We have become accustomed, for example, to a weather forecaster predicting that "there is a twenty percent risk of thundershowers."* Likewise, the likelihood that a person will be drenched if her umbrella malfunctions can be expressed probabilistically. For instance, one might say that there is a 80% chance that a one-year-old umbrella will work as designed. This probability is, of course, time dependent. The reliability of an umbrella would be expected to decrease with time; a two-year-old umbrella is more likely to fail than a one-year-old umbrella.

Reliability is by no means the only performance criterion by which a device such as an umbrella can be characterized. If it malfunctions or breaks, it can be repaired. Because the umbrella cannot be used while it is being repaired, one might also measure its performance in terms of availability, that is, the fraction of time it is available for use and functioning properly. Repairs cost money, so we also want to know the expected number of failures during any given time interval.

Intuitively, one feels that there are analytical relationships between descriptions such as reliability, availability, and expected number of failures. In this chapter, these relationships are developed. An accurate description of component failures and failure modes

*A comedian once asked whether this statement meant that if you stopped ten people in the street and asked them if it would rain, two of them would say "yes."

is central to the identification of system failures, because these are caused by combinations of component failures. If there are no system-dependent component failures, then the quantification of basic (component) failures is independent of a particular system, and generalizations can be made. Unfortunately that is not usually the case.

In this chapter, we first quantify basic events related to system components with binary states, that is, normal and failed states. By components, we mean elementary devices, equipment, subsystems, and so forth. Then this quantification is extended to components having plural failure modes. Finally, quantitative aspects of human errors and impacts from the environment are discussed.

We assume that the reader has some knowledge of statistics. Statistical concepts generic to reliability are developed in this chapter and additional material can be found in Appendix A.1 to this chapter. A useful glossary of definitions appears as Appendix A.6.

There are a seemingly endless number of sophisticated definitions and equations in this chapter, and the reader may wonder whether this degree of detail and complexity is justified or whether it is a purely academic indulgence.

The first version of this chapter, which was written in 1975, was considerably simpler and contained fewer definitions. When this material was distributed at the NATO Advanced Study Institute on Risk Analysis in 1978, it became clear during the ensuing discussion that the (historical) absence of very precise and commonly understood definitions for failure parameters had resulted in theories of limited validity and computer programs that purport to calculate identical parameters but don't. In rewriting this chapter, we tried to set things right, and to label all parameters so that their meanings are clear. Much existing confusion centers around the lack of rigor in defining failure parameters as being conditional or unconditional. Clearly, the probability of a person's living the day after their 30th birthday party is not the same as the probability of a person's living for 30 years and 1 day. The latter probability is unconditional, while the former is conditional on the person's having survived to age thirty.

As alluded to in the preface, the numerical precision in the example problems is not warranted in light of the normally very imprecise experimental failure data. The numbers are carried for ease of parameter identification.

6.2 PROBABILISTIC PARAMETERS

We assume that, at any given time, a component is either functioning normally or failed, and that the component state changes as time evolves. Possible transitions of state are shown in Figure 6.1. A new component "jumps" into a normal state and is there for some time, then fails and experiences a transition to the failed state. The failed state continues forever if the component is nonrepairable. A repairable component remains in the failed state for a period, then undergoes a transition to the normal state when the repair is completed. It is assumed that the component changes its state instantaneously when the transition takes place. It is further assumed that, at most, one transition occurs in a sufficiently small time interval and that the possibility of two or more transitions is negligible.

The transition to the normal state is called repair, whereas the transition to the failed state is failure. We assume that repairs restore the component to a condition as good as new, so we can regard the factory production of a component as a repair. The entire cycle thus consists of repetitions of the repair-to-failure and the failure-to-repair process. We first discuss the repair-to-failure process, then failure-to-repair process, and finally the combined process.

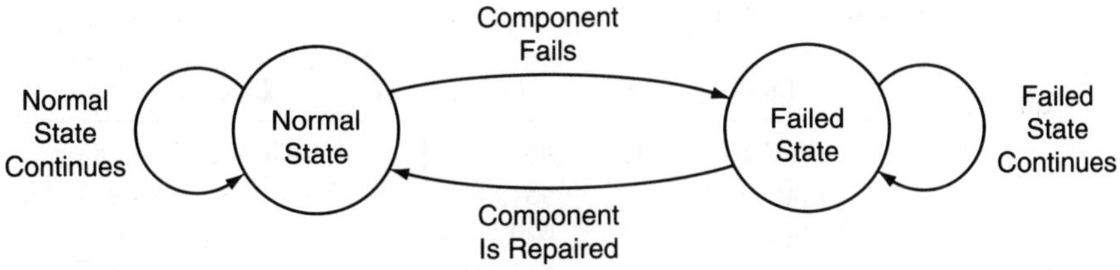

Figure 6.1. Transition diagram of component states.

6.2.1 A Repair-to-Failure Process

A life cycle is a typical repair-to-failure process. Here *repair* means birth and *failure* corresponds to death.

We cannot predict a person's exact lifetime, because death is a random variable whose characteristics must be established by considering a sample from a large population. Failure can be characterized only by the stochastic properties of the population as a whole.

The *reliability* $R(t)$, in this example, is the probability of survival to (inclusive or exclusive) age t, and is the number surviving at t divided by the total sample. Denote by random variable T the lifetime. Then,

$$R(t) = \Pr\{T \geq t\} = \Pr\{T > t\} \tag{6.1}$$

Similarly, the *unreliability* $F(t)$ is the probability of death to age t (inclusive or exclusive) and is obtained by dividing the total number of deaths before age t by the total population.

$$F(t) = \Pr\{T \leq t\} = \Pr\{T < t\} \tag{6.2}$$

Note that the inclusion or exclusion of equality in equations (6.1) and (6.2) yields no difference because variable T is continuous valued and hence in general

$$\Pr\{T = t\} = 0 \tag{6.3}$$

This book, for convenience, assumes that the equality is included and excluded for definitions of reliability and unreliability, respectively:

$$R(t) \equiv \Pr\{T \geq t\}, \quad F(t) \equiv \Pr\{T < t\} \tag{6.4}$$

From the mortality data in Table 6.1, which lists lifetimes for a population of 1,023,102, the reliability and the unreliability are calculated in Table 6.2 and plotted in Figure 6.2.

The curve of $R(t)$ versus t is a survival distribution, whereas the curve of $F(t)$ versus t is a failure distribution. The survival distribution represents both the probability of survival of an individual to age t and the proportion of the population expected to survive to any given age t. The failure distribution $F(t)$ is the probability of death of an individual before age t. It also represents the proportion of the population that is predicted to die before age t. The difference $F(t_2) - F(t_1)$, $(t_2 > t_1)$ is the proportion of the population expected to die between ages t_1 and t_2.

Because the number of deaths at each age is known, a histogram such as the one in Figure 6.3 can be drawn. The height of each bar in the histogram represents the number of deaths in a particular life band. This is proportional to the difference $F(t + \Delta) - F(t)$, where Δ is the width of the life band.

If the width is reduced, the steps in Figure 6.3 draw progressively closer, until a continuous curve is formed. This curve, when normalized by the total sample, is the *failure density* $f(t)$. This density is a probability density function. The probability of death during a small life band $[t, t + dt)$ is given by $f(t)dt$ and is equal to $F(t + dt) - F(t)$.

TABLE 6.1. Mortality Data [1]

t	$L(t)$	t	$L(t)$	t	$L(t)$	t	$L(t)$
0	1,023,102	15	962,270	50	810,900	85	78,221
1	1,000,000	20	951,483	55	754,191	90	21,577
2	994,230	25	939,197	60	677,771	95	3,011
3	990,114	30	924,609	65	577,822	99	125
4	986,767	35	906,554	70	454,548	100	
5	983,817	40	883,342	75	315,982	0	
10	971,804	45	852,554	80	181,765		

t = age in years
$L(t)$ = number living at age t

TABLE 6.2. Human Reliability

t	$L(t)$	$R(t) = L(t)/N$	$F(t) = 1 - R(t)$
0	1,023,102	1.0000	0.0000
1	1,000,000	0.9774	0.0226
2	994,230	0.9718	0.0282
3	990,114	0.9678	0.0322
4	986,767	0.9645	0.0355
5	983,817	0.9616	0.0384
10	971,804	0.9499	0.0501
15	962,270	0.9405	0.0595
20	951,483	0.9300	0.0700
25	939,197	0.9180	0.0820
30	924,609	0.9037	0.0963
35	906,554	0.8861	0.1139
40	883,342	0.8634	0.1366
45	852,554	0.8333	0.1667
50	810,900	0.7926	0.2074
55	754,191	0.7372	0.2628
60	677,771	0.6625	0.3375
65	577,822	0.5648	0.4352
70	454,548	0.4443	0.5557
75	315,982	0.3088	0.6912
80	181,765	0.1777	0.8223
85	78,221	0.0765	0.9235
90	21,577	0.0211	0.9789
95	3,011	0.0029	0.9971
99	125	0.0001	0.9999
100	0	0.0000	1.0000

t = age in years
$L(t)$ = number living at age t

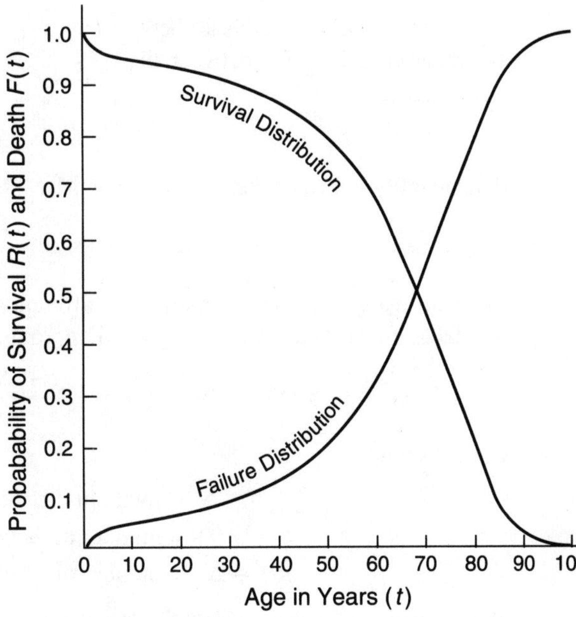

Figure 6.2. Survival and failure distributions.

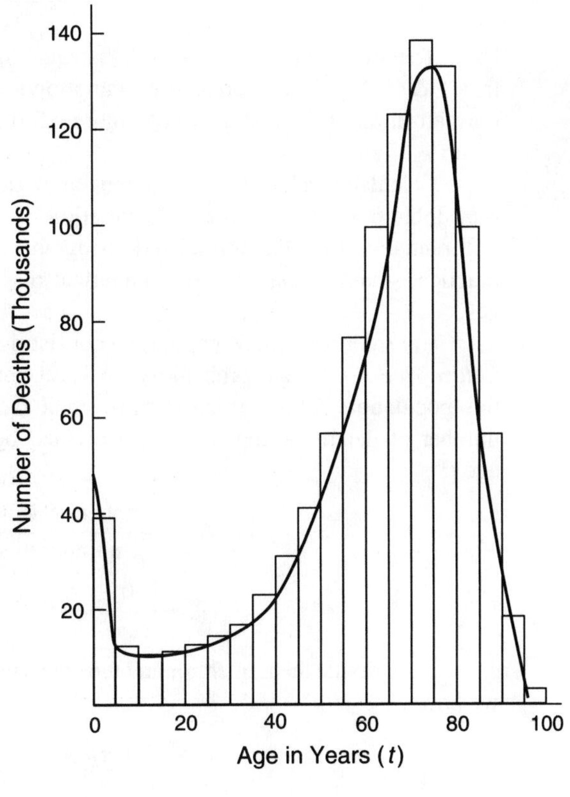

Figure 6.3. Histogram and smooth curve.

The probability of death between ages t_1 and t_2 is the area under the curve obtained by integrating the curve between the ages

$$F(t_2) - F(t_1) = \int_{t_1}^{t_2} f(t)dt \tag{6.5}$$

This identity indicates that the failure density $f(t)$ is

$$f(t) = \frac{dF(t)}{dt} \tag{6.6}$$

and can be approximated by numerical differentiation when a smooth failure distribution is available, for instance, by a polynomial approximation of discrete values of $F(t)$:

$$f(t) \simeq \frac{F(t+\Delta) - F(t)}{\Delta} \tag{6.7}$$

Letting

$$N = \text{total number of sample} = 1{,}023{,}102$$
$$n(t) = \text{number of deaths before age } t$$
$$n(t+\Delta) = \text{number of deaths before age } t+\Delta$$

the quantity $[n(t+\Delta) - n(t)]/N$ is the proportion of the population expected to die during $[t, t+\Delta)$ and equals $F(t+\Delta) - F(t)$. Thus

$$f(t) \simeq \frac{n(t+\Delta) - n(t)}{\Delta \cdot N} \tag{6.8}$$

The quantity $[n(t+\Delta) - n(t)]$ is equal to the height of the histogram in a life band $[t, t+\Delta)$. Thus the numerical differentiation formula of equation (6.8) is equivalent to the normalization of the histogram of Figure 6.3 divided by the total sample N and the band width Δ.

Calculated values for $f(t)$ are given in Table 6.3 and plotted in Figure 6.4. Column 4 of Table 6.3 is based on a differentiation of curve $F(t)$, and column 3 on a numerical differentiation (i.e., the normalized histogram). Ideally, the values should be identical; in practice, small sample size and numerical inaccuracies lead to differences in point values.

Consider now a new population consisting of the individuals surviving at age t. The *failure rate* $r(t)$ is the probability of death per unit time at age t for the individual in this population. Thus for sufficiently small Δ, the quantity $r(t) \cdot \Delta$ is estimated by the number of deaths during $[t, t+\Delta)$ divided by the number of individuals surviving at age t:

$$\begin{aligned} r(t) \cdot \Delta &= \frac{\text{number of deaths during } [t, t+\Delta)}{\text{number of survivals at age } t} \\ &= \frac{[n(t+\Delta) - n(t)]}{L(t)} \end{aligned} \tag{6.9}$$

If we divide the numerator and the denominator by the total sample ($N = 1{,}023{,}102$), we have

$$r(t)\Delta = \frac{f(t)\Delta}{R(t)} \tag{6.10}$$

TABLE 6.3. Failure Density Function $f(t)$

t	$n(t+\Delta)-n(t)$	$f(t)=\dfrac{n(t+\Delta)-n(t)}{N\cdot\Delta}$	$f(t)=\dfrac{dF(t)}{dt}$
0	23,102	0.0226	0.0054
1	5,770	0.0056	0.0045
2	4,116	0.0040	0.0028
3	3,347	0.0033	0.0033
4	2,950	0.0029	0.0029
5	12,013	0.0023	0.0019
10	9,534	0.0019	0.0020
15	10,787	0.0021	0.0022
20	12,286	0.0024	0.0026
25	14,588	0.0029	0.0036
30	18,055	0.0035	0.0039
35	23,212	0.0045	0.0044
40	30,788	0.0060	0.0064
45	41,654	0.0081	0.0096
50	56,709	0.0111	0.0137
55	76,420	0.0149	0.0180
60	99,949	0.0195	0.0220
65	123,274	0.0241	0.0249
70	138,566	0.0271	0.0261
75	134,217	0.0262	0.0246
80	103,544	0.0202	0.0195
85	56,644	0.0111	0.0097
90	18,566	0.0036	0.0021
95	2,886	0.0007	—
99	125	0.0001	—
100	—	—	—

t = age in years
$n(t+\Delta)-n(t)$ = number of failures (death)

because $R(t)$ is the number of survivals at age t divided by the population, and the numerator is equivalent to equation (6.8). This can also be written as

$$r(t)=\frac{f(t)}{R(t)}=\frac{f(t)}{1-F(t)} \tag{6.11}$$

This method of calculating the failure rate $r(t)$ results in the data summarized in Table 6.4 and plotted in Figure 6.5. The curve of $r(t)$ is known as a *bathtub curve*. It is characterized by a relatively high early failure rate (the burn-in period) followed by a fairly constant, prime-of-life period where failures occur randomly, and then a final wearout or burn-out phase. Ideally, critical hardware is put into service after a burn-in period and replaced before the wearout phase.

Example 1. Calculate, using the mortality data of Table 6.1, the reliability $R(t)$, unreliability $F(t)$, failure density $f(t)$, and failure rate $r(t)$ for:

1. A person's living to be 75 years old
2. A person on the day after their 75th birthday party

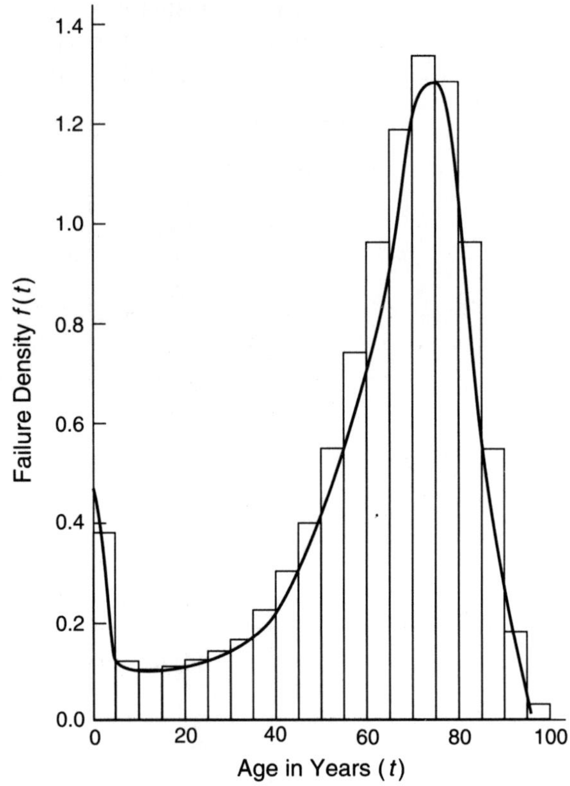

Figure 6.4. Failure density $f(t)$.

TABLE 6.4. Calculation of Failure Rate $r(t)$

Age in Years	Number of Failures (Death)	$r(t) = f(t)/R(t)$	Age in Years	Number of Failures (Death)	$r(t) = f(t)/R(t)$
0	23,102	0.0226	40	30,788	0.0070
1	5770	0.0058	45	41,654	0.0098
2	4116	0.0041	50	56,709	0.0140
3	3347	0.0034	55	76,420	0.0203
4	2950	0.0030	60	99,949	0.0295
5	12,013	0.0024	65	123,274	0.0427
10	9534	0.0020	70	138,566	0.0610
15	10,787	0.0022	75	134,217	0.0850
20	12,286	0.0026	80	103,544	0.1139
25	14,588	0.0031	85	56,644	0.1448
30	18,055	0.0039	90	18,566	0.1721
35	23,212	0.0051	95	2886	0.2396
			99	125	1.0000

Solution:

1. At age 75 (neglecting the additional day):

$$
\begin{aligned}
R(t) &= 0.3088, \quad F(t) = 0.6912 \text{ (Table 6.2)} \\
f(t) &= 0.02620 \quad \text{(Table 6.3)} \\
r(t) &= 0.08500 \quad \text{(Table 6.4)}
\end{aligned}
\tag{6.12}
$$

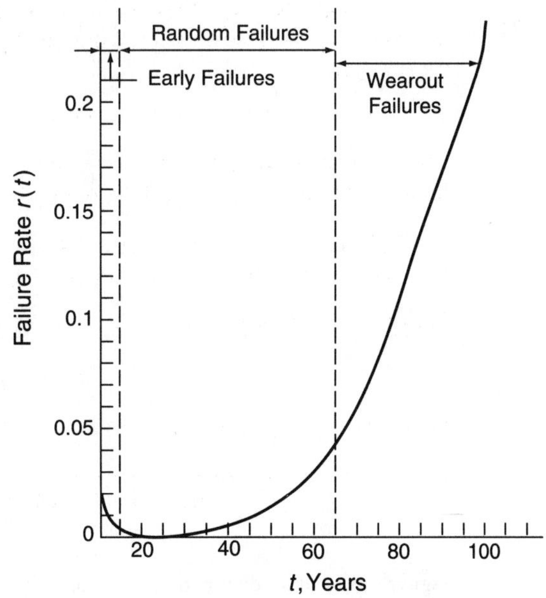

Figure 6.5. Failure rate $r(t)$ versus t.

2. In effect, we start with a new population of $N = 315{,}982$ having the following characteristics, where $t = 0$ means 75 years.

t	$L(t)$	$L(t)/N$ $R(t)$	$1 - R(t)$ $F(t)$	Table 6.3 $n(t+\Delta) - n(t)$	$\frac{n(t+\Delta)-n(t)}{N \cdot \Delta}$ $f(t)$	$f(t)/R(t)$ $r(t)$
0	315,982	1.0000	0.0000	134,217	0.0850	0.0850
5	181,765	0.5750	0.4250	103,554	0.0655	0.1139
10	78,221	0.2480	0.7520	56,634	0.0358	0.1444
15	21,577	0.0683	0.9317	18,566	0.0118	0.1728
20	3,011	0.0095	0.9905	2,886	0.0023	0.2421
24	125	0.0004	0.9996	125	0.0004	1.0000
25	0	0.0000	1.0000	0	0.0000	—

By linear interpolation techniques, at 75 years and 1 day.

$$\begin{aligned} R(t) &= 1 + \frac{0.575 - 1}{5 \times 365} = 0.9998 \\ F(t) &= 1 - R(t) = 0.0002 \\ f(t) &= 0.085 + \frac{0.0655 - 0.0850}{5 \times 365} = 0.0850 \\ r(t) &= 0.0850 \end{aligned} \tag{6.13}$$

Figure 6.6 shows the failure distribution for this population. ■

6.2.2 A Repair-Failure-Repair Process

A repairable component experiences repetitions of the repair-to-failure and failure-to-repair process. The characteristics of such components can be obtained by considering the component as a sample from a population of identical components undergoing similar

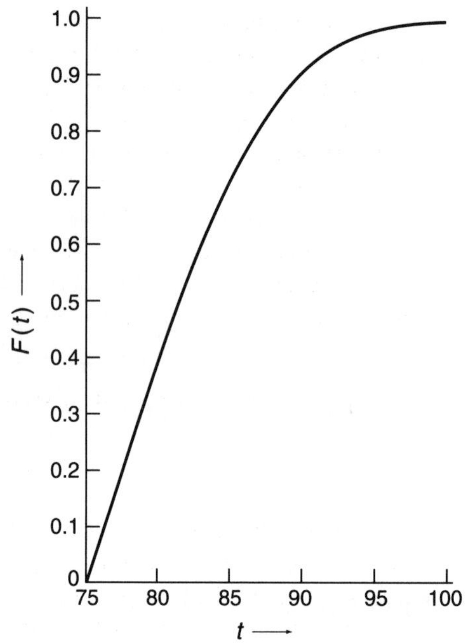

Figure 6.6. Failure distribution $F(t)$ for Example 1.

repetitions. The time-varying history of each sample in a population of 10 is illustrated in Figure 6.7. All samples are assumed to jump into the normal state at time zero; that is, each component is as good as new at $t = 0$. The following probabilistic parameters describe the population of Figure 6.7.

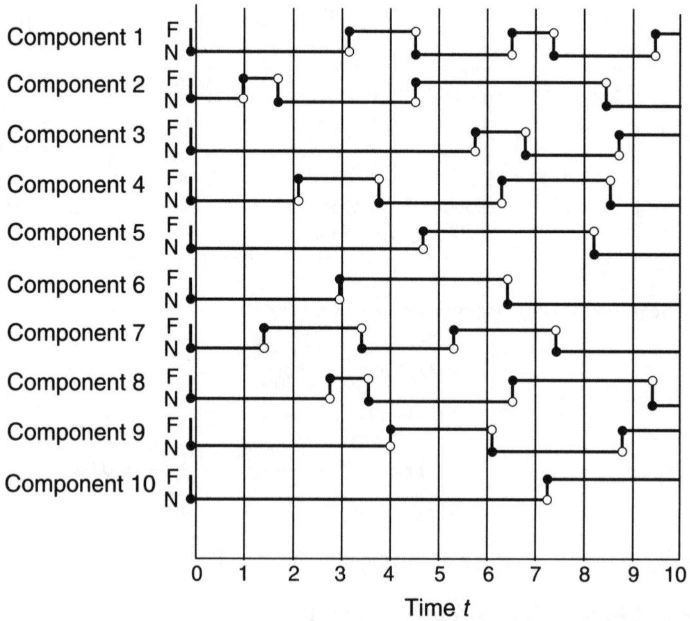

Figure 6.7. History of component states. F: failed; N: normal.

Availability $A(t)$ at time t is the probability of the component's being normal at time t. This is the number of the normal components at time t divided by the total sample. For our sample, we have $A(5) = 6/10 = 0.6$. Note that the normal components at time t have different ages, and that these differ from t. For example, component 1 in Figure 6.7 has age 0.5 at time 5, whereas component 4 has age 1.2.

Unavailability $Q(t)$ is the probability that the component is in the failed state at time t and is equal to the number of the failed components at time t divided by the total sample.

Unconditional failure intensity $w(t)$ is the probability that the component fails per unit time at time t. Figure 6.7 shows that components 3 and 7 fail during time period $[5, 6)$, so $w(5)$ is approximated by $2/10 = 0.2$.

The quantity $w(5) \times 1$ is equal to the *expected number of failures* $W(5, 6)$ during the time interval $[5, 6)$. The expected number of failures $W(0, 6)$ during $[0, 6)$ is evaluated by

$$W(0, 6) = w(0) \times 1 + \cdots + w(5) \times 1 \tag{6.14}$$

The exact value of $W(0, 6)$ is given by the integration

$$W(0, 6) = \int_0^6 w(t)dt \tag{6.15}$$

Unconditional repair intensity $v(t)$ and *expected number of repairs* $V(t_1, t_2)$ can be defined similarly to $w(t)$ and $W(t_1, t_2)$, respectively. The costs due to failures and repairs during $[t_1, t_2)$ can be related to $W(t_1, t_2)$ and $V(t_1, t_2)$, respectively, if the production losses for failure and cost-to-repair are known.

There is yet another failure parameter to be obtained. Consider another population of components that are normal at time t. When $t = 5$, this population consists of components 1, 3, 4, 7, 8, and 10. A *conditional failure intensity* $\lambda(t)$ is the proportion of the (normal) population expected to fail per unit time at time t. For example, $\lambda \times 1$ is estimated as $2/6$, because components 3 and 7 fail during $[5, 6)$. A *conditional repair intensity* $\mu(t)$ is defined similarly. Large values of $\lambda(t)$ mean that the component is about to fail, whereas large values of $\mu(t)$ state that the component will be repaired soon.

Example 2. Calculate values for $R(t)$, $F(t)$, $f(t)$, $r(t)$, $A(t)$, $Q(t)$, $w(t)$, $W(0, t)$, and $\lambda(t)$ for the 10 components of Figure 6.7 at 5 hr and 9 hr.

Solution: We need times to failures (i.e., lifetimes) to calculate $R(t)$, $F(t)$, $f(t)$, and $r(t)$, because these are parameters in the repair-to-failure process.

Component	Repair t	Failure t	TTF
1	0	3.1	3.1
1	4.5	6.6	2.1
1	7.4	9.5	2.1
2	0	1.05	1.05
2	1.7	4.5	2.8
3	0	5.8	5.8
3	6.8	8.8	2.0
4	0	2.1	2.1
4	3.8	6.4	2.6
5	0	4.8	4.8
6	0	3.0	3.0
7	0	1.4	1.4
7	3.5	5.4	1.9
8	0	2.85	2.85
8	3.65	6.7	3.05
9	0	4.1	4.1
9	6.2	8.95	2.75
10	0	7.35	7.35

The following mortality data is obtained from these times to failures.

t	$L(t)$	$R(t)$	$F(t)$	$n(t+\Delta)-n(t)$	$f(t)$	$r(t)=f(t)/R(t)$
0	18	1.0000	0.0000	0	0.0000	0.0000
1	18	1.0000	0.0000	3	0.1667	0.1667
2	15	0.8333	0.1667	10	0.5556	0.6667
3	7	0.3889	0.6111	3	0.1667	0.4286
4	4	0.2222	0.7778	2	0.1111	0.5000
5	2	0.1111	0.8889	1	0.0556	0.5005
6	1	0.0556	0.9444	0	0.0000	0.0000
7	1	0.0556	0.9444	1	0.0556	1.0000
8	0	0.0000	1.0000	0	0.0000	—
9	0	0.0000	1.0000	0	0.0000	—

Thus at age 5,

$$R(5) = 0.1111, \quad F(5) = 0.8889, \quad f(5) = 0.0556, \quad r(5) = 0.5005 \tag{6.16}$$

and at age 9,

$$R(9) = 0, \quad F(9) = 1, \quad f(9) = 0, \quad r(9)\text{: undefined} \tag{6.17}$$

Parameters $A(t)$, $Q(t)$, $w(t)$, $W(0, t)$, and $\lambda(t)$ are obtained from the combined repair-failure-repair process shown in Figure 6.7. At time 5,

$$A(5) = 6/10 = 0.6, \quad Q(5) = 0.4, \quad w(5) = 0.2 \tag{6.18}$$

$$W(0,5) = \frac{[2+2+2+3]}{10} = 0.9, \quad \lambda(5) = 2/6 = 1/3 \tag{6.19}$$

and at time 9,

$$A(9) = 6/10 = 0.6, \quad Q(9) = 0.4, \quad w(9) = 0.1 \tag{6.20}$$

$$W(0,9) = W(0,5) + \frac{[2+3+1+2]}{10} = 1.7, \quad \lambda(5) = 1/6 \tag{6.21}$$

■

6.2.3 Parameters of Repair-to-Failure Process

We return now to the problem of characterizing the reliability parameters for repair-to-failure processes. These processes apply to nonrepairable components and also to repairable components if we restrict our attention to times to the first failures. We first restate some of the concepts introduced in Section 6.2.1, in a more formal manner, and then deduce new relations.

Consider a process starting at a repair and ending in its first failure. Shift the time axis appropriately, and take $t = 0$ as the time at which the component is repaired, so that the component is then as good as new at time zero. The probabilistic definitions and their notations are summarized as follows:

$R(t)$ = reliability at time t:

The probability that the component experiences no failure during the time interval $[0, t]$, given that the component was repaired at time zero.

The curve $R(t)$ versus t is a survival distribution. The distribution is monotonically decreasing, because the reliability gets smaller as time increases. A typical survival distribution is shown in Figure 6.2.

The following asymptotic properties hold:

$$\lim_{t \to 0} R(t) = 1 \tag{6.22}$$

$$\lim_{t \to \infty} R(t) = 0 \tag{6.23}$$

Equation (6.22) shows that almost all components function near time zero, whereas equation (6.23) indicates a vanishingly small probability of a component's surviving forever.

$F(t)$ = unreliability at time t:

The probability that the component experiences the first failure during the time interval $[0, t)$, given that the component was repaired at time zero.

The curve $F(t)$ versus t is called a failure distribution and is a monotonically increasing function of t. A typical failure distribution is shown in Figure 6.2.

The following asymptotic properties hold:

$$\lim_{t \to 0} F(t) = 0 \tag{6.24}$$

$$\lim_{t \to \infty} F(t) = 1 \tag{6.25}$$

Equation (6.24) shows that few components fail just after repair (or birth), whereas (6.25) indicates an asymptotic approach to complete failure.

Because the component either remains normal or experiences its first failure during the time interval $[0, t)$,

$$R(t) + F(t) = 1 \tag{6.26}$$

Now let $t_1 \leq t_2$. The difference $F(t_2) - F(t_1)$ is the probability that the component experiences its first failure during the time interval $[t_1, t_2)$, given that it was as good as new at time zero. This probability is illustrated in Figure 6.8.

$f(t)$ = failure density of $F(t)$.

This was shown previously to be the first derivative of $F(t)$.

$$f(t) = \frac{dF(t)}{dt} \tag{6.27}$$

or, equivalently,

$$f(t)dt = F(t + dt) - F(t) \tag{6.28}$$

Thus, $f(t)dt$ is the probability that the first component failure occurs during the small interval $[t, t + dt)$, given that the component was repaired at time zero.

The unreliability $F(t)$ is obtained by integration,

$$F(t) = \int_0^t f(u)du \tag{6.29}$$

Similarly, the difference $F(\infty) - F(t) = 1 - F(t)$ in the unreliability is the reliability

$$R(t) = \int_t^\infty f(u)du \tag{6.30}$$

These relationships are illustrated in Figure 6.9.

$r(t)$ = failure rate:

The probability that the component experiences a failure per unit time at time t, given that the component was repaired at time zero and has survived to time t.

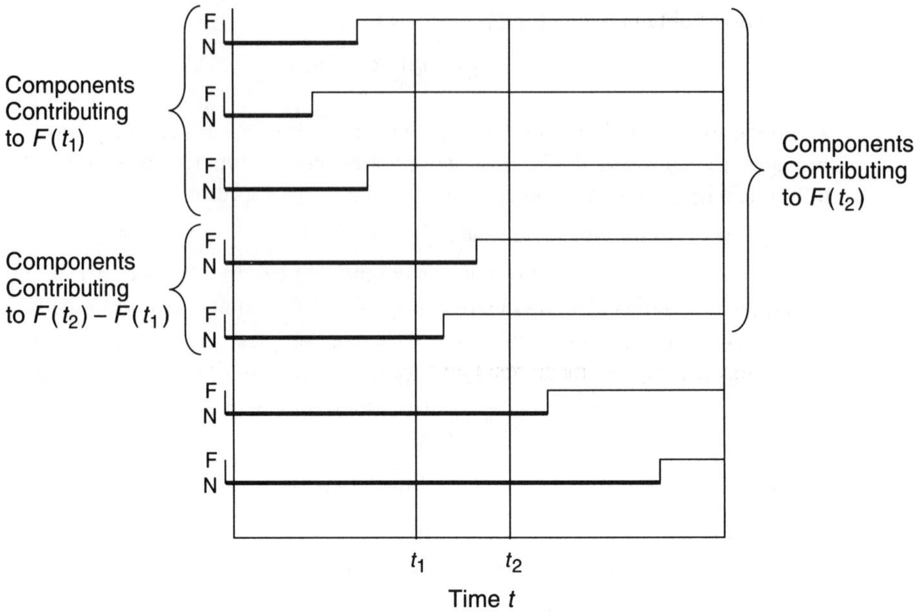

Figure 6.8. Illustration of probability $F(t_2) - F(t_1)$.

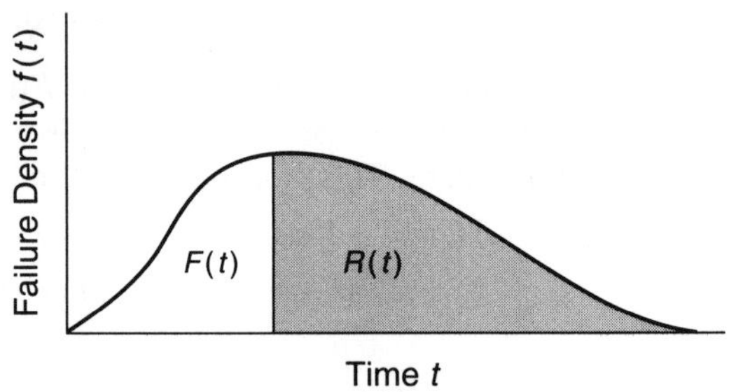

Figure 6.9. Integration of failure density $f(t)$.

The quantity $r(t)dt$ is the probability that the component fails during $[t, t+dt)$, given that the component age is t.† Here age t means that the component was repaired at time zero and has survived to time t. The rate is simply designated as r when it is independent of the age t. The component with a constant failure rate r is considered as good as new if it is functioning.

TTF = time to failure:

The span of time from repair to first failure.

The time to failure TTF is a random variable, because we cannot predict the exact time of the first failure.

MTTF = mean time to failure:

The expected value of the time to failure, TTF.

†The failure rate is called a *hazard rate function* in some texts.

This is obtained by

$$\text{MTTF} = \int_0^\infty t f(t) dt \tag{6.31}$$

The quantity $f(t)dt$ is the probability that the TTF is around t, so equation (6.31) is the average of all possible TTFs. If $R(t)$ decreases to zero, that is, if $R(\infty) = 0$, the above MTTF can be expressed as

$$\text{MTTF} = \int_0^\infty R(t) dt \tag{6.32}$$

This integral can be calculated more easily than (6.31).

Suppose that a component has been normal to time u. The residual life from u is also a random variable, and mean residual time to failure (MRTTF) is given by

$$\text{MRTTF} = \int_u^\infty \frac{(t-u)f(t)}{R(u)} dt \tag{6.33}$$

The MTTF is where $u = 0$.

Example 3. Table 6.5 shows failure data for 250 germanium transistors. Calculate the unreliability $F(t)$, the failure rate $r(t)$, the failure density $f(t)$, and the MTTF.

TABLE 6.5. Failure Data for Transistors

Time to Failure *t* (Days)	**Cumulative Failures**
0	0
20	9
40	23
60	50
90	83
160	113
230	143
400	160
900	220
1200	235
2500	240
∞	250

Solution: The unreliability $F(t)$ at a given time t is simply the number of transistors failed to time t divided by the total number (250) of samples tested. The results are summarized in Table 6.6 and the failure distribution is plotted in Figure 6.10.

The failure density $f(t)$ and the failure rate $r(t)$ are calculated in a similar manner to the mortality case (Example 1) and are listed in Table 6.6. The first-order approximation of the rate is a constant rate $r(t) = r = 0.0026$, the averaged value. In general, the constant failure rate describes solid-state components without moving parts, and systems and equipment that are in their prime of life, for example, an automobile having mileage of 3000 to 40,000 mi.

If the failure rate is constant then, as shown in Section 6.4, $\text{MTTF} = 1/r = 385$. Alternatively, equation (6.31) could be used, giving

$$\text{MTTF} = 10 \times 0.0018 \times 20 + 30 \times 0.0028 \times 20 + \cdots + 1850 \times 0.00002 \times 1300 = 501 \tag{6.34}$$

■

TABLE 6.6. Transistor Reliability, Unreliability, Failure Density, and Failure Rate

t	$L(t)$	$R(t)$	$F(t)$	$n(t+\Delta)-n(t)$	Δ	$f(t)=\frac{n(t+\Delta)-n(t)}{N\cdot\Delta}$	$r(t)=\frac{f(t)}{R(t)}$
0	250	1.0000	0.0000	9	20	0.00180	0.0018
20	241	0.9640	0.0360	14	20	0.00280	0.0029
40	227	0.9080	0.0920	27	20	0.00540	0.0059
60	200	0.8000	0.2000	33	30	0.00440	0.0055
90	167	0.6680	0.3320	30	70	0.00171	0.0026
160	137	0.5480	0.4520	30	70	0.00171	0.0031
230	107	0.4280	0.5720	17	170	0.00040	0.0009
400	90	0.3600	0.6400	60	500	0.00048	0.0013
900	30	0.1200	0.8800	15	300	0.00020	0.0017
1200	15	0.0600	0.9400	5	1300	0.00002	0.0003
2500	10	0.0400	0.9600	—	—	—	—

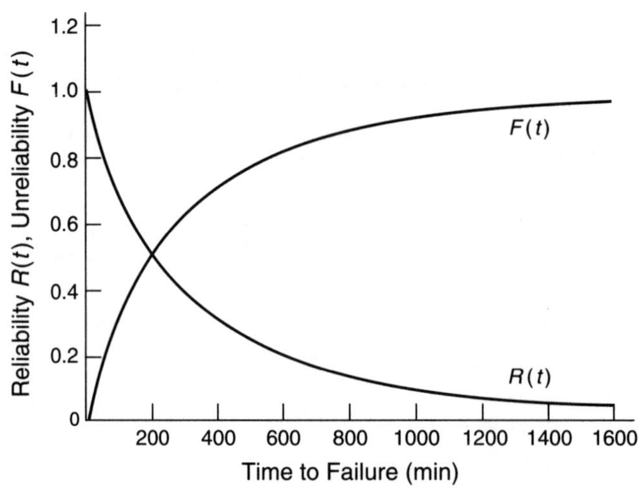

Figure 6.10. Transistor reliability and unreliability.

6.2.4 Parameters of Failure-to-Repair Process

Consider a process starting with a failure and ending at the completion of first repair. We shift the time axis and take $t = 0$ as the time at which the component failed. The probabilistic parameters are conditioned by the fact that the component failed at time zero.

$G(t)$ = repair distribution at time t:

The probability that the repair is completed before time t, given that the component failed at time zero.

The curve $G(t)$ versus t is a repair distribution and has properties similar to that of the failure distribution $F(t)$. A nonrepairable component has $G(t)$ identically equal to zero. The repair distribution $G(t)$ is a monotonically increasing function for the repairable component, and the following asymptotic property holds:

$$\lim_{t \to 0} G(t) = 0 \tag{6.35}$$

$$\lim_{t \to \infty} G(t) = 1 \tag{6.36}$$

$g(t) =$ repair density of $G(t)$.

This can be written as

$$g(t) = \frac{dG(t)}{dt} \tag{6.37}$$

or, equivalently,

$$g(t)dt = G(t + dt) - G(t) \tag{6.38}$$

Thus, the quantity $g(t)dt$ is the probability that component repair is completed during $[t, t + dt)$, given that the component failed at time zero.

The repair density is related to the repair distribution in the following way:

$$G(t) = \int_0^t g(u)du \tag{6.39}$$

$$G(t_2) - G(t_1) = \int_{t_1}^{t_2} g(u)du \tag{6.40}$$

Note that the difference $G(t_2) - G(t_1)$ is the probability that the first repair is completed during $[t_1, t_2)$, given that the component failed at time zero.

$m(t) =$ repair rate:

The probability that the component is repaired per unit time at time t, given that the component failed at time zero and has been failed to time t.

The quantity $m(t)dt$ is the probability that the component is repaired during $[t, t+dt)$, given that the component's failure age is t. Failure age t means that the component failed at time zero and has been failed to time t. The rate is designated as m when it is independent of the failure age t. A component with a constant repair rate has the same chance of being repaired whenever it is failed, and a nonrepairable component has a repair rate of zero.

TTR = time to repair:

The span of time from failure to repair completion.

The time to repair is a random variable because the first repair occurs randomly.

MTTR = mean time to repair:

The expected value of the time to repair, TTR.

The mean time to repair is given by

$$\text{MTTR} = \int_0^\infty tg(t)dt \tag{6.41}$$

If $G(\infty) = 1$, then the MTTR can be written as

$$\text{MTTR} = \int_0^\infty [1 - G(t)]dt \tag{6.42}$$

Suppose that a component has been failed to time u. A mean residual time to repair can be calculated by an equation analogous to equation (6.33).

Example 4. The following repair times (i.e., TTRs) for the repair of electric motors have been logged in:

Repair No.	Time (hr)	Repair No.	Time (hr)
1	3.3	10	0.8
2	1.4	11	0.7
3	0.8	12	0.6
4	0.9	13	1.8
5	0.8	14	1.3
6	1.6	15	0.8
7	0.7	16	4.2
8	1.2	17	1.1
9	1.1		

Using these data, obtain the values for $G(t)$, $g(t)$, $m(t)$, and MTTR.

Solution: $N = 17$ = total number of repairs.

TTR t	Number of Completed Repairs $M(t)$	$\frac{M(t)}{N}$ $G(t)$	$\frac{G(t+\Delta)-G(t)}{\Delta}$ $g(t)$	$\frac{g(t)}{1-G(t)}$ $m(t)$
0.0	0	0.0000	0.0000	0.0000
0.5	0	0.0000	0.9412	0.9412
1.0	8	0.4706	0.5882	1.1100
1.5	13	0.7647	0.2354	1.0004
2.0	15	0.8824	0.0000	0.0000
2.5	15	0.8824	0.0000	0.0000
3.0	15	0.8824	0.1176	1.0000
3.5	16	0.9412	0.0000	0.0000
4.0	16	0.9412	0.1176	2.0000
4.5	17	1.0000	—	—

Equation (6.41) gives

$$\text{MTTR} = (0.25 \times 0 + 0.75 \times 0.9412 + \cdots + 4.25 \times 0.1176) \times 0.5 = 1.4 \tag{6.43}$$

The average repair times also give MTTR:

$$\text{MTTR} = \frac{3.3 + 1.4 + \cdots + 1.1}{17} = 1.4 \tag{6.44}$$

■

6.2.5 Probabilistic Combined-Process Parameters

Consider a process consisting of repetitions of the repair-to-failure and the failure-to-repair processes. Assume that the component jumped into the normal state at time zero so that it is as good as new at $t = 0$. A number of failures and repairs may occur to time $t > 0$. Figure 6.11 shows that time t for the combined process differs from the time t for the repair-to-failure process because the latter time is measured from the latest repair before time t of the combined process. Both time scales coincide if and only if the component has been normal to time t. In this case, the time scale of the repair-to-failure is measured from time zero of the combined process because the component is assumed to jump into the normal state at time zero. Similarly, time t for the combined process differs from the time t of the failure-to-repair process. The probabilistic concepts for the combined process are summarized as follows.

$A(t)$ = availability at time t:

The probability that the component is normal at time t, given that it was as good as new at time zero.

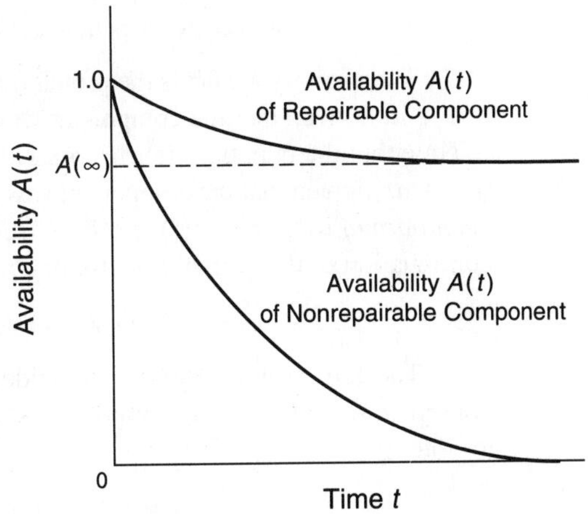

Figure 6.11. Schematic curves of availability $A(t)$.

Reliability generally differs from availability because the reliability requires the continuation of the normal state over the whole interval $[0, t]$. A component contributes to the availability $A(t)$ but not to the reliability $R(t)$ if the component failed before time t, is then repaired, and is normal at time t. Thus the availability $A(t)$ is larger than or equal to the reliability $R(t)$:

$$A(t) \geq R(t) \tag{6.45}$$

The equality in equation (6.45) holds for a nonrepairable component because the component is normal at time t if and only if it has been normal to time t. Thus

$$A(t) = R(t), \quad \text{for nonrepairable components} \tag{6.46}$$

The availability of a nonrepairable component decreases to zero as t becomes larger, whereas the availability of the repairable component converges to a nonzero positive number. Typical curves of $A(t)$ are shown in Figure 6.11.

$Q(t)$ = unavailability at time t:

The probability that the component is in the failed state at time t, given that it was as good as new at time zero.

Because a component is either in the normal state or in the failed state at time t, the unavailability $Q(t)$ is obtained from the availability and vice versa:

$$A(t) + Q(t) = 1 \tag{6.47}$$

From equations (6.26), (6.45), and (6.47), we have the inequality

$$Q(t) \leq F(t) \tag{6.48}$$

In other words, the unavailability $Q(t)$ is less than or equal to the unreliability $F(t)$. The equality holds for nonrepairable components:

$$Q(t) = F(t), \quad \text{for nonrepairable components} \tag{6.49}$$

The unavailability of a nonrepairable component approaches unity as t gets larger, whereas the unavailability of a repairable component remains smaller than unity.

$\lambda(t) =$ conditional failure intensity at time t:

The probability that the component fails per unit time at time t, given that it was as good as new at time zero and is normal at time t.

The quantity $\lambda(t)dt$ is the probability that a component fails during the small interval $[t, t + dt)$, given that the component was as good as new at time zero and normal at time t. Note that the quantity $r(t)dt$ represents the probability that the component fails during $[t, t + dt)$, given that the component was repaired (or as good as new) at time zero and *has been normal* to time t. $\lambda(t)dt$ differs from $r(t)dt$ because the latter quantity assumes the continuation of the normal state to time t, that is, no failure in the interval $[0, t]$.

$$\lambda(t) \neq r(t), \quad \text{for the general case} \tag{6.50}$$

The failure intensity $\lambda(t)$ coincides with the failure rate $r(t)$ if the component is nonrepairable because the component is normal at time t if and only if it has been normal to time t:

$$\lambda(t) = r(t), \quad \text{for nonrepairable component} \tag{6.51}$$

Also, it is proven in Appendix A.2 at the end of this chapter that the conditional failure intensity $\lambda(t)$ is the failure rate if the rate is a constant r:

$$\lambda(t) = r, \quad \text{for constant failure rate } r \tag{6.52}$$

$w(t) =$ unconditional failure intensity:

The probability that the component fails per unit time at time t, given that it was as good as new at time zero.

In other words, the quantity $w(t)dt$ is the probability that the component fails during $[t, t + dt)$, given that the component was as good as new at time zero. For a nonrepairable component, the unconditional failure intensity $w(t)$ coincides with the failure density $f(t)$.

Both the quantities $\lambda(t)$ and $w(t)$ refer to the failure per unit time at time t. These quantities, however, assume different populations. The conditional failure intensity $\lambda(t)$ presumes a set of components as good as new at time zero and normal at time t, whereas the unconditional failure intensity $w(t)$ assumes components as good as new at time zero. Thus they are different quantities. For example, using Figure 6.12

$$\begin{aligned} \lambda(t)dt &= \frac{0.7dt}{70} = 0.01dt \\ w(t)dt &= \frac{0.7dt}{100} = 0.007dt \end{aligned} \tag{6.53}$$

$W(t, t + dt) =$ expected number of failures (ENF) during $[t, t + dt)$:

Expected number of failures during $[t, t + dt)$, given that the component was as good as new at time zero.

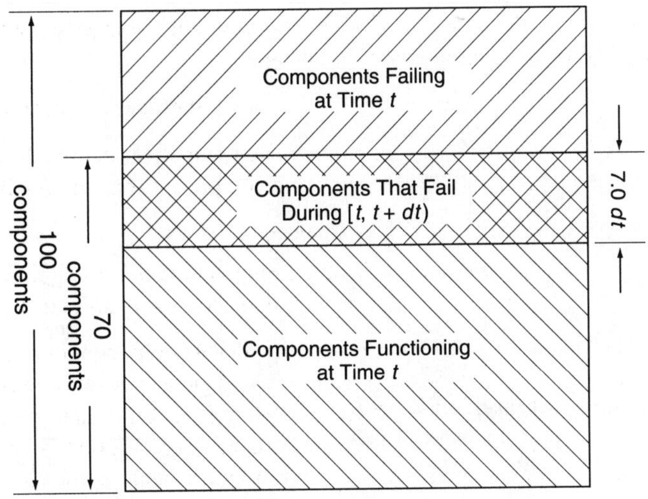

Figure 6.12. Conditional intensity $\lambda(t)$ and unconditional intensity $w(t)$.

From the definition of the expected values, we have

$$W(t, t + dt) = \sum_{i=1}^{\infty} i \cdot \Pr\{i \text{ failures during } [t, t + dt)|C\} \tag{6.54}$$

where condition C means that the component was as good as new at time zero. At most, one failure occurs during $[t, t + dt)$ and we obtain

$$W(t, t + dt) = \Pr\{\text{one failure during } [t, t + dt)|C\} \tag{6.55}$$

or, equivalently,

$$W(t, t + dt) = w(t)dt \tag{6.56}$$

The expected number of failures during $[t_1, t_2)$ is calculated from the unconditional failure intensity $w(t)$ by integration.

$W(t_1, t_2)$ = ENF over interval $[t_1, t_2)$:

Expected number of failures during $[t_1, t_2)$, given that the component was as good as new at time zero.

$W(t_1, t_2)$ is the integration of $W(t, t + dt)$ over the interval $[t_1, t_2)$. Thus wc have

$$W(t_1, t_2) = \int_{t_1}^{t_2} w(t)dt \tag{6.57}$$

The $W(0, t)$ of a nonrepairable component is equal to $F(t)$ and approaches unity as t gets larger. The $W(0, t)$ of a repairable component goes to infinity as t becomes infinite. Typical curves of $W(0, t)$ are shown in Figure 6.13. The asymptotic behavior of W and other parameters are summarized in Table 6.9.

$\mu(t)$ = conditional repair intensity at time t:

The probability that the component is repaired per unit time at time t, given that the component was as good as new at time zero and is failed at time t.

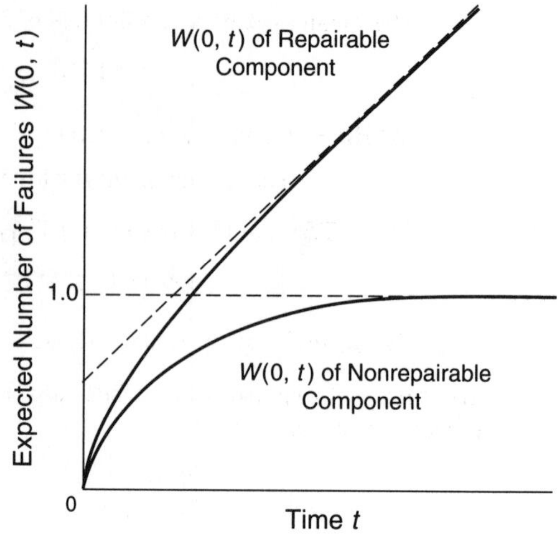

Figure 6.13. Schematic curves of expected number of failures $W(0, t)$.

The repair intensity generally differs from the repair rate $m(t)$. Similarly, to the relationship between $\lambda(t)$ and $r(t)$ we have the following special cases:

$$\mu(t) = m(t) = 0, \quad \text{for a nonrepairable component} \tag{6.58}$$

$$\mu(t) = m, \quad \text{for constant repair rate } m \tag{6.59}$$

$v(t) =$ unconditional repair intensity at time t:

The probability that the component is repaired per unit time at time t, given that the component was as good as new at time zero.

The intensities $v(t)$ and $\mu(t)$ are different quantities because they involve different populations.

$V(t, t + dt) =$ expected number of repairs during $[t, t + dt)$:

Expected number of repairs during $[t, t + dt)$, given that the component was as good as new at time zero.

Similar to equation (6.56), the following relation holds:

$$V(t, t + dt) = v(t)dt \tag{6.60}$$

$V(t_1, t_2) =$ expected number of repairs over interval $[t_1, t_2)$:

Expected number of repairs during $[t_1, t_2)$, given that the component was as good as new at time zero.

Analogous to equation (6.57), we have

$$V(t_1, t_2) = \int_{t_1}^{t_2} v(t)dt \tag{6.61}$$

The expected number of repairs $V(0, t)$ is zero for a nonrepairable component. For a repairable component, $V(0, t)$ approaches infinity as t gets larger. It is proven in the next section that the difference $W(0, t) - V(0, t)$ equals the unavailability $Q(t)$.

MTBF = mean time between failures:

The expected value of the time between two consecutive failures.

The mean time between failures is equal to the sum of MTTF and MTTR:

$$\text{MTBF} = \text{MTTF} + \text{MTTR} \tag{6.62}$$

MTBR = mean time between repairs:

The expected value of the time between two consecutive repairs.

The MTBR equals the sum of MTTF and MTTR and hence MTBF:

$$\text{MTBR} = \text{MTBF} = \text{MTTF} + \text{MTTR} \tag{6.63}$$

Example 5. For the data of Figure 6.7, calculate $\mu(7)$, $v(7)$, and $V(0, 5)$.

Solution: Six components are failed at $t = 7$. Among them, only two components are repaired during unit interval $[7, 8)$. Thus

$$\begin{aligned}
\mu(7) &= 2/6 = 1/3 \\
v(7) &= 2/10 = 0.2 \\
V(0, 5) &= \frac{1}{10}\sum_{i=0}^{4} \{\text{total number of repairs in } [i, i+1)\} \\
&= \frac{1}{10} \times (0 + 1 + 0 + 3 + 1) = 0.5
\end{aligned} \tag{6.64}$$

■

6.3 FUNDAMENTAL RELATIONS AMONG PROBABILISTIC PARAMETERS

In the previous section, we defined various probabilistic parameters and their interrelationships. These relations and the characteristics of the probabilistic parameters are summarized in Tables 6.7, 6.8, and 6.9. Table 6.7 refers to the repair-to-failure process, Table 6.8 to the failure-to-repair process, and Table 6.9 to the combined process. These tables include some new and important relations that are deduced in this section.

6.3.1 Repair-to-Failure Parameters

We shall derive the following relations:

$$r(t) = \frac{f(t)}{1 - F(t)} = \frac{f(t)}{R(t)} \tag{6.65}$$

$$F(t) = 1 - \exp\left[-\int_0^t r(u)du\right] \tag{6.66}$$

$$R(t) = \exp\left[-\int_0^t r(u)du\right] \tag{6.67}$$

$$f(t) = r(t)\exp\left[-\int_0^t r(u)du\right] \tag{6.68}$$

The first identity is used to obtain the failure rate $r(t)$ when the unreliability $F(t)$ and the failure density $f(t)$ are given. The second through the fourth identities can be used to calculate $F(t)$, $R(t)$, and $f(t)$ when the failure rate $r(t)$ is given.

The flow chart of Figure 6.14 shows general procedures for calculating the probabilistic parameters for the repair-to-failure process. The number adjacent to each arrow

TABLE 6.7. Relations Among Parameters for Repair-to-Failure Process

General Failure Rate $r(t)$	
1. $R(t) + F(t) = 1$	7. $R(t) = \int_t^{\infty} F(u)du$
2. $R(0) = 1,\ R(\infty) = 0$	8. $\text{MTTF} = \int_0^{\infty} tf(t)dt = \int_0^{\infty} R(t)dt$
3. $F(0) = 0,\ F(\infty) = 1$	9. $r(t) = \dfrac{f(t)}{1 - F(t)} = \dfrac{f(t)}{R(t)}$
4. $f(t) = \dfrac{dF(t)}{dt}$	10. $R(t) = \exp\left[-\int_0^t r(u)du\right]$
5. $f(t)dt = F(t + dt) - F(t)$	11. $F(t) = 1 - \exp\left[-\int_0^t r(u)du\right]$
6. $F(t) = \int_0^t f(u)du$	12. $f(t) = r(t)\exp\left[-\int_0^t r(u)du\right]$
Constant Failure Rate $r(t) = \lambda$	
13. $R(t) = e^{-\lambda t}$	15. $f(t) = \lambda e^{-\lambda t}$
14. $F(t) = 1 - e^{-\lambda t}$	16. $\text{MTTF} = \dfrac{1}{\lambda}$

TABLE 6.8. Relations Among Parameters for Failure-to-Repair Process

General Repair Rate $m(t)$	
1. $G(0) = 0, \quad G(\infty) = 1$	6. $\text{MTTR} = \int_0^{\infty} tg(t)dt = \int_0^{\infty} [1 - G(t)]dt$
2. $g(t) = \dfrac{dG(t)}{dt}$	7. $m(t) = \dfrac{g(t)}{1 - G(t)}$
3. $g(t)dt = G(t + dt) - G(t)$	8. $G(t) = 1 - \exp\left[-\int_0^t m(u)du\right]$
4. $G(t) = \int_0^t g(u)du$	9. $g(t) = m(t)\exp\left[-\int_0^t m(u)du\right]$
5. $G(t_2) - G(t_1) = \int_{t_1}^{t_2} g(u)du$	
Constant Repair Rate $m(t) = \mu$	
10. $G(t) = 1 - e^{-\mu t}$	12. $g(t) = \mu e^{-\mu t}$
11. $\text{MTTR} = \dfrac{1}{\mu}$	13. $\mu = 0$ (nonrepairable)

TABLE 6.9. Relations Among Parameters for the Combined Process

	Repairable	Nonrepairable
	Fundamental Relations	
1.	$A(t) + Q(t) = 1$	$A(t) + Q(t) = 1$
2.	$A(t) > R(t)$	$A(t) = R(t)$
3.	$Q(t) < F(t)$	$Q(t) = F(t)$
4.	$w(t) = f(t) + \int_0^t f(t-u)v(u)du$	$w(t) = f(t)$
5.	$v(t) = \int_0^t g(t-u)w(u)du$	$v(t) = 0$
6.	$W(t, t+dt) = w(t)dt$	$W(t, t+dt) = w(t)dt$
7.	$V(t, t+dt) = v(t)dt$	$V(t, t+dt) = 0$
8.	$W(t_1, t_2) = \int_{t_1}^{t_2} w(u)du$	$W(t_1, t_2) = F(t_2) - F(t_1)$
9.	$V(t_1, t_2) = \int_{t_1}^{t_2} v(u)du$	$V(t_1, t_2) = 0$
10.	$Q(t) = W(0, t) - V(0, t)$	$Q(t) = W(0, t) = F(t)$
11.	$\lambda(t) = \dfrac{w(t)}{1 - Q(t)}$	$\lambda(t) = \dfrac{w(t)}{1 - Q(t)}$
12.	$\mu(t) = v(t)/Q(t)$	$\mu(t) = 0$
	Stationary Values	
13.	MTBF = MTBR = MTTF + MTTR	MTBF = MTBR = ∞
14.	$0 < A(\infty) < 1$, $0 < Q(\infty) < 1$	$A(\infty) = 0$, $Q(\infty) = 1$
15.	$0 < w(\infty) < \infty$, $0 < v(\infty) < \infty$	$w(\infty) = 0$, $v(\infty) = 0$
16.	$w(\infty) = v(\infty)$	$w(\infty) = v(\infty) = 0$
17.	$W(0, \infty) = \infty$, $V(0, \infty) = \infty$	$W(0, \infty) = 1$, $V(0, \infty) = 0$
	Remarks	
18.	$w(t) \neq \lambda(t)$, $v(t) \neq \mu(t)$	$w(t) \neq \lambda(t)$, $v(t) = \mu(t) = 0$
19.	$\lambda(t) \neq r(t)$, $\mu(t) \neq m(t)$	$\lambda(t) = r(t)$, $\mu(t) = m(t) = 0$
20.	$w(t) \neq f(t)$, $v(t) \neq g(t)$	$w(t) = f(t)$, $v(t) = g(t) = 0$

corresponds to the relation identified in Table 6.7. Note that the first step in processing failure data (such as the data in Tables 6.1 and 6.5) is to plot it as a histogram (Figure 6.3) or to fit it, by parameter estimation techniques, to a standard distribution (exponential, normal, etc.). Parameter-estimation techniques and failure distributions are discussed later in this chapter. The flow chart indicates that $R(t)$, $F(t)$, $f(t)$, and $r(t)$ can be obtained if any one of the parameters is known.

We now begin the derivation of identities (6.65) through (6.68) with a statement of the definition of a conditional probability [see equation (A.14), Appendix of Chapter 3].

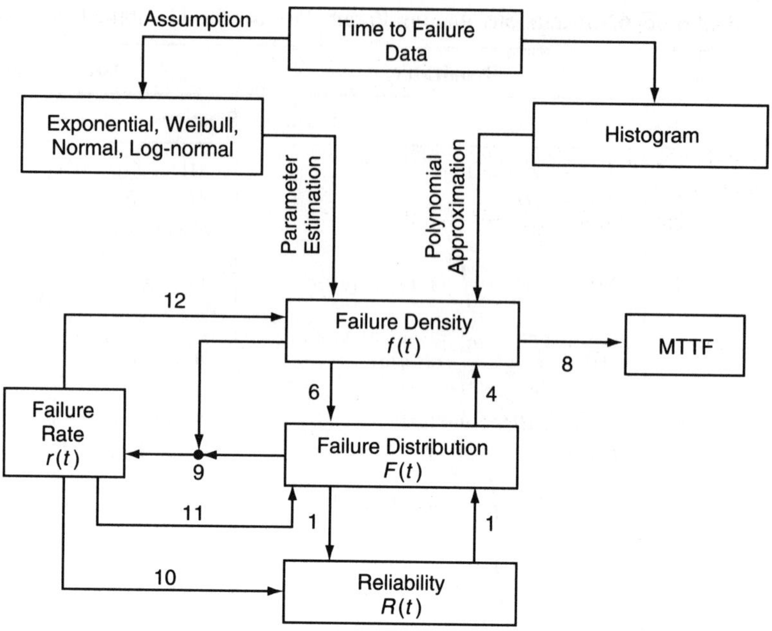

Figure 6.14. Flow chart for repair-to-failure process parameters.

$$\Pr\{A|C, W\} = \frac{\Pr\{A, C|W\}}{\Pr\{C|W\}} \tag{6.69}$$

The quantity $r(t)dt$ coincides with the conditional probability $\Pr\{A|C, W\}$ where

$$\begin{aligned} A &= \text{the component fails during } [t, t+dt), \\ C &= \text{the component has been normal to time } t, \text{ and} \\ W &= \text{the component was repaired at time zero} \end{aligned} \tag{6.70}$$

The probability $\Pr\{C|W\}$ is the reliability $R(t) = 1 - F(t)$, and $\Pr\{A, C|W\}$ is given by $f(t)dt$. Thus from equation (6.69), we have

$$r(t)dt = \frac{f(t)dt}{1 - F(t)} \tag{6.71}$$

yielding equation (6.65). Note that $f(t) = dF/dt$, so we obtain

$$r(t) = \frac{dF/dt}{1 - F(t)} \tag{6.72}$$

We can rewrite equation (6.72) as

$$r(t) = -\frac{d}{dt}\ln[1 - F(t)] \tag{6.73}$$

Integrating both sides of equation (6.73),

$$\int_0^t r(u)du = \ln[1 - F(0)] - \ln[1 - F(t)] \tag{6.74}$$

Substituting $F(0) = 0$ into equation (6.74)

$$\int_0^t r(u)du = -\ln[1 - F(t)] \tag{6.75}$$

yields equation (6.66). The remaining two identities are obtained from equations (6.26) and (6.27).

Consider, for example, failure density $f(t)$.

$$f(t) = \begin{cases} t/2, & 0 \le t < 2 \\ 0, & 2 \le t \end{cases} \tag{6.76}$$

Failure distribution $F(t)$, reliability $R(t)$, and failure rate $r(t)$ become

$$F(t) = \begin{cases} t^2/4, & 0 \le t < 2 \\ 1, & 2 \le t \end{cases} \tag{6.77}$$

$$R(t) = 1 - F(t) = \begin{cases} 1 - (t^2/4), & 0 \le t < 2 \\ 0, & 2 \le t \end{cases} \tag{6.78}$$

$$r(t) = f(t)/R(t) = \begin{cases} \dfrac{t/2}{1 - (t^2/4)}, & 0 \le t < 2 \\ \text{not defined}, & 2 \le t \end{cases} \tag{6.79}$$

Mean time to failure MTTF is

$$\text{MTTF} = \int_0^2 tf(t)dt = \int_0^2 (t^2/2)dt = \left[t^3/6\right]_0^2 = 4/3 \tag{6.80}$$

This is also obtained from

$$\text{MTTF} = \int_0^2 R(t)dt = \int_0^2 1 - (t^2/4)dt = \left[t - (t^3/12)\right]_0^2 = 4/3 \tag{6.81}$$

6.3.2 Failure-to-Repair Parameters

Similar to the case of the repair-to-failure process, we obtain the following relations for the failure-to-repair process:

$$m(t) = \frac{g(t)}{1 - G(t)} \tag{6.82}$$

$$G(t) = 1 - \exp\left[-\int_0^t m(u)du\right] \tag{6.83}$$

$$g(t) = m(t)\exp\left[-\int_0^t m(u)du\right] \tag{6.84}$$

The first identity is used to obtain the repair rate $m(t)$ when the repair distribution $G(t)$ and the repair density $g(t)$ are given. The second and third identities calculate $G(t)$ and $g(t)$ when the repair rate $m(u)$ is given.

The flow chart, Figure 6.15, shows the procedures for calculating the probabilistic parameters related to the failure-to-repair process. The number adjacent to each arrow corresponds to Table 6.8. We can calculate $G(t)$, $g(t)$, and $m(t)$ if any one of them is known.

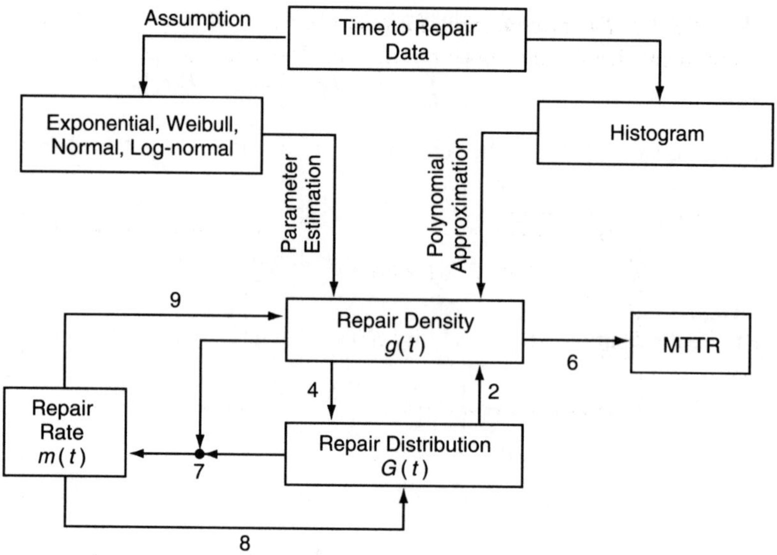

Figure 6.15. Flow chart for failure-to-repair process parameters.

6.3.3 Combined-Process Parameters

General procedures for calculating combined-process probabilistic parameters are shown in Figure 6.16. The identification numbers in the flow chart are listed in Table 6.9. The chart includes some new and important relations that we now derive.

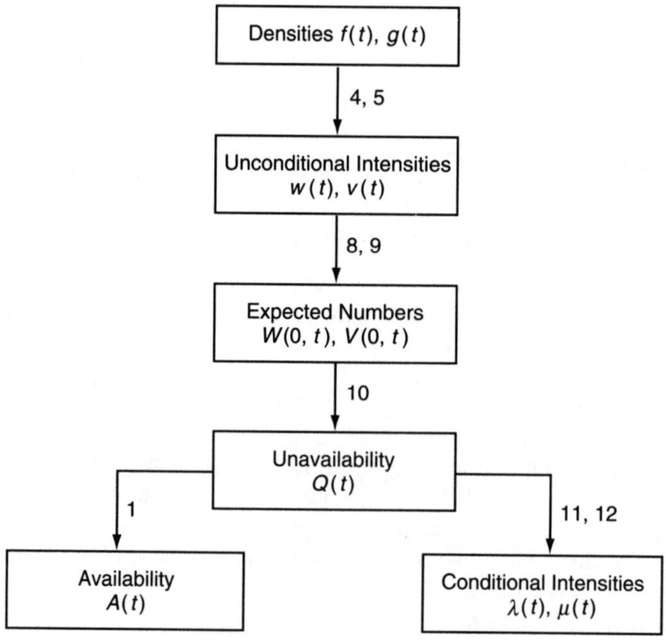

Figure 6.16. Flow chart for the combined-process parameters.

***6.3.3.1 The unconditional intensities* w(t) *and* v(t).** As shown in Figure 6.17, the components that fail during $[t, t + dt)$ are classified into two types.

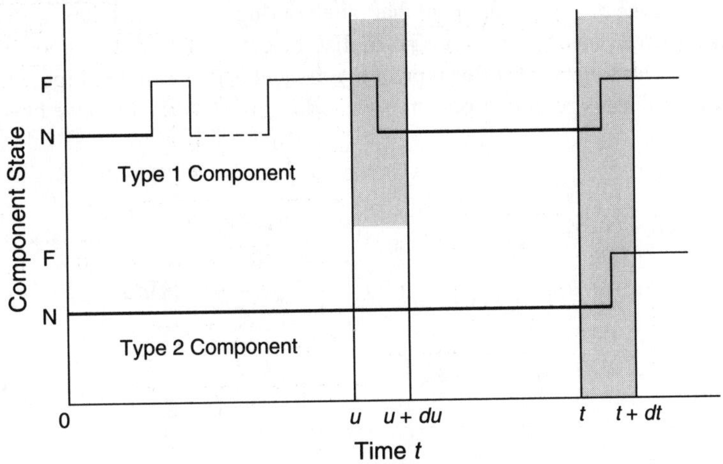

Figure 6.17. Component that fails during $[t, t + dt)$.

Type 1. A component that was repaired during $[u, u+du)$, has been normal to time t, and fails during $[t, t + dt)$, given that the component was as good as new at time zero.

Type 2. A component that has been normal to time t and fails during $[t, t + dt)$, given that it was as good as new at time zero.

The probability for the first type of component is $v(u)du \cdot f(t - u)dt$, because

$v(u)du =$ the probability that the component is repaired during $[u, u + du)$, given that it was as good as new at time zero.

and

$f(t - u)dt =$ the probability that the component has been normal to time t and failed during $[t, t + dt)$, given that it was as good as new at time zero and was repaired at time u.

Notice that we add the condition "as good as new at time zero" to the definition of $f(t-u)dt$ because the component-failure characteristics depend only on the survival age $t - u$ at time t and are independent of the history before u.

The probability for the second type of component is $f(t)dt$, as shown by equation (6.28). The quantity $w(t)dt$ is the probability that the component fails during $[t, t+dt)$, given that it was as good as new at time zero. Because this probability is a sum of the probabilities for the first and second type of components, we have

$$w(t)dt = f(t)dt + dt \int_0^t f(t - u)v(u)du \tag{6.85}$$

or, equivalently,

$$w(t) = f(t) + \int_0^t f(t - u)v(u)du \tag{6.86}$$

On the other hand, the components that are repaired during $[t, t + dt)$ consist of components of the following type.

Type 3. A component that failed during $[u, u + du)$, has been failed till time t, and is repaired during $[t, t + dt)$, given that the component was as good as new at time zero.

The behavior for this type of component is illustrated in Figure 6.18. The probability for the third type of component is $w(u)du \cdot g(t - u)dt$. Thus we have

$$v(t)dt = dt \int_0^t g(t - u)w(u)du \tag{6.87}$$

or, equivalently,

$$v(t) = \int_0^t g(t - u)w(u)du \tag{6.88}$$

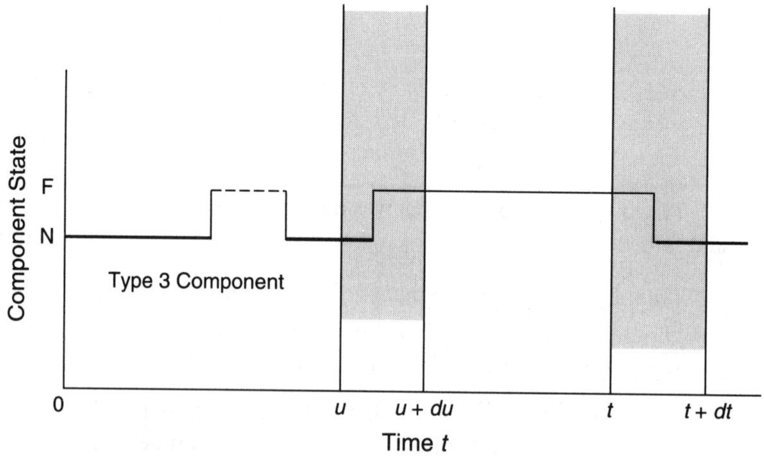

Figure 6.18. Component that is repaired during $[t, t + dt)$.

From equations (6.86) and (6.88), we have the following simultaneous identity:

$$\left.\begin{aligned} w(t) &= f(t) + \int_0^t f(t - u)v(u)du \\ v(t) &= \int_0^t g(t - u)w(u)du \end{aligned}\right\} \tag{6.89}$$

The unconditional failure intensity $w(t)$ and the repair intensity $v(t)$ are calculated by an iterative numerical integration of equation (6.89) when densities $f(t)$ and $g(t)$ are given. If a rigorous, analytical solution is required, Laplace transforms can be used.

If a component is nonrepairable, then the repair density is zero, $g(t) \equiv 0$, and the above equation becomes

$$\left.\begin{aligned} w(t) &= f(t) \\ v(t) &= 0 \end{aligned}\right\} \tag{6.90}$$

Thus the unconditional failure intensity coincides with the failure density.

When a failed component can be repaired instantly, then the corresponding combined process is called a *renewal process*, which is the converse of a nonrepairable combined process. For the instant repair, the repair density becomes a delta function, $g(t-u)=\delta(t-u)$. Thus equation (6.89) becomes a so-called *renewal equation*, and the expected number of renewals $W(0,t)=V(0,t)$ can be calculated accordingly.

$$\left.\begin{aligned} w(t) &= f(t)+\int_0^t f(t-u)w(u)du \\ v(t) &= w(t) \end{aligned}\right\} \tag{6.91}$$

6.3.3.2 *Relations for calculating unavailability* Q(t). Let $x(t)$ be an indicator variable defined by

$$x(t)=1, \quad \text{if the component is in a failed state, and} \tag{6.92}$$

$$x(t)=0, \quad \text{if the component is in a normal state} \tag{6.93}$$

Represent by $x_{0,1}(t)$ and $x_{1,0}(t)$ the numbers of failures and repairs to time t, respectively. Then we have

$$x(t)=x_{0,1}(t)-x_{1,0}(t) \tag{6.94}$$

For example, if the component has experienced three failures and two repairs to time t, the component state $x(t)$ at time t is given by

$$x(t)=3-2=1 \tag{6.95}$$

As shown in Appendix A.3 of this chapter, we have

$$Q(t)=W(0,t)-V(0,t) \tag{6.96}$$

In other words, the unavailability $Q(t)$ is given by the difference between the expected number of failures $W(0,t)$ and repairs $V(0,t)$ to time t. The expected numbers are obtained from the unconditional failure intensity $w(u)$ and the repair intensity $v(u)$, according to equations (6.57) and (6.61). We can rewrite equation (6.96) as

$$Q(t)=\int_0^t [w(u)-v(u)]du \tag{6.97}$$

6.3.3.3 *Calculating the conditional failure intensity* λ(t). The simultaneous occurrence of events A and C is equivalent to the occurrence of event C followed by event A [see equation (A.14), Appendix of Chapter 3]:

$$\Pr\{A,C|W\}=\Pr\{C|W\}P\{A|C,W\} \tag{6.98}$$

Substitute the following events into equation (6.98):

$$\left.\begin{aligned} C &= \text{the component is normal at time } t, \\ A &= \text{the component fails during } [t,t+dt), \\ W &= \text{the component was as good as new at time zero} \end{aligned}\right. \tag{6.99}$$

At most, one failure occurs during a small interval, and the event A implies event C. Thus the simultaneous occurrence of A and C reduces to the occurrence of A, and equation (6.98) can be written as

$$\Pr\{A|W\}=\Pr\{C|W\}P\{A|C,W\} \tag{6.100}$$

According to the definition of availability $A(t)$, conditional failure intensity $\lambda(t)$, and unconditional failure intensity $w(t)$, we have

$$\Pr\{A|W\}=w(t)dt \tag{6.101}$$

$$\Pr\{A|C, W\} = \lambda(t)dt \tag{6.102}$$

$$\Pr\{C|W\} = A(t) \tag{6.103}$$

Thus from equation (6.100),

$$w(t) = \lambda(t)A(t) \tag{6.104}$$

or, equivalently,

$$w(t) = \lambda(t)[1 - Q(t)] \tag{6.105}$$

and

$$\lambda(t) = \frac{w(t)}{1 - Q(t)} \tag{6.106}$$

Identity (6.106) is used to calculate the conditional failure intensity $\lambda(t)$ when the unconditional failure intensity $w(t)$ and the unavailability $Q(t)$ are given. Parameters $w(t)$ and $Q(t)$ can be obtained by equations (6.89) and (6.97), respectively.

In the case of a constant failure rate, the conditional failure intensity coincides with the failure rate r as shown by equation (6.52). Thus $\lambda(t)$ is known and equation (6.105) is used to obtain $w(t)$ from $\lambda(t) = r$ and $Q(t)$.

***6.3.3.4 Calculating* $\mu(t)$.** As in the case of $\lambda(t)$, we have the following identities for the conditional repair intensity $\mu(t)$:

$$\mu(t) = \frac{v(t)}{Q(t)} \tag{6.107}$$

$$v(t) = \mu(t)Q(t) \tag{6.108}$$

Parameter $\mu(t)$ can be calculated using equation (6.107) when the unconditional repair intensity $v(t)$ and the unavailability $Q(t)$ are known. Parameters $v(t)$ and $Q(t)$ can be obtained by equations (6.89) and (6.97), respectively.

When the component has a constant repair rate $m(t) = m$, the conditional repair intensity is m and is known. In this case, equation (6.108) is used to calculate the unconditional repair intensity $v(t)$, given $\mu(t) = m$ and $Q(t)$.

If the component has a time-varying failure rate $r(t)$, the conditional failure intensity $\lambda(t)$ does not coincide with $r(t)$. Similarly, a time-varying repair rate $m(t)$ is not equal to the conditional repair intensity $\mu(t)$. Thus in general,

$$w(t) \neq r(t)[1 - Q(t)] \tag{6.109}$$

$$v(t) \neq m(t)Q(t) \tag{6.110}$$

Example 6. Use the results of Examples 2 and 5 to confirm, in Table 6.9, relations (2), (3), (4), (5), (10), (11), and (12). Obtain the TTFs, TTRs, TBFs and TBRs for component 1.

Solution:

1. Inequality (2): From Example 2,

$$A(5) = 0.6 > R(5) = 0.1111 \tag{6.111}$$

2. Inequality (3):

$$Q(5) = 0.4 < F(5) = 0.8889 \text{ (Example 2)} \tag{6.112}$$

3. Equality (4): We shall show that

$$w(5) = f(5) + \int_0^5 f(5 - u)v(u)du \tag{6.113}$$

From Example 2,

$$w(5) = 0.2 \tag{6.114}$$

The probability $f(5) \times 1$ refers to the component that has been normal to time 5 and failed during $[5, 6)$, given that it was as good as new at time zero. Component 3 is identified, and we have

$$f(5) = \frac{1}{10} \tag{6.115}$$

The integral on the right-hand side of (6.113) refers to the components shown below.

Repaired	Normal	Failed	Components
[0, 1)	[1,5)	[5,6)	None
[1, 2)	[2,5)	[5,6)	None
[2, 3)	[3,5)	[5,6)	None
[3, 4)	[4,5)	[5,6)	Component 7
[4, 5)	—	[5,6)	None

Therefore,

$$\int_0^5 f(5-u)v(u)du = 1/10 \tag{6.116}$$

Equation (4) is confirmed because

$$0.2 = \frac{1}{10} + \frac{1}{10} \tag{6.117}$$

4. Equality (5): We shall show that

$$v(7) = \int_0^7 g(5-u)w(u)du \tag{6.118}$$

From Example 5,

$$v(7) = 0.2 \tag{6.119}$$

The integral on the right-hand side refers to the components listed below.

Fails	Failed	Repaired	Components
[0, 1)	[1,7)	[7,8)	None
[1, 2)	[2,7)	[7,8)	None
[2, 3)	[3,7)	[7,8)	None
[3, 4)	[4,7)	[7,8)	None
[4, 5)	[5,7)	[7,8)	None
[5, 6)	[6,7)	[7,8)	Component 7
[6, 7)	—	[7,8)	Component 1

Thus the integral is $2/10 = 0.2$, and we confirm the equality.

5. Equality (10): We shall show that

$$Q(5) = W(0,5) - V(0,5) \tag{6.120}$$

From Example 2,

$$Q(5) = 0.4, \qquad W(0,5) = 0.9 \tag{6.121}$$

From Example 5,

$$V(0,5) = 0.5 \tag{6.122}$$

Thus

$$0.4 = 0.9 - 0.5 \tag{6.123}$$

6. Equality (11): From Example 2,

$$Q(5) = 0.4, \qquad w(5) = 0.2, \qquad \lambda(5) = 1/3 \tag{6.124}$$

Thus

$$\frac{1}{3} = \frac{0.2}{1 - 0.4} \tag{6.125}$$

and

$$\lambda(5) = \frac{w(5)}{1 - Q(5)} \tag{6.126}$$

is confirmed.

7. Equality (12): We shall show that

$$\mu(7) = \frac{v(7)}{Q(7)} \tag{6.127}$$

From Example 5,

$$\mu(7) = 1/3, \qquad v(7) = 0.2 \tag{6.128}$$

From Figure 6.7,

$$Q(7) = 6/10 = 0.6 \tag{6.129}$$

This is now confirmed, because

$$\frac{1}{3} = \frac{0.2}{0.6} \tag{6.130}$$

8. TTFs, TTRs, TBFs, and TBRs are shown in Figure 6.19. ■

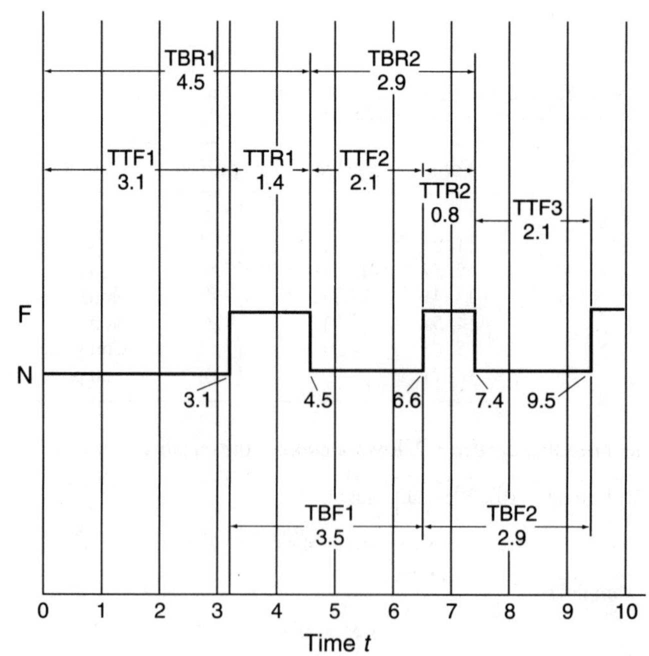

Figure 6.19. Time history of component 1.

6.4 CONSTANT-FAILURE RATE AND REPAIR-RATE MODEL

An example of a pseudo-constant failure rate process was given in Example 3, Section 6.2.3. We now extend and generalize the treatment of these processes.

6.4.1 Repair-to-Failure Process

Constant-failure rates greatly simplify systems analysis and are, accordingly, very popular with mathematicians, systems analysts, and optimization specialists.

The assumption of the constant rate is viable if

1. the component is in its prime of life,
2. the component in question is a large one with many subcomponents having different rates or ages, or
3. the data are so limited that elaborate mathematical treatments are unjustified.

Identity (6.52) shows that there is no difference between the failure rate $r(t)$ and the conditional failure intensity $\lambda(t)$ when the rate r is constant. Therefore, we denote by λ both the constant-failure rate and the constant conditional failure intensity.

Substituting λ into equations (6.66), (6.67), and (6.68), and we obtain

$$F(t) = 1 - e^{-\lambda t} \tag{6.131}$$

$$R(t) = e^{-\lambda t} \tag{6.132}$$

$$f(t) = \lambda e^{-\lambda t} \tag{6.133}$$

The distribution (6.131) is called an *exponential distribution*, and its characteristics are given in Table 6.10.

The MTTF is defined by equation (6.31),

$$\text{MTTF} = \int_0^\infty t\lambda e^{-\lambda t}\, dt = \frac{1}{\lambda} \tag{6.134}$$

Equivalently, the MTTF can be calculated by equation (6.32):

$$\text{MTTF} = \int_0^\infty e^{-\lambda t}\, dt = \frac{1}{\lambda} \tag{6.135}$$

The MTTF is obtained from an arithmetical mean of the time-to-failure data. The conditional failure intensity λ is the reciprocal of the MTTF.

The mean residual time to failure (MRTTF) at time u is calculated by equation (6.33), and becomes

$$\text{MRTTF} = \int_u^\infty (t-u)\lambda e^{-\lambda(t-u)} dt = \int_0^\infty t\lambda e^{-\lambda t} dt = \frac{1}{\lambda} \tag{6.136}$$

When a component failure follows the exponential distribution, a normal component at time t is always as good as new. Thus the MRTTF is equal to the MTTF.

On a plot of $F(t)$ versus t, the value of $F(t)$ at t = MTTF is $(1 - e^{-1}) = 0.63$ (Figure 6.20). When the failure distribution is known, we can obtain MTTF by finding the time t that satisfies the equality

$$F(t) = 0.63 \tag{6.137}$$

The presence or absence of a constant-failure rate can be detected by plotting procedures discussed in the parameter-identification section later in this chapter.

TABLE 6.10. Summary of Constant Rate Model

	Repairable	Nonrepairable
	Repair-to-Failure Process	
1.	$r(t) = \lambda$	$r(t) = \lambda$
2.	$R(t) = e^{-\lambda t}$	$R(t) = e^{-\lambda t}$
3.	$F(t) = 1 - e^{-\lambda t}$	$F(t) = 1 - e^{-\lambda t}$
4.	$f(t) = \lambda e^{-\lambda t}$	$f(t) = \lambda e^{-\lambda t}$
5.	$\mathrm{MTTF} = \frac{1}{\lambda}$	$\mathrm{MTTF} = \frac{1}{\lambda}$
	Failure-to-Repair Process	
6.	$m(t) = \mu$	$m(t) = \mu$
7.	$G(t) = 1 - e^{-\mu t}$	$G(t) = 1 - e^{-\mu t}$
8.	$g(t) = \mu e^{-\mu t}$	$g(t) = \mu e^{-\mu t}$
9.	$\mathrm{MTTR} = \frac{1}{\mu}$	$\mathrm{MTTR} = \frac{1}{\mu}$
	Dynamic System Behavior	
10.	$Q(t) = \frac{\lambda}{\lambda+\mu}\left[1 - e^{-(\lambda+\mu)t}\right]$	$Q(t) = 1 - e^{-\lambda t} = F(t)$
11.	$A(t) = \frac{\mu}{\lambda+\mu} + \frac{\lambda}{\lambda+\mu}e^{-(\lambda+\mu)t}$	$A(t) = e^{-\lambda t} = R(t)$
12.	$w(t) = \frac{\lambda\mu}{\lambda+\mu} + \frac{\lambda^2}{\lambda+\mu}e^{-(\lambda+\mu)t}$	$w(t) = \lambda e^{-\lambda t} = f(t)$
13.	$v(t) = \frac{\lambda\mu}{\lambda+\mu}\left[1 - e^{-(\lambda+\mu)t}\right]$	$v(t) = 0$
14.	$W(0, t) = \frac{\lambda\mu}{\lambda+\mu}t + \frac{\lambda^2}{(\lambda+\mu)^2}\left[1 - e^{-(\lambda+\mu)t}\right]$	$W(0, t) = 1 - e^{-\lambda t} = F(t)$
15.	$V(0, t) = \frac{\lambda\mu}{\lambda+\mu}t - \frac{\lambda\mu}{(\lambda+\mu)^2}\left[1 - e^{-(\lambda+\mu)t}\right]$	$V(0, t) = 0$
16.	$\frac{dQ(t)}{dt} = -(\lambda+\mu)Q(t) + \lambda, \quad Q(0) = 0$	$\frac{dQ(t)}{dt} = -\lambda Q(t) + \lambda, \quad Q(0) = 0$
	Stationary System Behavior	
17.	$Q(\infty) = \frac{\lambda}{\lambda+\mu} = \frac{\mathrm{MTTR}}{\mathrm{MTTF}+\mathrm{MTTR}}$	$Q(\infty) = 1$
18.	$A(\infty) = \frac{\mu}{\lambda+\mu} = \frac{\mathrm{MTTF}}{\mathrm{MTTF}+\mathrm{MTTR}}$	$A(\infty) = 0$
19.	$w(\infty) = \frac{\lambda\mu}{\lambda+\mu} = \frac{1}{\mathrm{MTTF}+\mathrm{MTTR}}$	$w(\infty) = 0$
20.	$v(\infty) = \frac{\lambda\mu}{\lambda+\mu} = w(\infty)$	$v(\infty) = 0 = w(\infty)$
21.	$\frac{Q(t)}{Q(\infty)} = 0.63, \quad \text{for } t = \frac{1}{\lambda+\mu}$	$\frac{Q(t)}{Q(\infty)} = 0.63, \quad \text{for } t = \frac{1}{\lambda}$
22.	$0 = -(\lambda+\mu)Q(\infty) + \lambda$	$0 = -\lambda Q(\infty) + \lambda$

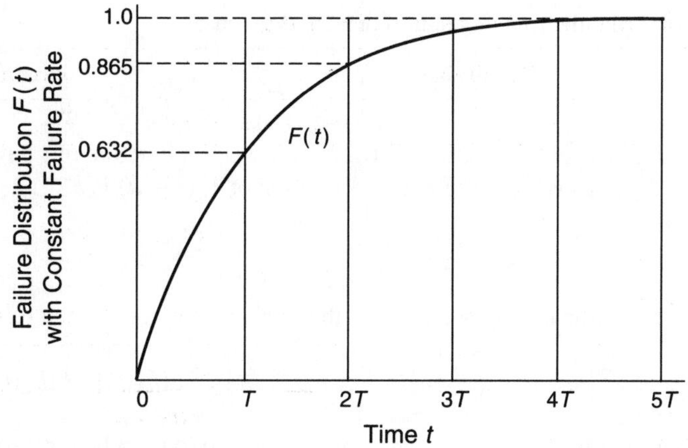

Figure 6.20. Determination of mean time to failure T.

6.4.2 Failure-to-Repair Process

When the repair rate is constant, it coincides with the conditional repair intensity and is designated as μ.

Substituting μ into equations (6.83) and (6.84), we obtain

$$G(t) = 1 - e^{-\mu t} \tag{6.138}$$

$$g(t) = \mu e^{-\mu t} \tag{6.139}$$

The distribution described by equation (6.138) is an exponential repair distribution. The MTTR is given by

$$\text{MTTR} = \int_0^\infty t\mu e^{-\mu t}\, dt = \frac{1}{\mu} \tag{6.140}$$

The MTTR can be estimated by an arithmetical mean of the time-to-repair data, and the constant repair rate μ is the reciprocal of the MTTR.

When the repair distribution $G(t)$ is known, the MTTR can also be evaluated by noting the time t satisfying

$$G(t) = 0.63 \tag{6.141}$$

The assumption of a constant-repair rate can be verified by suitable plotting procedures, as will be shown shortly.

6.4.3 Laplace Transform Analysis

When constant-failure rate and constant-repair rate apply we can simplify the analysis of the combined process to such an extent that analytical solutions become possible. The solutions, summarized in Table 6.10, are now derived. First, we make a few comments regarding Laplace transforms.

A Laplace transform $L[h(t)]$ of $h(t)$ is a function of a complex variable $s = \alpha + j\omega$ and is defined by

$$L[h(t)] = \int_0^\infty e^{-st} h(t) dt \tag{6.142}$$

For example, the transformation of e^{-at} is given by

$$L[e^{-at}] = \int_0^{\infty} e^{-st} e^{-at} dt = \frac{1}{s+a} \tag{6.143}$$

An inverse Laplace transform $L^{-1}[H(s)]$ is a function of t having the Laplace transform $H(s)$. Thus the inverse transformation of $1/(s+a)$ is e^{-at}:

$$L^{-1}\left[\frac{1}{s+a}\right] = e^{-at} \tag{6.144}$$

A significant characteristic of the Laplace transform is the following identity:

$$L\left[\int_0^t h_1(t-u)h_2(u)du\right] = L[h_1(t)] \cdot L[h_2(t)] \tag{6.145}$$

In other words, the transformation of the convolution can be represented by the product of the two Laplace transforms $L[h_1(t)]$ and $L[h_2(t)]$. The convolution integral is treated as an algebraic product in the Laplace-transformed domain.

Now we take the Laplace transform of equation (6.89):

$$\left.\begin{aligned} L[w(t)] &= L[f(t)] + L[f(t)] \cdot L[v(t)] \\ L[v(t)] &= L[g(t)] \cdot L[w(t)] \end{aligned}\right\} \tag{6.146}$$

The constant-failure rate λ and the repair rate μ give

$$L[f(t)] = L[\lambda e^{-\lambda t}] = \lambda \cdot L[e^{-\lambda t}] = \frac{\lambda}{s+\lambda} \tag{6.147}$$

$$L[g(t)] = \frac{\mu}{s+\mu} \tag{6.148}$$

Thus equation (6.146) becomes

$$\left.\begin{aligned} L[w(t)] &= \frac{\lambda}{s+\lambda} + \frac{\lambda}{s+\lambda} L[v(t)] \\ L[v(t)] &= \frac{\mu}{s+\mu} L[w(t)] \end{aligned}\right\} \tag{6.149}$$

Equation (6.149) is a simultaneous algebraic equation for $L[w(t)]$ and $L[v(t)]$ and can be solved:

$$L[w(t)] = \frac{\lambda\mu}{\lambda+\mu}\left(\frac{1}{s}\right) + \frac{\lambda^2}{\lambda+\mu}\left(\frac{1}{s+\lambda+\mu}\right) \tag{6.150}$$

$$L[v(t)] = \frac{\lambda\mu}{\lambda+\mu}\left(\frac{1}{s}\right) - \frac{\lambda\mu}{\lambda+\mu}\left(\frac{1}{s+\lambda+\mu}\right) \tag{6.151}$$

Taking the inverse Laplace transform of equations (6.150) and (6.151) we have:

$$w(t) = \frac{\lambda\mu}{\lambda+\mu} L^{-1}\left(\frac{1}{s}\right) + \frac{\lambda^2}{\lambda+\mu} L^{-1}\left(\frac{1}{s+\lambda+\mu}\right) \tag{6.152}$$

$$v(t) = \frac{\lambda\mu}{\lambda+\mu} L^{-1}\left(\frac{1}{s}\right) - \frac{\lambda\mu}{\lambda+\mu} L^{-1}\left(\frac{1}{s+\lambda+\mu}\right) \tag{6.153}$$

From equation (6.144),

$$w(t) = \frac{\lambda\mu}{\lambda+\mu} + \frac{\lambda^2}{\lambda+\mu}e^{-(\lambda+\mu)t} \tag{6.154}$$

$$v(t) = \frac{\lambda\mu}{\lambda+\mu} - \frac{\lambda\mu}{\lambda+\mu}e^{-(\lambda+\mu)t} \tag{6.155}$$

The expected number of failures $W(0, t)$ and the expected number of repairs $V(0, t)$ are given by the integration of equations (6.57) and (6.61) from $t_1 = 0$ to $t_2 = t$:

$$W(0,t) = \frac{\lambda\mu}{\lambda+\mu}t + \frac{\lambda^2}{(\lambda+\mu)^2}\left[1 - e^{-(\lambda+\mu)t}\right] \tag{6.156}$$

$$V(0,t) = \frac{\lambda\mu}{\lambda+\mu}t - \frac{\lambda\mu}{(\lambda+\mu)^2}\left[1 - e^{-(\lambda+\mu)t}\right] \tag{6.157}$$

The unavailability $Q(t)$ is obtained by equation (6.96):

$$Q(t) = W(0,t) - V(0,t) = \frac{\lambda}{\lambda+\mu}\left[1 - e^{-(\lambda+\mu)t}\right] \tag{6.158}$$

The availability is given by equation (6.47):

$$A(t) = 1 - Q(t) = \frac{\mu}{\lambda+\mu} + \frac{\lambda}{\lambda+\mu}e^{-(\lambda+\mu)t} \tag{6.159}$$

The stationary unavailability $Q(\infty)$ and the stationary availability $A(\infty)$ are

$$Q(\infty) = \frac{\lambda}{\lambda+\mu} = \frac{1/\mu}{1/\lambda + 1/\mu} \tag{6.160}$$

$$A(\infty) = \frac{\mu}{\lambda+\mu} = \frac{1/\lambda}{1/\lambda + 1/\mu} \tag{6.161}$$

Equivalently, the steady-state unavailability and availability are expressed as

$$Q(\infty) = \frac{\text{MTTR}}{\text{MTTF} + \text{MTTR}} \tag{6.162}$$

$$A(\infty) = \frac{\text{MTTF}}{\text{MTTF} + \text{MTTR}} \tag{6.163}$$

We also have

$$\frac{Q(t)}{Q(\infty)} = 1 - e^{(\lambda+\mu)t} \tag{6.164}$$

Thus 63% and 86% of the stationary steady-state unavailability is attained at time T and $2T$, respectively, where

$$T = \frac{1}{\lambda+\mu} = \frac{\text{MTTF} \cdot \text{MTTR}}{\text{MTTF} + \text{MTTR}} \tag{6.165}$$

$$\simeq \text{MTTR}, \quad \text{if MTTR} << \text{MTTF} \tag{6.166}$$

For a nonrepairable component, the repair rate is zero, that is, $\mu \equiv 0$. Thus the unconditional failure intensity of equation (6.154) becomes the failure density.

$$w(t) = \lambda e^{-\lambda t} = f(t) \tag{6.167}$$

If component repair is made instantaneously, the combined process becomes a renewal process. This corresponds to an infinite repair intensity ($\mu = \infty$), and $w(t)$ and $W(0, t)$ are given by

$$w(t) = \lambda, \quad W(0, t) = \lambda t \tag{6.168}$$

The expected number of renewals $W(0, t)$ are proportional to the time span t. This property holds asymptotically for most distributions.

Example 7. Assume constant failure and repair rates for the components shown in Figure 6.7. Obtain $Q(t)$ and $w(t)$ at $t = 5$ and $t = \infty$ (stationary values).

Solution: TTFs in Example 2 give

$$\text{MTTF} = \frac{54.85}{18} = 3.05 \tag{6.169}$$

Further, we have the following TTR data

Component	Fails At	Repaired At	TTR
1	3.1	4.5	1.4
1	6.6	7.4	0.8
2	1.05	1.7	0.65
2	4.5	8.5	4.0
3	5.8	6.8	1.0
4	2.1	3.8	1.7
4	6.4	8.6	2.2
5	4.8	8.3	3.5
6	3.0	6.5	3.5
7	1.4	3.5	2.1
7	5.4	7.6	2.2
8	2.85	3.65	0.8
8	6.7	9.5	2.8
9	4.1	6.2	2.1

Thus

$$\text{MTTR} = \frac{28.75}{14} = 2.05$$

$$\lambda = \frac{1}{\text{MTTF}} = 0.328$$

$$\mu = \frac{1}{\text{MTTR}} = 0.488$$

$$Q(t) = \frac{0.328}{0.328 + 0.488}\left[1 - e^{-(0.328+0.488)t}\right]$$

$$= 0.402 \times (1 - e^{-0.816t})$$

$$w(t) = \frac{0.328 \times 0.488}{0.328 + 0.488} + \frac{0.328^2}{0.328 + 0.488} e^{-(0.328+0.488)t}$$

$$= 0.196 + 0.131e^{-0.816t}$$

and, finally

$$\begin{aligned} Q(5) &= 0.395, \quad Q(\infty) = 0.402 \\ w(5) &= 0.198, \quad w(\infty) = 0.196 \end{aligned} \tag{6.170}$$

yielding a good agreement with the results in Example 2. ■

6.4.4 Markov Analysis

We now present a Markov analysis approach for analyzing the combined process for the case of constant failure and repair rates.

Let $x(t)$ be the indicator variable defined by equations (6.92) and (6.93). The definition of the conditional failure intensity λ can be used to give

$$\left.\begin{aligned} \Pr\{1|0\} &\equiv \Pr\{x(t+dt)=1|x(t)=0\} = \lambda dt \\ \Pr\{0|0\} &\equiv \Pr\{x(t+dt)=0|x(t)=0\} = 1-\lambda dt \\ \Pr\{1|1\} &\equiv \Pr\{x(t+dt)=1|x(t)=1\} = 1-\mu dt \\ \Pr\{0|1\} &\equiv \Pr\{x(t+dt)=0|x(t)=1\} = \mu dt \end{aligned}\right\} \tag{6.171}$$

Term $\Pr\{x(t+dt)=1|x(t)=0\}$ is the probability of failure at $t+dt$, given that the component is working at time t, and so forth. The quantities $\Pr\{1|0\}$, $\Pr\{0|0\}$, $\Pr\{1|1\}$, and $\Pr\{0|1\}$ are called *transition probabilities*. The state transitions are summarized by the Markov diagram of Figure 6.21.

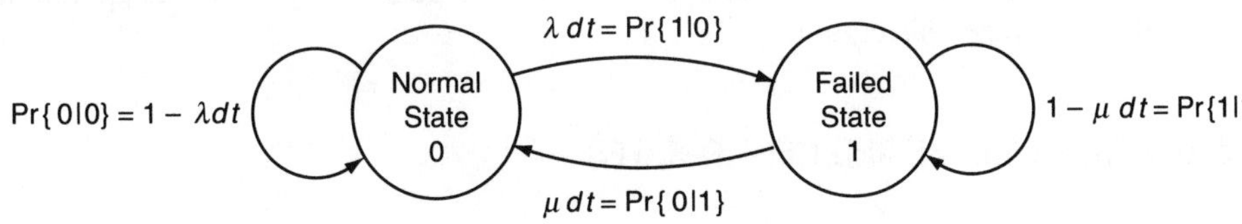

Figure 6.21. Markov transition diagram.

The conditional intensities λ and μ are the known constants r and m, respectively. A Markov analysis cannot handle the time-varying rates $r(t)$ and $m(t)$, because the conditional intensities are time-varying unknowns.

The unavailability $Q(t+dt)$ is the probability of $x(t+dt)=1$, which is, in turn, expressed in terms of the two possible states of $x(t)$ and the corresponding transitions to $x(t+dt)=1$:

$$\begin{aligned} Q(t+dt) &= \Pr\{x(t+dt)=1\} \\ &= \Pr\{1|0\}\Pr\{x(t)=0\} + \Pr\{1|1\}\Pr\{x(t)=1\} \\ &= \lambda dt[1-Q(t)] + (1-\mu dt)Q(t) \end{aligned} \tag{6.172}$$

This identity can be rewritten as

$$Q(t+dt) - Q(t) = dt(-\lambda-\mu)Q(t) + \lambda dt \tag{6.173}$$

yielding

$$\frac{dQ(t)}{dt} = -(\lambda+\mu)Q(t) + \lambda \tag{6.174}$$

with the initial condition at $t=0$ of

$$Q(0) = 0 \tag{6.175}$$

The solution of this linear differential equation is

$$Q(t) = \frac{\lambda}{\lambda+\mu}\left(1-e^{-(\lambda+\mu)t}\right) \tag{6.176}$$

Thus we reach the result given by equation (6.158).

The unconditional intensities $w(t)$ and $v(t)$ are obtained from equations (6.105) and (6.108) because $Q(t)$, λ, and μ are known. We have the results previously obtained: equations (6.154) and (6.155).

The expected number of failures $W(0,t)$ and $V(0,t)$ can be calculated by equations (6.57) and (6.61), yielding (6.156) and (6.157), respectively.

6.5 STATISTICAL DISTRIBUTIONS

The commonly used distributions are listed and pictorialized in Tables 6.11 and 6.12, respectively. For components that have an increasing failure rate with time, the normal, log-normal, or the Weibull distribution with shape parameter β larger than unity apply. The normal distributions arise by pure chance, resulting from a sum of a large number of small disturbances. Repair times are frequently best fitted by the log-normal distribution because some repair times can be much greater than the mean (some repairs take a long time due to a lack of spare parts or local expertise). A detailed description of these distributions is given in Appendix A.1 of this chapter and in most textbooks on statistics or reliability.

When enough data are available, a histogram similar to Figure 6.3 can be constructed. The density can be obtained analytically through a piecewise polynomial approximation of the normalized histogram.

6.6 GENERAL FAILURE AND REPAIR RATES

Consider a histogram such as Figure 6.4. This histogram was constructed from the mortality data shown in Figure 6.3 after dividing by the total number of individuals, 1,023,102. A piecewise polynomial interpolation of the histogram yields the following failure density:

$$f(t) = \begin{cases} 0.00638 - 0.001096t + 0.951 \times 10^{-4}t^2 - 0.349 \times 10^{-5}t^3 \\ \quad +0.478 \times 10^{-7}t^4, \quad \text{for } t \le 30 \\ 0.0566 - 0.279 \times 10^{-2}t + 0.259 \times 10^{-4}t^2 + 0.508 \times 10^{-6}t^3 \\ \quad -0.573 \times 10^{-8}t^4, \quad \text{for } 30 < t \le 90 \\ -0.003608 + 0.777 \times 10^{-3}t - 0.755 \times 10^{-5}t^2, \quad \text{for } t > 90 \end{cases} \tag{6.177}$$

The failure density is plotted in Figure 6.4. Assume now that the repair data are also available and have been fitted to a log-normal distribution.

$$g(t) = \frac{1}{\sqrt{2\pi}\,\sigma t} \exp\left[-\frac{1}{2}\left(\frac{\ln t - \mu}{\sigma}\right)^2\right] \tag{6.178}$$

with parameter values of

$$\mu = 1.0, \qquad \sigma = 0.5 \tag{6.179}$$

We now differentiate the fundamental identity of equation (6.89):

$$\left.\begin{aligned} w(t)/dt &= f'(t) + f(0)v(t) + \int_0^t f'(t-u)v(u)du \\ v(t)/dt &= g(0)w(t) + \int_0^t g'(t-u)w(u)du \end{aligned}\right\} \tag{6.180}$$

where $f'(t)$ and $g'(t)$ are defined by

$$f'(t) = \frac{f(t)}{dt}, \qquad g'(t) = \frac{g(t)}{dt} \tag{6.181}$$

Table 6.11. Summary of Typical Distributions

Distributions → **Descriptions ↓**	**Exponential**	**Normal**	**Log-Normal**	**Weibull**
Name	$\exp^*(\lambda)$	$\text{gau}^*(\mu, \sigma^2)$	$\log - \text{gau}^*(\mu, \sigma^2)$	$\text{wei}^*(\beta, \sigma, \gamma)$
Variable	$0 \leq t$	$-\infty < t < \infty$	$0 < t$	$\max\{0, \gamma\} \leq t$
Parameter	$0 < \lambda$	$-\infty < \mu < \infty, \quad 0 < \sigma$	$-\infty < \mu < \infty, \quad 0 < \sigma$	$-\infty < \gamma < \infty, \quad 0 < \beta, \quad 0 < \sigma$
$Pdf.\ f(t)$	$\lambda \exp(-\lambda t)$	$\frac{1}{\sqrt{2\pi}\sigma} \exp\left[-\frac{1}{2}\left(\frac{t-\mu}{\sigma}\right)^2\right]$	$\frac{1}{\sqrt{2\pi}\sigma t} \exp\left[-\frac{1}{2}\left(\frac{\ln t-\mu}{\sigma}\right)^2\right]$	$\frac{\beta}{\sigma}\left(\frac{t-\gamma}{\sigma}\right)^{\beta-1} \exp\left[-\left(\frac{t-\gamma}{\sigma}\right)^{\beta}\right]$
Unreliability $F(t)$	$1 - \exp(-\lambda t)$	$\int_0^t f(u)du$	$\int_0^t f(u)du$	$1 - \exp\left[-\left(\frac{t-\gamma}{\sigma}\right)^{\beta}\right]$
Failure rate $r(t)$	λ	$\frac{f(t)}{1-F(t)}$	$\frac{f(t)}{1-F(t)}$	$\frac{\beta}{\sigma}\left(\frac{t-\gamma}{\sigma}\right)^{\beta-1}$
Mean	$1/\lambda$	μ	$\exp[\mu + 0.5\sigma^2]$	$\gamma + \sigma\Gamma(\frac{1+\beta}{\beta})$
Variance	$(1/\lambda)^2$	σ^2	$\exp(2\mu^2 + 2\sigma^2) - \exp(2\mu + \sigma^2)$	$\sigma^2\left\{\Gamma(\frac{2+\beta}{\beta}) - \left[\Gamma(\frac{1+\beta}{\beta})\right]^2\right\}$

Table 6.11. *Continued*

Distributions → **Descriptions ↓**	**Poisson**	**Binomial**	**Gumbel**
Name	$\text{poi}^*(\lambda)$	$\text{bin}^*(P, N)$	$\text{gum}^*(\theta, b)$
Variable	$0 \le n$: integer	$0 \le n$: integer $\le N$	$-\infty < t < \infty$
Parameter	$0 < \lambda, \quad 0 \le t$	$1 \le N$: integer, $\quad 0 \le P \le 1$	$-\infty < \theta < \infty, \quad 0 < b$
Pdf. $f(t)$	$f(n) = \dfrac{\exp(-\lambda t)(\lambda t)^n}{n!}$	$f(n) = \dfrac{N!}{n!(N-n)!} P^n (1-P)^{N-n}$	$\dfrac{1}{b} \exp\left[\left(\dfrac{t-\theta}{b}\right) - \exp\left(\dfrac{t-\theta}{b}\right)\right]$
Unreliability $F(t)$	$F(n) = \sum_{i=0}^{i=n} \dfrac{(\lambda t)^i}{i!} \exp(-\lambda t)$	$F(n) = \sum_{i=0}^{n} \dfrac{N!}{i!(N-i)!} P^i (1-P)^{N-i}$	$1 - \exp\left[-\exp\left(\dfrac{t-\theta}{b}\right)\right]$
Failure rate $r(t)$	—	—	$\dfrac{1}{b} \exp\left(\dfrac{t-\theta}{b}\right)$
Mean	$\overline{n} = \lambda t$	$\overline{n} = NP$	—
Variance	$\sigma_n^2 = \lambda t$	$\sigma_n^2 = NP(1-P)$	—

Table 6.11. *Continued*

Distributions → **Descriptions ↓**	**Inverse Gaussian**	**Gamma**	**Beta**
Name	$\text{inv} - \text{gau}^*(\rho, k)$	$\text{gam}^*(\beta, \eta)$	$\text{beta}^*(\alpha, \beta)$
Variable	$0 < t$	$0 < t$	$0 < x < 1$
Parameter	$\rho \neq 0, \quad 0 < k$	$0 < \beta, \quad 0 < \eta$	$-1 < \alpha, \quad -1 < \beta$
Pdf. $f(t)$	$\left(\frac{k}{2\pi\rho t^3}\right)^{1/2} \exp\left[\frac{-k\rho\left(t - \frac{1}{\rho}\right)^2}{2t}\right]$	$\frac{1}{\eta\Gamma(\beta)}\left(\frac{t}{\eta}\right)^{\beta-1} e^{-t/\eta}$	$f(x) = \frac{\Gamma(\alpha+\beta+2)}{\Gamma(\alpha+1)\Gamma(\beta+1)} x^{\alpha}(1-x)^{\beta}$
Unreliability $F(t)$	$\int_0^t f(u)du$	$\int_0^t f(u)du$	$F(x) = \int_0^x f(u)du$
Failure rate $r(t)$	$\frac{f(t)}{1 - F(t)}$	$\frac{f(t)}{1 - F(t)}$	$r(x) = \frac{f(x)}{1 - F(x)}$
Mean	$\bar{t} = 1/\rho$	$\eta\beta$	$(\alpha + 1)/(\alpha + \beta + 2)$
Variance	$\sigma_t^2 = 1/(k\rho^2)$	$\eta^2\beta$	$\sigma_x^2 = \frac{(\alpha+1)(\beta+1)}{(\alpha+\beta+2)^2(\alpha+\beta+3)}$

TABLE 6.12. Graphs of Typical Distributions

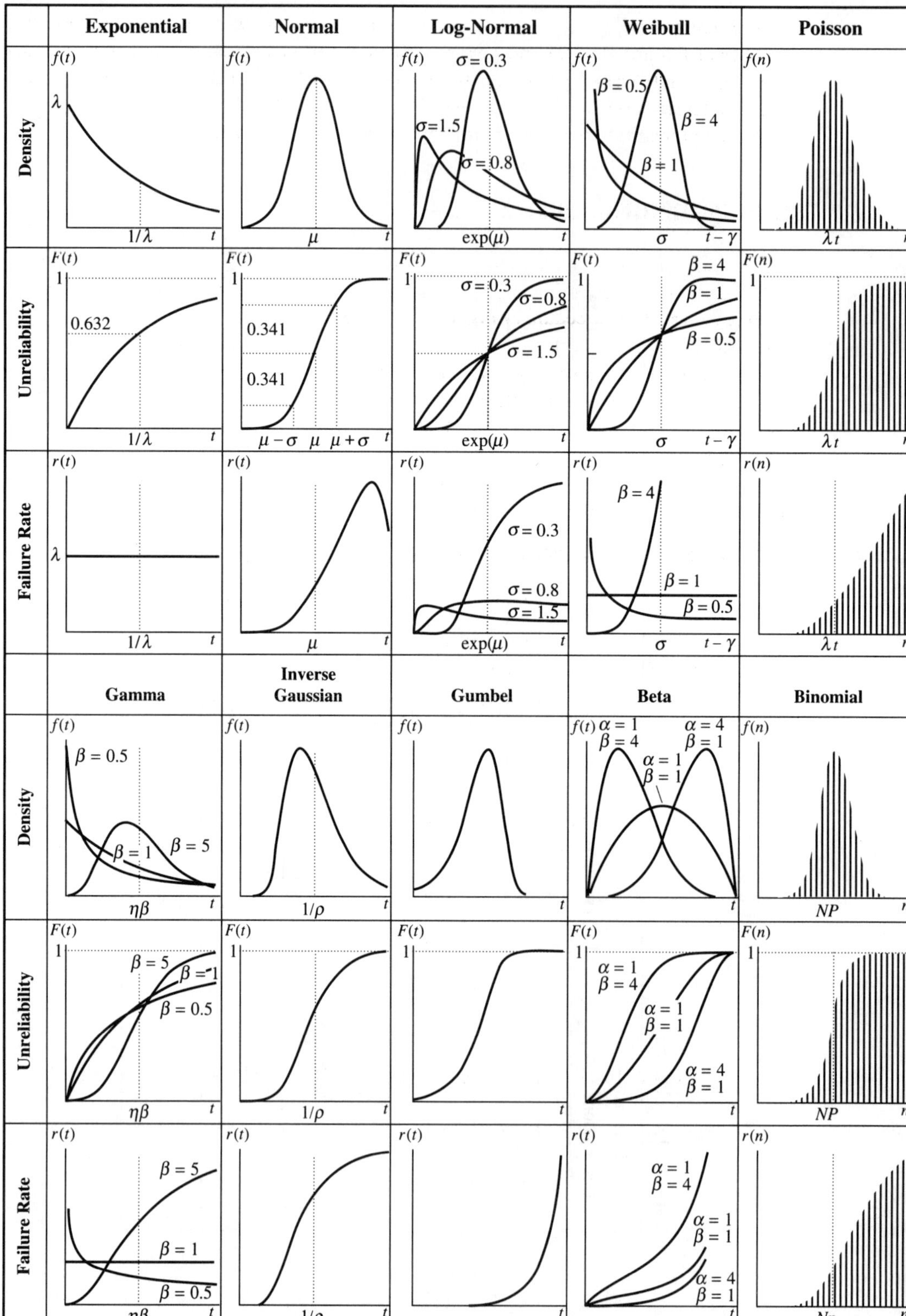

The differential equation (6.180) is now integrated, yielding $w(t)$ and $v(t)$. The expected number of failures $W(0, t)$ and repairs $V(0, t)$ can be calculated by integration of equations (6.57) and (6.61). The unavailability $Q(t)$ is given by equation (6.96). The conditional failure intensity $\lambda(t)$ can be calculated by equation (6.106). Given failure and repair densities, the probabilistic parameters for any process can be obtained in this manner.

6.7 ESTIMATING DISTRIBUTION PARAMETERS

Given sufficient data, a histogram such as Figure 6.4 can be constructed and the failure or repair distribution determined by a piecewise polynomial approximation, as demonstrated in Section 6.6. The procedure of Figure 6.16 is then applied, and the probabilistic concepts are quantified.

When only fragmentary data are available we cannot construct the complete histogram. In such a case, an appropriate distribution must be assumed and its parameters evaluated from the data. The component quantification can then be made using the flow chart of Figure 6.16.

In this section, parameter estimation (or identification) methods for the repair-to-failure and the failure-to-repair process are presented.

6.7.1 Parameter Estimation for Repair-to-Failure Process

In parameter estimation based on test data, three cases arise:

1. All components concerned proceed to failure and no component is taken out of use before failure. (All samples fail.)
2. Not all components being tested proceed to failure because they have been taken out of service before failure. (Incomplete failure data.)
3. Only a small portion of the sample is tested to failure. (Early failure data.)

Case 1: All samples fail. Consider the failure data for the 250 germanium transistors in Table 6.5. Assume a constant failure rate λ. The existence of the constant λ can be checked as follows.

The survival distribution is given by

$$R(t) = e^{-\lambda t} \tag{6.182}$$

This can be written as

$$\ln\left[\frac{1}{R(t)}\right] = \lambda t \tag{6.183}$$

So, if the natural ln of $1/R(t)$ is plotted against t, it should be a straight line with slope λ.

Values of $\ln[1/R(t)]$ versus t from Table 6.5 are plotted in Figure 6.22. The best straight line is passed through the points and the slope is readily calculated:

$$\lambda = \frac{y_2 - y_1}{x_2 - x_1} = \frac{1.08 - 0.27}{400 - 100} = 0.0027 \tag{6.184}$$

Note that this λ is consistent with constant rate $r = 0.0026$ in Example 3.

Case 2: Incomplete failure data. In some tests, components are taken out of service for reasons other than failures. This will affect the number of components exposed to failure

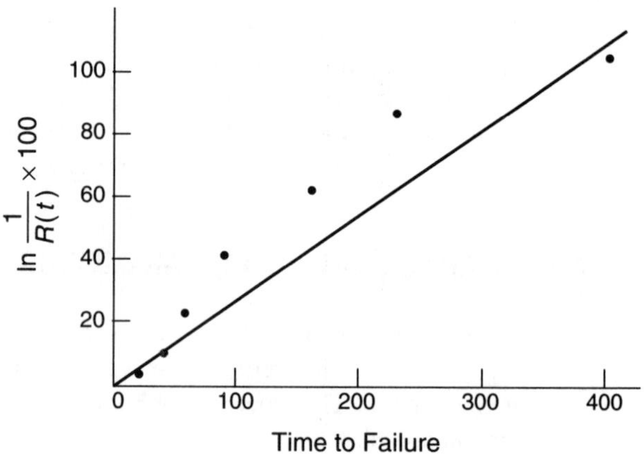

Figure 6.22. Test for constant λ.

at any given time and a correction factor must be used in calculating the reliability. As an example, consider the lifetime to failure for bearings given in Table 6.13 [1]. The original number of bearings exposed to failure is 202; however, between each failure some of the bearings are taken out of service before failure has occurred.

TABLE 6.13. Bearing Test Data

1	2	3	4	5	6	7
Lifetime to Failure (hr)	**Number of Failures**	**Number Exposed to Failure**	**Number of Failures Expected if Original Population Had Been Allowed to Proceed to Failure**	**Cumulative Number of Failures Expected**	***F*(*t*)**	***R*(*t*)**
141	1	202		1.00	0.005	0.995
337	1	177	$1 \times \frac{202 - 1.00}{177} = 1.14$	2.14	0.011	0.989
364	1	176	$1 \times \frac{202 - 2.14}{176} = 1.14$	3.27	0.016	0.984
542	1	165	$1 \times \frac{202 - 3.27}{165} = 1.20$	4.47	0.022	0.978
716	1	156	$1 \times \frac{202 - 4.47}{156} = 1.27$	5.74	0.028	0.972
765	1	153	$1 \times \frac{202 - 5.74}{153} = 1.28$	7.02	0.035	0.965
940	1	144	$1 \times \frac{202 - 7.02}{144} = 1.35$	8.37	0.041	0.959
986	1	143	$1 \times \frac{202 - 8.37}{143} = 1.35$	9.72	0.048	0.952

The unreliability $F(t)$ is calculated by dividing the cumulative number of failures expected if all original components had been allowed to proceed to failure by the original number of components exposed to failure (202). The failure distribution $F(t)$ for data of Table 6.13 is plotted in Figure 6.23. (See the discussion in Appendix A.4 of this chapter for a description of the computational procedure.) The curve represents only the portion of the mortality curve that corresponds to early wearout failures.

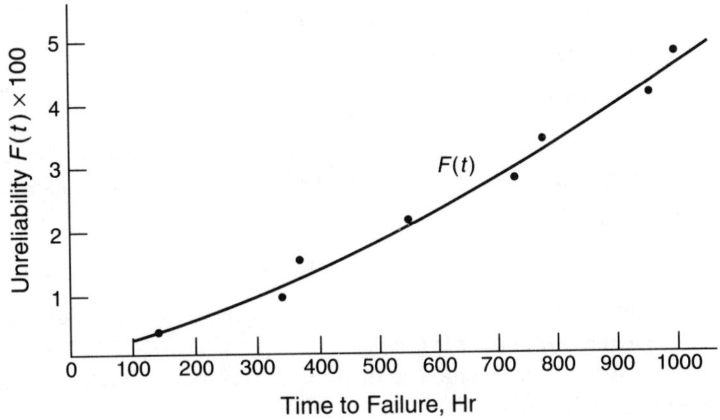

Figure 6.23. Bearing failure distribution.

Case 3: Early failure data. Generally, when n items are being tested for failure, the test is terminated before all of the n items have failed, either because of limited time available for testing or for economical reasons. For such a situation the failure distribution can still be estimated from the available data by assuming a particular distribution and plotting the data for the assumed distribution. The closeness of the plotted data to a straight line indicates whether the model represents the data reasonably. As an example, consider the time to failure for the first seven failures (failure-terminated data) of 20 guidance systems ($n = 20$) given in Table 6.14 [2].

TABLE 6.14. Failure Data for Guidance Systems

Failure Number	Time to Failure (hr)
1	1
2	4
3	5
4	6
5	15
6	20
7	40

Suppose it is necessary to estimate the number of failures to $t = 100$ hr and $t = 300$ hr. First, let us assume that the data can be described by a three-parameter Weibull distribution for which the equation is (see Table 6.11) as follows.

1. For nonnegative $\gamma \geq 0$,

$$F(t) = \begin{cases} 0, & \text{for } 0 \leq t < \gamma \\ 1 - \exp\left[-\left(\dfrac{t-\gamma}{\sigma}\right)^{\beta}\right], & \text{for } t \geq \gamma \end{cases} \tag{6.185}$$

2. For negative $\gamma < 0$,

$$F(t) = 1 - \exp\left[-\left(\frac{t-\gamma}{\sigma}\right)^{\beta}\right], \quad \text{for } t \geq 0 \tag{6.186}$$

where σ = scale parameter (characteristic life, positive)
β = shape parameter (positive), and
γ = location parameter.

Some components fail at time zero when γ is negative. There is some failure-free period of time when γ is positive. The Weibull distribution becomes an exponential distribution when $\gamma = 0$ and $\beta = 1$.

$$F(t) = 1 - e^{t/\sigma} \tag{6.187}$$

Thus parameter σ is a mean time to failure of the exponential distribution, and hence is given the name *characteristic life*.

The Weibull distribution with $\beta = 2$ becomes a Rayleigh distribution with time proportional failure rate $r(t)$.

$$r(t) = \frac{2}{\sigma}\frac{t-\gamma}{\sigma}, \quad \text{for } t \geq \gamma \tag{6.188}$$

For practical reasons, it is frequently convenient to assume that $\gamma = 0$, which reduces the above equation to

$$F(t) = 1 - \exp\left[-\left(\frac{t}{\sigma}\right)^{\beta}\right] \tag{6.189}$$

or

$$\frac{1}{1-F(t)} = \exp\left[\left(\frac{t}{\sigma}\right)^{\beta}\right] \tag{6.190}$$

and

$$\ln\ln\frac{1}{1-F(t)} = \beta\ln t - \beta\ln\sigma \tag{6.191}$$

This is the basis for the Weibull probability plots, where $\ln\ln\{1/[1-F(t)]\}$ plots as a straight line against $\ln t$ with slope β and y-intersection $\tilde{y}$ of $-\beta\ln\sigma$:

$$\text{slope} = \beta \tag{6.192}$$

$$\tilde{y} = -\beta\ln\sigma \quad \text{or} \quad \sigma = \exp\left(\frac{-\tilde{y}}{\beta}\right) \tag{6.193}$$

To use this equation to extrapolate failure probabilities, it is necessary to estimate the two parameters σ and β from the time to failure data. This is done by plotting the data of Table 6.15 in Figure 6.24. The median-rank plotting position is obtained by the method described in Appendix A.5 of this chapter.

From the graph, the parameters β and σ are

$$\beta = \text{slope} = \frac{y_2 - y_1}{x_2 - x_1} = \frac{2.0-(-3.0)}{7.25-0.06} = 0.695 \tag{6.194}$$

$$\sigma = e^{-(\tilde{y})/\beta} = e^{-(3.4/0.695)} = 132.85 \tag{6.195}$$

Thus

$$F(100) = 1 - \exp\left[-\left(\frac{100}{132.85}\right)^{0.695}\right] = 0.56 \tag{6.196}$$

TABLE 6.15. Plotting Points

Failure Number i	Time to Failure	Plotting Points (%) $F(t) = (i - 0.5) \times 100/n$
1	1	2.5
2	4	7.5
3	5	12.5
4	6	17.5
5	15	22.5
6	20	27.5
7	40	32.5

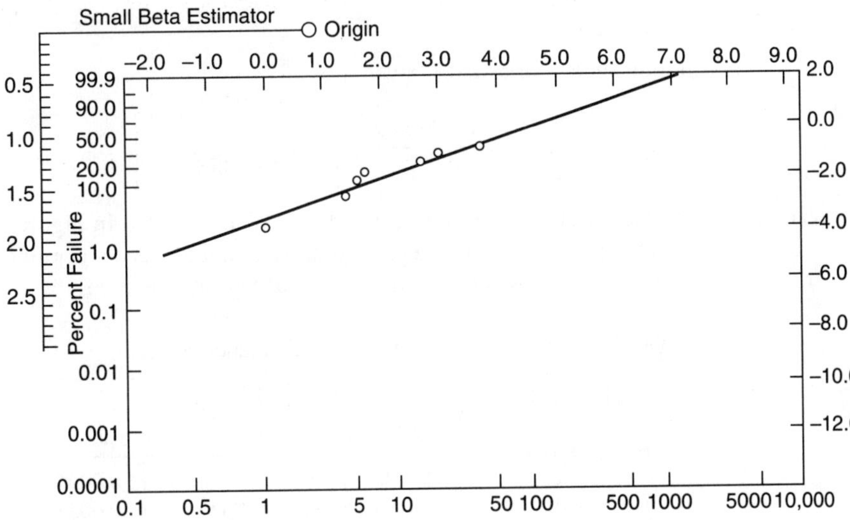

Figure 6.24. Test data plot.

The number of failures to time $t = 100$ is $0.56 \times 20 = 11.2$. Also,

$$F(300) = 1 - \exp\left[-\left(\frac{300}{132.85}\right)^{0.695}\right] = 0.828 \tag{6.197}$$

or, the number of failures to time $t = 300$ is $0.828 \times 20 = 16.6$.

Table 6.16 gives the time to failure for all 20 components. The comparison of the above results with the actual number of failures to 100 hr and 300 hr demonstrates our serendipity in choosing the Weibull distribution with $\gamma = 0$.

Once the functional form of the failure distribution has been established and the constants determined, other reliability factors of the repair-to-failure process can be obtained. For example, to calculate the failure density, the derivative of the Weibull mortality equation is employed.

$$F(t) = 1 - \exp\left[-\left(\frac{t}{\sigma}\right)^{\beta}\right] \tag{6.198}$$

Then

$$f(t) = \frac{dF(t)}{dt} = \frac{\beta \cdot t^{\beta-1}}{\sigma^{\beta}} \exp\left[-\left(\frac{t}{\sigma}\right)^{\beta}\right] \tag{6.199}$$

TABLE 6.16. More Data for Guidance System

Failure Number	Time to Failure (hr)	Failure Number	Time to Failure (hr)
1	1	11	95
2	4	12	106
3	5	13	125
4	6	14	151
5	15	15	200
6	20	16	268
7	40	17	459
8	41	18	827
9	60	19	840
10	93	20	1089

Substituting values for σ and β gives

$$f(t) = \frac{0.02324}{t^{0.305}} \exp\left[-\left(\frac{t}{132.85}\right)^{0.695}\right] \tag{6.200}$$

The calculated values of $f(t)$ are given in Table 6.17 and plotted in Figure 6.25. These values represent the probability that the first component failure occurs per unit time at time t, given that the component was operating as good as new at time zero.

TABLE 6.17. Failure Density for Guidance System

Time to Failure (hr)	f(t)	Time to Failure (hr)	f(t)
1	0.0225	95	0.0026
4	0.0139	106	0.0024
5	0.0128	125	0.0020
6	0.0120	151	0.0017
15	0.0082	200	0.0012
20	0.0071	268	0.0008
40	0.0049	459	0.0003
40	0.0049	827	0.0001
60	0.0037	840	—
93	0.0027	1089	—

The expected number of times the failures occur in the interval t to $t + dt$ is $w(t)dt$, and its integral over an interval is the expected number of failures. Once the failure density and the repair density are known, the unconditional failure intensity $w(t)$ may be obtained from equation (6.89).

Assume that the component is as good as new at time zero. Assume further that once the component fails at time $t > 0$ it cannot be repaired (nonrepairable component). Then the repair density is identically equal to zero, and the unconditional repair intensity $v(t)$ of equation (6.89) becomes zero. Thus

$$w(t) = f(t) = \frac{0.02324}{t^{0.305}} \exp\left[-\left(\frac{t}{132.85}\right)^{0.695}\right] \tag{6.201}$$

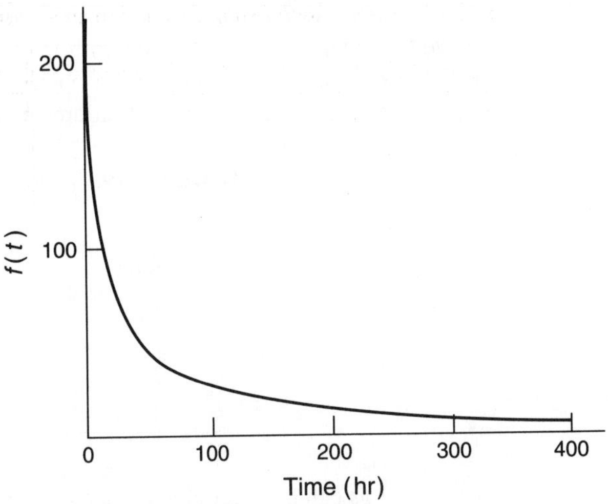

Figure 6.25. Failure density for guidance system.

The unconditional failure intensity is also the failure density for the nonrepairable component. The values of $f(t)$ in Figure 6.25 represent $w(t)$ as well.

The expected number of failures $W(t_1, t_2)$ can be obtained by integrating the above equation over the t_1 to t_2 time interval and is equal to $F(t_2) - F(t_1)$:

$$W(t_1, t_2) = \int_{t_1}^{t_2} w(t)dt$$

$$= \int_{t_1}^{t_2} f(t)dt = F(t_2) - F(t_1) \tag{6.202}$$

$$= \left\{1 - \exp\left[-\left(\frac{t}{\sigma}\right)^{\beta}\right]\right\}_{t_1}^{t_2}$$

The ENF (expected number of failures) values $W(0, t)$ for the data of Figure 6.25 are given in Table 6.18. In this case, because no repairs can be made, $W(0, t) = F(t)$, and equation (6.202) is equivalent to equation (6.198).

TABLE 6.18. Expected Number of Failures of Guidance System

$[\phi, t)$, t	ENF×20	$[\phi, t)$, t	ENF×20
1	0.66	95	10.94
4	1.68	106	11.49
5	1.95	125	12.33
6	2.19	151	13.30
15	2.94	200	14.70
20	4.71	268	16.08
40	7.04	459	18.13
40	7.04	827	19.43
60	8.75	840	19.46
93	10.84	1089	19.73

Parameter estimation in a wearout situation. This example concerns a retrospective Weibull analysis carried out on an Imperial Chemicals Industries Ltd. (ICI) furnace. The furnace was commissioned in 1962 and had 176 tubes. Early in 1963, tubes began to fail after 475 days on-line, the first four failures being logged at the times listed in Table 6.19.

TABLE 6.19. Times to Failure of First Four Reformer Tubes

Failure	On-Line (days)
1	475
2	482
3	541
4	556

As far as can be ascertained, operation up to the time of these failures was perfectly normal; there had been no unusual excursions of temperature or pressure. Hence, it appears that tubes were beginning to wear out, and if normal operations were continued it should be possible to predict the likely number of failures in a future period on the basis of the pattern of failures that these early failures establish. In order to make this statement, however, it is necessary to make one further assumption.

It may well be that the wearout failures occurred at a weak weld in the tubes; one would expect the number of tubes with weak welds to be limited. If, for example, six tubes had poor welds, then two further failures would clear this failure mode out of the system, and no further failures would take place until another wearout failure mode such as corrosion became significant.

If we assume that all 176 tubes can fail for the same wearout phenomenon, then we are liable to make a pessimistic prediction of the number of failures in a future period. However, without being able to shut the furnace down to determine the failure mode, this is the most useful assumption that can be made. The problem, therefore, is to predict future failures based on this assumption.

The median-rank plotting positions $(i - 0.3) \times 100/(n + 0.4)$ for the first four failures are listed in Table 6.20. The corresponding points are then plotted and the best straight line is drawn through the four points: line (a) of Figure 6.26.

TABLE 6.20. Median Rank Plotting Positions for the First Four Failures

Failure i	On-Line (days)	Median Rank (%)
1	475	0.40
2	482	0.96
3	541	1.53
4	556	2.10

The line intersects the time axis at around 400 days and is extremely steep, corresponding to an apparent Weibull shape parameter β of around 10. Both of these observations suggest that if we were able to plot the complete failure distribution, it would curve over

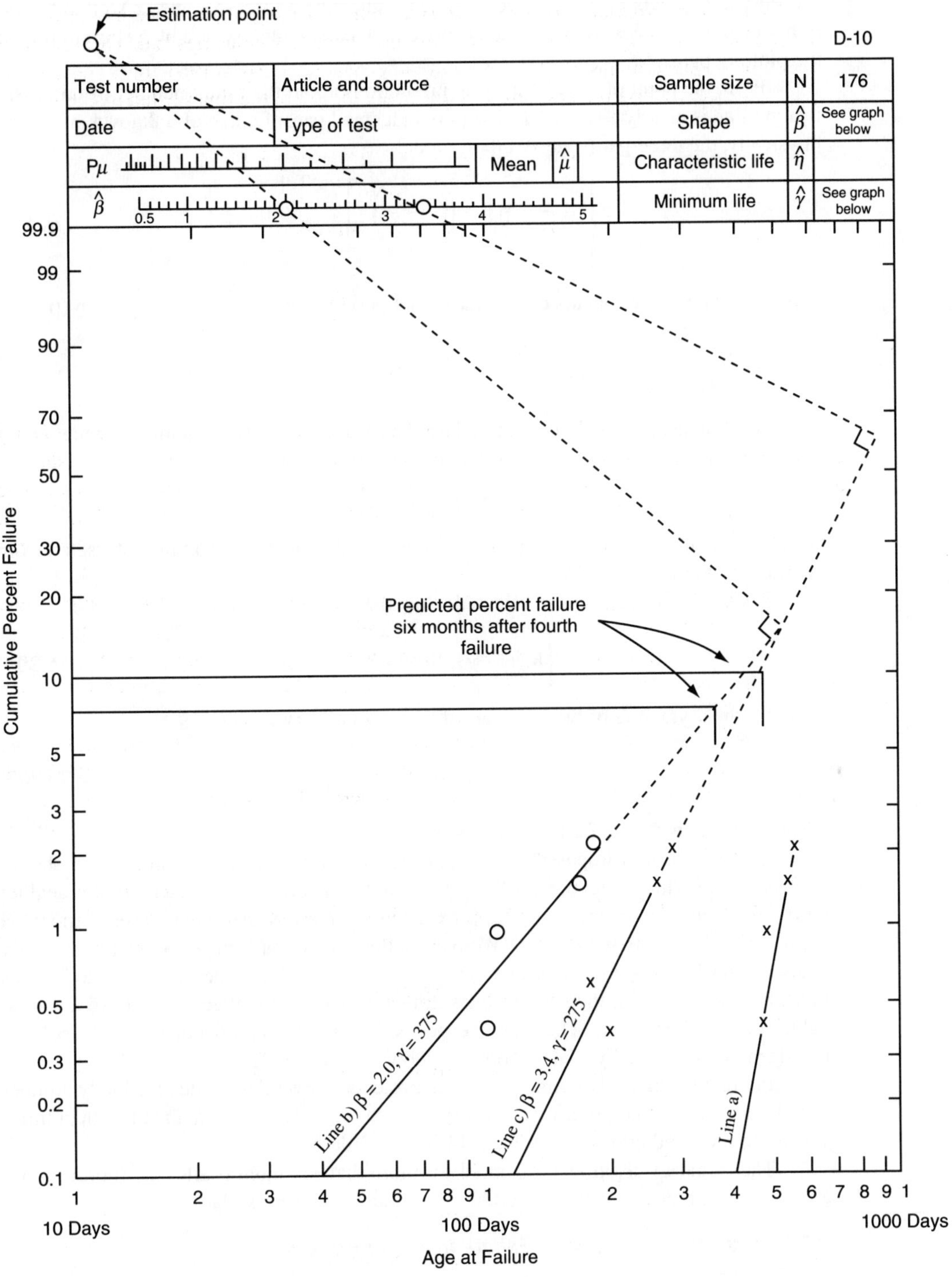

Figure 6.26. Weibull plots of reformer tube failures.

toward the time axis as failures accumulated, indicating a three-parameter Weibull model rather than the simplest two-parameter model that can be represented by a straight line on the plotting paper.

From the point of view of making predictions about the future number of failures, a straight line is clearly easier to deal with than a small part of a line of unknown curvature. Physically, the three-parameter Weibull model

$$F(t) = \begin{cases} 1 - \exp\left[-\left(\dfrac{t-\gamma}{\sigma}\right)^{\beta}\right], & \text{for } t \geq \gamma \geq 0 \\ 0, & \text{for } 0 \leq t < \gamma \end{cases} \tag{6.203}$$

implies that no failure occurs during the initial period $[0, \gamma)$. Similar to equation (6.191), we have for $t \geq \gamma$,

$$\ln\ln\frac{1}{1-F(t)} = \beta\ln(t-\gamma) - \beta\ln\sigma \tag{6.204}$$

Thus mathematically, the Weibull model can be reduced to the two-parameter model and is represented by a straight line by making the transformation

$$t' = t - \gamma \tag{6.205}$$

Graphically, this is equivalent to plotting the failure data with a fixed time subtracted from the times to failure.

The correct time has been selected when the transformed plot

$$\left\{\ln(t-\gamma),\ \ln\ln\left[\frac{1}{1-F(t)}\right]\right\} \tag{6.206}$$

becomes the asymptote of the final part of the original curved plot

$$\left\{\ln t,\ \ln\ln\left[\frac{1}{1-F(t)}\right]\right\} \tag{6.207}$$

because $\ln t \simeq \ln(t-\gamma)$ for large values of t.

In this case it is impossible to decide empirically what the transformation should be because only the initial part of the curved plot is available. However, we are dealing with a wearout phenomenon, and from experience we know that when these phenomena are represented by a two-parameter Weibull model, the Weibull shape parameter generally takes a value $2 \leq \beta \leq 3.4$. Hence fixed times are subtracted from the four times to failures until, by trial and error, the straight lines drawn through the plotted points have apparent values of β of 2 and 3.4. These are, respectively, lines (b) and (c) of Figure 6.26. The transformation formed by trial and error is shown in Table 6.21.

In Figure 6.26, the two lines have been projected forward to predict the likely number of failures in the six months after the fourth failure (i.e., to 182 days after the fourth failure). The respective predictions are of 9 and 14 further failures.

The furnace was, in fact, operated for more than six months after the fourth failure and, in the six-month period referred to, 11 further failures took place.

6.7.2 Parameter Estimation for Failure-to-Repair Process

Time to repair (TTR), or downtime, consists not only of the time it takes to repair a failure but also of waiting time for spare parts, personnel, and so on. The availability

TABLE 6.21. Transformation to Yield Apparent Values of β of 2 and 3.4

Failure	On-Line (days)	$\beta = 2.0$ $\gamma = 375$ (days)	$\beta = 3.4$ $\gamma = 275$ (days)	Median Rank (%)
1	475	100	200	0.40
2	482	107	207	0.96
3	541	166	266	1.53
4	556	181	281	2.10

$A(t)$ is the proportion of population of the components expected to function at time t. This availability is related to the "population ensemble." We can consider another availability based on an average over a "time ensemble." It is defined by

$$\overline{A} = \frac{\sum_{i=1}^{N} \mathrm{TTF}_i}{\sum_{i=1}^{N}[\mathrm{TTF}_i + \mathrm{TTR}_i]} \tag{6.208}$$

where $(\mathrm{TTF}_i, \mathrm{TTR}_i)$, $i = 1, \ldots, N$ are consecutive pairs of times to failure and times to repair of a particular component. The number N of the cycles $(\mathrm{TTF}_i, \mathrm{TTR}_i)$ is assumed sufficiently large. The time-ensemble availability represents percentiles of the component functioning in one cycle. The so-called *ergodic theorem* states that the time-ensemble availability $\overline{A}$ coincides with the stationary values of the population-ensemble availability $A(\infty)$.

As an example, consider the 20 consecutive sets of TTF and TTR given in Table 6.22 [3]. The time-ensemble availability is

$$\overline{A} = \frac{1102}{1151.8} = 0.957 \tag{6.209}$$

TABLE 6.22. Time to Failure and Time to Repair Data

TTF (hr)	TTR (hr)	TTF (hr)	TTR (hr)
125	1.0	58	1.0
44	1.0	53	0.8
27	9.8	36	0.5
53	1.0	25	1.7
8	1.2	106	3.6
46	0.2	200	6.0
5	3.0	159	1.5
20	0.3	4	2.5
15	3.1	79	0.3
12	1.5	27	9.8
Subtotal		1102	49.8
Total		1151.8	

The mean time to failure and the mean time to repair are

$$\text{MTTF} = \frac{1102}{20} = 55.10 \tag{6.210}$$

$$\text{MTTR} = \frac{49.8}{20} = 2.49 \tag{6.211}$$

As with the failure parameters, the TTR data of Table 6.22 form a distribution for which parameters can be estimated. Table 6.23 is an ordered listing of the repair times in Table 6.22 (see Appendix A.5, this chapter, for the method used for plotting points in Table 6.23).

TABLE 6.23. Ordered Listing of Repair Times

Repair No. i	TTR	Plotting Points (%) $(i - 0.5) \times 100/n$
1	0.2	2.5
2	0.3	7.5
3	0.3	12.5
4	0.5	17.5
5	0.8	22.5
6	1.0	27.5
7	1.0	32.5
8	1.0	37.5
9	1.0	42.5
10	1.2	47.5
11	1.5	52.5
12	1.5	57.5
13	1.7	62.5
14	2.5	67.5
15	3.0	72.5
16	3.1	77.5
17	3.6	82.5
18	6.0	87.5
19	9.8	92.5
20	9.8	97.5

Let us assume that these data can be described by a log-normal distribution where the natural log of times to repair are distributed according to a normal distribution with mean μ and variance σ^2. The mean μ may then be best estimated by plotting the TTR data on a log-normal probability paper against the plotting points (Figure 6.27) and finding the TTR of the plotted 50th percentile. The 50th percentile is 1.43, so the parameter $\mu = \ln 1.43 = 0.358$.

The μ is not only the median (50th percentile) of the normal distribution of ln(TTR) but also a mean value of ln(TTR). Thus the parameter μ may also be estimated by the arithmetical mean of the natural log of TTRs in Table 6.22. This yields $\overline{\mu} = 0.368$, almost the same result as 0.358 obtained from the log-normal probability paper.

Notice that the $T = 1.43$ satisfying $\ln T = \mu = 0.358$ is not the expected value of the time to repair, although it is a 50th percentile of the log-normal distribution. The expected value, or the mean time to repair, can be estimated by averaging observed times to repair data in Table 6.22, and was given as 2.49 by equation (6.211). This is considerably larger

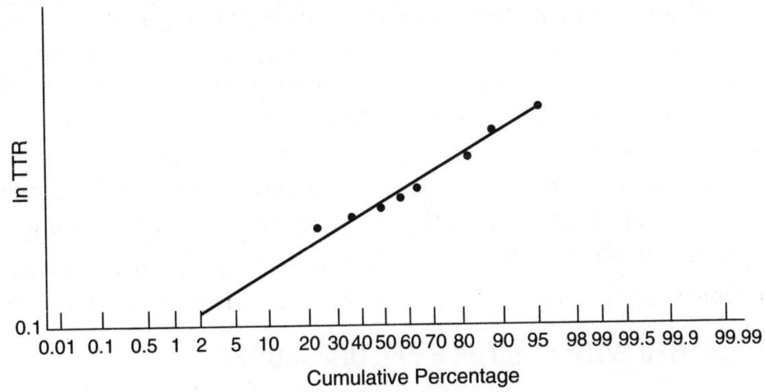

Figure 6.27. Plot of TTR data.

than the 50th percentile ($T = 1.43$) because, in practice, there are usually some unexpected breakdowns that take a long time to repair. A time to repair distribution with this property frequently follows a log-normal density that decreases gently for large values of TTR.

The parameter σ^2 is a variance of ln(TTR) and can be estimated by

$$\begin{aligned} \overline{\mu} &= \sum_{i=1}^{N} \ln \text{TTR}_i, \quad \text{(sample mean)} \\ \sigma^2 &= \frac{\sum_{i=1}^{N} (\ln \text{TTR}_i - \overline{\mu})^2}{N-1}, \quad \text{(sample variance)} \\ N &= \text{total number of sample} \end{aligned} \tag{6.212}$$

Table 6.22 gives $\sigma = 1.09$. See Appendix A.1.6 of this chapter for more information about sample mean and sample variance.

Assume that the TTF is distributed with constant failure rate $\lambda = 1/\text{MTTF} = 1/55.1 = 0.0182$. Because both of the distributions for repair-to-failure and failure-to-repair processes are known, the general procedure of Figure 6.16 can be used. The results are shown in Figure 6.28. Note that the stationary unavailability $Q(\infty) = 0.043$ agrees with the time-ensemble availability $\overline{A} = 0.957$ of equation (6.209).

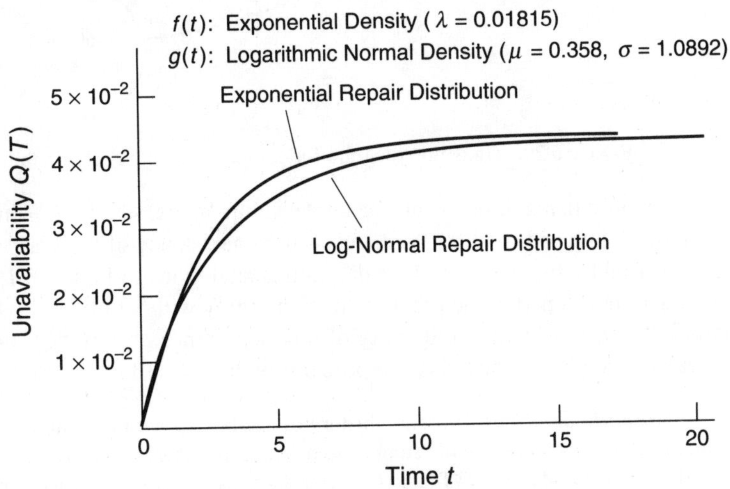

Figure 6.28. Unavailability $Q(t)$.

Consider now the case where the repair distribution is approximated by a constant repair rate model. The constant m is given by $m = 1/\text{MTTR} = 1/2.49 = 0.402$. The unavailabilities $Q(t)$ as calculated by equation (6.158) are plotted in Figure 6.28. This $Q(t)$ is a good approximation to the unavailability obtained by the log-normal repair assumption. This is not an unusual situation. The constant rate model frequently gives a first-order approximation and should be tried prior to more complicated distributions. We can ascertain trends by using the constant rate model and recognize system improvements. Usually, the constant rate model itself gives sufficiently accurate results.

6.8 COMPONENTS WITH MULTIPLE FAILURE MODES

Many components have more than one failure mode. In any practical application of fault trees, if a basic event is a component failure, then the exact failure modes must be stated. When the basic event refers to more than one failure mode, it can be developed through OR gates to more basic events, each of which refers to a single failure mode. Thus, we can assume that every basic event has associated with it only one failure mode, although a component itself may suffer from multiple failure modes. The state transition for such components is represented by Figure 6.29.

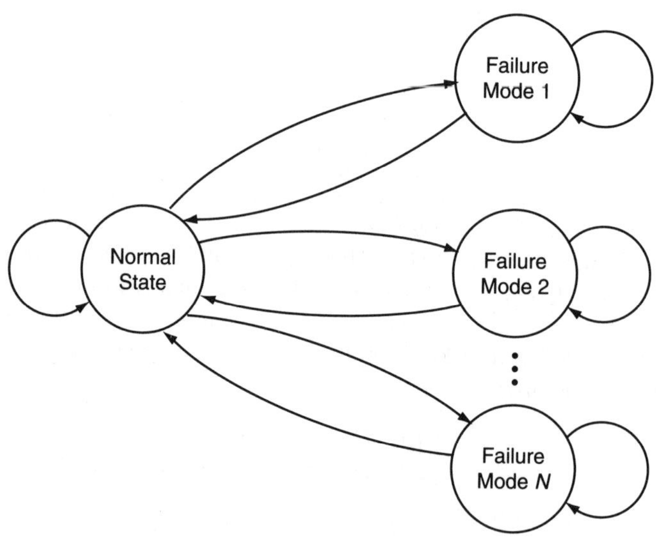

Figure 6.29. Transition diagram for components with multiple failure modes.

Suppose that a basic event is a single-failure mode, say mode 1 in Figure 6.29. Then the normal state and modes 2 to N result in nonexistence of the basic event, and this can be expressed by Figure 6.30. This diagram is analogous to Figure 6.1, and quantification techniques developed in the previous sections apply without major modifications: the reliability $R(t)$ becomes the probability of non-occurrence of a mode 1 failure to time t, the unavailability $Q(t)$ is the existence probability of mode 1 failure at time t, and so forth.

Example 8. Consider a time history of a valve, shown in Figure 6.31. The valve has two failure modes, "stuck open" and "stuck closed." Assume a basic event with the failure mode "stuck closed." Calculate MTTF, MTTR, $R(t)$, $F(t)$, $A(t)$, $Q(t)$, $w(t)$, and $W(0, t)$ by assuming constant failure and repair rates.

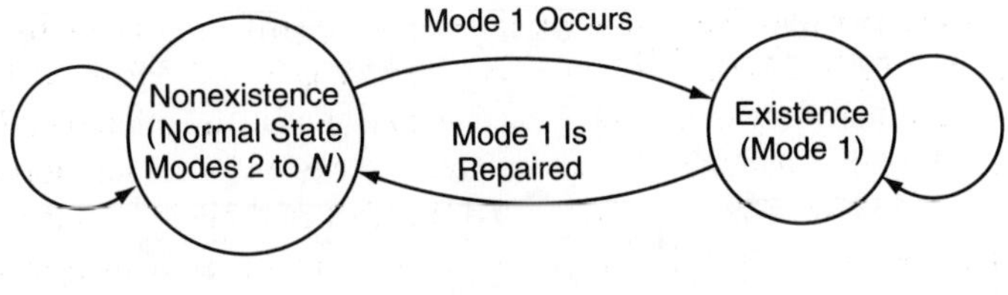

Figure 6.30. Transition diagram for a basic event.

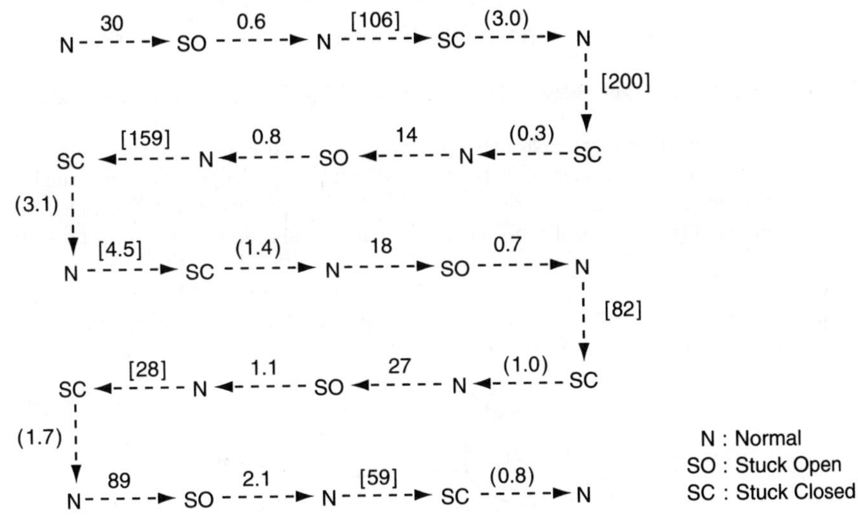

Figure 6.31. A time history of a valve.

Solution: The "valve normal" and "valve stuck open" denote nonexistence of the basic event. Thus Figure 6.31 can be rewritten as Figure 6.32, where the symbol NON denotes the nonexistence.

$$
\begin{aligned}
\text{MTTF} &= \frac{136.6 + 200 + 173.8 + 4.5 + 100.7 + 56.1 + 150.1}{7} = 117.4 \\
\text{MTTR} &= \frac{3.0 + 0.3 + 3.1 + 1.4 + 1.0 + 1.7 + 0.8}{7} = 1.61 \\
\lambda &= \frac{1}{\text{MTTF}} = 0.0085, \qquad \mu = \frac{1}{\text{MTTR}} = 0.619
\end{aligned} \tag{6.213}
$$

Table 6.10 yields

$$
\begin{aligned}
F(t) &= 1 - e^{-0.0085t}, \qquad R(t) = e^{-0.0085t} \\
Q(t) &= \frac{0.0085}{0.0085 + 0.619}[1 - e^{-(0.0085+0.619)t}] \\
&= 0.0135 \times [1 - e^{-0.6275t}] \\
A(t) &= 0.9865 + 0.0135e^{-0.6275t} \\
w(t) &= \frac{0.0085 \times 0.619}{0.0085 + 0.619} + \frac{0.0085^2}{(0.0085 + 0.619)}[1 - e^{-(0.0085+0.619)t}] \\
&= 0.0084 + 0.0001e^{-0.6275t} \\
W(0, t) &= \frac{0.0085 \times 0.619}{0.0085 + 0.619}t + \frac{0.0085^2}{(0.0085 + 0.619)^2}[1 - e^{-(0.0085+0.619)t}] \\
&= 0.0002 + 0.0084t - 0.0002e^{-0.6275t}
\end{aligned} \tag{6.214}
$$

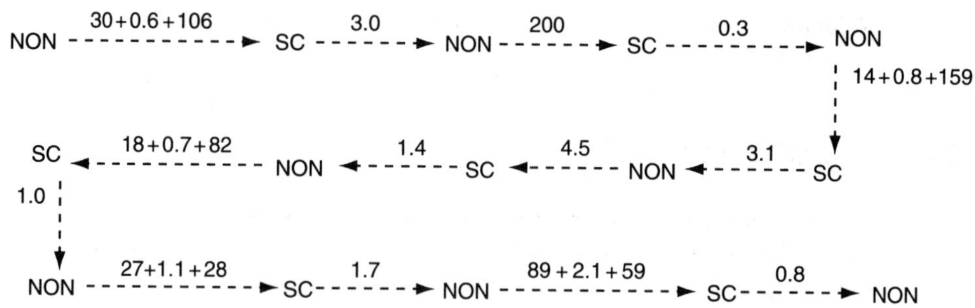

Figure 6.32. TTFs and TTRs of "stuck closed" event for the valve.

These calculations hold only approximately because the three-state valve is modeled by the two-state diagram of Figure 6.32. However, MTTR for "stuck open" is usually small, and the approximation error is negligible. If rigorous analysis is required, we can start with the Markov transition diagram of Figure 6.33 and apply the differential equations described in Chapter 9 for the calculation of $R(t)$, $Q(t)$, $w(t)$, and so on. ■

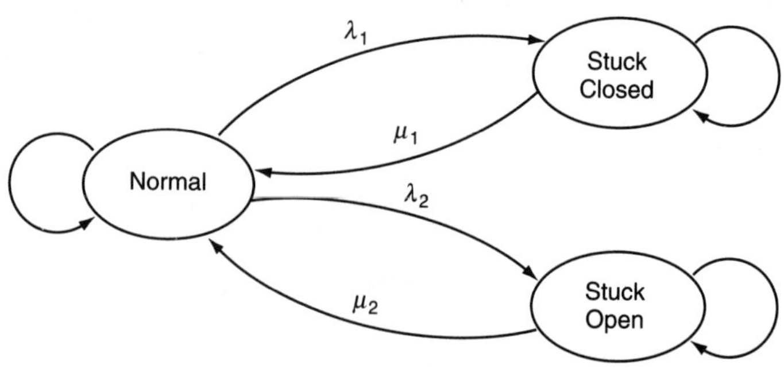

Figure 6.33. Markov transition diagram for the valve.

Some data on *repairable* component failure modes are available in the form of "frequency = failures/period." The frequency can be converted into the constant failure intensity λ in the following way.

From Table 6.10, the stationary value of the frequency is

$$w(\infty) = \frac{\lambda\mu}{\lambda + \mu} \tag{6.215}$$

Usually, MTTF is much greater than MTTR; that is,

$$\lambda << \mu \tag{6.216}$$

Thus

$$w(\infty) = \lambda \tag{6.217}$$

The frequency itself can be used as the conditional failure intensity λ, provided that MTTR is sufficiently small. When this is not true, equation (6.215) is used to calculate λ for given MTTR and frequency data.

Example 9. The frequency $w(t)$ in Example 8 yields $w(\infty) = 0.0084$ ("stuck closed" failures/time unit). Recalculate the unconditional failure intensity λ.

Solution: $\lambda = w(\infty) = 0.0084$ by equation (6.217). This gives good agreement with $\lambda = 0.0085$ in Example 8. ■

6.9 ENVIRONMENTAL INPUTS

System failures are caused by one or a set of system components generating failure events. The environment, plant personnel, and aging can affect the system only through the system components.

As to the environmental inputs, we have two cases.

1. Environmental causes of component command failures
2. Environmental causes of component secondary failures

6.9.1 Command Failures

Commands such as "area power failure" and "water supply failure" appear as basic events in fault trees, and can be quantified in the same way as components.

Example 10. Assume MTTF $= 0.5$ yr and MTTR $= 30$ min for an area power failure. Calculate $R(t)$ and $Q(t)$ at $t = 1$ yr.

Solution:

$$
\begin{aligned}
\lambda &= \frac{1}{0.5} = 2/\text{year} \\
\text{MTTR} &= \frac{30}{365 \times 24 \times 60} = 5.71 \times 10^{-5} \text{ year} \\
\mu &= \frac{1}{\text{MTTR}} = 1.75 \times 10^{4}/\text{year} \\
R(1) &= e^{-2\times 1} = 0.135 \\
Q(1) &= \frac{2}{2 + 17500}[1 - e^{-(2+17500)\times 1}] = 1.14 \times 10^{-4}
\end{aligned}
\tag{6.218}
$$

■

6.9.2 Secondary Failures

In qualitative fault-tree analysis, a primary failure and the corresponding secondary failure are sometimes aggregated into a single basic event. The event occurs if the primary failure or secondary failure occurs. If we assume constant failure and repair rates for the two failures, we have the transition diagram of Figure 6.34. Here $\lambda_{(P)}$ and $\lambda_{(S)}$ are conditional failure intensities for primary and secondary failures, respectively, and μ is the repair intensity that is assumed to be the same for primary and secondary failures. The diagram can be used to quantify basic events, including secondary component failures resulting from environmental inputs.

Example 11. Assume that an earthquake occurs once in 60 yr. When it occurs, there is a 50% chance of a tank being destroyed. Assume that MTTF $= 30$ (yr) for the tank under normal environment. Assume further that it takes 0.1 yr to repair the tank. Calculate $R(10)$ and $Q(10)$ for the basic event, obtained by the aggregation of the primary and secondary tank failure.

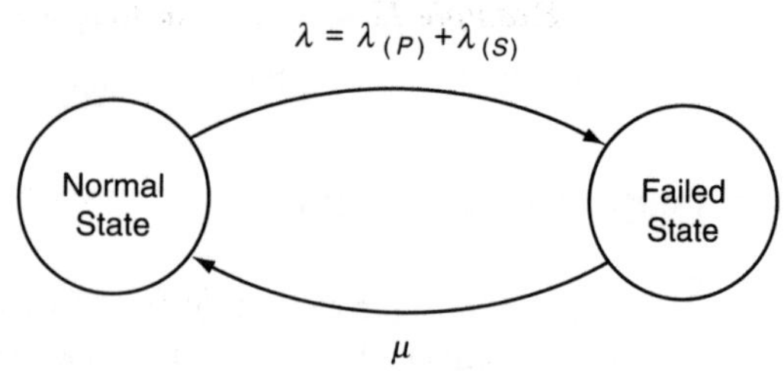

Figure 6.34. Transition diagram for primary and secondary failures.

Solution: The tank is destroyed by the earthquakes once in 120 yr. Thus

$$\lambda_{(S)} = \frac{1}{120} = 8.33 \times 10^{-3}/\text{yr} \tag{6.219}$$

Further,

$$\lambda_{(P)} = \frac{1}{30} = 3.33 \times 10^{-2}/\text{yr}$$
$$\lambda = \lambda_{(P)} + \lambda_{(S)} = 4.163 \times 10^{-2}/\text{yr} \tag{6.220}$$
$$\mu = \frac{1}{0.1} = 10/\text{yr}$$

Thus at 10 years

$$R(10) = e^{-4.163\times 10^{-2}\times 10} = 0.659$$
$$Q(10) = \frac{4.163 \times 10^{-2}}{4.163 \times 10^{-2} + 10}[1 - e^{-(4.163\times 10^{-2}+10)\times 10}] \tag{6.221}$$
$$= 4.15 \times 10^{-3}$$

■

In most cases, environmental inputs act as common causes. The quantification of basic events involved in common causes is developed in Chapter 9.

6.10 HUMAN ERROR

In a similar fashion to environmental inputs, human errors are causes of a component command failure or secondary failure. Plant operators act in response to demands. A typical fault-tree representation is shown in Figure 4.2. The operator error is included in Figures 4.24 and 4.30. As explained in Chapter 4, various conditions are introduced by OR and AND gates. We may use these conditions to quantify operator error because the operator may be 99.99% perfect at a routine job, but useless if he panics in an emergency. Probabilities of operator error are usually time invariant and can be expressed as "error per demand." Human-error quantification is described in more detail in Chapter 10.

6.11 SYSTEM-DEPENDENT BASIC EVENT

Finally, we come to so-called *system-dependent basic events*, typified by the "secondary fuse failure" of Figure 4.18. This failure can also be analyzed by a diagram similar to Figure 6.34. The parameter $\lambda_{(S)}$ is given by the sum of conditional failure intensities for "wire shorted" and "generator surge" because "excessive current to fuse" is expressed by Figure 4.19.

Example 12. Assume the following conditional failure intensities:

$$\begin{aligned}\text{Wire shorted} &= \frac{1}{10,000}\ (\text{hr}^{-1})\\ \text{Generator surge} &= \frac{1}{50,000}\ (\text{hr}^{-1})\\ \text{Primary fuse failure} &= \frac{1}{25,000}\ (\text{hr}^{-1})\\ \text{Repair rate } \mu &= \frac{1}{2}\ (\text{hr})^{-1}\end{aligned} \tag{6.222}$$

To obtain conservative results, the mean repair time, $1/\mu$, should be that to repair "broken fuse," "shorted wire," and "generator surge" because, without repairing all of them, we cannot return the fuse to the system. Calculate $R(1000)$ and $Q(1000)$.

Solution:

$$\lambda = \frac{1}{10,000} + \frac{1}{50,000} + \frac{1}{25,000} = 0.00016\ (\text{hr})^{-1}$$

$$R(1000) = e^{-0.00016\times 1000} = 0.852 \tag{6.223}$$

$$Q(1000) = \frac{0.00016}{0.00016 + 0.5}[1 - e^{-(0.00016+0.5)\times 1000}] = 3.20 \times 10^{-4}$$

■

REFERENCES

[1] Bompas-Smith, J. H. *Mechanical Survival: The Use of Reliability Data*. New York: McGraw-Hill, 1971.

[2] Hahn, G. J., and S. S. Shapiro. *Statistical Methods in Engineering*. New York: John Wiley & Sons, 1967.

[3] Locks, M. O. *Reliability, Maintainability, and Availability Assessment*. New York: Hayden Book Co., 1973.

[4] Kapur, K. C., and L. R. Lamberson. *Reliability in Engineering Design*. New York: John Wiley & Sons, 1977.

[5] Weilbull, W. "A statistical distribution of wide applicability," *J. of Applied Mechanics*, vol. 18, pp. 293–297, 1951.

[6] Shooman, M. L. *Probabilistic Reliability: An Engineering Approach*. New York: McGraw Hill, 1968.

CHAPTER SIX APPENDICES

A.1 DISTRIBUTIONS

For a continuous random variable X, the distribution $F(x)$ is defined by

$$\begin{aligned}F(x) &= \Pr\{X \le x\} = \Pr\{X < x\}\\ &= \text{probability of } X \text{ being less than (or equal to) } x.\end{aligned}$$

The probability density is defined as the first derivative of $F(x)$.

$$f(x) = \frac{dF(x)}{dx} \tag{A.1}$$

The small quantity $f(x)dx$ is the probability that a random variable takes a value in the interval $[x, x+dx)$.

For a discrete random variable, the distribution $F(x)$ is defined by

$$\begin{aligned} F(x) &= \Pr\{X \le x\} \\ &= \text{probability of } X \text{ being less than or equal to } x. \end{aligned}$$

The probability mass $\Pr\{X = x_i\}$ is denoted by $\Pr\{x_i\}$ and is given by

$$\Pr\{x_i\} = F(x_{i+1}) - F(x_i) \tag{A.2}$$

provided that

$$x_1 < x_2 < x_3 \cdots \tag{A.3}$$

Different families of distribution are described by their particular parameters. However, as an alternative one may use the values of certain related measures such as the mean, median, or mode.

A.1.1 Mean

The mean, sometimes called the expected value $E\{X\}$, is the average of all values that make up the distribution. Mathematically, it may be defined as

$$E\{X\} = \int_{-\infty}^{\infty} x f(x)dx \tag{A.4}$$

if X is a continuous random variable with probability density function $f(x)$, and

$$E\{X\} = \sum_i x_i \Pr\{x_i\} \tag{A.5}$$

if X is a discrete random variable with probability mass $\Pr\{x_i\}$.

A.1.2 Median

The median is midpoint z of the distribution. For a continuous Pdf, $f(x)$, this is

$$\int_{-\infty}^{z} f(x)dx = 0.5 \tag{A.6}$$

and for a discrete random variable it is the largest z satisfying

$$\sum_{i=1}^{z} \Pr\{x_i\} \le 0.5 \tag{A.7}$$

A.1.3 Mode

The mode for a continuous variable is the value associated with the maximum of the probability density function, and for a discrete random variable it is that value of the random variable that has the highest probability mass.

The approximate relationship among mean, median, and mode is shown graphically for three different probability densities in Figure A6.1.

A.1.4 Variance and Standard Deviation

In addition to the measures of tendency discussed above, it is often necessary to describe the distribution spread, symmetry, and peakedness. One such measure is the

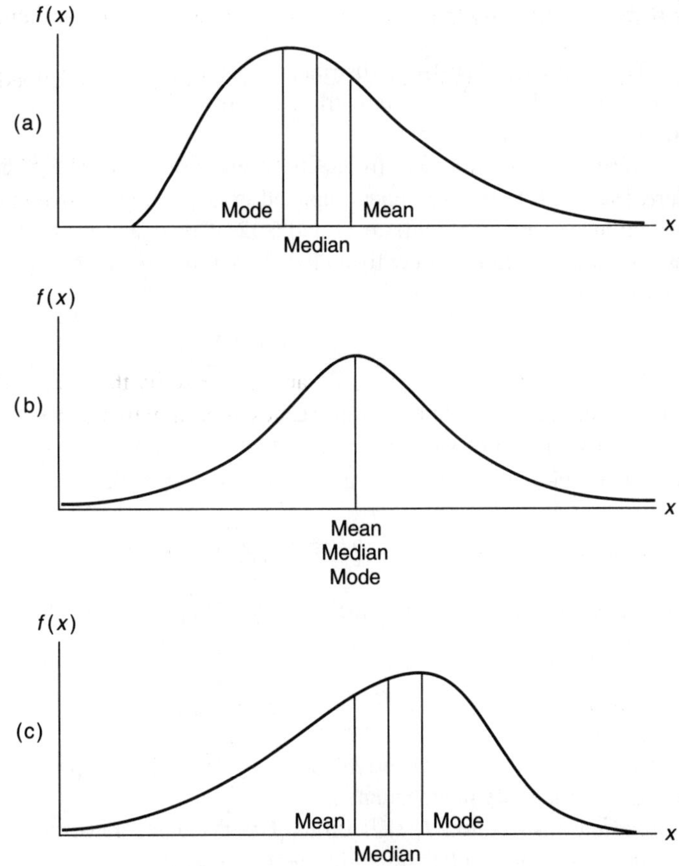

Figure A6.1. Mean, median, and mode.

moment that is defined for the kth moment about the mean as

$$\mu_k = E\{[X - E\{X\}]^k\} \tag{A.8}$$

where μ_k is the kth moment and $E\{\cdot\}$ is the mean or expected value. The second moment about the mean and its square root are measures of dispersion and are the variance σ^2 and standard deviation σ, respectively. Hence the variance is given by

$$\sigma^2 = E\{[X - E\{X\}]^2\} \tag{A.9}$$

which may be proved to be

$$\sigma^2 = E\{X^2\} - [E\{X\}]^2 \tag{A.10}$$

The standard deviation is the square root of the above expression.

A.1.5 Exponential Distribution

Exponential distributions are used frequently for the analysis of time-dependent data when the rate at which events occur does not vary. The defining equations for $f(t)$, $F(t)$, $r(t)$, and their graphs for the exponential distribution and other distributions discussed here are shown in Tables 6.11 and 6.12.

A.1.6 Normal Distribution

The normal (or Gaussian) distribution is the best-known two-parameter distribution. All normal distributions are symmetric, and the two distribution parameters, μ and σ, are its mean and standard deviation.

Normal distributions are frequently used to describe equipment that has increasing failure rates with time. The equations and graphs for $f(t)$, $F(t)$, and $r(t)$ for a normal distribution are shown in Tables 6.11 and 6.12. The mean time to failure, μ, is obtained by simple averaging and is frequently called the *first moment*. The sample average $\overline{\mu}$ is called a *sample mean*.

$$\overline{\mu} = n^{-1} \sum_{i=1}^{n} t_i \tag{A.11}$$

where t_i is the time to failure for sample i, and n is the total number of samples.

The estimation of variance σ^2 or standard deviation σ depends on whether mean μ is known or unknown. For a known mean μ, variance estimator $\overline{\sigma^2}$ is given by

$$\overline{\sigma^2} = n^{-1} \sum_{i=1}^{n} (t_i - \mu)^2 \tag{A.12}$$

For unknown mean μ, the sample mean $\overline{\mu}$ is used in place of μ, and sample size n is replaced by $n - 1$.

$$\overline{\sigma^2} = (n-1)^{-1} \sum_{i=1}^{n} (t_i - \overline{\mu})^2 \tag{A.13}$$

This sample variance is frequently denoted by S^2. It can be proven that random variables $\overline{\mu}$ and S^2 are mutually independent.

Normal distribution $F(t)$ is difficult to evaluate; however, there are tabulations of integrals in statistics and/or reliability texts. Special graph paper, which can be used to transform an S-shaped $F(t)$ curve to a straight line function, is available.

A.1.7 Log-Normal Distribution

A log-normal distribution is similar to a normal distribution with the exception that the logarithm of the values of random variables, rather than the values themselves, are assumed to be normally distributed. Thus all values are positive, the distribution is skewed to the right, and the skewness is a function of σ. The availability of log-normal probability paper makes it relatively easy to test experimental data to see whether they are distributed log-normally.

Log-normal distributions are encountered frequently in metal-fatigue testing, maintainability data (time to repair), and chemical-process equipment failures and repairs. This distribution is used for uncertainty propagation in Chapter 11.

A.1.8 Weibull Distribution

Among all the distributions available for reliability calculations, the Weibull distribution is the only one unique to the field. In his original paper, "A distribution of wide applicability," Professor Weibull [5], who was studying metallurgical failures, argued that normal distributions require that initial metallurgical strengths be normally distributed and that what was needed was a function that could embrace a great variety of distributions (including the normal).

The Weibull distribution is a three-parameter (γ, σ, β) distribution (unlike the normal, which has only two), where:

γ = the time until $F(t) = 0$, and is a datum parameter; that is, failures start occurring at time t
σ = the characteristic life, and is a scale parameter
β = a shape parameter

As can be seen from Table 6.12, the Weibull distribution assumes a great variety of shapes. If $\gamma = 0$, that is, failures start occurring at time zero, or if the time axis is shifted to conform to this requirement, then we see that

1. for $\beta < 1$, we have a decreasing failure rate (such as may exist at the beginning of a bathtub curve);
2. for $\beta = 1$, $r(t) \equiv \lambda = \beta/\sigma = 1/\sigma$, and we have an exponential reliability curve;
3. for $1 < \beta < 2$ (not shown), we have a skewed normal distribution (failure rate increases at a decreasing rate as t increases);
4. for $\beta > 2$, the curve approaches a normal distribution.

The gamma function $\Gamma(\cdot)$ for the Weibull mean and variance in Table 6.11 is a generalization of a factorial [$\Gamma(x + 1) = x!$ for integer x], and is defined by

$$\Gamma(x) = \int_0^\infty t^{x-1} e^{-t} dt \tag{A.14}$$

By suitable arrangement of the variables, σ can be obtained by reading the value of $(t - \gamma)$ at $F(t) = 0.63$. Methods for obtaining γ, which must frequently be guessed, have been published [2].

A.1.9 Binomial Distribution

Denote by P the probability of failure for a component. Assume N identical components are tested. Then the number of failures y is a random variable with probability

$$\Pr\{y = n\} = \frac{N!}{n!(N-n)!} P^n (1 - P)^{N-n} \tag{A.15}$$

The binomial distribution has mean NP and variance $NP(1 - P)$.

A generalization of this distribution is a multinomial distribution. Suppose that type i event occurs with probability P_i. Assume k types of events and that a total of m trials are performed. Denote by y_i the total number of type i events observed. Then, random vector $(y_1, \ldots, y_k)$ follows a multinomial distribution

$$\Pr\{y_1, \ldots, y_k\} = \frac{m!}{y_1! \cdots y_k!} P_1^{y_1} \cdots P_k^{y_k} \tag{A.16}$$

A.1.10 Poisson Distribution

Consider a component that fails according to an exponential distribution. Assume that the failed component can be repaired instantaneously, that is, a renewal process. The number of failures n to time t is a random variable with a Poisson distribution probability (Tables 6.11 and 6.12).

$$\Pr\{n\} = \frac{(\lambda t)^n e^{-\lambda t}}{n!}, \qquad n = 0, 1, \ldots \tag{A.17}$$

The Poisson distribution is an approximation to the binomial distribution function for a large number of samples N, and small failure probability P with a constraint $NP = \lambda t$.

$$\Pr\{y = n\} = \frac{N!}{n!(N-n)!} P^n (1-P)^n \simeq \frac{(\lambda t)^n e^{-\lambda t}}{n!} \tag{A.18}$$

Equation (A.18) is called a Poisson approximation.

The Poisson distribution is used to calculate the probability of a certain number of events occurring in a large system, given a constant failure rate λ and a time t.

One would use the $F(n)$ in Table 6.11 that is, the probability of having n or less failures in time t. In an expansion for $F(n)$,

$$F(n) = e^{-\lambda t} + \lambda t e^{-\lambda t} + \frac{(\lambda t)^2}{2} e^{-\lambda t} + \cdots + \frac{(\lambda t)^n}{n!} e^{-\lambda t} \tag{A.19}$$

the first term defines the probability of no component failures, the second term defines the probability of one component failure, and so forth.

A.1.11 Gamma Distribution

The gamma distribution probability density is (Table 6.11)

$$\frac{1}{\eta \Gamma(\beta)} \left(\frac{t}{\eta}\right)^{\beta-1} e^{-t/\eta}, \qquad \beta > 0, \qquad \eta > 0 \tag{A.20}$$

Assume an instantaneously repairable component that fails according to an exponential distribution with failure rate $1/\eta$. Consider for integer β an event that the component fails β or more times. This event is equivalent to the occurrence of β or more shocks with rate $1/\eta$. Then the density $f(t)$ for such an event at time t is given by the gamma distribution with integer β

$$f(t) = \frac{e^{-\lambda t}(\lambda t)^{\beta-1}}{(\beta-1)!} \lambda \tag{A.21}$$

This is called an *Erlang probability density*. The gamma density of (A.20) is a mathematical generalization of (A.21) because

$$\Gamma(\beta) = (\beta - 1)!, \qquad \beta\text{: integer} \tag{A.22}$$

A.1.12 Other Distributions

Tables 6.11 and 6.12 include Gumbel, inverse Gaussian, and beta distributions.

A.2 A CONSTANT-FAILURE-RATE PROPERTY

We first prove equation (6.52). The failure during $[t, t+dt)$ occurs in a repair-to-failure process. Let s be a survival age of the component that is normal at time t. In other words, assume that the component has been normal since time $t - s$ and is normal at time t. The bridge rule of equation (A.29), appendix of Chapter 3, can be written in integral form as

$$\Pr\{A|C\} = \int \Pr\{A|s, C\} p\{s|C\} ds \tag{A.23}$$

where $p\{s|C\}$ is the conditional probability density of s, given that event C occurs. The term $p\{s|C\}ds$ is the probability of "bridge $[s, s+ds)$," and the term $\Pr\{A|s, C\}$ is the probability of the occurrence of event A when we have passed through the bridge. The integral in (A.23) is the representation of $\Pr\{A|C\}$ by the sum of all possible bridges. Define the following events and parameter s.

A = Failure during $[t, t + dt)$
s = The normal component has survival age s at time t
C = The component was as good as new at time zero and is normal at time t

Because the component failure characteristics at time t are assumed to depend only on the survival age s at time t, we have

$$\Pr\{A|s, C\} = \Pr\{A|s\} = r(s)dt \tag{A.24}$$

From the definition of $\lambda(t)$, we obtain

$$\Pr\{A|C\} = \lambda(t)dt \tag{A.25}$$

Substituting equations (A.24) and (A.25) into equation (A.23), we have

$$\lambda(t)dt = dt \cdot \int r(s)p\{s|C\}ds \tag{A.26}$$

For the constant-failure rate r,

$$\lambda(t)dt = dt \cdot r \cdot \int p\{s|C\}ds = dt \cdot r \cdot 1 \tag{A.27}$$

yielding equation (6.52).

A.3 DERIVATION OF UNAVAILABILITY FORMULA

We now prove equation (6.96). Denote by $E\{\cdot\}$ the operation of taking the expected value. In general,

$$E\{x(t)\} = E\{x_{0,1}(t)\} - E\{x_{1,0}(t)\} \tag{A.28}$$

holds. The expected value $E\{x(t)\}$ of $x(t)$ is

$$\begin{aligned} E\{x(t)\} &= 1 \times \Pr\{x(t) = 1\} + 0 \times \Pr\{x(t) = 0\} \\ &= \Pr\{x(t) = 1\} \end{aligned} \tag{A.29}$$

yielding

$$E\{x(t)\} = Q(t) \tag{A.30}$$

Because $x_{01}(t)$ is the number of failures to time t, $E\{x_{0,1}(t)\}$ is the expected number of failures to that time.

$$E\{x_{0,1}(t)\} = W(0, t) \tag{A.31}$$

Similarly,

$$E\{x_{1,0}(t)\} = V(0, t) \tag{A.32}$$

Equations (A.28), (A.30), (A.31), and (A.32) yield (6.96).

A.4 COMPUTATIONAL PROCEDURE FOR INCOMPLETE TEST DATA

Suppose that N items fail, in turn, at discrete lives $t_1, t_2, \ldots, t_m$. Denote by r_i the number of failures at lifetime t_i. The probability of failure at lifetime t_1 can be approximated by $P(t_1) = r_1/N$, at lifetime t_2 by $P(t_2) = r_2/N$, and, in general, by $P(t_i) = r_i/N$.

The above approximation is applicable when all the items concerned continue to fail. In many cases, however, some items are taken out of use for reasons other than failures, hence affecting the numbers exposed to failures at different lifetimes. Therefore a correction to take this into account must be included in the calculation.

Suppose that N items have been put into use and failure occurs at discrete lives $t_1, t_2, t_3, \ldots,$ the number of failures occurring at each lifetime are $r_1, r_2, r_3, \ldots,$ and the number of items actually exposed to failure at each lifetime are $N_1, N_2, N_3, \ldots.$

Because r_1 failed at t_1, the original number has been reduced to $N_1 - r_1$. The proportion actually failing at t_2 is r_2/N_2, so the number that would have failed, had N_1 proceeded to failure, is

$$(N_1 - r_1)\frac{r_2}{N_2} \tag{A.33}$$

and the proportion of N_1 expected to fail at t_2 is

$$P(t_2) = (N_1 - r_1)\frac{r_2}{N_1 N_2} \tag{A.34}$$

We now proceed in the same manner to estimate the proportion of N_1 that would fail at t_3.

If the original number had been allowed to proceed to failure, the number exposed to failure at t_3 would be

$$N_1 - \left[r_1 + (N_1 - r_1)\frac{r_2}{N_2}\right] \tag{A.35}$$

and the proportion of N_1 expected to fail at t_3 is

$$P(t_3) = \left\{N_1 - \left[r_1 + (N_1 - r_1)\frac{r_2}{N_2}\right]\right\}\frac{r_3}{N_1 N_3} \tag{A.36}$$

The same process can be repeated for subsequent values.

A.5 MEDIAN-RANK PLOTTING POSITION

Suppose that n times to failure are arranged in increasing order: $t_1, \ldots, t_i, \ldots, t_n$. Abscissa values for plotting points are obtained from these times to failures. We also need the corresponding estimate P_i of the cumulative distribution function $F(t)$. A primitive estimator i/n is unsuitable because it indicates that 100% of the population would fail prior to the largest time to failure t_5 for the sample size $n = 5$.

For an unknown distribution function $F(t)$, define P_i by $P_i = F(t_i)$. This P_i is a random variable because t_i varies from sample to sample. It can be shown that the probability density function $g(P_i)$ of P_i is given by [4]

$$g(P_i) = \frac{n!}{(i-1)!(n-i)!} P_i^{i-1}(1 - P_i)^{n-i} \tag{A.37}$$

In other words, random variable P_i follows a beta distribution.

The median $\hat{P}_i$ value of this beta distribution is its median rank.

$$\int_0^{\hat{P}_i} g(P_i)dP_i = 0.5 \tag{A.38}$$

These values can be obtained from tables of incomplete beta functions.

$$B_x(m,n) = \int_0^x y^{m-1}(1-y)^{n-1}dy \tag{A.39}$$

An approximation to the median-rank value is given by

$$\hat{P}_i = \frac{i-0.3}{n+0.4} \tag{A.40}$$

A simpler form is

$$\hat{P}_i = \frac{i-0.5}{n} \tag{A.41}$$

A.6 FAILURE AND REPAIR BASIC DEFINITIONS

Table A6.1 provides a summary of basic failure and repair definitions.

PROBLEMS

6.1. Calculate, using the mortality data of Table 6.1, the reliability $R(t)$, failure density $f(t)$, and failure rate $r(t)$ for:

(a) a man living to be 60 years old ($t = 0$ means zero years);

(b) a man living to be 15 years and 1 day after his 60th birthday ($t = 0$ means 60 years).

6.2. Calculate values for $R(t)$, $F(t)$, $r(t)$, $A(t)$, $Q(t)$, $w(t)$, $W(0,t)$, and $\lambda(t)$ for the ten components of Figure 6.7 at 3 hr and 8 hr.

6.3. Prove MTTF equation (6.32).

6.4. Using the values shown in Figure 6.7, calculate $G(t)$, $g(t)$, $m(t)$, and MTTR.

6.5. Use the data of Figure 6.7 to obtain $\mu(t)$ and $v(t)$ at $t = 3$ and also $V(0,t)$.

6.6. Obtain $f(t)$, $r(t)$, $g(t)$, and $m(t)$, assuming

$$F(t) = 1 - \frac{8}{7}e^{-t} + \frac{1}{7}e^{-8t}, \qquad G(t) = 1 - e^{-6t}$$

6.7. Suppose that

$$f(t) = \frac{1}{2}\left(e^{-t} + 3e^{-3t}\right), \qquad g(t) = 1.5e^{-1.5t}$$

(a) Show that the following $w(t)$ and $v(t)$ satisfy the (6.89) equations .

$$w(t) = \frac{1}{4}\left(3 + 5e^{-4t}\right), \qquad v(t) = \frac{3}{4}\left(1 - e^{-4t}\right)$$

(b) Obtain $W(0,t)$, $V(0,t)$, $Q(t)$, $\lambda(t)$, and $\mu(t)$.

(c) Obtain $r(t)$ to confirm (6.109).

6.8. A device has a constant failure rate of $\lambda = 10^{-5}$ failures per hour.

(a) What is its reliability for an operating period of 1000 hr?

(b) If there are 1000 such devices, how many will fail in 1000 hr?

(c) What is the reliability for an operating time equal to the MTTF?

TABLE A6.1. Basic Failure and Repair Definitions

		Repair-to-Failure Process
$R(t)$	Reliability	Probability that the component experiences no failure during the time interval $[0, t]$, given that the component was repaired (as good as new) at time zero.
$F(t)$	Unreliability (Failure distribution)	Probability that the component experiences the first failure during the time interval $[0, t)$, given that the component was repaired at time zero.
$f(t)$	Failure density	Probability that the first component failure occurs per unit time at time t, given that the component was repaired at time zero.
$r(t)$	Failure rate	Probability that the component experiences a failure per unit time at time t, given that the component was repaired at time zero and has survived to time t.
TTF	Time to failure	Span of time from repair to the first failure.
MTTF	Mean time to failure	Expected value of the time to failure, TTF.
		Failure-to-Repair Process
$G(t)$	Repair distribution	Probability that the repair is completed before time t, given that the component failed at time zero.
$g(t)$	Repair density	Probability that component repair is completed per unit time at time t, given that the component failed at time zero.
$m(t)$	Repair rate	Probability that the component is repaired per unit time at time t, given that the component failed at time zero and has been failed to time t
TTR	Time to repair	Span of time from failure to repair completion.
MTTR	Mean time to repair	Expected value of the time to repair, TTR.
		Combined Process
$A(t)$	Availability	Probability that the component is normal at time t, given that it was as good as new at time zero.
$w(t)$	Unconditional failure intensity	Probability that the component fails per unit time at time t, given that it was as good as new at time zero.
$W(t_1, t_2)$	Expected number of failures	Expected number of failures during $[t_1, t_2)$, given that the component was as good as new at time zero.
$\lambda(t)$	Conditional failure intensity	Probability that the component fails per unit time at time t, given that it was as good as new at time zero and is normal at time t.
MTBF	Mean time between failures	Expected value of the time between two consecutive failures.
$Q(t)$	Unavailability	Probability that the component is in the failed state at time t, given that it was as good as new at time zero.
$v(t)$	Unconditional repair intensity	Probability that the component is repaired per unit time at time t, given that the component was as good as new at time zero.
$V(t_1, t_2)$	Expected number of repairs	Expected number of repairs during $[t_1, t_2)$, given that the component was as good as new at time zero.
$\mu(t)$	Conditional repair intensity	Probability that the component is repaired per unit time at time t, given that the component was as good as new at time zero and is failed at time t.
MTBR	Mean time between repairs	Expected value of the time between two consecutive repairs.

(d) What is the probability of its surviving for an additional 1000 hr, given it has survived for 1000 hr?

6.9. Suppose that

$$f(t) = \frac{1}{2}\left(e^{-t} + 3e^{-3t}\right), \qquad g(t) = 1.5e^{-1.5t}$$

Obtain $w(t)$ and $v(t)$, using the inverse Laplace transforms.

$$L^{-1}\left[\frac{1}{(s+a)(s+b)}\right] = \frac{1}{b-a}\left(e^{-at} - e^{-bt}\right)$$

$$L^{-1}\left[\frac{s+z}{(s+a)(s+b)}\right] = \frac{1}{b-a}\left[(z-a)e^{-at} - (z-b)e^{-bt}\right]$$

6.10. Given a component for which the failure rate is 0.001 hr^{-1} and the mean time to repair is 20 hr, calculate the parameters of Table 6.10 at 10 hr and 1000 hr.

6.11. **(a)** Using the failure data for 1000 B-52 aircraft given below, obtain $R(t)$ [6].

Time to Failure (hr)	Number of Failures
0–2	222
2–4	45
4–6	32
6–8	27
8–10	21
10–12	15
12–14	17
14–16	7
16–18	14
18–20	9
20–22	8
22–24	3

(b) Determine if the above data can be approximated by an exponential distribution, plotting $\ln[1/R(t)]$ against t.

6.12. **(a)** Determine a Weibull distribution for the data in Problem 6.11, assuming that $\gamma = 0$.
(b) Estimate the number of failures to $t = 0.5$ (hr) and $t = 30$ (hr), assuming that the aircraft were nonrepairable.

6.13. A thermocouple fails 0.35 times per year. Obtain the failure rate λ, assuming that 1) $\mu = 0$ and 2) $\mu = 1$ day^{-1}, respectively.

7

Confidence Intervals

7.1 CLASSICAL CONFIDENCE LIMITS

7.1.1 Introduction

When the statistical distribution of a failure or repair characteristic (time to failure or time to repair) of a population is known, the probability of a population member's having a particular characteristic can be calculated. On the other hand, as mentioned in the preceding chapter, measurement of the characteristic of every member in a population is seldom possible because such a determination would be too time-consuming and expensive, particularly if the measurement destroys the member. Thus methods for estimating the characteristics of a population from sample data are required.

It is difficult to generalize about a given population when we measure only the characteristic of a sample because that sample may not be representative of the population. As the sample size increases, the sample parameters and those of the population will, of course, agree more closely.

Although we cannot be certain that a sample is representative of a population, it is usually possible to associate a degree of assurance with a sample characteristic. That degree of assurance is called confidence, and can be defined as the level of certainty associated with a conclusion based on the results of sampling.

To illustrate the above statements, suppose that a set of ten identical components are life-tested for a specified length of time. At the end of the test, there are five survivors. Based on these experiments, we would expect that the components have an average reliability of 0.5 for the test time span. However, that is far from certain. We would not be surprised if the true reliability was 0.4, but we would deem it unlikely that the reliability was 0.01 or 0.99.

7.1.2 General Principles

We can associate a confidence interval to probabilistic parameters such as reliability. That is, we can say we are $(1-\alpha)$ confident the true reliability is at least (or at most) a certain value, where α is a small positive number.

Figure 7.1 illustrates one-sided and two-sided confidence limits or intervals (note that for single-sidedness the confidence is $1-\alpha$ and for double-sidedness it is $1-2\alpha$). We see that 19 out of 20 single-sided confidence intervals include the true reliability, whereas 18 out of 20 double-sided intervals contain the reliability. Note that the confidence interval varies according to the results of life-tests. For example, if we have no test survivors, the reliability confidence interval would be located around zero; if there are no failures, the interval would be around unity. The leftmost and rightmost points of a (horizontal) double-sided confidence interval are called lower and upper confidence limits, respectively.

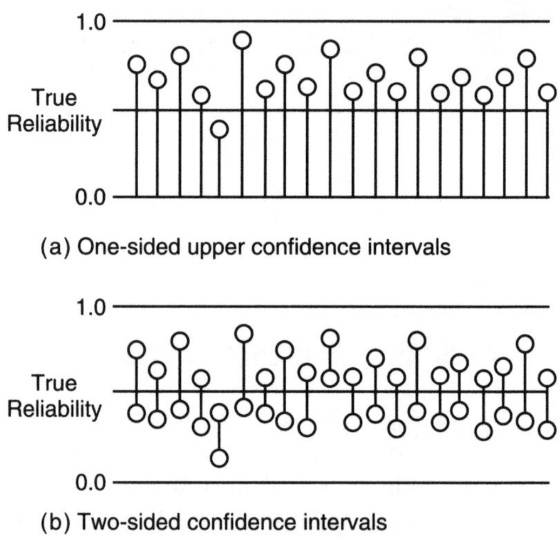

Figure 7.1. Illustration of confidence limit.

Suppose that N random samples $X_1, X_2, \ldots, X_N$ are taken from a population with unknown parameters (for example, mean and standard deviation). Let the population be represented by an unknown constant parameter θ. Measured characteristic $S = g(X_1, \ldots, X_N)$ has a probability distribution $F(s;\theta)$ or density $f(s;\theta)$ that depends on θ, so we can say something about θ on the basis of this dependence. Probability distribution $F(s;\theta)$ is the sampling distribution for S.

The classical approach uses the sampling distribution to determine two values, $s_\alpha(\theta)$ and $s_{1-\alpha}(\theta)$, as a function of θ, such that

$$\int_{s_\alpha(\theta)}^{\infty} f(s;\theta)ds = \alpha \tag{7.1}$$

$$\int_{s_{1-\alpha}(\theta)}^{\infty} f(s;\theta)ds = 1-\alpha \tag{7.2}$$

Values $s_\alpha(\theta)$ and $s_{1-\alpha}(\theta)$ are called the 100α and $100(1-\alpha)$ percentage points of the sampling distribution $F(s;\theta)$. respectively;* These values are also called α and $1-\alpha$ points.

---

*Note that 100α percentage point corresponds to the $100(1-\alpha)$th percentile.

Figure 7.2 illustrates this definition of $s_\alpha(\theta)$ and $s_{1-\alpha}(\theta)$ for a particular θ. Note that equations (7.1) and (7.2) are equivalent, respectively, to

$$\Pr\{S \le s_\alpha(\theta)\} = 1 - \alpha \tag{7.3}$$

and

$$\Pr\{s_{1-\alpha}(\theta) \le S\} = 1 - \alpha \tag{7.4}$$

Because constant α is generally less than 0.5, we have

$$s_{1-\alpha}(\theta) < s_\alpha(\theta) \tag{7.5}$$

Equations (7.3) and (7.4) yield another probability expression,

$$\Pr\{s_{1-\alpha}(\theta) \le S \le s_\alpha(\theta)\} = 1 - 2\alpha \tag{7.6}$$

Although equations (7.3), (7.4), and (7.6) do not include explicit inequalities for θ, they can be rewritten to express confidence limits for θ.

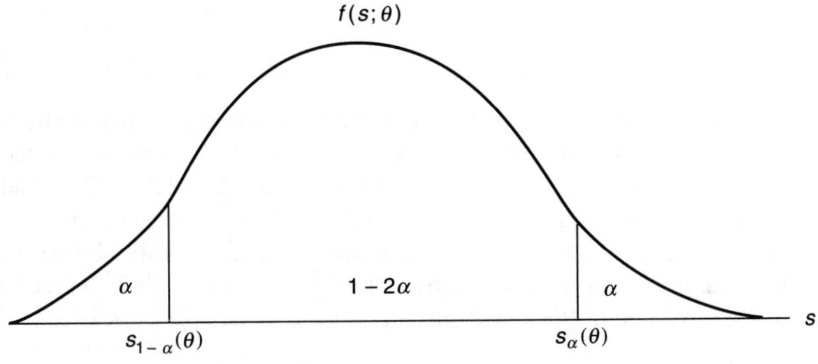

Figure 7.2. Quantities $s_\alpha(\theta)$ and $s_{1-\alpha}(\theta)$ for a given θ.

Example 1—Sample mean of normal population. Table 7.1 lists 20 samples, $X_1, \ldots, X_{20}$, from a normal population with *unknown* mean θ and *known* standard deviation $\sigma = 1.5$. Let $S = g(X_1, \ldots, X_{20})$ be the arithmetical mean $\overline{X}$ of $N = 20$ samples $X_1, \ldots, X_{20}$ from the population:

$$S = \overline{X} = \frac{1}{N}\sum_{i=1}^{N} X_i = 0.647 \tag{7.7}$$

Obtain $s_\alpha(\theta)$ and $s_{1-\alpha}(\theta)$ for $\alpha = 0.05$.

Solution: Sample $\overline{X}$ is a normal random variable with mean θ and standard deviation $\sigma/\sqrt{N} = 1.5/\sqrt{20} = 0.335$. Normal distribution tables indicate that it is 95% certain that the sample mean is not more than $(\theta + 1.65\sigma/\sqrt{N}) = \theta + 0.553$:

$$\Pr\{\overline{X} \le \theta + 0.553\} = 0.95 \tag{7.8}$$

Similarly, we are also 95% confident that $\overline{X}$ is not less than $(\theta - 1.65\sigma/\sqrt{N})$:

$$\Pr\{\theta - 0.553 \le \overline{X}\} = 0.95 \tag{7.9}$$

In other words,

$$\Pr\{\theta - 0.553 \le \overline{X} \le \theta + 0.553\} = 0.9 \tag{7.10}$$

TABLE 7.1. Twenty Samples from a Normal Population (θ: unknown, $\sigma = 1.5$)

X_1	0.090	X_{11}	0.049
X_2	−0.105	X_{12}	0.588
X_3	2.280	X_{13}	−0.693
X_4	−0.051	X_{14}	5.310
X_5	0.182	X_{15}	1.280
X_6	−1.610	X_{16}	1.790
X_7	1.100	X_{17}	0.405
X_8	−1.200	X_{18}	0.916
X_9	1.130	X_{19}	−1.200
X_{10}	0.405	X_{20}	2.280

Thus $s_{1-\alpha}(\theta)$ and $s_\alpha(\theta)$ are given by

$$s_{1-\alpha}(\theta) = \theta - 0.553 \tag{7.11}$$

$$s_\alpha(\theta) = \theta + 0.553 \tag{7.12}$$

■

Assume that $s_{1-\alpha}(\cdot)$ and $s_\alpha(\cdot)$ are the monotonically increasing functions of θ shown in Figure 7.3 (similar representations are possible for monotonically decreasing cases or more general cases). Consider now rewriting equations (7.3), (7.4), and (7.6) in a form suitable for expressing confidence intervals. Equation (7.3) shows that the random variable $S = g(X_1, \ldots, X_N)$ is not more than $s_\alpha(\theta)$ with probability $(1 - \alpha)$ when we repeat a large number of experiments, each of which yields possibly different sets of N observations $X_1, \ldots, X_N$ and S. We now define a new random variable Θ_α related to S, such that

$$s_\alpha(\Theta_\alpha) = S \tag{7.13}$$

where S is the observed characteristic and $s_\alpha(\cdot)$ the known function of θ. Or equivalently,

$$\Theta_\alpha = s_\alpha^{-1}(S) \tag{7.14}$$

Variable Θ_α is illustrated in Figure 7.3. The inequality $S \le s_\alpha(\cdot)$ describes the fact that variable Θ_α, thus defined, falls on the left-hand side of constant θ:

$$S \le s_\alpha(\theta) \Leftrightarrow \Theta_\alpha \le \theta \tag{7.15}$$

Hence from equation (7.3),

$$\Pr\{\Theta_\alpha \le \theta\} = 1 - \alpha \tag{7.16}$$

This shows that *random* variable Θ_α determined by S and curve $s_\alpha(\cdot)$ is a $(1 - \alpha)$ lower confidence limit; variable $\Theta_\alpha = s_\alpha^{-1}(S)$ becomes a lower confidence limit for unknown *constant* θ, with probability $(1 - \alpha)$.

Similarly, we define another random variable $\Theta_{1-\alpha}$ by

$$s_{1-\alpha}(\Theta_{1-\alpha}) = S \tag{7.17}$$

where S is the observed characteristic and $s_{1-\alpha}(\cdot)$ is the known function of θ; or, equivalently,

$$\Theta_{1-\alpha} = s_{1-\alpha}^{-1}(S) \tag{7.18}$$

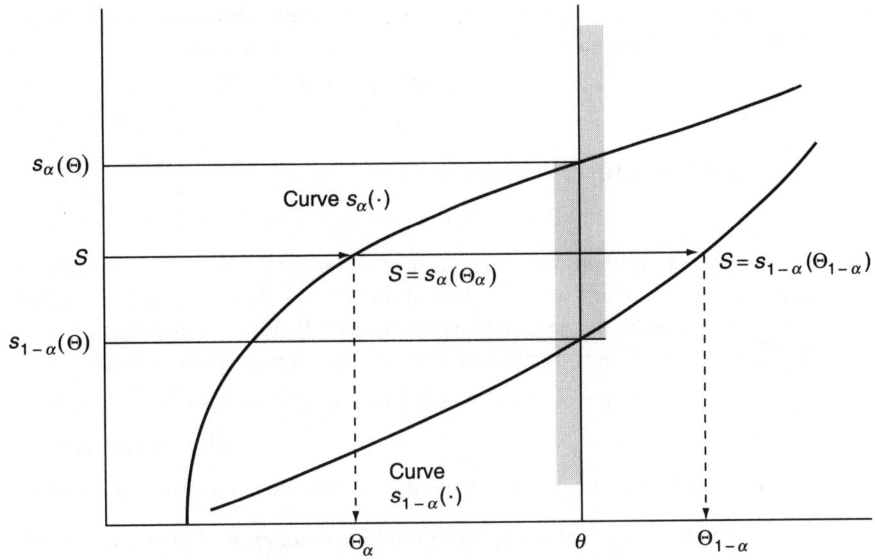

Figure 7.3. Variable Θ determined from S and curves $s_\alpha(\cdot)$ and $s_{1-\alpha}(\cdot)$.

Random variable $\Theta_{1-\alpha}$ is illustrated in Figure 7.3. Equation (7.4) yields

$$\Pr\{\theta \le \Theta_{1-\alpha}\} = 1 - \alpha \tag{7.19}$$

Thus variable $\Theta_{1-\alpha}$ gives an upper confidence limit for constant θ.

Combining equations (7.16) and (7.19), we have

$$\Pr\{\Theta_\alpha \le \theta \le \Theta_{1-\alpha}\} = 1 - 2\alpha \tag{7.20}$$

Random interval $[\Theta_\alpha, \Theta_{1-\alpha}]$ becomes the $100(1 - 2\alpha)\%$ confidence interval. In other words, the interval includes true parameter θ with probability $1 - 2\alpha$. Note that inequalities are reversed for confidence limits and percentage points.

$$\Theta_\alpha < \Theta_{1-\alpha}, \qquad s_{1-\alpha} < s_\alpha \tag{7.21}$$

For monotonically decreasing $s_\alpha(\theta)$ and $s_{1-\alpha}(\theta)$, the confidence interval is $[\Theta_{1-\alpha}, \Theta_\alpha]$:

	Increasing s_α, $s_{1-\alpha}$	**Decreasing s_α, $s_{1-\alpha}$**
Interval	$[\Theta_\alpha, \Theta_{1-\alpha}]$	$[\Theta_{1-\alpha}, \Theta_\alpha]$

Example 2—Confidence interval of population mean. Obtain the 95% single-sided upper and lower limits and the 90% double-sided interval for the population mean θ in Example 1.

Solution: Equations (7.11) and (7.12) and the definition of $\Theta_{1-\alpha}$ and Θ_α [see equations (7.13) and (7.17)] yield

$$\Theta_{1-\alpha} - 0.553 = \overline{X} \Rightarrow \Theta_{1-\alpha} = \overline{X} + 0.553 = 0.647 + 0.553 = 1.20 \tag{7.22}$$

$$\Theta_\alpha + 0.553 = \overline{X} \Rightarrow \Theta_\alpha = \overline{X} - 0.553 = 0.647 - 0.553 = 0.094 \tag{7.23}$$

Variable $\Theta_{1-\alpha}$ and Θ_α are the 95% upper and lower single-sided confidence limits, respectively. The double-sided confidence interval is

$$[\Theta_\alpha, \Theta_{1-\alpha}] = [0.094, 1.20] \tag{7.24}$$

■

Equation (7.10) can be rewritten as

$$\Pr\{\overline{X} - 0.553 \le \theta \le \overline{X} + 0.553\} = 0.90 \tag{7.25}$$

Although θ is an unknown constant in the classical approach, this expression is correct because $\overline{X}$ is a random variable. This shows that random interval $[\overline{X} - 0.553, \overline{X} + 0.553]$ contains the unknown constant with probability 0.9. When sample value 0.647 is substituted for $\overline{X}$, the expression is not correct any more because there is no random variable, that is,

$$\begin{aligned}\Pr\{0.647 - 0.553 \le \theta \le 0.647 + 0.553\} &= \Pr\{0.094 \le \theta \le 1.20\} \\ &= 0.90, \quad \text{(incorrect)}\end{aligned} \tag{7.26}$$

This expression is, however, convenient for confidence interval manipulations.

Example 3—Normal population with unknown variance. Assume that the $N = 20$ samples in Example 1 are drawn from a normal population with *unknown* mean θ and *unknown* standard deviation σ. Obtain the 90% confidence interval for the mean θ.

Solution: Sample mean $\overline{X}$ and sample standard deviation $\overline{\sigma}$ are given by (Section A.1.6, Appendix of Chapter 6)

$$\overline{X} = \frac{1}{N}\sum_{i=1}^{N} X_i = 0.647 \tag{7.27}$$

$$\overline{\sigma} = \sqrt{\frac{1}{N-1}\sum_{i=1}^{N}(X_i - \overline{X})^2} = 1.54 \tag{7.28}$$

It is well known that the following variable t follows a Student's t distribution* with $N - 1$ degrees of freedom (see Case 3, Student's t column of Table A.2 in Appendix A.1 to this chapter; note that sample variance $\overline{\sigma}^2$ is denoted by S^2 in this table).

$$t \equiv \sqrt{N}\,(\overline{X} - \theta)/\overline{\sigma} \sim \text{stu}^*(N-1) = \text{stu}^*(19) \tag{7.29}$$

Denote by $t_{\alpha,19}$ and $t_{1-\alpha,19}$ the α and $1 - \alpha$ points of the Student's distribution, that is,

$$\begin{aligned}\Pr\{t_{\alpha,19} \le t\} &= \alpha = 0.05 \\ \Pr\{t_{1-\alpha,19} \le t\} &= 1 - \alpha = 0.95\end{aligned} \tag{7.30}$$

Then

$$\Pr\{t_{1-\alpha,19} \le \sqrt{N}(\overline{X} - \theta)/\overline{\sigma} \le t_{\alpha,19}\} = 1 - 2\alpha \tag{7.31}$$

or, in terms of the sampling distribution percentage points of $\overline{X}$,

$$\Pr\{s_{1-\alpha(\theta)} \le \overline{X} \le s_\alpha(\theta)\} = 1 - 2\alpha \tag{7.32}$$

where

$$s_{1-\alpha}(\theta) \equiv \theta + \frac{\overline{\sigma} t_{1-\alpha,19}}{\sqrt{N}}, \qquad s_\alpha(\theta) \equiv \theta + \frac{\overline{\sigma} t_{\alpha,19}}{\sqrt{N}} \tag{7.33}$$

---

*These properties were first investigated by W. S. Gosset, who was one of the first industrial statisticians. He worked as a chemist for the Guinness Brewing Company. Because Guinness would not allow him to publish his work, it appeared under the pen name "Student."[1]

Because function $s_\alpha(\theta)$ and $s_{1-\alpha}(\theta)$ are monotonically increasing, we have the $(1-2\alpha)$ confidence interval

$$[\Theta_\alpha,\ \Theta_{1-\alpha}],\ \Theta_\alpha \equiv \overline{X} - \frac{\overline{\sigma} t_{\alpha,19}}{\sqrt{N}}, \qquad \Theta_{1-\alpha} \equiv \overline{X} - \frac{\overline{\sigma} t_{1-\alpha,19}}{\sqrt{N}} \tag{7.34}$$

Equation (7.31) can be rewritten as

$$\Pr\left\{\overline{X} - \frac{t_{\alpha,19}\overline{\sigma}}{\sqrt{N}} \le \theta \le \overline{X} - \frac{t_{1-\alpha,19}\overline{\sigma}}{\sqrt{N}}\right\} = 1 - 2\alpha, \tag{7.35}$$

yielding the same confidence interval as equation (7.34).

From a Student's t table we have $t_{\alpha,19} = 1.729$. The Student's t distribution is symmetric around $t = 0$, and we have $t_{1-\alpha,19} = -1.729$. From sample values of $\overline{X}$ and $\overline{\sigma}$, we have a 90% confidence interval for mean θ under an unknown standard deviation.

$$[0.052,\ 1.2] \tag{7.36}$$

Notice that this interval is wider than that of Example 2 where the true standard deviation σ is known. ■

Example 4—Student's* t *approximation by a normal distribution. For large degrees of freedom ν, say $\nu \ge 30$, the Student's t distribution can be approximated by a normal distribution with mean zero and variance unity. Repeat Example 3 for this approximation.

Solution: From normal distribution tables, we have $t_{\alpha,19} = -t_{1-\alpha,19} = 1.65$, yielding the 90% confidence interval for mean θ

$$\theta \in [0.079,\ 1.22] \tag{7.37}$$

Although the degrees of freedom, $\nu = 19$, is smaller than 30, this interval gives an approximation of the interval calculated in Example 3. ■

Example 5—Hypothesis test of equal means. Consider the 20 samples of Example 1. Assume that the first ten samples come from a normal population with mean θ_1 and standard deviation σ_1, while the remaining ten samples come from a second normal population with mean θ_2 and standard deviation σ_2. Evaluate the hypothesis that the two mean values are equal, that is,

$$H:\ \theta_1 = \theta_2 \tag{7.38}$$

Solution: From the two sets of samples, sample means ($\overline{X_1}$ and $\overline{X_2}$) and sample standard deviations ($\overline{\sigma_1}$ and $\overline{\sigma_2}$) are calculated as follows.

$$\overline{X_1} = 0.222, \qquad \overline{X_2} = 1.07 \tag{7.39}$$

$$\overline{\sigma_1} = 1.13, \qquad \overline{\sigma_2} = 1.83 \tag{7.40}$$

From Case 2 of the Student's t column of Table A.2, Appendix A.1, we observe that, under hypothesis H, random variable

$$t = \frac{\overline{X_1} - \overline{X_2}}{\left[\dfrac{(n_1-1)\overline{\sigma_1}^2 + (n_2-1)\overline{\sigma_2}^2}{n_1+n_2-2}\right]^{\frac{1}{2}} \left[\dfrac{1}{n_1} + \dfrac{1}{n_2}\right]^{\frac{1}{2}}} \qquad (n_1 = n_2 = 10) \tag{7.41}$$

has a Student's t distribution with $n_1 + n_2 - 2$ degrees of freedom. Therefore, we are 90% confident that variable t lies in interval $[t_{1-\alpha,18},\ t_{\alpha,18}]$, $\alpha = 0.05$. From a Student's t distribution table, $t_{0.05,18} = 1.734 = -t_{0.95,18}$. Thus

$$\Pr\{-1.734 \le t \le 1.734\} = 0.90 \tag{7.42}$$

On the other hand, a sample value of t is calculated as

$$t = \frac{0.222 - 1.07}{\left[\dfrac{(10-1)(1.13)^2 + (10-1)(1.83)^2}{10+10-2}\right]^{\frac{1}{2}} [(1/10) + (1/10)]^{\frac{1}{2}}} = -1.25 \qquad (7.43)$$

This value lies in the 90% interval of equation (7.42), and the hypothesis cannot be rejected; if a t value is not included in the interval, the hypothesis is rejected because the observed t value is too large or too small in view of the hypothesis. ■

Example 6—Hypothesis test of equal variances. For two normal populations, equal variance hypothesis can be tested by an F distribution. From the Case 2 row of the F distribution column of Table A.3, Appendix A.1, we see that a ratio of two sample variances follow an F distribution. An equal variance hypothesis can be evaluated similarly to the equal mean hypothesis. ■

Example 7—Variance confidence interval. Obtain the 90% confidence interval for unknown variance σ^2 in Example 3.

Solution: As shown in Case 2 of the χ^2 distribution column of Table A7.1, Appendix A.1, random variable $(N-1)\overline{\sigma}^2/\sigma^2$ is χ^2 distributed with $N-1$ degrees of freedom, that is,

$$\frac{(N-1)\overline{\sigma}^2}{\sigma^2} \sim \text{csq}^*(n-1) = \text{csq}^*(19) \qquad (7.44)$$

or

$$\frac{19 \times 1.54^2}{\sigma^2} = 45.1/\sigma^2 \sim \text{csq}^2(19) \qquad (7.45)$$

Let $\chi^2_{0.05,19}$ and $\chi^2_{0.95,19}$ be the 5 and 95 percentage points of the chi-square distribution, respectively. Then from standard chi-square tables $\chi^2_{0.05,19} = 30.14$ and $\chi^2_{0.95,19} = 10.12$. Thus

$$\Pr\{10.12 \leq 45.1/\sigma^2 \leq 30.14\} = 0.9 \qquad (7.46)$$

or, equivalently,

$$\Pr\{1.22 \leq \sigma \leq 2.11\} = 0.9 \qquad (7.47)$$

Again, expressions (7.45), (7.46), and (7.47) are used only for convenience because they involve no random variables. This interval includes the true standard variation, $\sigma = 1.5$ of Example 1. ■

7.1.3 Types of Life-Tests

Suppose N identical components are placed on life-tests and no components are taken out for service before test termination. The two test options are [2]:

1. Time-terminated test. Life-test is terminated at time T before all N components have failed.
2. Failure-terminated test. Test is terminated at the time of the rth, $r \leq N$ failure.

In time-terminated tests, T is fixed, and the number of failures r and all the failure times $t_1 \leq t_2 \leq \cdots \leq t_r \leq T$ are random variables. In failure-terminated tests, the number of failures r is fixed, and the r failure times and $T = t_r$ are random variables.

7.1.4 Confidence Limits for Mean Time to Failure

Assume failure-terminated test for N components, with an exponential time-to-failure distribution for each component. A point estimate $\hat{\theta}$ for the true mean time to failure $\theta = 1/\lambda$, is

$$\hat{\theta} = \frac{(N-r)t_r + \sum_{i=1}^{r} t_i}{r} \tag{7.48}$$

$$= S, \quad \text{the observed characteristic} \tag{7.49}$$

This estimate is called the maximum-likelihood estimator for MTTF. It can be shown that $2rS/\theta$ follows a chi-square distribution with $2r$ degrees of freedom [2,3] (see the last expression in Case 3 of the χ^2 distribution column of Table A7.1, Appendix A.1). Let $\chi^2_{\alpha,2r}$ and $\chi^2_{1-\alpha,2r}$ be the 100α and $100(1-\alpha)$ percentage points of the chi-square distribution obtained from standard chi-square tables [2–5]. From the definition of percentage points,

$$\Pr\left\{\chi^2_{\alpha,2r} \le \frac{2rS}{\theta}\right\} = \alpha, \qquad \Pr\left\{\chi^2_{1-\alpha,2r} \le \frac{2rS}{\theta}\right\} = 1-\alpha \tag{7.50}$$

These two expressions can be rewritten as

$$\Pr\left\{s_{1-\alpha}(\theta) \equiv \frac{\chi^2_{1-\alpha,2r}\theta}{2r} \le S \le \frac{\chi^2_{\alpha,2r}\theta}{2r} \equiv s_\alpha(\theta)\right\} = 1-2\alpha \tag{7.51}$$

yielding

$$\Theta_\alpha = \frac{2rS}{\chi^2_\alpha(2r)}, \qquad \Theta_{1-\alpha} = \frac{2rS}{\chi^2_{1-\alpha}(2r)} \tag{7.52}$$

Quantities Θ_α and $\Theta_{1-\alpha}$ give $100(1-\alpha)\%$ the lower and upper confidence limits, whereas the range $[\Theta_\alpha, \Theta_{1-\alpha}]$ becomes the $100(1-2\alpha)\%$ confidence interval.

Example 8—MTTF of exponential distribution. Assume 30 identical components are placed on failure-terminated test with $r = 20$. The 20th failure has a time to failure of 39.89 min., that is, $T = 39.89$, and the other 19 times to failure are listed in Table 7.2, along with times to failure that would occur if the test were to continue after the 20th failure, assuming the failures follow an exponential distribution. Find the 95% two-sided confidence interval for the MTTF.

Solution: $N = 30, r = 20, T = 39.89, \alpha = 0.025$.

$$\hat{\theta} = S = \frac{(30-20)\times 39.89 + 291.09}{20} = 34.5 \tag{7.53}$$

From the chi-square table in reference [3]:

$$\chi^2_{\alpha,2r} = \chi^2_{0.025,40} = 59.34 \tag{7.54}$$

$$\chi^2_{1-\alpha,2r} = \chi^2_{0.975,40} = 24.43 \tag{7.55}$$

Equation (7.52) yields

$$\Theta_\alpha = 2\times 30 \times \frac{34.5}{59.34} = 23.3 \tag{7.56}$$

$$\Theta_{1-\alpha} = 2\times 30 \times \frac{34.5}{24.43} = 56.5 \tag{7.57}$$

Then

$$23.3 \le \theta \le 56.5 \tag{7.58}$$

that is, we are 95% confident that the mean time to failure (θ) is in the interval [23.3, 56.5]. As a matter of fact, TTFs in Table 7.2 were generated from an exponential distribution with the MTTF = 26.6. The confidence interval includes this true MTTF. ■

TABLE 7.2. TTF Data for Example 8

TTFs up to 20th Failure				TTFs after 20th Failure	
t_1	0.26	t_{11}	11.04	t_{21}	40.84
t_2	1.49	t_{12}	12.07	t_{22}	47.02
t_3	3.65	t_{13}	13.61	t_{23}	54.75
t_4	4.25	t_{14}	15.07	t_{24}	61.08
t_5	5.43	t_{15}	19.28	t_{25}	64.36
t_6	6.97	t_{16}	24.04	t_{26}	64.45
t_7	8.09	t_{17}	26.16	t_{27}	65.92
t_8	9.47	t_{18}	31.15	t_{28}	70.82
t_9	10.18	t_{19}	38.70	t_{29}	97.32
t_{10}	10.29	t_{20}	39.89	t_{30}	164.26

Example 9—Reliability and failure rate. The reliability of components with exponential distributions was shown to be

$$R(t) = e^{-\lambda t} = e^{-t/\theta} \tag{7.59}$$

Confidence intervals can be obtained by substituting $\Theta_{1-\alpha}$ and Θ_α for θ; hence

$$e^{-t/\Theta_\alpha} \le R(t) \le e^{-t/\Theta_{1-\alpha}} \tag{7.60}$$

Thus for the data in Example 8,

$$e^{-t/23.3} \le R(t) \le e^{-t/56.5} \tag{7.61}$$

Similarly, the confidence interval for failure rate λ is given by

$$\frac{1}{\Theta_{1-\alpha}} \le \lambda \le \frac{1}{\Theta_\alpha} \tag{7.62}$$

■

Example 10—All components fail. Calculate the 95% confidence interval from the 30 TTFs in Table 7.2 where all 30 components failed.

Solution: Let $t_1, \ldots, t_n$ be a sequence of n independent and identically distributed exponential random variables. As shown in Case 3 of the χ^2 column of Table A.1, the quantity $(2/\theta)\sum_{i=1}^{n} t_i$ is chi-square distributed with $2n$ degrees of freedom, where $\theta = 1/\lambda$ is a true mean time to failure of the exponential distribution. From a chi-square table, we have $\chi^2_{0.975,60} = 40.47$ and $\chi^2_{0.0025,60} = 83.30$. Thus

$$\Pr\{40.47 \le (2/\theta) \times 1021.8 \le 83.30\} = 0.9 \tag{7.63}$$

yielding a slightly narrower confidence interval than Example 8 because all 30 TTFs are utilized.

$$[24.5,\ 50.5] \tag{7.64}$$

■

Example 11—Abnormally long failure times. Consider independently and identically distributed exponential random variables TTFs denoted by $T_1, \ldots, T_n$. Suppose that these variables have not been ordered. Then, as shown in row Case 3 and F distribution column of Table A.3, a ratio of these random variables follows an F distribution. Abnormally long failure times such as T_1 can be evaluated by checking whether the F variable is excluded from a confidence interval. In a similar way, failure rates for two sets of exponential TTFs can be evaluated. Note that TTFs should not be ordered because an increased order violates the independence assumption. ■

7.1.5 Confidence Limits for Binomial Distributions

Assume N identical components placed in a time-terminated test with r failures in test period T. We wish to obtain confidence limits for the component reliability $R(T)$ at time T. We begin by replacing static S by discrete random variable r, where

$$S = r \tag{7.65}$$

The S sampling distribution is given by the binomial distribution

$$\Pr\{S = s;\, R\} = \frac{N!}{(N-s)!s!} R^{N-s}[1-R]^s \tag{7.66}$$

with $R = R(T)$ corresponding to unknown parameter θ in Section 7.1.2.

Equation (7.3) thus becomes

$$\Pr\{S \le s_\alpha(R)\} = \sum_{s=0}^{s_\alpha(R)} \frac{N!}{(N-s)!s!} R^{N-s}[1-R]^s \ge 1-\alpha \tag{7.67}$$

Here inequality $\ge 1-\alpha$ is necessary because S is discrete. The parameter $s_\alpha(R)$ is defined as the smallest satisfying equation (7.67).

A schematic graph of $s_\alpha(R)$ is shown in Figure 7.4. Notice that the graph is a monotonically decreasing step function in R. We can define R_α for any observed characteristic S, as shown in Figure 7.4, with the exception that R_α is defined as unity when $S = 0$ is observed. This R_α corresponds to the Θ_α in Figure 7.3, where function $s_\alpha(\theta)$ is monotonically increasing. The event $S \le s_\alpha(R)$ occurs if and only if R_α falls on the right-hand side of R.

$$S \le s_\alpha(R) \Leftrightarrow R \le R_\alpha \tag{7.68}$$

Thus

$$\Pr\{R \le R_\alpha\} \ge 1-\alpha \tag{7.69}$$

and R_α gives $1-\alpha$, the upper confidence limit for reliability R.

Point $(R_\alpha, S-1)$ is represented by A in Figure 7.4. We notice that, at point A, inequality (7.67) reduces to an equality for $S \ne 0$ because the value $s_\alpha(R)$ decreases by one. Thus the value of R_α can be obtained for any given S by solving the following equation.

$$\sum_{s=S}^{N} \frac{N!}{(N-s)!s!} R_\alpha^{N-s}[1-R_\alpha]^s = \alpha, \quad \text{for } S \ne 0 \tag{7.70}$$

$$R_\alpha = 1, \quad \text{for } S = 0 \tag{7.71}$$

The above equation can be solved for R by iterative methods, although tables have been compiled [6]. (See also Problems 7.8 to 7.10.)

Similar to equation (7.70), the lower confidence limit $R_{1-\alpha}$ for R is given by the solution of the equation

$$\sum_{s=0}^{S} \frac{N!}{(N-s)!s!} R_{1-\alpha}^{N-s}[1-R_{1-\alpha}]^s = \alpha, \quad \text{for } S \ne N \tag{7.72}$$

$$R_{1-\alpha} = 0, \quad \text{for} S = N \tag{7.73}$$

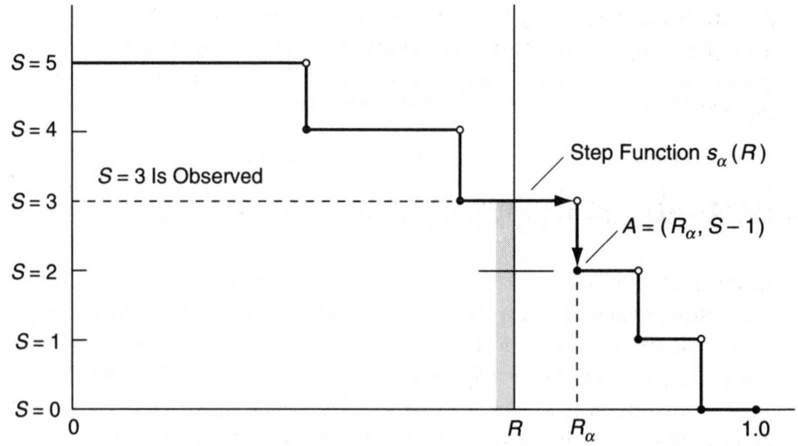

Figure 7.4. Quantity R_α determined by S and step function $s_\alpha(R)$.

Example 12—Reliability of binomial distribution. Assume a test situation that is go-no-go with only two possible outcomes, success or failure. Suppose no failures have occurred during the life-test of N components to a specified time T. (This situation would apply, for example, to the calculation of the probability of having a major plant disaster, given that none had ever occurred.)

Solution: Because $S = 0$ in equation (7.72)

$$R_{1-\alpha}^N = \alpha \tag{7.74}$$

Thus the lower confidence limit is $R_{1-\alpha} = \alpha^{1/N}$. If $\alpha = 0.05$ and $N = 1000$, then $R_{1-\alpha} = 0.997$. That is, we are 95% confident that the reliability is not less than 0.997. ■

Example 13—Reliability of binomial distribution. Assume that $r = 1$, $N = 20$, and $\alpha = 0.1$ in Example 12. Obtain upper and lower confidence limits.

Solution: Because $S = 1$, equations (7.70) and (7.72) yield

$$R_\alpha^N = 1 - \alpha, \qquad R_\alpha^{20} = 0.9 \tag{7.75}$$

$$R_{1-\alpha}^N + NR_{1-\alpha}^{N-1}[1 - R_{1-\alpha}] = \alpha, \qquad R_{1-\alpha}^{20} + 20R_{1-\alpha}^{19}[1 - R_{1-\alpha}] = 0.1 \tag{7.76}$$

Thus

$$R_\alpha = 0.9^{0.05} = 0.995 \tag{7.77}$$

$$R_{1-\alpha} = 0.819 \text{ (from reference [6])} \tag{7.78}$$

Thus we are 80% sure that the true reliability is between 0.819 and 0.995. ■

Assume that variable S follows the binomial distribution of equation (7.66). For large N, we have an asymptotic approximation.

$$\frac{S - NR}{\sqrt{NR(1-R)}} \sim \text{gau}^*(0, 1) \tag{7.79}$$

This property can be used to calculate an approximate confidence interval for reliability R from its observation $1 - (S/N)$.

A multinomial distribution (Chapter 6) is a generalization of the binomial distribution. Coin throwing (heads or tails) yields a binomial distribution while die casting yields a multinomial distribution. An average number of i-die events divided by their standard deviation asymptotically follows a normal distribution. Thus the sum of squares of these asymptotically normal variables follows a χ^2 distribution (see Case 1, Table A.1), and a die hypothesis can be evaluated accordingly. This is an example of a goodness-of-fit problem [2].

7.2 BAYESIAN RELIABILITY AND CONFIDENCE LIMITS

In the previous sections, classical statistics were applied to test data to demonstrate the reliability parameter of a system or component to a calculated degree of confidence. In many design situations, however, the designer uses test data, combined with past experience, to meet or exceed a reliability specification. Because the application of classical statistics for predicting reliability parameters does not make use of past experience, an alternate approach is desirable. An example of where this new approach would be required is the case where a designer is redesigning a component to achieve an improved reliability. Here, if we use the classical approach to predict a failure rate (with a given level of confidence) that is higher than the failure rate for the previous component, then the designer has obtained no really useful information; indeed, he may simply reject the premise and its result. So a method is needed that takes into consideration the designer's past experience.

One such method is based on Bayesian statistics, which combines a priori experience with hard posterior data to provide estimates similar to those obtained using the classical approach.

7.2.1 Discrete Bayes Theorem

To illustrate the application of Bayes theorem, let us consider a hypothetical example. Suppose that we are concerned about the reliability of a new untested system. The Bayesian approach regards reliability as a random variable, while the classical approach treats it as an unknown constant. Based on past experience, we believe there is an 80% chance that the system's reliability is $R_1 = 0.95$ and a 20% chance it is $R_2 = 0.75$. Now suppose that we test one system and find that it operates successfully. We would like to know the probability that the reliability level is R_1.

If we define S_i as the event in which system test i results in a success, then for the first success S_1, we want $\Pr\{R_1 | S_1\}$, using Bayes equation (see Section A.1.6, Chapter 3):

$$\Pr\{R_1 | S_1\} = \frac{\Pr\{R_1\}\Pr\{S_1 | R_1\}}{\Pr\{R_1\}\Pr\{S_1 | R_1\} + \Pr\{R_2\}\Pr\{S_1 | R_2\}} \tag{7.80}$$

Substituting numerical values, we find that

$$\Pr\{R_1 | S_1\} = \frac{(0.80)(0.95)}{(0.80)(0.95) + (0.20)(0.75)} = 0.835 \tag{7.81}$$

Let us assume that a second system was tested and it also was successful. Then

$$\Pr\{R_1 | S_1, S_2\} = \frac{\Pr\{R_1\}\Pr\{S_1, S_2 | R_1\}}{\Pr\{R_1\}\Pr\{S_1, S_2 | R_1\} + \Pr\{R_2\}\Pr\{S_1, S_2 | R_2\}} \tag{7.82}$$

which gives

$$\Pr\{R_1 | S_1, S_2\} = \frac{(0.80)(0.95 \times 0.95)}{(0.80)(0.95 \times 0.95) + (0.20)(0.75 \times 0.75)} = 0.865 \tag{7.83}$$

Here the probability of event $R_1 = 0.95$ was updated by applying Bayes theorem as new information became available.

7.2.2 Continuous Bayes Theorem

Bayes theorem for continuous variables is given in Section A.1.7, Chapter 3.

Example 14—Reliability with uniform a priori distribution. Suppose N components are placed in a time-terminated test, where $r(\leq N)$ components failed before specified time T. Define y_i by

$$y_i = \begin{cases} 1, & \text{if component } i \text{ failed} \\ 0, & \text{if component } i \text{ survived} \end{cases} \tag{7.84}$$

Obviously, $\sum y_i = r$. Obtain a posteriori density $p\{R|\mathbf{y}\} \equiv p\{R|y_1, \ldots, y_N\}$ for component reliability R at time T, assuming a uniform a priori distribution in interval [0, 1].

Solution:

$$p\{R\} = \begin{cases} 1, & \text{for } 0 \leq R \leq 1 \\ 0, & \text{otherwise} \end{cases} \tag{7.85}$$

$$p\{y|R\} = R^{N-r}[1-R]^r \tag{7.86}$$

The binomial coefficient $N!/[r!(N-r)!]$ is not necessary in the above equation because the sequence $y_1, \ldots, y_N$ along with total failures r are given. In other words, observation $(1, 0, 1)$ is treated separately from $(1, 1, 0)$ or $(0, 1, 1)$.

$$p\{R|y\} = \frac{R^{N-r}[1-R]^r}{\int [\text{numerator}] dR}, \quad \text{for } 0 \leq R \leq 1 \tag{7.87}$$

This a posteriori density is a beta probability distribution [2,3] (see Chapter 6). Note that the denominator of equation (7.87) is a constant when $\mathbf{y}$ is given (see Problem 7.5). It is known that if the a priori distribution is a beta distribution, then the a posteriori distribution is also a beta distribution; in this sense, the beta distribution is conserved in the Bayes transformation. ■

Example 15—Reliability with uniform a priori distribution. Assume that three components are placed in a 10 hr test, and that two components, 1 and 3, fail. Calculate the a posteriori probability density for the component reliability at 10 hr, assuming a uniform a priori distribution.

Solution: Because components 1 and 3 failed,

$$\mathbf{y} = (1, 0, 1), \qquad N = 3, \qquad r = 2 \tag{7.88}$$

Equation (7.87) gives

$$p\{R|\mathbf{y}\} = \frac{R^{3-2}[1-R]^2}{\text{const.}} = \frac{R[1-R]^2}{\text{const.}}, \quad \text{for } 0 \leq R \leq 1 \tag{7.89}$$

The normalizing constant in the above equation can be found by

$$\int_0^1 \frac{R[1-R]^2}{\text{const.}} dR = \frac{1}{\text{const.}} \times \frac{1}{12} = 1 \tag{7.90}$$

or

$$\text{const.} = 1/12 \tag{7.91}$$

Thus

$$p\{R|\mathbf{y}\} = \begin{cases} 12R[1-R]^2, & \text{for } 0 \leq R \leq 1 \\ 0, & \text{otherwise} \end{cases} \tag{7.92}$$

The a posteriori and a priori densities are plotted in Figure 7.5. We see that the a posteriori density approaches zero reliability because two out of three components failed. ■

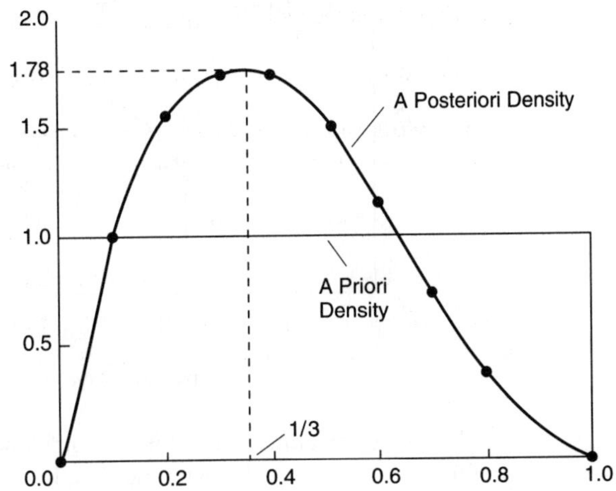

Figure 7.5. A priori and a posteriori densities.

7.2.3 Confidence Limits

The Bayesian one-sided confidence limits $L(\mathbf{y})$ and $U(\mathbf{y})$ for parameter x based on hard evidence $\mathbf{y}$ may be defined as the $(1-\alpha)$ and α points of a posteriori probability density $p\{x|\mathbf{y}\}$

$$\int_{L(\mathbf{y})}^{\infty} p\{x|\mathbf{y}\}dx = 1-\alpha \tag{7.93}$$

$$\int_{U(\mathbf{y})}^{\infty} p\{x|\mathbf{y}\}dx = \alpha \tag{7.94}$$

Quantities $L(\mathbf{y})$ and $U(\mathbf{y})$ are illustrated in Figure 7.6 and are constants when hard evidence $\mathbf{y}$ is given. Obviously, $L(\mathbf{y})$ is the Bayesian $(1-\alpha)$ lower confidence limit for x, and $U(\mathbf{y})$ is the Bayesian $(1-\alpha)$ upper confidence limit for x.

An interesting application of the Bayesian approach is in binomial testing, where a number of components are placed on test and the results are successes or failures (as described in Section 7.2.2). The Bayesian approach to the problem is to find the smallest $R_{1-\alpha} = L(\mathbf{y})$ in a table of beta probabilities for $N-r$ successes and r failures, such that the Bayesian can say, "the probability that the true reliability is greater than $R_{1-\alpha}$ is $100(1-\alpha)\%$." Similar procedures yield upper bound $R_{\alpha} = U(\mathbf{y})$ for the reliability.

Example 16—Confidence limit for reliability. To illustrate the Bayesian confidence limits, consider Example 13 in Section 7.1.5. Assume a uniform a priori distribution for reliability R. Obtain the 90% Bayesian lower confidence limit.

Solution: From equation (7.87) we see that equation (7.93) can be written as

$$\int_{0}^{R_{1-\alpha}} \frac{R^{19}[1-R]}{\text{const.}} dR = 0.1 \tag{7.95}$$

The beta probability value in reference [7] gives $R_{1-\alpha} = 0.827$. That is, the probability that the true reliability is greater than 0.827 is 90%. Notice that the reliability obtained in Example 13 by applying the binomial distribution was 0.819 with 90% confidence. We achieved an improved lower confidence limit by applying Bayesian techniques. ■

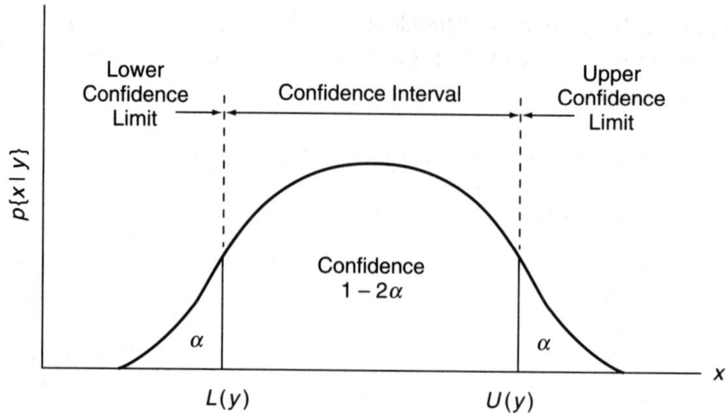

Figure 7.6. Bayesian confidence limits.

The Bayesian approach applies to confidence limits for reliability parameters such as reliability, failure rate, and mean time to failure. The reader is referred to [3,8] for details.

REFERENCES

[1] John, P. W. M. *Statistical Methods in Engineering and Quality Assurance.* New York: John Wiley & Sons, 1990.

[2] Kececioglu, D. *Reliability & Life Testing Handbook, Volume 1.* Englewood Cliffs, NJ: Prentice Hall, 1993.

[3] Mann, N. R. R., R. E. Schafer, and N. D. Singpurwalla. *Methods for Statistical Analysis of Reliability and Life Data.* New York: John Wiley & Sons, 1974.

[4] Catherine, M. T. "Tables of the percentage points of the χ^2 distribution," *Biometrika*, vol. 32, pp. 188–189, 1941.

[5] Bayer, W. H. (ed.). *Handbook of Tables for Probability and Statistics* (2d ed.). Cleveland, OH: The Chemical Rubber Company, 1968.

[6] Burington, M. *Handbook of Probability and Statistics, with Tables.* New York: McGraw-Hill, 1953.

[7] Harter, H. L. *New Tables of the Incomplete Gamma-Function Ratio and of Percentage Points of the Chi-Square and Beta Distribution.* Washington, D.C.: U.S. Government Printing Office, 1964.

[8] Martz, H. F., and R. A. Waller. *Bayesian Reliability Analysis.* New York: John Wiley & Sons, 1992.

CHAPTER SEVEN APPENDIX

A.1 THE χ^2, STUDENT'S *t*, AND *F* DISTRIBUTIONS

These three distributions are summarized in Tables A7.1, A7.2, and A7.3, which show the headings of distribution, random variable, degrees of freedom, probability density function ($Pdf.$), mean, variance, three application modes (Case 1 to Case 3), and asymptotic distribution for large degrees of freedom. For the application mode rows, random variables are assumed to be independent. Figures A7.1, A7.2, and A7.3 show probability density graphs and percentage points.

TABLE A7.1. Summary of χ^2 Distributions

Distributions → Descriptions ↓	χ^2 Distribution
Name	$\text{csq}^*(\nu)$
Variable	$0 \le \chi^2$
Degrees of freedom	$0 < \nu$: integer
Pdf.	$\frac{1}{2^{\nu/2}\Gamma(\nu/2)}(\chi^2)^{\frac{\nu}{2}-1}e^{-(\chi^2)/2}$
Mean	$\overline{\chi^2} = \nu$
Variance	$\sigma^2_{\chi^2} = 2\nu$
Case 1	$X_1, \ldots, X_n \sim \text{gau}^*(0, 1)$ $\Downarrow$ $\chi^2 \equiv X_1^2 + \cdots + X_n^2 \sim \text{csq}^*(n)$
Case 2	$X_1, \ldots, X_n \sim \text{gau}^*(\mu, \sigma)$ $\overline{X} \equiv \frac{1}{n}\sum_{i=1}^n X_i$: sample mean $S^2 \equiv \frac{1}{n-1}\sum_{i=1}^n (X_i - \overline{X})^2$: sample var. $\Downarrow$ $(n-1)S^2/\sigma^2 \sim \text{csq}^*(n-1)$
Case 3	$T_1, \ldots, T_n \sim \exp^*(\lambda)$ $\Downarrow$ $2\lambda T_1 \sim \text{csq}^*(2)$ $2\lambda \sum_{i=2}^n T_i \sim \text{csq}^*(2n-2)$ $2\lambda \sum_{i=1}^n T_i \sim \text{csq}^*(2n)$ $2\lambda\left[(n-r)T_r + \sum_{i=1}^r T_i\right] \sim \text{csq}^*(2r)$, T_i : ordered
$\nu \to \infty$	$\left(\frac{\chi^2}{\nu}\right)^{1/3} \sim \text{gau}^*\left(1 - \frac{2}{9\nu}, \frac{2}{9\nu}\right)$ $(2\chi^2)^{1/2} \sim \text{gau}^*((2\nu-1)^{1/2}, 1)$, $\nu \ge 100$

A.1.1 χ^2 Distribution Application Modes

Case 1. The sum of squares of normal random variables follows a χ^2 distribution. This fact is used, for example, for a goodness-of-fit problem. Note that many random variables are approximated asymptotically by a normal random variable. Variable symbol χ^2 suggests the random variable squared.

Case 2. A ratio of sample variance to true variance for a normal population follows a χ^2 distribution. A confidence interval of the true variance is obtained.

Case 3. The sum of an exponentially distributed random variable follows a χ^2 distribution. A confidence interval of the mean time to failure is obtained. Notice that the exponential variables in the first three equations are not ordered in ascending order. On

TABLE A7.2. Summary of Student's t Distributions

Distributions → **Descriptions ↓**	**Student's t Distribution**
Name Variable Degrees of freedom *Pdf.* Mean Variance	$\text{stu}^*(\nu)$ $-\infty < t < \infty$ $0 < \nu$: integer $\dfrac{\Gamma(\frac{\nu+1}{2})}{(\pi\nu)^{1/2}\Gamma(\nu/2)}\left(1+\dfrac{t^2}{\nu}\right)^{-\frac{\nu+1}{2}}$ $\bar{t} = 0$ $\sigma_t^2 = \nu/(\nu-2), \qquad \nu > 2$
Case 1	$X \sim \text{gau}^*(0, 1),\ \chi^2 \sim \text{csq}^*(\nu)$ $\Downarrow$ $\dfrac{X}{(\chi^2/\nu)^{1/2}} \sim \text{stu}^*(\nu)$
Case 2	$X_1, \ldots, X_{n_x} \sim \text{gau}^*(\mu_x, \sigma_x)$ $Y_1, \ldots, Y_{n_y} \sim \text{gau}^*(\mu_y, \sigma_y)$ $\overline{X},\ \overline{Y}$: sample means $S_x^2,\ S_y^2$: sample variances $\Downarrow$ $\dfrac{(\overline{X}-\overline{Y})-(\mu_x-\mu_y)}{\left[\dfrac{(n_x-1)S_x^2+(n_y-1)S_y^2}{n_x+n_y-2}\right]^{1/2}\left(\dfrac{1}{n_x}+\dfrac{1}{n_y}\right)^{1/2}}$ $\sim \text{stu}^*(n_x+n_y-2)$
Case 3	$X_1, \ldots, X_n \sim \text{gau}^*(\mu, \sigma)$ $\overline{X}$: sample mean S^2: sample variance $\Downarrow$ $\sqrt{n}(\overline{X}-\mu)/S \sim \text{stu}^*(n-1)$
$\nu \to \infty$	$t \sim \text{gau}^*(0, 1), \qquad \nu \geq 30$

the other hand, n exponential variables are ordered in the fourth equation. The ordering is accepted in the third relation because the sum equals the sum of the original independent variables.

As shown in the last row, for large degrees of freedom—say $\nu \geq 100$—conversions of χ^2 can be approximated by normal distribution variables. This property is conveniently used for calculating $\chi_{\alpha,\nu}$ and $\chi_{1-\alpha,\nu}$ from a normal distribution table.

Two independent χ^2 variables have an additive property, that is,

$$\chi_1^2 \sim \text{chi}^*(\nu_1) \quad \text{and} \quad \chi_2^2 \sim \text{chi}^*(\nu_2) \Rightarrow \chi_1^2 + \chi_2^2 \sim \text{chi}^*(\nu_1+\nu_2) \tag{A.1}$$

A.1.2 Student's t Distribution Application Modes

Case 1. A ratio of a normal random variable to a χ^2 variable square root follows a Student's t distribution. This gives the theoretical background for Cases 2 and 3.

Case 2. Given two normal populations, the ratio of a difference of two sample mean errors to a square root of a sum of two sample variances follows a Student's t distribution. This property is used, for instance, to evaluate an equal mean hypothesis.

TABLE A7.3. Summary of F Distributions

Distributions → **Descriptions ↓**	***F* Distribution**
Name	$\text{fis}^*(\nu_1, \nu_2)$
Variable	$0 \le F$
Degrees of freedom	$0 < \nu_1,\ 0 < \nu_2$: integer
Pdf.	$\dfrac{\Gamma(\frac{\nu_1+\nu_2}{2})(\nu_1/\nu_2)^{\nu_1/2}}{\Gamma(\nu_1/2)\Gamma(\nu_2/2)} \dfrac{F^{(\nu_1/2)-1}}{[1+(\nu_1/\nu_2)F]^{\frac{\nu_1+\nu_2}{2}}}$
Mean	$\overline{F} = \nu_2/(\nu_2-2),\ \nu_2 > 2$
Variance	$\sigma_F^2 = \dfrac{2\nu_2^2(\nu_2+\nu_1-2)}{\nu_1(\nu_2-2)^2(\nu_2-4)}, \quad \nu_2 > 4$
Case 1	$\chi_1^2 \sim \text{csq}^*(\nu_1),\ \chi_2^2 \sim \text{csq}^*(\nu_2)$ ⇓ $\dfrac{\chi_1^2/\nu_1}{\chi_2^2/\nu_2} \sim \text{fis}^*(\nu_1, \nu_2)$
Case 2	$X_1, \ldots, X_{n_x} \sim \text{gau}^*(\mu_x, \sigma_x)$ $Y_1, \ldots, Y_{n_y} \sim \text{gau}^*(\mu_y, \sigma_y)$ $S_x^2,\ S_y^2$: sample variances ⇓ $\dfrac{S_x^2}{S_y^2}\dfrac{\sigma_y^2}{\sigma_x^2} \sim \text{fis}^*(n_x-1, n_y-1)$
Case 3	$T_1, \ldots, T_n \sim \exp^*(\lambda)$ ⇓ $(n-1)T_1/\sum_{i=2}^n T_i \sim \text{fis}^*(2, 2n-2)$ $(n-r)\sum_{i=1}^r T_i/\left[r\sum_{i=r+1}^n T_i\right] \sim \text{fis}^*(2r, 2n-2r)$

Case 3. A ratio of sample mean minus true mean to sample standard deviation follows a Student's t distribution. A confidence interval of the true mean is obtained.

For large degrees of freedom, the Student's t variable asymptotically follows a normal distribution. This is a convenient way to calculate $t_{\alpha,\nu}$. The Student's t distribution is symmetrical with respect to $t = 0$, and hence $t_{1-\alpha,\nu} = -t_{\alpha,\nu}$.

A.1.3 F Distribution Application Modes

Case 1. A ratio of a χ^2 variable to another χ^2 variable follows an F distribution. This is the theoretical background for Cases 2 and 3.

Case 2. Given two normal populations, a ratio of one sample variance to another sample variance follows an F distribution. An equal variance hypothesis is evaluated accordingly.

Case 3. A ratio of a sum of independent exponential variables to another sum of independent exponential variables follows an F distribution. An abnormally long or short time to failure or a failure rate change can be evaluated accordingly. Note that the n exponential variables $T_1, \ldots, T_n$ are not arranged in ascending order.

Given an α point F_{α,ν_1,ν_2}, a $(1-\alpha)$ point $F_{1-\alpha,\nu_1,\nu_2}$ is given by the reciprocal,

$$F_{1-\alpha,\nu_1,\nu_2} = 1/F_{\alpha,\nu_1,\nu_2} \tag{A.2}$$

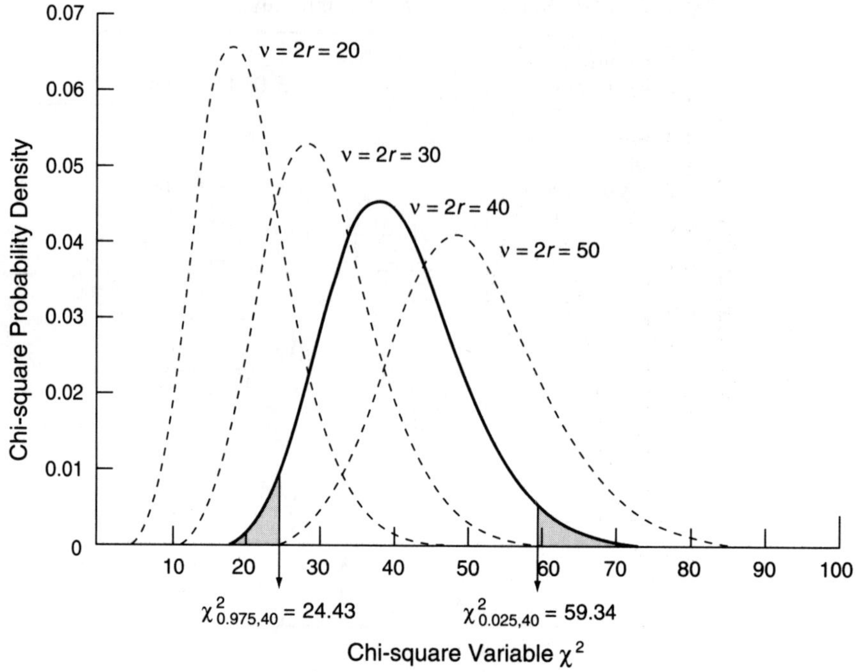

Figure A7.1. Densities and percentage points of χ^2 distribution.

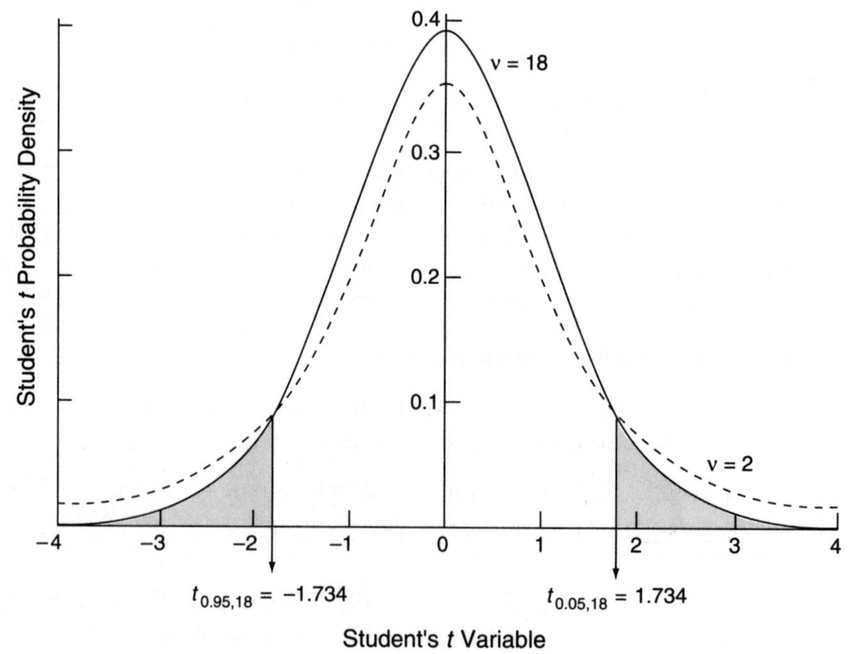

Figure A7.2. Densities and percentiles of Student's t distribution.

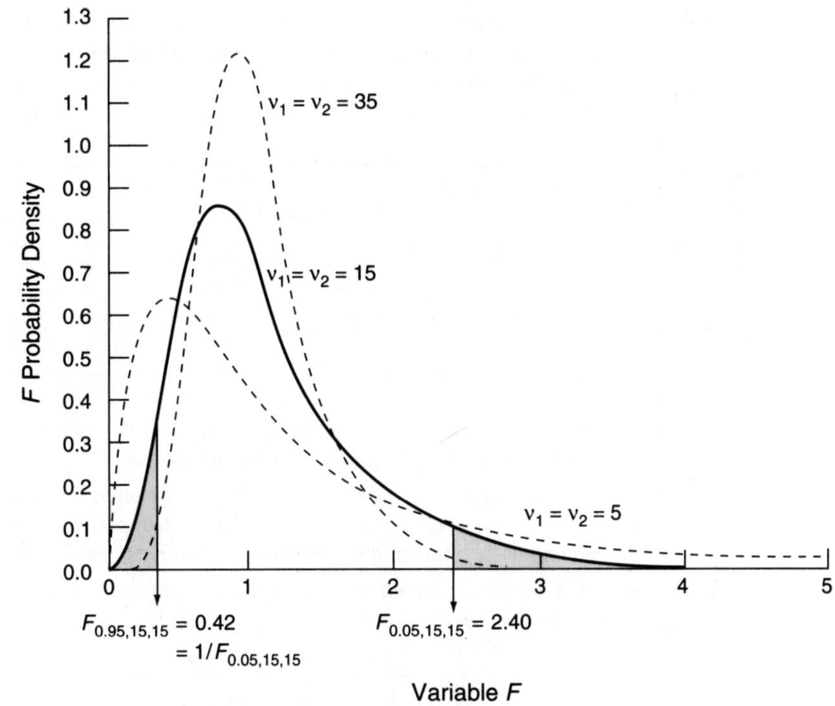

Figure A7.3. Densities and percentage points of F distribution.

PROBLEMS

7.1. Assume 30 samples, X_i, $i = 1, \ldots, 30$, from a normal population with unknown mean θ and unknown standard deviation σ:

−0.112,	−0.265,	−0.937,	0.064,	1.236
−1.317,	−1.239,	−0.061,	1.508,	−1.165
−0.082,	0.254,	1.742,	1.706,	−1.659
1.211,	−1.532,	1.127,	−0.741,	−0.097
−1.736,	0.252,	−0.379,	−0.875,	−0.598
1.600,	0.694,	0.401,	−1.098,	−0.430

(a) Obtain $\bar{\theta}$ and $\bar{\sigma}$, the estimates of mean θ and standard deviation σ, respectively.
(b) Obtain $s_\alpha(\theta)$ and $s_{1-\alpha}(\theta)$ for $\alpha = 0.05$, using $\bar{\sigma}$ as the true standard deviation σ.
(c) Determine the 90% two-sided confidence interval for mean θ.

7.2. A test of 15 identical components produced the following times to failures (hr):

118.2,	128.4,	17.0,	161.6,	33.8
55.1,	68.5,	74.7,	15.0,	0.7
25.5,	158.5,	335.5,	306.8,	15.2

(a) Obtain the times to failures for time-terminated test with $T = 70$.
(b) Obtain the times to failures for failure-terminated test with $r = 10$.
(c) Find the 90% two-sided confidence interval of MTTF for failure-terminated test, assuming an exponential failure distribution and the chi-square table:

	$\Pr\{\chi^2 \geq \chi^2_\alpha(\nu)\} = \alpha$			
	$\alpha = 0.975$	$\alpha = 0.950$	$\alpha = 0.05$	$\alpha = 0.025$
$\nu = 10$	3.247	3.940	18.31	20.48
$\nu = 15$	6.262	7.261	25.00	27.49
$\nu = 20$	9.591	10.851	31.41	34.17

(d) Obtain 90% confidence intervals for the component failure rate λ and component reliability at $t = 100$, assuming a failure-terminated test.

7.3. A total of ten identical components were tested using time-terminated test with $T = 40$ (hr). Four components failed during the test. Obtain algebraic equations for 95% upper and lower confidence limits of the component reliability at $t = 40$ (hr).

7.4. Assume that we are concerned about the reliability of a new system. Past experience gives the following a priori information.

Reliability	Probability
$R_1 = 0.98$	0.6
$R_2 = 0.78$	0.3
$R_3 = 0.63$	0.1

Now suppose that we test the two systems and find that the first system operates successfully and the second one fails. Determine the probability that the reliability level is R_i $(i = 1, 2, 3)$, based on these two test results.

7.5. An a priori probability density of reliability R is given by

$$p\{R\} = \frac{R^{N-r}[1-R]^r}{\text{const.}}, \qquad 0 \leq r \leq N, \qquad 1 \leq N$$

Prove that the constant is

$$\frac{r!}{(N+1)N(N-1) \times \cdots \times (N-r+1)}$$

7.6. A failure-terminated test of 100 components resulted in a component failure within 200 hr.

(a) Obtain an a posteriori probability density $p\{R|y\}$ of the component reliability at 200 hr, assuming an a priori density information:

$$p\{R\} = \frac{R^{28}[1-R]^2}{\text{const.}}$$

(b) Obtain the mean values of the reliability that distributes according to $p\{R\}$ and $p\{R|y\}$, respectively.
(c) Obtain reliabilities $\hat{R}$ and $\hat{R}|y$ that maximize $p\{R\}$ and $p\{R|y\}$, respectively.
(d) Graph $p\{R\}$ and $p\{R|y\}$.

7.7. Consider an a posteriori probability density

$$p\{R|\mathbf{y}\} = \frac{R^{N-r}[1-R]^r}{\text{const.}}$$

Prove that:

(a) The mean value $\bar{R}|\mathbf{y}$ of R is

$$\bar{R}|\mathbf{y} = \frac{N-r+1}{N+2}$$

(b) The value $\hat{R}|\mathbf{y}$ that maximizes $p\{R|\mathbf{y}\}$ is

$$\hat{R}|\mathbf{y} = \frac{N-r}{N}$$

7.8. Prove the identities

$$1 - \sum_{s=S}^{N} \frac{N!}{(N-s)!s!} R_\alpha^{N-s}[1-R_\alpha]^s$$

$$= \frac{N!}{(N-S)!(S-1)!} \int_0^{R_\alpha} u^{N-S}(1-u)^{S-1}du, \quad (S \neq 0)$$

$$1 - \sum_{s=0}^{S} \frac{N!}{(N-s)!s!} R_{1-\alpha}^{N-s}[1-R_{1-\alpha}]^s$$

$$= \frac{N!}{S!(N-S-1)!} \int_0^{1-R_{1-\alpha}} u^{S}(1-u)^{N-S-1}du, \quad (S \neq N)$$

7.9. The beta probability density with integer parameters α, β is defined by

$$p\{u\} = \frac{(\alpha+\beta+1)!}{\alpha!\beta!} u^\alpha[1-u]^\beta, \qquad 0 < u < 1$$

Prove that:

(a) The upper confidence limit R_α in (7.70) satisfies the following probability equation, where X is a beta distribution variable with parameters $[N-S, S-1]$. (For upper bound R_α for Problem 7.3, the beta distribution has parameters 6 and 3.)

$$\Pr\{X \leq R_\alpha\} = 1 - \alpha$$

(b) The lower confidence limit $R_{1-\alpha}$ in (7.72) satisfies the following probability equation, where X is a beta distribution variable with parameters $[S, N-S-1]$. (For lower bound $R_{1-\alpha}$ for Problem 7.3, the beta distribution has parameters 4 and 5.)

$$\Pr\{X \leq 1 - R_{1-\alpha}\} = 1 - \alpha$$

7.10. The F distribution with $2k$ and $2l$ degrees of freedom has the probability density

$$p\{F\} = \frac{(k+l-1)!}{(k-1)!(l-1)!} \left(\frac{k}{l}\right)^k F^{k-1}(1+\frac{k}{l}F)^{-k-l}$$

Show that when V is distributed with the beta distribution with parameters $k-1$ and $l-1$, then the distribution of the new random variable

$$U = \frac{l}{k} \times \frac{V}{1-V}$$

is an F distribution with $2k$ and $2l$ degrees of freedom.

7.11. Obtain the upper and lower bounds of the component reliability in Problem 7.3, using the results of Problems 7.9 and 7.10. Assume an F distribution table with ν_1 and ν_2 degrees of freedom. Interpolate $F_{0.05}$ values if necessary:

	$\Pr\{F \geq F_{0.05}\} = 0.05$		
	$\nu_1 = 10$	$\nu_1 = 12$	$\nu_1 = 15$
$\nu_2 = 8$	3.347	3.284	3.218
$\nu_2 = 10$	2.978	2.913	2.845
$\nu_2 = 12$	2.753	2.687	2.617

7.12. A component reliability has the a posteriori distribution

$$p\{R|y\} = \frac{R^5(1-R)^4}{\text{const.}}$$

Obtain the 90% confidence reliability for R.

8

Quantitative Aspects of System Analysis

8.1 INTRODUCTION

Chapters 6 and 7 deal with the quantification of basic events. We now extend these methods to systems.

System success or failure can be described by a combination of top events defined by an OR combination of all system hazards into a composite fault tree (Figure 8.1). The non-occurrence of all system hazards implies system success. In general, we can analyze either a particular system hazard or a system success by an appropriate top event and its corresponding fault tree.

The following probabilistic parameters describe the system. Their interpretation depends on whether the top event refers to a system hazard or an OR combination of these hazards.

1. System availability $A_s(t)$ = probability that the top event does not exist at time t. Subscript s stands for system. This is the probability of the system's operating successfully when the top event refers to an OR combination of all system hazards. It is the probability of the non-occurrence of a particular hazard when the top event is a single system hazard.
2. System unavailability $Q_s(t)$ = probability that the top event exists at time t. This is either the probability of system failure or the probability of a particular system hazard at time t, depending on the definition of the top event. The system unavailability is complementary to the availability, and the following identity holds:

$$A_s(t) + Q_s(t) = 1 \tag{8.1}$$

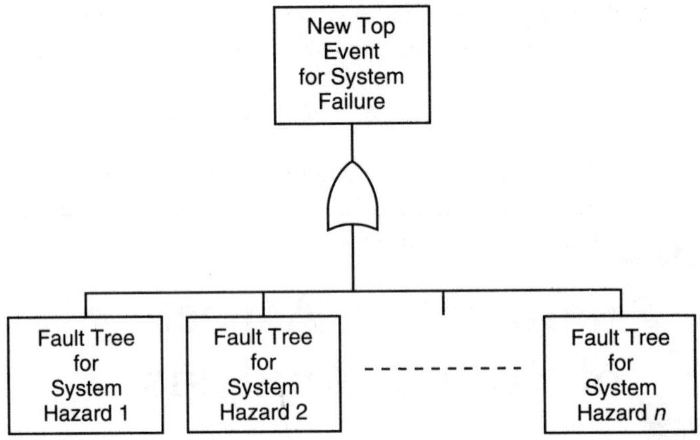

Figure 8.1. Defining a new fault tree by an OR configuration of fault trees.

3. System reliability $R_s(t)$ = probability that the top event does not occur over the time interval [0, t]. The system reliability $R_s(t)$ requires continuation of the nonexistence of the top event and differs from the system availability $A_s(t)$. Inequality (8.2) holds. Reliability is used to characterize catastrophic or unrepairable system failures.

$$R_s(t) \leq A_s(t) \tag{8.2}$$

4. System unreliability $F_s(t)$ = probability that the top event occurs before time t. This is the complement of the system reliability, and the identity

$$R_s(t) + F_s(t) = 1 \tag{8.3}$$

holds. The system unreliability $F_s(t)$ is larger than or equal to the system unavailability:

$$F_s(t) \geq Q_s(t) \tag{8.4}$$

5. System failure density $f_s(t)$ = first-order derivative of the system failure distribution $F_s(t)$:

$$f_s(t) = \frac{dF_s(t)}{dt} \tag{8.5}$$

The term $f_s(t)dt$ is the probability that the first top event occurs during $[t, t+dt)$.

6. System conditional failure intensity $\lambda_s(t)$ = probability that the top event occurs per unit time at time t, given that it does not exist at time t. A large value of $\lambda_s(t)$ means that the system is about to fail.
7. System unconditional failure intensity $w_s(t)$ = probability that the top event occurs per unit time at time t. The term $w_s(t)dt$ is the probability that the top event occurs during $[t, t + dt)$.
8. $W_s(t, t + dt)$ = expected number of top events during $[t, t + dt)$. The following relation holds.

$$W_s(t, t + dt) = w_s(t)dt \tag{8.6}$$

9. $W_s(t_1, t_2)$ = expected number of top events during $[t_1, t_2)$. This is given by integration of the unconditional failure intensity $w_s(t)$:

$$W_s(t_1, t_2) = \int_{t_1}^{t_2} w_s(t)dt \tag{8.7}$$

10. MTTF_s = mean time to failure = expected length of time to the first occurrence of the top event. The MTTF_s corresponds to average lifetime and is a suitable parameter for catastrophic system hazards. It is given by

$$\text{MTTF}_s = \int_0^{\infty} t f_s(t)dt \tag{8.8}$$

or

$$\text{MTTF}_s = \int_0^{\infty} R_s(t)dt, \quad \text{if } R_s(\infty) = 0 \tag{8.9}$$

In this chapter we discuss mainly the system availability and unavailability: system reliability and unreliability is quantified by Markov methods in Chapter 9. Unless otherwise stated, all basic events are assumed to be mutually independent. Dependent failures are also described in Chapter 9. We first demonstrate availability $A_s(t)$ or unavailability $Q_s(t) = 1 - A_s(t)$ calculations, given relatively simple fault trees. Quantification methods apply to reliability block diagrams and fault trees because both are modeled by Boolean functions. Next we discuss methods for calculating lower and upper bounds for the system unavailability $Q_s(t)$. Then we give a brief summary of the so-called *kinetic tree theory* [1], which is used to quantify system parameters for large and complex fault trees. Two types of sensor system-failure probabilities, that is, failed-safe and failed-dangerous probabilities are developed.

As shown in Figure 4.16, each basic event is a component primary failure, a component secondary failure, or a command failure.

To simplify the nomenclature, we use capital letters B, B_1, C, and so on, to represent both the basic events and their existence at time t. When event B is a component failure, the probability $\Pr\{B\}$ is the component unavailability $Q(t)$.

Failure modes should be defined for component failures. Primary failures are caused by natural aging (random or wearout) within the design envelope. Environmental impacts, human error, or system-dependent stresses should be identified as possible causes of the secondary failures that create transitions to the failed state. These failure modes and possible causes clarify the basic events and are necessary for successful reliability quantification.

8.2 SIMPLE SYSTEMS

8.2.1 Independent Basic Events

The usual assumption regarding basic events $B_1, \ldots, B_n$ is that they are independent, which means that the occurrence of a given basic event is in no way affected by the occurrence of any other basic event. For independent basic events, the simultaneous existence probability $\Pr\{B_1 \cap B_2 \cap \cdots \cap B_n\}$ reduces to

$$\Pr\{B_1 \cap B_2 \cap \cdots \cap B_n\} = \Pr\{B_1\}\Pr\{B_2\} \cdots \Pr\{B_n\} \tag{8.10}$$

where the symbol $\cap$ represents the intersection of events $B_1, \ldots, B_n$.

8.2.2 AND Gate

Consider the fault tree of Figure 8.2. Simultaneous existence of basic events $B_1, \ldots,$ B_n results in the top event. Thus the system unavailability $Q_s(t)$ is given by the probability that all basic events exist at time t:

$$Q_s(t) = \Pr\{B_1 \cap B_2 \cap \cdots \cap B_n\} \tag{8.11}$$

$$= \Pr\{B_1\}\Pr\{B_2\}\cdots\Pr\{B_n\} \tag{8.12}$$

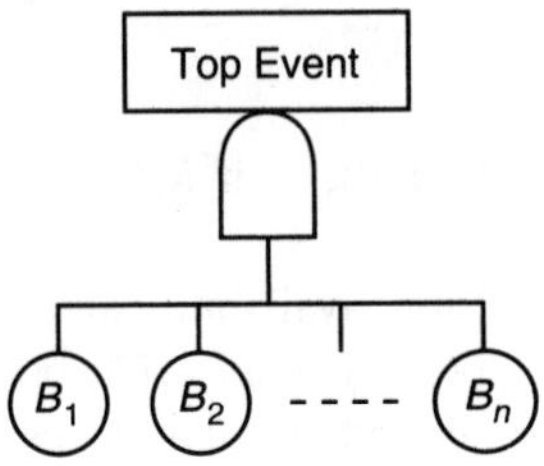

Figure 8.2. Gated AND fault tree.

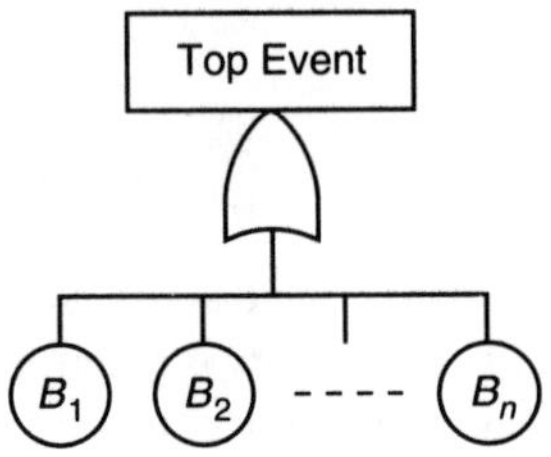

Figure 8.3. Gated OR fault tree.

8.2.3 OR Gate

With reference to Figure 8.3, the top event exists at time t if and only if at least one of the n basic events exists at time t. Thus the system availability $A_s(t)$ and the system unavailability $Q_s(t)$ are given by

$$A_s(t) = \Pr\{\overline{B}_1 \cap \overline{B}_2 \cap \cdots \cap \overline{B}_n\} \tag{8.13}$$

$$Q_s(t) = \Pr\{B_1 \cup B_2 \cup \cdots \cup B_n\} \tag{8.14}$$

where the symbol $\cup$ denotes a union of the events, and $\overline{B}_i$ represents the complement of the event B_i; that is, the event $\overline{B}_i$ means nonexistence of event B_i at time t. Independence of basic events $B_1, \ldots, B_n$ implies independence of the complementary events $\overline{B}_1, \overline{B}_2, \ldots, \overline{B}_n$. Thus $A_s(t)$ in (8.13) can be rewritten as

$$\begin{aligned} A_s(t) &= \Pr\{\overline{B}_1\}\Pr\{\overline{B}_2\}\cdots\Pr\{\overline{B}_n\} \\ &= [1 - \Pr\{B_1\}][1 - \Pr\{B_2\}]\cdots[1 - \Pr\{B_n\}] \end{aligned} \tag{8.15}$$

Unavailability $Q_s(t)$ is calculated using (8.1):

$$\begin{aligned} Q_s(t) &= \Pr\{B_1 \cup B_2 \cup \cdots \cup B_n\} \\ &= 1 - A_s(t) \\ &= 1 - [1 - \Pr\{B_1\}][1 - \Pr\{B_2\}]\cdots[1 - \Pr\{B_n\}] \end{aligned} \tag{8.16}$$

Another derivation of $Q_s(t)$ is based on de Morgan's law by which we rewrite OR operations in terms of AND and complement operations (see Section A.2, appendix of Chapter 3):

$$B_1 \cup B_2 \cup \cdots \cup B_n = \overline{\overline{B}_1 \cap \overline{B}_2 \cap \cdots \cap \overline{B}_n} \tag{8.17}$$

Thus

$$\begin{aligned} Q_s(t) &= \Pr\{\overline{\overline{B}_1 \cap \overline{B}_2 \cap \cdots \cap \overline{B}_n}\} \\ &= 1 - \Pr\{\overline{B}_1 \cap \overline{B}_2 \cap \cdots \cap \overline{B}_n\} \\ &= 1 - [1 - \Pr\{B_1\}][1 - \Pr\{B_2\}] \cdots [1 - \Pr\{B_n\}] \end{aligned} \tag{8.18}$$

For $n = 2$,

$$Q_s(t) = \Pr\{B_1 \cup B_2\} \tag{8.19}$$

$$= \Pr\{B_1\} + \Pr\{B_2\} - \Pr\{B_1\}\Pr\{B_2\} \tag{8.20}$$

In other words, the probability $Q_s(t)$ that at least one of the events B_1 and B_2 exists is equal to the sum of the probabilities of each event minus the probability of both events existing simultaneously. This is shown by the Venn diagram of Figure 8.4. For $n = 3$,

$$\begin{aligned} Q_s(t) &= \Pr\{B_1 \cup B_2 \cup B_3\} \\ &= \Pr\{B_1\} + \Pr\{B_2\} + \Pr\{B_3\} - \Pr\{B_1\}\Pr\{B_2\} - \Pr\{B_2\}\Pr\{B_3\} \\ &\quad - \Pr\{B_3\}\Pr\{B_1\} + \Pr\{B_1\}\Pr\{B_2\}\Pr\{B_3\} \end{aligned} \tag{8.21}$$

This unavailability is depicted in Figure 8.5. Equations (8.20) and (8.21) are special cases of the inclusion-exclusion formula described in Section 8.5.4.

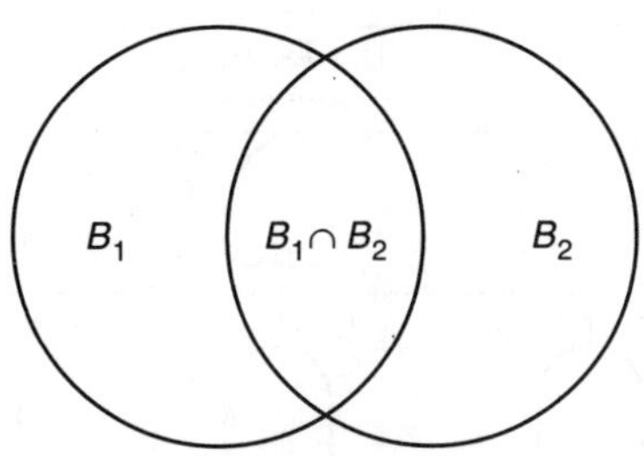

Figure 8.4. $\Pr\{B_1\} + \Pr\{B_2\} - \Pr\{B_1\}\Pr\{B_2\}$.

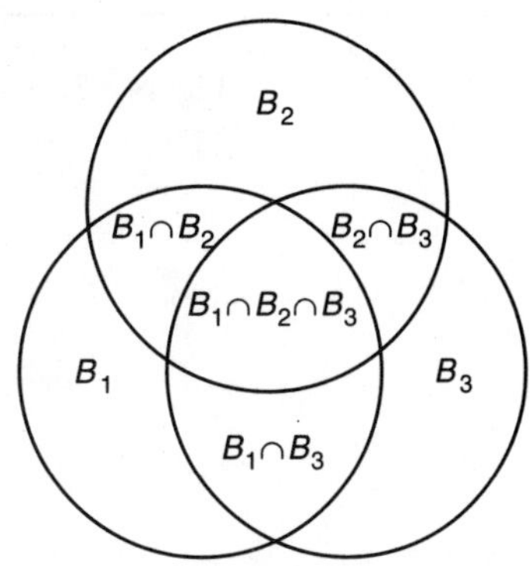

Figure 8.5. Illustration of formula for $\Pr\{B_1 \cup B_2 \cup B_3\}$.

8.2.4 Voting Gate

The fault tree of Figure 8.6 appears in a voting system that produces an output if m or more components out of n generate a command signal. A common application of the m-out-of-n system is in safety systems, where it is desirable to avoid expensive plant shutdowns by a spurious signal from a single safety monitor.

As an example, consider the two-out-of-three shutdown device of Figure 8.7. Plant shutdown occurs when two out of three safety monitors generate shutdown signals. Consider a case where the plant is normal and requires no shutdown. An unnecessary shutdown occurs if two or more safety monitors produce spurious signals. Denote by B_i a false signal from monitor i. The resulting fault tree is shown in Figure 8.8, which is a special case of Figure 8.6.

Although an m-out-of-n gate such as Figure 8.6 can always be decomposed into equivalent AND and OR gates, direct application of the binomial Bernoulli distribution equations represents an alternative analytical approach.

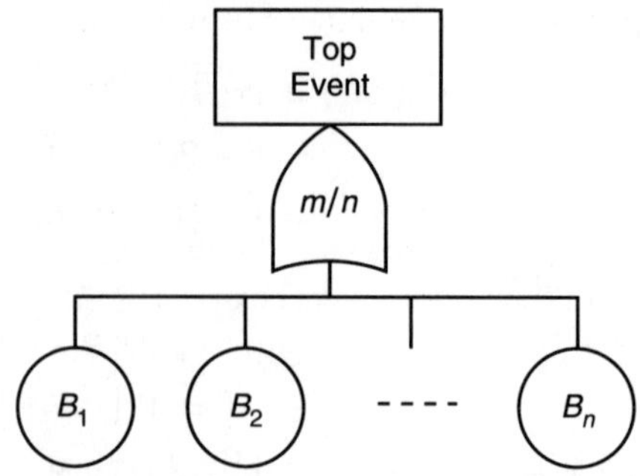

Figure 8.6. m-out-of-n voting system.

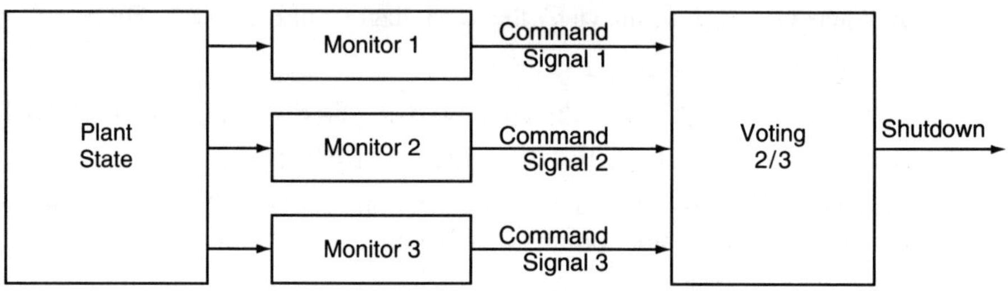

Figure 8.7. Two-out-of-three shutdown system.

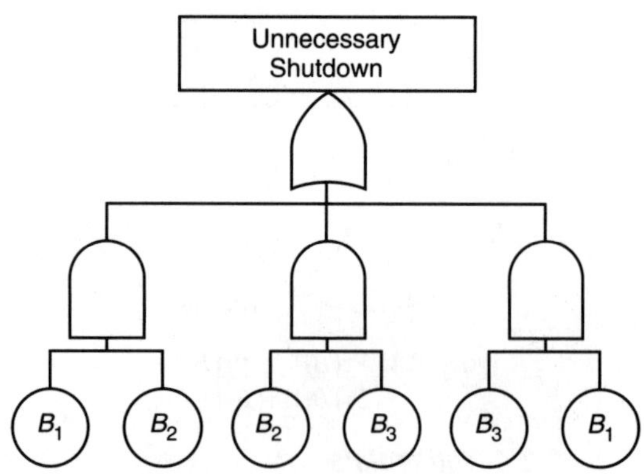

Figure 8.8. Fault tree for two-out-of-three shutdown system.

Assume that all basic events have the probability Q.

$$\Pr\{B_1\} = \Pr\{B_2\} = \cdots = \Pr\{B_n\} = Q \tag{8.22}$$

The binomial distribution gives the probability that a total of m outcomes will occur, given the outcome probability Q of any one trial and the number of trials n:

$$\Pr\{m; n, Q\} = \binom{n}{m} Q^m (1 - Q)^{n-m} \tag{8.23}$$

This equation is derived by considering that one way of achieving m outcomes is to have m consecutive occurrences, then $(n-m)$ consecutive non-occurrences. The probability of this sequence is $Q^m(1 - Q)^{n-m}$. The total number of sequences is the number of combinations of n things taken m at a time:

$$\binom{n}{m} \equiv \frac{n!}{m!(n-m)!} \tag{8.24}$$

Therefore, $\Pr\{m; n, Q\}$ is the sum of all these probabilities and equation (8.23) is proven. In applying it to reliability problems, it is necessary to recognize that the top event will exist if m or more basic events exist. Thus it is necessary to sum equation (8.23) over all $k = m$ to n.

$$Q_s(t) = \sum_{k=m}^{n} \Pr\{k; n, Q\} = \sum_{k=m}^{n} \binom{n}{k} Q^k (1-Q)^{n-k} \tag{8.25}$$

Simple examples follow that demonstrate the application of the methodology developed in the preceding subsections.

Example 1—Two-out-of-three system. Compare the unavailability $Q_s(t)$ for the two-out-of-three configuration of Figure 8.9 and the OR configuration of Figure 8.10.

Solution: The unavailability $Q_{s,1}(t)$ for Figure 8.9 is given by (8.25):

$$Q_{s,1}(t) = \binom{3}{2} Q^2(1-Q) + \binom{3}{3} Q^3(1-Q)^0 = 3Q^2 - 2Q^3 \tag{8.26}$$

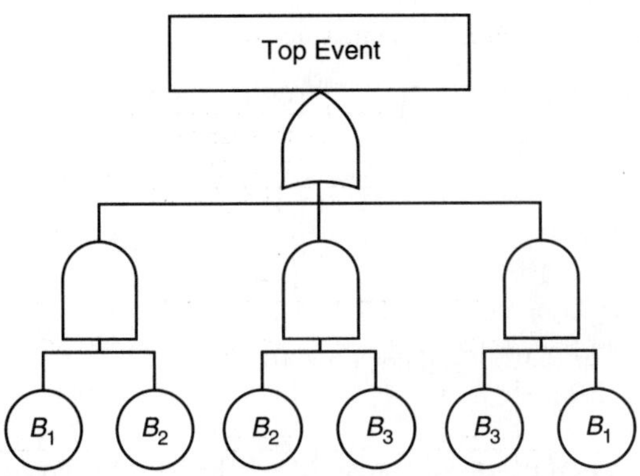

Figure 8.9. Fault tree for two-out-of-three system ($\Pr\{B_i\} = Q$).

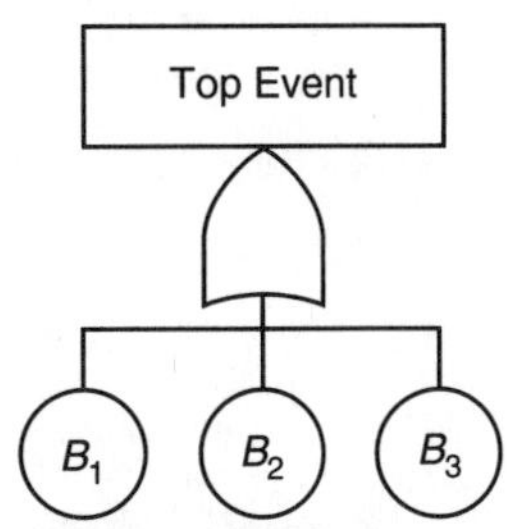

Figure 8.10. Gated OR fault tree ($\Pr\{B_i\} = Q$).

The unavailability $Q_{s,2}(t)$ for Figure 8.10 is obtained from (8.16) or (8.21).

$$Q_{s,2}(t) = 1 - (1-Q)^3 = 3Q - 3Q^2 + Q^3 \tag{8.27}$$

Thus

$$Q_{s,2}(t) - Q_{s,1}(t) = 3Q(1-Q)^3 > 0, \quad \text{for } 0 < Q < 1 \tag{8.28}$$

and we conclude that the safety system with a two-out-of-three configuration has a smaller probability of spurious shutdowns than the system with the simple OR configuration. ■

Example 2—Simple combination of gates. Calculate the unavailability of the system described by the fault tree of Figure 8.11, given the basic events probabilities shown in the tree.

Solution: Using (8.16) for OR gate $G1$:

$$\Pr\{G1\} = 1 - (1-0.05)(1-0.07)(1-0.1) = 0.20 \tag{8.29}$$

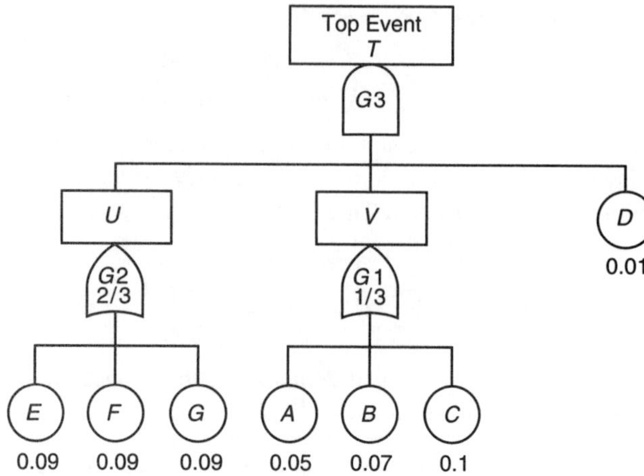

Figure 8.11. Simple combination of gates.

For the two-out-of-three gate $G2$, by (8.25):

$$\begin{aligned} \Pr\{G2\} &= \sum_{k=2}^{3} \binom{3}{k} 0.09^k (1-0.09)^{3-k} \\ &= \binom{3}{2} 0.09^2 (1-0.09) + \binom{3}{3} 0.09^3 (1-0.09)^0 && (8.30) \\ &= 0.023 && (8.31) \end{aligned}$$

Using (8.12) for AND gate $G3$:

$$\begin{aligned} Q_s(t) &= \Pr\{G3\} = \Pr\{G1\}\Pr\{G2\}\Pr\{D\} \\ &= (0.20)(0.023)(0.01) = 4.6 \times 10^{-5} \end{aligned} \quad (8.32)$$

■

Example 3—Tail-gas quench and clean-up system [2]. The system in Figure 8.12 is designed to: 1) decrease the temperature of a hot gas by a water quench, 2) saturate the gas with water vapor, and 3) remove solid particles entrained in the gas.

A hot "tail" gas from a calciner is first cooled by contacting it with water supplied by quench pumps B or C. It then passes to a prescrubber where it is contacted with more fresh water supplied by feedwater pump D. Water from the bottom of the prescrubber is either recirculated by pumps E or F or removed as a purge stream. Mesh pad G removes particulates from the gases that flow to an absorber after they leave the prescrubber.

A simplified fault tree is shown in Figure 8.13. The booster fan (A), both of the quench pumps (B and C), the feedwater pump (D), both of the circulation pumps (E and F), or the filter system (G) must fail for the top event T to occur. The top event expression for this fault tree is

$$T = A \cup (B \cap C) \cup D \cup (E \cap F) \cup G \quad (8.33)$$

Calculate the system unavailability $Q_s(t) = \Pr\{T\}$ using as data:

$$\begin{aligned} &\Pr\{A\} = 0.9, \quad \Pr\{B\} = 0.8, \quad \Pr\{C\} = 0.7, \quad \Pr\{D\} = 0.6, \\ &\Pr\{E\} = 0.5, \quad \Pr\{F\} = 0.4, \quad \Pr\{G\} = 0.3 \end{aligned} \quad (8.34)$$

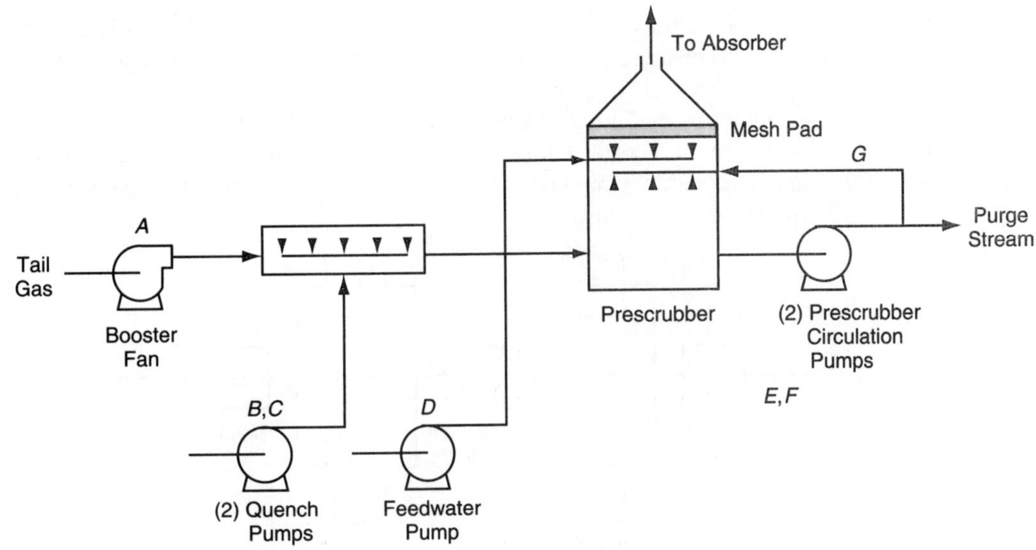

Figure 8.12. Schematic diagram of tail-gas quench and clean-up system.

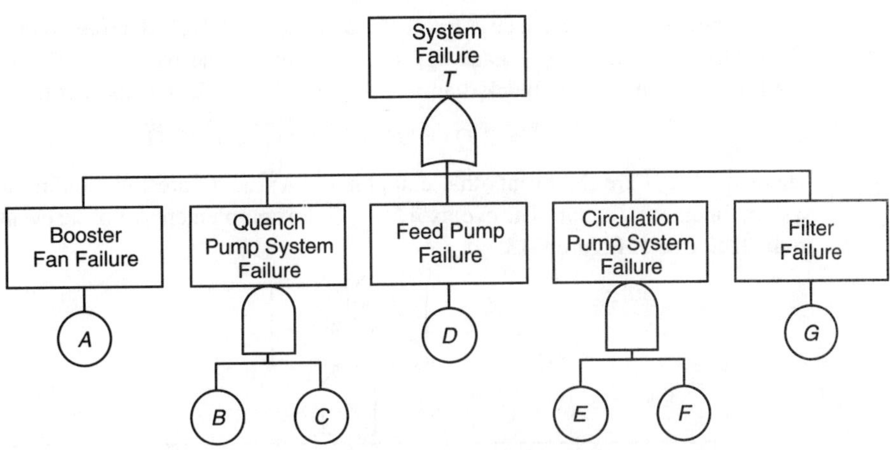

Figure 8.13. Fault tree for tail-gas quench and clean-up system.

Solution: We proceed in a stepwise fashion:

$$
\begin{aligned}
\Pr\{B \cap C\} &= (0.8)(0.7) = 0.56 \\
\Pr\{A \cup (B \cap C)\} &= 0.9 + 0.56 - (0.9)(0.56) = 0.96 \\
\Pr\{A \cup (B \cap C) \cup D\} &= 0.96 + 0.6 - (0.96)(0.6) = 0.98 \\
\Pr\{E \cap F\} &= (0.5)(0.4) = 0.2 \\
\Pr\{A \cup (B \cap C) \cup D \cup (E \cap F)\} &= 0.98 + 0.2 - (0.98)(0.2) = 0.98 \\
Q_s(t) = \Pr\{T\} &= 0.98 + 0.3 - (0.98)(0.3) = 0.99
\end{aligned}
\tag{8.35}
$$

■

8.2.5 Reliability Block Diagrams

Reliability block diagrams are an alternative way of representing events and gates, as are success trees, which are the mathematical duals of fault trees in which the top of the tree represents system success, and the events are success rather than failure states. The relationship between these three forms of system representation can best be shown by example.

Consider again the system of Figure 8.12. The reliability block diagram is given as Figure 8.14, where the booster fan ($\overline{A}$), either quench pump ($\overline{B}$ or $\overline{C}$), the feedwater pump ($\overline{D}$), either circulation pump ($\overline{E}$ or $\overline{F}$), and the filter system ($\overline{G}$) must be operating successfully for the system to work.

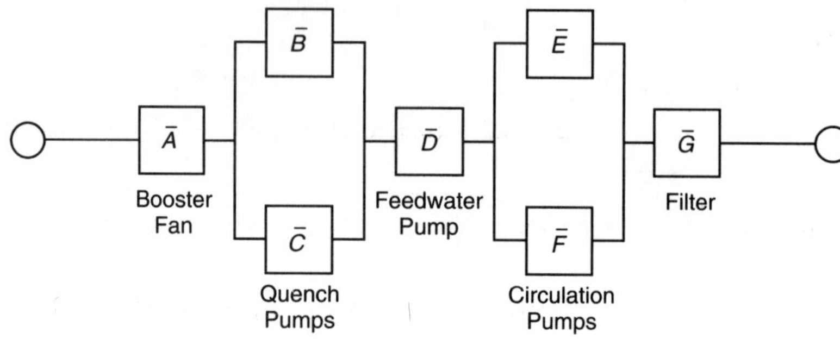

Figure 8.14. Reliability block diagram for tail-gas quench and clean-up system.

Figure 8.15 is the success-tree equivalent to the block diagram representation in Figure 8.14. Boolean logic gates are used to indicate the parallel (OR) and the series (AND) connections in the block diagram. The expression for the success tree is

$$\overline{T} = \overline{A} \cap (\overline{B} \cup \overline{C}) \cap \overline{D} \cap (\overline{E} \cup \overline{F}) \cap \overline{G} \tag{8.36}$$

where $\overline{A}, \ldots, \overline{G}$ are the events that components $A, \ldots, G$ are functioning, and $\overline{T}$ is the system functioning event. The events $\overline{A}, \ldots, \overline{G}$ are complements of basic events $A, \ldots, G$ in the fault tree of Figure 8.13.

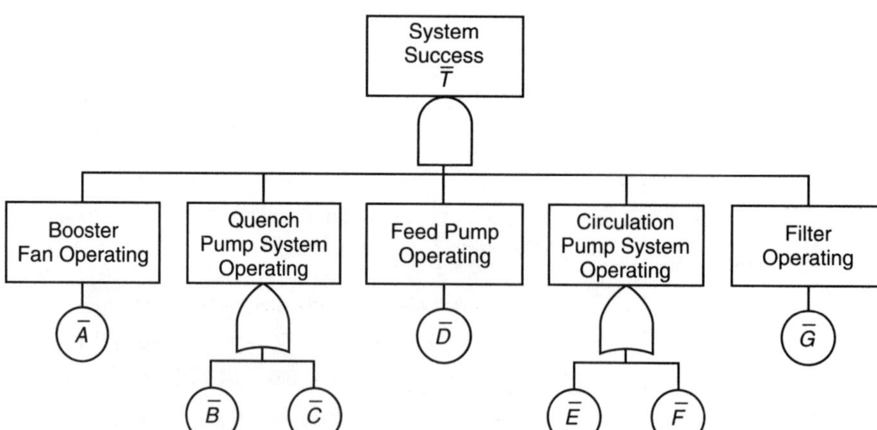

Figure 8.15. Success tree for tail-gas quench and clean-up system.

Because the system is either functioning or failed at time t, the $\overline{T}$ of (8.36) is the complement of event T of (8.33). This complementary relation between (8.36) and (8.33) can also be stated in terms of de Morgan's law, which—for systems such as Figures 8.13 and 8.15—states that if $\overline{T}$ is complementary to T, we can obtain $\overline{T}$ from the negation of the Boolean expression for T, that is, by interchanging ANDs and ORs and replacing A by $\overline{A}$,

B by $\overline{B}$, and so forth. This is proven by examining (8.33) and (8.36) or Figures 8.13 and 8.15.

The system availability $A_s(t)$ is calculated from the probability $\Pr\{\overline{T}\}$ in the following way.

From (8.34) in Example 3:

$$\begin{aligned} &\Pr\{\overline{A}\} = 0.1, \quad \Pr\{\overline{B}\} = 0.2, \quad \Pr\{\overline{C}\} = 0.3, \quad \Pr\{\overline{D}\} = 0.4, \\ &\Pr\{\overline{E}\} = 0.5, \quad \Pr\{\overline{F}\} = 0.6, \quad \Pr\{\overline{G}\} = 0.7 \end{aligned} \tag{8.37}$$

Hence

$$\begin{aligned} A_s(t) &= \Pr\{\overline{T}\} \\ &= (0.1)[0.3 + 0.2 - (0.3)(0.2)](0.4)[0.6 + 0.5 - (0.6)(0.5)](0.7) \\ &= 0.0099 \end{aligned} \tag{8.38}$$

The availability and the unavailability in the preceding example agree with identity (8.1) within round-off errors:

$$A_s(t) + Q_s(t) = 0.0099 + 0.99 = 0.9999 \simeq 1 \tag{8.39}$$

The foregoing examples show that:

1. A parallel reliability block diagram corresponds to a gated AND fault tree, and a series block diagram to a gated OR fault tree (Table 8.1).

TABLE 8.1. Reliability Block Diagram Versus Fault Tree

	Reliability Block Diagram	Fault Tree
Series System	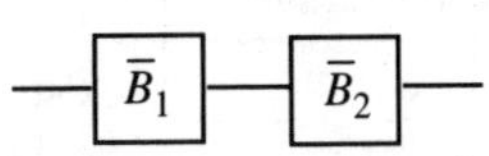 $\Pr\{\overline{B}_1 \cap \overline{B}_2\} = \Pr\{\overline{B}_1\}\Pr\{\overline{B}_2\}$	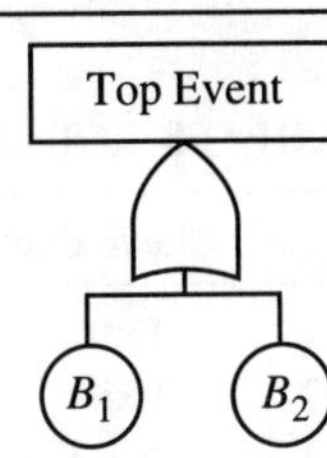 $\Pr\{B_1 \cup B_2\} = \Pr\{B_1\} + \Pr\{B_2\} - \Pr\{B_1\}\Pr\{B_2\}$
Parallel System	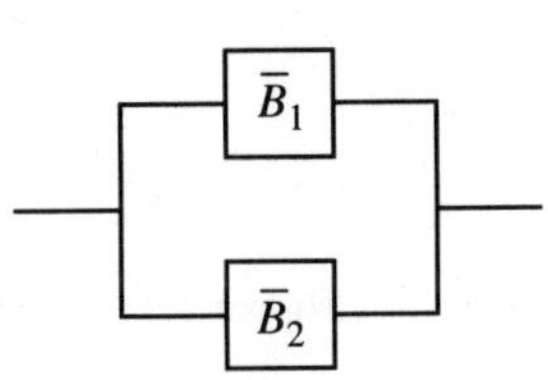 $\Pr\{\overline{B}_1 \cup \overline{B}_2\} = \Pr\{\overline{B}_1\} + \Pr\{\overline{B}_2\} - \Pr\{\overline{B}_1\}\Pr\{\overline{B}_2\}$	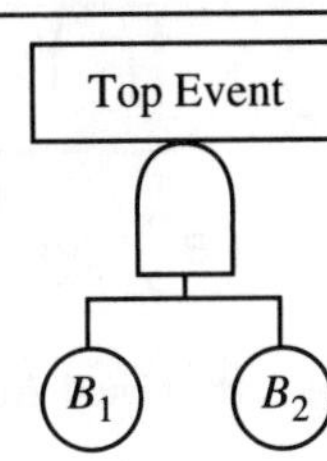 $\Pr\{B_1 \cap B_2\} = \Pr\{B_1\}\Pr\{B_2\}$

2. The unavailability calculation methods for fault trees can be extended directly to availability calculations for success trees when basic events $B_1, \ldots, B_n$ are replaced by their complementary events $\overline{B}_1, \ldots, \overline{B}_n$ in (8.10) and (8.16):

$$\Pr\{\overline{B}_1 \cap \overline{B}_2 \cap \cdots \cap \overline{B}_n\} = \prod_{i=1}^{n} \Pr\{\overline{B}_i\} \tag{8.40}$$

$$\Pr\{\overline{B}_1 \cup \overline{B}_2 \cup \cdots \cup \overline{B}_n\} = 1 - \prod_{i=1}^{n}[1 - \Pr\{\overline{B}_i\}] \tag{8.41}$$

$$= 1 - \prod_{i=1}^{n} \Pr\{B_i\} \tag{8.42}$$

8.3 TRUTH-TABLE APPROACH

A truth table is a listing of all combinations of basic event states, the resulting existence or nonexistence of a top event, and the corresponding probabilities for these combinations. A summation of a set of probabilities in the table yields the system unavailability $Q_s(t)$, and a complementary summation gives the system availability $A_s(t)$.

8.3.1 AND Gate

Table 8.2 is a truth table for the system of Figure 8.16. The system unavailability $Q_s(t)$ is given by row 1:

$$Q_s(t) = \Pr\{B_1\}\Pr\{B_2\} \tag{8.43}$$

TABLE 8.2. Truth Table for Gated AND Fault Tree

	Basic Event B_1	Basic Event B_2	Top Event	Probability
1	Exists	Exists	Exists	$\Pr\{B_1\}\Pr\{B_2\}$
2	Exists	Not Exist	Not Exist	$\Pr\{B_1\}\Pr\{\overline{B}_2\}$
3	Not Exist	Exists	Not Exist	$\Pr\{\overline{B}_1\}\Pr\{B_2\}$
4	Not Exist	Not Exist	Not Exist	$\Pr\{\overline{B}_1\}\Pr\{\overline{B}_2\}$

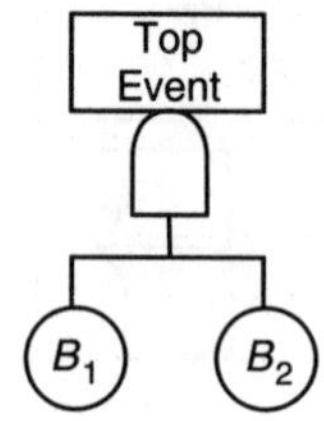

Figure 8.16. Gated AND fault tree.

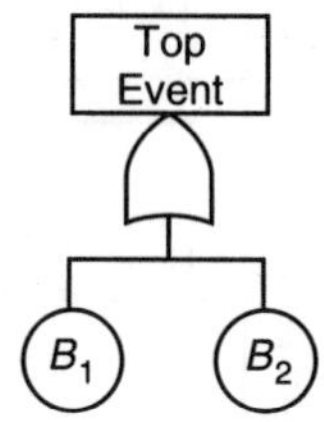

Figure 8.17. Gated OR fault tree.

8.3.2 OR Gate

The system of Figure 8.17 is represented by the truth table of Table 8.3. The unavailability $Q_s(t)$ is obtained by a summation of the probabilities of the mutually exclusive rows 1, 2, and 3.

TABLE 8.3. Truth Table for Gated OR Fault Tree

	Basic Event B_1	Basic Event B_2	Top Event	Probability
1	Exists	Exists	Exists	$\Pr\{B_1\}\Pr\{B_2\}$
2	Exists	Not Exist	Exists	$\Pr\{B_1\}\Pr\{\overline{B}_2\}$
3	Not Exist	Exists	Exists	$\Pr\{\overline{B}_1\}\Pr\{B_2\}$
4	Not Exist	Not Exist	Not Exist	$\Pr\{\overline{B}_1\}\Pr\{\overline{B}_2\}$

$$\begin{aligned} Q_s(t) &= \Pr\{B_1\}\Pr\{B_2\} + \Pr\{B_1\}\Pr\{\overline{B}_2\} + \Pr\{\overline{B}_1\}\Pr\{B_2\} \\ &= \Pr\{B_1\}\Pr\{B_2\} + \Pr\{B_1\}[1 - \Pr\{B_2\}] + [1 - \Pr\{B_1\}]\Pr\{B_2\} \\ &= \Pr\{B_1\} + \Pr\{B_2\} - \Pr\{B_1\}\Pr\{B_2\} \end{aligned} \tag{8.44}$$

This confirms equation (8.20).

Example 4—Pump-filter system. A truth table provides a tedious but reliable technique for calculating the availability and unavailability for moderately complicated systems, as illustrated by the following example.*

A plant has two identical, parallel streams, A and B, consisting of one transfer pump and one rotary filter (Figure 8.18). The failure rate of the pumps and filters are, respectively, 0.04 and 0.08 failures per day, whether equipment is in operation or standby. Assume MTTRs for the pumps and filters of 5 and 10 hr, respectively.

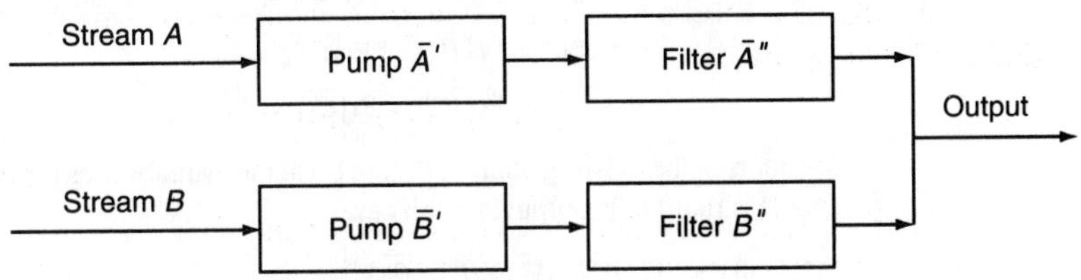

Figure 8.18. Two parallel process streams.

Two alternative schemes to increase plant availability are:

1. Add a third identical stream, C (Figure 8.19).
2. Install a third transfer pump capable of pumping slurry to either filter (Figure 8.20).

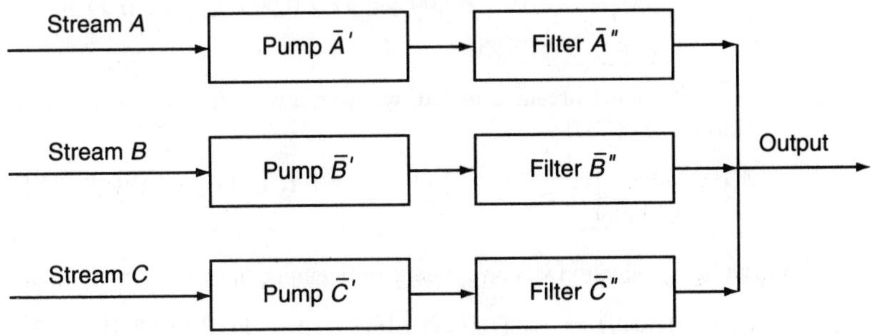

Figure 8.19. Three parallel process streams.

*Courtesy of B. Bulloch, ICI Ltd., Runcorn, England.

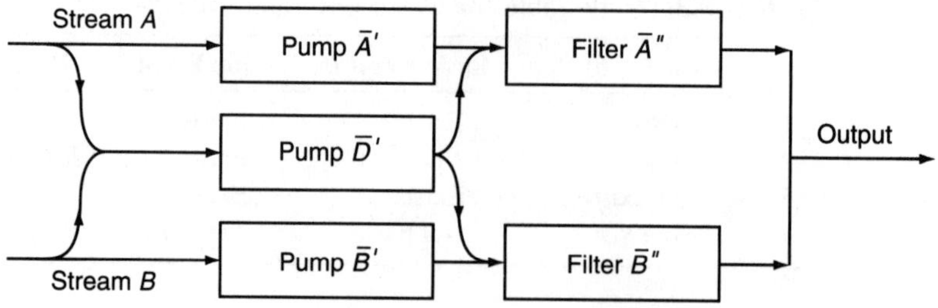

Figure 8.20. Additional spare pump $\overline{D}$.

Compare the effect of these two schemes on the ability of the plant to maintain: a) full output; b) not less than half output.

Solution:

1. Making the usual constant-failure and repair rates assumption, the steady-state availabilities for the filter and the pump become (see Table 6.10)

$$A(\text{filter}) = \frac{\text{MTTF}}{\text{MTTF} + \text{MTTR}} = \frac{1/0.08}{1/0.08 + 10/24} = 0.97$$
$$A(\text{pump}) = \frac{\text{MTTF}}{\text{MTTF} + \text{MTTR}} = \frac{1/0.04}{1/0.04 + 5/24} = 0.99$$

Thus the steady-state event probabilities are given by

$$\Pr\{\overline{A''}\} = \Pr\{\overline{B''}\} = \Pr\{\overline{C''}\} = 0.97$$
$$\Pr\{\overline{A'}\} = \Pr\{\overline{B'}\} = \Pr\{\overline{C'}\} = \Pr\{\overline{D'}\} = 0.99$$

Considering the existing plant of Figure 8.18, the availabilities for full output A_s(full) and for (not less than) half output A_s(half) are

$$\begin{aligned}
A_s(\text{full}) &= \Pr\{\overline{A'} \cap \overline{A''} \cap \overline{B'} \cap \overline{B''}\} \\
&= \Pr\{\overline{A'}\}\Pr\{\overline{A''}\}\Pr\{\overline{B'}\}\Pr\{\overline{B''}\} \\
&= 0.97^2 \times 0.99^2 = 0.92 \\
A_s(\text{half}) &= \Pr\{[\overline{A'} \cap \overline{A''}] \cup [\overline{B'} \cap \overline{B''}]\} \\
&= \Pr\{\overline{A'} \cap \overline{A''}\} + \Pr\{\overline{B'} \cap \overline{B''}\} - \Pr\{\overline{A'} \cap \overline{A''}\}\Pr\{\overline{B'} \cap \overline{B''}\} \\
&= \Pr\{\overline{A'}\}\Pr\{\overline{A''}\} + \Pr\{\overline{B'}\}\Pr\{\overline{B''}\} - \Pr\{\overline{A'}\}\Pr\{\overline{A''}\}\Pr\{\overline{B'}\}\Pr\{\overline{B''}\} \\
&= 0.97 \times 0.99 + 0.97 \times 0.99 - 0.97^2 \times 0.99^2 \\
&= 0.9984
\end{aligned}$$

If a third stream is added, we have a two-out-of-three system for full production. Thus using (8.25)

$$\begin{aligned}
A_s(\text{full}) &= 3 \cdot [\Pr\{\overline{A'}\}\Pr\{\overline{A''}\}]^2[1 - \Pr\{\overline{A'}\}\Pr\{\overline{A''}\}] + [\Pr\{\overline{A'}\}\Pr\{\overline{A''}\}]^3[1 - \Pr\{\overline{A'}\}\Pr\{\overline{A''}\}]^0 \\
&= 0.9954
\end{aligned}$$

For half production we have three parallel units, thus:

$$\begin{aligned}
A_s(\text{half}) &= 1 - [1 - \Pr\{\overline{A'}\}\Pr\{\overline{A''}\}][1 - \Pr\{\overline{B'}\}\Pr\{\overline{B''}\}][1 - \Pr\{\overline{C'}\}\Pr\{\overline{C''}\}] \\
&= 0.99994
\end{aligned}$$

2. Calculation of the availability of the configuration shown as Figure 8.20 represents a problem because this is a bridged network and cannot be reduced to a simple parallel system. A

truth table is used to enumerate all possible component states and select the combinations that give full and half output (Table 8.4). The availability for full production is given by

$$\begin{aligned}
A_s(\text{full}) &= \sum \Pr\{\text{rows } 1, 2, 5, 17\} \\
&= \Pr\{\overline{A'}\}\Pr\{\overline{A''}\}\Pr\{\overline{B'}\}\Pr\{\overline{B''}\}\Pr\{\overline{D'}\} + \Pr\{\overline{A'}\}\Pr\{\overline{A''}\}\Pr\{\overline{B'}\}\Pr\{\overline{B''}\}[1 - \Pr\{\overline{D'}\}] \\
&\quad + \Pr\{\overline{A'}\}\Pr\{\overline{A''}\}[1 - \Pr\{\overline{B'}\}]\Pr\{\overline{B''}\}\Pr\{\overline{D'}\} \\
&\quad + [1 - \Pr\{\overline{A'}\}]\Pr\{\overline{A''}\}\Pr\{\overline{B'}\}\Pr\{\overline{B''}\}\Pr\{\overline{D'}\} \\
&= 0.94
\end{aligned}$$

TABLE 8.4. State Enumeration for System with Additional Spare Pump D'

State	$\overline{A'}$	$\overline{A''}$	$\overline{B'}$	$\overline{B''}$	$\overline{D'}$	Full Output	Half Output
1	W	W	W	W	W	W	W
2	W	W	W	W	F	W	W
3	W	W	W	F	W	F	W
4	W	W	W	F	F	F	W
5	W	W	F	W	W	W	W
6	W	W	F	W	F	F	W
7	W	W	F	F	W	F	W
8	W	W	F	F	F	F	W
9	W	F	W	W	W	F	W
10	W	F	W	W	F	F	W
11	W	F	W	F	W	F	F
12	W	F	W	F	F	F	F
13	W	F	F	W	W	F	W
14	W	F	F	W	F	F	F
15	W	F	F	F	W	F	F
16	W	F	F	F	F	F	F
17	F	W	W	W	W	W	W
18	F	W	W	W	F	F	W
19	F	W	W	F	W	F	W
20	F	W	W	F	F	F	F
21	F	W	F	W	W	F	W
22	F	W	F	W	F	F	F
23	F	W	F	F	W	F	W
24	F	W	F	F	F	F	F
25	F	F	W	W	W	F	W
26	F	F	W	W	F	F	W
27	F	F	W	F	W	F	F
28	F	F	W	F	F	F	F
29	F	F	F	W	W	F	W
30	F	F	F	W	F	F	F
31	F	F	F	F	W	F	F
32	F	F	F	F	F	F	F

W: working, F: failed

There are so many states leading to half production that it is easier to work with the unavailability Q_s(half).

$$Q_s(\text{half}) = \sum \Pr\{\text{rows } 11, 12, 14, 15, 16, 20, 22, 24, 27, 28, 30, 31, 32\}$$
$$= 0.001$$

yielding

$$A_s(\text{half}) = 1 - Q_s(\text{half}) = 0.999 \tag{8.45}$$

The results are summarized in columns 2 and 3 of Table 8.5. The availabilities, when coupled with economic data on the equipment capital costs and the cost of lost production, permit economic assessments to be made. If, for example, the full cost of a pump (including maintenance, installation, etc.) is \$15 per day and a filter costs \$60 per day and the costs of full- and half-production lost are \$10,000 per day and \$2,000 per day, respectively, then the expected loss can be calculated by the following formula.

$$\text{expected loss/day (dollars)} = n' \times 15 + n'' \times 60 + [1 - A_s(\text{half})] \times 10{,}000 + [A_s(\text{half}) - A_s(\text{full})] \times 2{,}000 \tag{8.46}$$

where n' = the number of pumps,
n'' = the number of filters.

TABLE 8.5. Comparison of Costs for Three Plants

Plant	A_s(full)	A_s(half)	Expected Cost
Existing Plant	0.92	0.9984	\$323/day
Plant with spare stream	0.9954	0.9994	\$239/day
Plant with spare pump	0.94	0.999	\$293/day

The formula is illustrated by Figure 8.21. Note that $1 - A_s$(half) is the proportion of the plant operation time expected to result in full-production lost, and $A_s(\text{half}) - A_s(\text{full})$ is the proportion resulting in half-production lost. The expected costs are summarized in Table 8.5. We observe that the plant with the spare stream is the best choice. ■

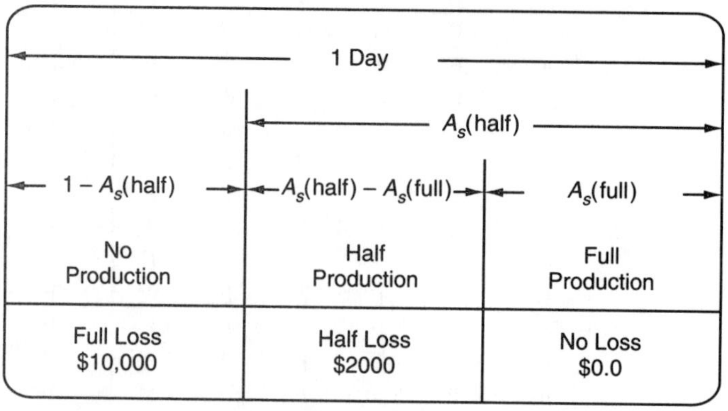

Figure 8.21. Illustration of expected loss per day.

8.4 STRUCTURE-FUNCTION APPROACH

8.4.1 Structure Functions

It is possible to describe the state of the basic event or the system by a binary indicator variable. If we assign a binary indicator variable Y_i to the basic event i, then

$$Y_i = \begin{cases} 1, & \text{when the basic event exists} \\ 0, & \text{when the event does not exist} \end{cases} \tag{8.47}$$

Similarly, the top event is associated with a binary indicator variable $\psi(Y)$ related to the state of the system by

$$\psi(Y) = \begin{cases} 1, & \text{when the top event exists} \\ 0, & \text{when the top event does not exist} \end{cases} \tag{8.48}$$

Here $Y = (Y_1, Y_2, \ldots, Y_n)$ is the vector of basic event states. The function $\psi(Y)$ is known as the structure function for the top event.

8.4.2 System Representation

8.4.2.1 Gated AND tree. The top event of the gated AND tree in Figure 8.2 exists if and only if all basic events $B_1, \ldots, B_n$ exist. In terms of the system structure function,

$$\psi(Y) = \psi(Y_1, Y_2, \ldots, Y_n) = \bigwedge_{i=1}^{n} Y_i = Y_1 \wedge Y_2 \wedge \cdots \wedge Y_n \tag{8.49}$$

where Y_i is an indicator variable for the basic event B_i.

The structure function can be expressed in terms of algebraic operators (see Table A.2, appendix of Chapter 3):

$$\psi(Y) = \prod_{i=1}^{n} Y_i = Y_1 Y_2 \cdots Y_n \tag{8.50}$$

8.4.2.2 Gated OR tree. The gated OR tree of Figure 8.3 fails (the top event exists) if any of the basic events $B_1, B_2, \ldots, B_n$ exist. The structure function is

$$\psi(Y) = \bigvee_{i=1}^{n} Y_i = Y_1 \vee Y_2 \vee \cdots \vee Y_n \tag{8.51}$$

and its algebraic form is

$$\psi(Y) = 1 - \prod_{i=1}^{n} [1 - Y_i] \tag{8.52}$$

$$= 1 - [1 - Y_1][1 - Y_2] \cdots [1 - Y_n] \tag{8.53}$$

If the n in Figure 8.3 is two, that is, for a two-event series structure

$$\psi(Y) = Y_1 \vee Y_2 = 1 - [1 - Y_1][1 - Y_2] \tag{8.54}$$

$$= Y_1 + Y_2 - Y_1 Y_2 \tag{8.55}$$

This result is analogous to (8.20): Here $Y_1 Y_2$ represent the probability of the intersecting portion of the two events B_1 and B_2.

8.4.2.3 Two-out-of-three system. A slightly more sophisticated example is the two-out-of-three voting system of Figure 8.8. The structure function is

$$\psi(Y) = (Y_1 \wedge Y_2) \vee (Y_2 \wedge Y_3) \vee (Y_3 \wedge Y_1) \tag{8.56}$$

and its algebraic expression is obtained in the following way:

$$\psi(Y) = 1 - [1 - (Y_1 \wedge Y_2)][1 - (Y_2 \wedge Y_3)][1 - (Y_3 \wedge Y_1)] \tag{8.57}$$

$$= 1 - [1 - Y_1 Y_2][1 - Y_2 Y_3][1 - Y_3 Y_1] \tag{8.58}$$

This equation can be expanded and simplified by the absorption law of Table A.3, Chapter 3:

$$\begin{aligned}\psi(Y) = 1 - [1 &- Y_1Y_2 - Y_2Y_3 - Y_3Y_1 + Y_1Y_2Y_2Y_3 + Y_2Y_3Y_3Y_1 \\ &+ Y_3Y_1Y_1Y_2 - Y_1Y_2Y_2Y_3Y_3Y_1]\end{aligned} \tag{8.59}$$

$$= Y_1Y_2 + Y_2Y_3 + Y_3Y_1 - 2Y_1Y_2Y_3 \tag{8.60}$$

where the absorption law

$$Y_1Y_2Y_2Y_3 = Y_2Y_3Y_3Y_1 = Y_3Y_1Y_1Y_2 = Y_1Y_2Y_2Y_3Y_3Y_1 = Y_1Y_2Y_3 \tag{8.61}$$

was used in going from (8.59) to (8.60).

8.4.2.4 Tail-gas quench and clean-up system. Structure functions can be obtained in a stepwise way. Denote by $\psi_1(Y)$ and $\psi_2(Y)$ the structure functions for the first and second AND gates of Figure 8.13:

$$\psi_1(Y) = Y_B \wedge Y_C = Y_B Y_C, \qquad \psi_2(Y) = Y_E \wedge Y_F = Y_E Y_F \tag{8.62}$$

Here, Y_B is an indicator variable for basic event B, and so on. The structure function for the fault tree is

$$\begin{aligned}\psi(Y) &= Y_A \vee \psi_1(Y) \vee Y_D \vee \psi_2(Y) \vee Y_G \\ &= 1 - [1 - Y_A][1 - \psi_1(Y)][1 - Y_D][1 - \psi_2(Y)][1 - Y_G] \\ &= 1 - [1 - Y_A][1 - Y_B Y_C][1 - Y_D][1 - Y_E Y_F][1 - Y_G]\end{aligned} \tag{8.63}$$

8.4.3 Unavailability Calculations

It is of significance to recognize the probabilistic nature of expressions such as (8.55), (8.60), and (8.63). If we examine the system at some point in time, and the state of the basic event Y_i is assumed to be a Bernoulli or zero-one random variable, then $\psi(Y)$ is also a Bernoulli random variable. The probability of existence of state $Y_i = 1$ is equal to the expected value of Y_i and to the event B_i probability.

$$\Pr\{Y_i = 1\} = \Pr\{B_i\} = E\{Y_i\} \tag{8.64}$$

Notice that this probability is the unavailability $Q_i(t)$, or existence probability, depending on whether basic event B_i is a component failure or human error or environmental impact. The probability of the top event, that is, the unavailability $Q_s(t)$ is the probability $\Pr\{\psi(Y) = 1\}$, or expectation $E\{\psi(Y)\}$. An alternative way of stating this is as follows:

$$Q_s(t) = \Pr\{\text{top event}\} \tag{8.65}$$

$$= \Pr\{\psi(Y) = 1\} = E\{\psi(Y)\} \tag{8.66}$$

$$= \sum_Y \psi(Y)\Pr\{Y\} \tag{8.67}$$

The next three examples demonstrate the use of structure functions in system analysis.

Example 5—Two-out-of-three system. Compare the unavailability for a two-out-of-three voting system with that of a two-component series system for

$$E\{Y_1\} = E\{Y_2\} = E\{Y_3\} = Q = 0.6 \tag{8.68}$$

Solution: For the two-out-of-three system, according to (8.60)

$$\begin{aligned} Q_s(t) &= E\{\psi(Y)\} \\ &= E\{Y_1Y_2\} + E\{Y_2Y_3\} + E\{Y_3Y_1\} - 2E\{Y_1Y_2Y_3\} && (8.69) \\ &= E\{Y_1\}E\{Y_2\} + E\{Y_2\}E\{Y_3\} + E\{Y_3\}E\{Y_1\} - 2E\{Y_1\}E\{Y_2\}E\{Y_3\} && (8.70) \\ &= 3 \times 0.6^2 - 2 \times 0.6^3 = 0.65 && (8.71) \end{aligned}$$

Note that the expectation of the product of independent variables is equal to the product of expectation of these variables. This property is used in going from (8.69) to (8.70).

For the series system, from equation (8.55),

$$\begin{aligned} Q_s(t) &= E\{\psi(Y)\} = E\{Y_1\} + E\{Y_2\} - E\{Y_1\}E\{Y_2\} \\ &= 2 \times 0.6 - 0.6^2 = 0.84 \end{aligned}$$

Hence a one-out-of-two system has an 84% chance of being in the top event state, and the two-out-of-three system has a smaller, 64.8% probability. ■

Example 6—Tail-gas quench and clean-up system. Calculate the system unavailability $Q_s(t)$ for the fault tree of Figure 8.13, assuming component unavailabilities of (8.34).

Solution: According to (8.63) we have

$$\begin{aligned} Q_s(t) &= E\{\psi(Y)\} \\ &= 1 - E\{[1 - Y_A][1 - Y_BY_C][1 - Y_D][1 - Y_EY_F][1 - Y_G]\} \end{aligned} \tag{8.72}$$

Each factor in the expected value operator E of this equation has different indicator variables, and these factors are independent because the indicator variables are assumed to be independent. Thus (8.72) can be written as

$$\begin{aligned} Q_s(t) &= 1 - E\{1 - Y_A\}E\{1 - Y_BY_C\}E\{1 - Y_D\}E\{1 - Y_EY_F\}E\{1 - Y_G\} && (8.73) \\ &= 1 - [1 - E\{Y_A\}][1 - E\{Y_B\}E\{Y_C\}] \\ &\quad \times [1 - E\{Y_D\}][1 - E\{Y_E\}E\{Y_F\}][1 - E\{Y_G\}] && (8.74) \end{aligned}$$

The component unavailabilities of (8.34) give

$$\begin{aligned} Q_s(t) &= 1 - [1 - 0.9][1 - (0.8)(0.7)][1 - 0.6][1 - (0.5)(0.4)][1 - 0.3] \\ &= 0.99 \end{aligned} \tag{8.75}$$

This confirms the result of (8.35).

Contrary to (8.72), each indicator variable appears more than once in the products of (8.58), the structure function for a two-out-of-three system. For example, the variable Y_2 appears in $[1 - Y_1Y_2]$ and $[1 - Y_2Y_3]$. Here we cannot proceed as we did in going from (8.72) to (8.74) because these factors are no longer independent. This is confirmed by the following derivation, which gives an incorrect result:

$$\begin{aligned} Q_s(t) &= 1 - E\{1 - Y_1Y_2\}E\{1 - Y_2Y_3\}E\{1 - Y_3Y_1\} \\ &= 1 - [1 - E\{Y_1\}E\{Y_1\}][1 - E\{Y_2\}E\{Y_3\}][1 - E\{Y_3\}E\{Y_1\}] \end{aligned}$$

Substituting (8.68) into the above,

$$Q_s(t) = 1 - [1 - 0.6^2]^3 = 0.74 \tag{8.76}$$

This contradicts (8.71). ■

If $\psi_1(Y)$ and $\psi_2(Y)$ have one or more common variables, then in general

$$E\{\psi_1(Y)\psi_2(Y)\} \neq E\{\psi_1(Y)\}E\{\psi_2(Y)\} \tag{8.77}$$

On the other hand, the following equation always holds regardless of the common variables.

$$E\{\psi_1(Y) + \psi_2(Y)\} = E\{\psi_1(Y)\} + E\{\psi_2(Y)\} \tag{8.78}$$

A structure function can be expanded into a sum of products (sop) expression, where each product has no common variables. An extreme version is a truth table expansion given by

$$\psi(Y) = \sum_u \psi(u)\left[\prod_{i=1}^{n} Y_i^{u_i}(1-Y_i)^{1-u_i}\right] \tag{8.79}$$

$$E\{\psi(Y)\} = \sum_u \psi(u)\left[\prod_{i=1}^{n} Q_i^{u_i}(1-Q_i)^{1-u_i}\right] \tag{8.80}$$

where

$$Y_i^{u_i}(1-Y_i)^{1-u_i} = \begin{cases} Y_i, & \text{if } u_i = 1, \\ 1-Y_i, & \text{if } u_i = 0 \end{cases} \tag{8.81}$$

$$Q_i^{u_i}(1-Q_i)^{1-u_i} = \begin{cases} Q_i, & \text{if } u_i = 1, \\ 1-Q_i, & \text{if } u_i = 0 \end{cases} \tag{8.82}$$

Expression (8.79) is the canonical form of $\psi(y)$.

Example 7—Bridged circuit. Draw a fault tree for the case of full production for the bridged circuit of Figure 8.20, and calculate the system unavailability.

Solution: The condensed fault tree is shown as Figure 8.22.

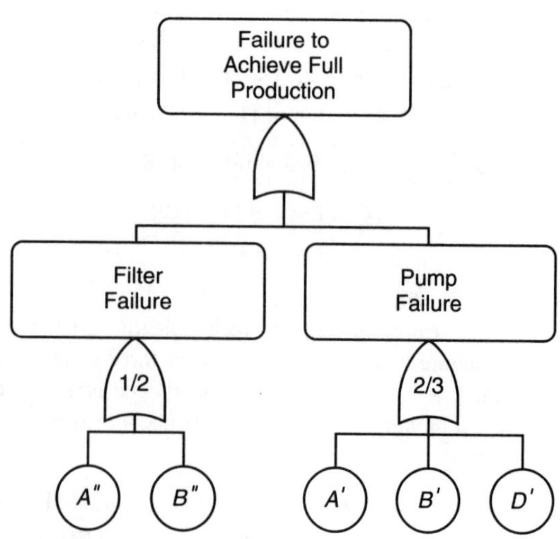

Figure 8.22. Condensed fault tree for full production.

$$\begin{aligned} \Pr\{A''\} &= \Pr\{B''\} = 0.032 \\ \Pr\{A'' \cup B''\} &= 0.032 + 0.032 - (0.032)(0.032) = 0.063 \\ \Pr\{A'\} &= \Pr\{B'\} = \Pr\{D'\} = 0.008 \\ Q_s(t) &= \Pr\{A'' \cup B'' \cup (A' \cap D') \cup (D' \cap B') \cup (A' \cap B')\} \end{aligned} \tag{8.83}$$

The three pumps constitute a two-out-of-three voting system, so we can use the results of equation (8.60).

$$\begin{aligned}\Pr\{(A' \cap D') \cup (D' \cap B') \cup (A' \cap B')\} &= Y_{A'}Y_{B'} + Y_{B'}Y_{D'} + Y_{D'}Y_{A'} - 2Y_{A'}Y_{B'}Y_{D'} \\ &= 3Q^2 - 2Q^3 = 3(0.008)^2 - 2(0.008)^3 \\ &= 0.00019\end{aligned} \tag{8.84}$$

Thus

$$Q_s(t) = (0.063) + (0.00019) - (0.063)(0.00019) = 0.063 \tag{8.85}$$

This confirms the result of Table 8.5. ■

8.5 APPROACHES BASED ON MINIMAL CUTS OR MINIMAL PATHS

8.5.1 Minimal Cut Representations

The preceding section gave a method for constructing structure functions for calculating system unavailability. In this section another approach, based on minimal cut or path sets, is developed.

Consider a fault tree having the following m minimal cut sets.

$$\begin{aligned}&\{B_{1,1}, B_{2,1}, \ldots, B_{n_1,1}\}: \quad \text{cut set } 1\\ &\qquad\vdots\\ &\{B_{1,j}, B_{2,j}, \ldots, B_{n_j,j}\}: \quad \text{cut set } j\\ &\qquad\vdots\\ &\{B_{1,m}, B_{2,m}, \ldots, B_{n_m,m}\}: \quad \text{cut set } m\end{aligned}$$

Denote by $Y_{i,j}$ the indicator variable for the event $B_{i,j}$. Subscript j refers to a particular cut set, and subscript i to an event in the cut set. Variables m and n denote the number of cut sets and the number of components in the cut set, respectively. The top event exists if and only if all basic events in a minimal cut set exist simultaneously. Thus the minimal-cut-set fault tree of Figure 8.23 is equivalent to the original fault tree. The structure function of this fault tree is

$$\psi(Y) = \bigvee_{j=1}^{m}\left[\bigwedge_{i=1}^{n_j} Y_{i,j}\right] \tag{8.86}$$

and its algebraic form is

$$\psi(Y) = \bigvee_{j=1}^{m}\left[\prod_{i=1}^{n_j} Y_{i,j}\right] \tag{8.87}$$

$$= 1 - \prod_{j=1}^{m}\left[1 - \prod_{i=1}^{n_j} Y_{i,j}\right] \tag{8.88}$$

Let $\kappa_j(Y)$ be a structure function for the AND gate G_j of Figure 8.23:

$$\kappa_j(Y) = \prod_{i=1}^{n_j} Y_{i,j} \tag{8.89}$$

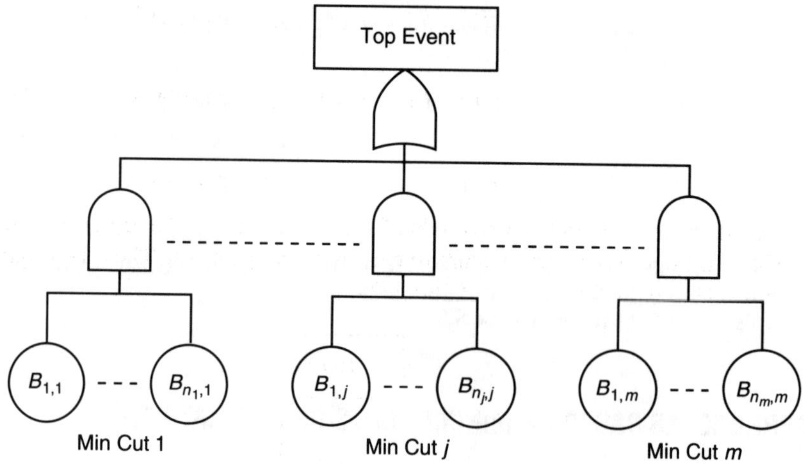

Figure 8.23. Minimal cut representation of fault tree.

The function $\kappa_j(Y)$ is the jth minimal cut structure to express the cut set existence. Equation (8.88) can be rewritten as

$$\psi(Y) = 1 - \prod_{j=1}^{m} [1 - \kappa_j(Y)] \tag{8.90}$$

This equation is important because it gives a structure function of the fault tree in terms of minimal cut structures $\kappa_j(Y)$'s. The structure function $\psi(Y)$ can be expanded and simplified by the absorption law, resulting in a polynomial similar to (8.60). The system unavailability $Q_s(t)$ is calculated using (8.66), as shown in the following example.

Example 8—Two-out-of-three system. Calculate the system unavailability for the two-out-of-three voting system in Figure 8.8. Unavailabilities for the three components are as given by (8.68).

Solution: The voting system has three minimal cut sets:

$$\{B_1, B_2\}, \qquad \{B_2, B_3\}, \qquad \{B_3, B_1\} \tag{8.91}$$

The minimal cut structures $\kappa_1(Y), \kappa_2(Y), \kappa_3(Y)$, are

$$\kappa_1(Y) = Y_1Y_2, \qquad \kappa_2(Y) = Y_2Y_3, \qquad \kappa_3(Y) = Y_3Y_1 \tag{8.92}$$

Thus the minimal cut representation of the structure function $\psi(Y)$ is

$$\psi(Y) = 1 - [1 - Y_1Y_2][1 - Y_2Y_3][1 - Y_3Y_1] \tag{8.93}$$

The expansion of $\psi(Y)$ is

$$\psi(Y) = Y_1Y_2 + Y_2Y_3 + Y_3Y_1 - 2Y_1Y_2Y_3 \tag{8.94}$$

which is identical to (8.60). The system unavailability is as given by (8.71). ■

8.5.2 Minimal Path Representations

Consider a fault tree with m minimal path sets:

$$\{B_{1,1}, B_{2,1}, \ldots, B_{n_1,1}\}: \quad \text{path set } 1$$

$$\vdots$$

$$\{B_{1,j}, B_{2,j}, \ldots, B_{n_j,j}\}: \quad \text{path set } j$$

$$\vdots$$

$$\{B_{1,m}, B_{2,m}, \ldots, B_{n_m,m}\}: \quad \text{path set } m$$

Denote by $Y_{i,j}$ the indicator variable for the event $B_{i,j}$. The top event occurs if and only if at least one basic event occurs in each minimal path set. Thus the original fault tree is equivalent to the fault tree of Figure 8.24.

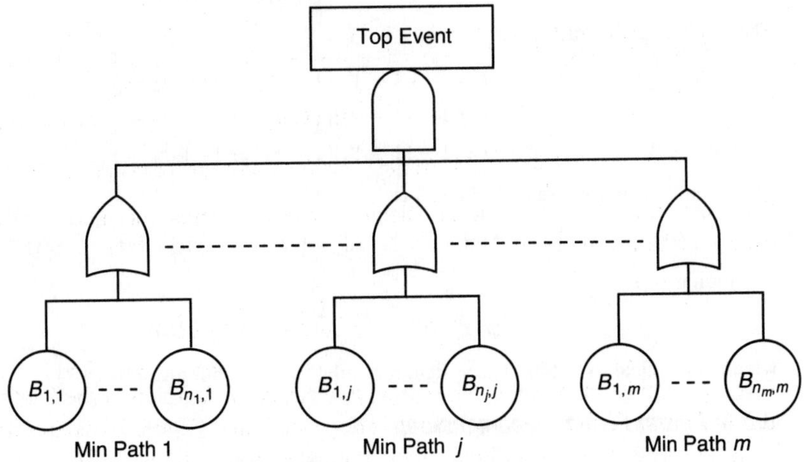

Figure 8.24. Minimal path representation of fault trees.

The structure function for this tree is

$$\psi(Y) = \bigwedge_{j=1}^{m} \left[\bigvee_{i=1}^{n_j} Y_{i,j} \right] \tag{8.95}$$

An algebraic form for this function is

$$\psi(Y) = \bigwedge_{j=1}^{m} \left[1 - \prod_{i=1}^{n_j} (1 - Y_{i,j}) \right] \tag{8.96}$$

$$= \prod_{j=1}^{m} \left[1 - \prod_{i=1}^{n_j} (1 - Y_{i,j}) \right] \tag{8.97}$$

Let $\rho_j(Y)$ be a structure function for the OR gate G_j of Figure 8.24:

$$\rho_j(Y) = 1 - \prod_{i=1}^{n_j} [1 - Y_{i,j}] \tag{8.98}$$

The structure function (8.97) can be written as

$$\psi(Y) = \prod_{j=1}^{m} \rho_j(Y) \tag{8.99}$$

This $\psi(Y)$ is a minimal path representation, and the $\rho_j(Y)$ is the jth minimal path structure to express the existence of path set failure. The minimal path representation $\psi(Y)$ can be expanded and simplified via the absorption law. The system unavailability $Q_s(t)$ can be calculated by using (8.66), as shown in the next example.

Example 9—Two-out-of-three system. Calculate the system unavailability for the two-out-of-three voting system of Figure 8.8. Unavailabilities for the three components are given by (8.68).

Solution: The voting system has three minimal path sets:

$$\{B_1, B_2\}, \qquad \{B_2, B_3\}, \qquad \{B_3, B_1\} \tag{8.100}$$

The minimal path structures are

$$\begin{aligned} \rho_1(Y) &= 1 - [1 - Y_1][1 - Y_2] = Y_1 + Y_2 - Y_1Y_2 \\ \rho_2(Y) &= 1 - [1 - Y_2][1 - Y_3] = Y_2 + Y_3 - Y_2Y_3 \\ \rho_3(Y) &= 1 - [1 - Y_3][1 - Y_1] = Y_3 + Y_1 - Y_3Y_1 \end{aligned} \tag{8.101}$$

The minimal path representation $\psi(Y)$ is

$$\psi(Y) = [Y_1 + Y_2 - Y_1Y_2][Y_2 + Y_3 - Y_2Y_3][Y_3 + Y_1 - Y_3Y_1] \tag{8.102}$$

Expanding $\psi(Y)$,

$$\psi(Y) = Y_1Y_2 + Y_2Y_3 + Y_3Y_1 - 2Y_1Y_2Y_3 \tag{8.103}$$

which is identical to (8.60). The system unavailability is again given by (8.71). ■

8.5.3 Partial Pivotal Decomposition

If basic events appear in more than one minimal cut set, factors $[1 - \kappa_j(Y)]$'s in (8.90) are no longer independent, and the equality

$$E\{\psi(Y)\} = 1 - \prod_{j=1}^{m} [1 - E\{\kappa_j(Y)\}] \tag{8.104}$$

does not hold. For the same reason, (8.99) does not imply that

$$E\{\psi(Y)\} = \prod_{j=1}^{m} E\{\rho_j(Y)\} \tag{8.105}$$

One way of calculating $E\{\psi(Y)\}$ is to expand $\psi(Y)$ and simplify the results by the absorption law. This is a tedious process, however, when the expansion contains a large number of terms. The process can be simplified by partial pivotal decomposition.

The structure function $\psi(Y)$ is first rewritten as

$$\psi(Y) = Y_i\psi(1_i, Y) + (1 - Y_i)\psi(0_i, Y) \tag{8.106}$$

where $\psi(1_i, Y)$ and $\psi(0_i, Y)$ are binary functions obtained by setting the ith indicator variable Y_i to unity and zero, respectively. These binary functions can be pivoted around other indicator variables until the resulting binary functions consist only of independent factors; then $E\{\psi(Y)\}$ can be easily calculated.

In terms of Boolean operators, equation (8.106) becomes

$$\begin{aligned} \psi(Y) &= [Y_i \wedge \psi(1_i, Y)] \vee [\overline{Y}_i \wedge \psi(0_i, Y)] && (8.107) \\ &= Y_i \cdot \psi(\text{true}_i, Y) \vee \overline{Y}_i \cdot \psi(\text{false}_i, Y) && (8.108) \end{aligned}$$

A Boolean AND operation is denoted by symbol $\wedge$, which is often replaced by the equivalent multiplication operation, that is, $Y_1 \wedge Y_2 = Y_1 \cdot Y_2 = Y_1 Y_2$. Values 1_i and 0_i denote *true* and *false* values of ith indicator variable Y_i, respectively.

These algebraic or Boolean pivotal decomposition techniques are demonstrated by the following example.

Example 10—Two-out-of-three system. Consider the minimal path representation of (8.102).

$$\begin{aligned}\psi(Y) &= Y_1[Y_2 + Y_3 - Y_2Y_3] \\ &\quad + [1 - Y_1]Y_2[Y_2 + Y_3 - Y_2Y_3]Y_3 \\ &= Y_1[Y_2 + Y_3 - Y_2Y_3] \\ &\quad + [1 - Y_1]Y_2Y_3 \\ &\quad + [1 - Y_1][1 - Y_2]\cdot 0\end{aligned} \qquad \begin{aligned}\psi(Y) &= Y_1\psi(1_1, Y) \\ &\quad + [1 - Y_1]\psi(0_1, Y) \\ &= Y_1\psi(1_1, Y) \\ &\quad + [1 - Y_1]Y_2\psi(0_1, 1_2, Y) \\ &\quad + [1 - Y_1][1 - Y_2]\psi(0_1, 0_2, Y)\end{aligned}$$

Thus

$$\psi(Y) = Y_1[Y_2 + Y_3 - Y_2Y_3] + [1 - Y_1]Y_2Y_3 \tag{8.109}$$

Note that Y_1 and $[Y_2 + Y_3 - Y_2Y_3]$ have different indicator variables. Similarly, $[1 - Y_1]$, Y_2, and Y_3 have no common variables. Thus each product in (8.109) consists of independent factors, and the expected value $E\{\psi(Y)\}$ is given by

$$E\{\psi(Y)\} = E\{Y_1\}[E\{Y_2\} + E\{Y_3\} - E\{Y_2\}E\{Y_3\}] + [1 - E\{Y_1\}]E\{Y_2\}E\{Y_3\} \tag{8.110}$$

To confirm (8.110), we substitute (8.68)

$$\begin{aligned}Q_s(t) = E\{\psi(Y)\} &= (0.6)[0.6 + 0.6 - 0.6^2] + [1 - 0.6](0.6)^2 \\ &= 0.65\end{aligned} \tag{8.111}$$

The results of (8.71) are obtained; thus the methodology is confirmed.

A Boolean decomposition yields

$$\psi(Y) = Y_1Y_2 \vee Y_2Y_3 \vee Y_3Y_1 \tag{8.112}$$

$$= Y_1(Y_2 \vee Y_2Y_3 \vee Y_3) \vee \overline{Y}_1(Y_2Y_3) \tag{8.113}$$

$$= Y_1(Y_2 \vee Y_3) \vee \overline{Y}_1(Y_2Y_3) \tag{8.114}$$

Because the two terms in the last equation are mutually exclusive, we have

$$\begin{aligned}\Pr\{Y_1(Y_2 \vee Y_3) = 1\} &= \Pr\{Y_1\overline{\overline{Y}_2\overline{Y}_3} = 1\} \\ &= Q_1[1 - (1 - Q_2)(1 - Q_3)]\end{aligned} \tag{8.115}$$

$$\Pr\{\overline{Y}_1(Y_2Y_3) = 1\} = (1 - Q_1)Q_2Q_3 \tag{8.116}$$

$$\Pr\{\psi(Y) = 1\} = Q_1[1 - (1 - Q_2)(1 - Q_3)] + (1 - Q_1)Q_2Q_3 \tag{8.117}$$

$$Q_s(t) = \Pr\{\psi(Y) = 1\} = (0.6)[1 - 0.4^2] + [1 - 0.6](0.6)^2 \tag{8.118}$$

$$= 0.65 \tag{8.119}$$

The results of (8.71) are obtained again. ■

8.5.4 Inclusion-Exclusion Formula

Define event d_j by

d_j = all basic events exist in the jth minimal cut set at time t.

The top event T can be expressed in terms of d_j as

$$T = \bigcup_{j=1}^{m} d_j, \quad (m = \text{ total number of minimal cuts}) \tag{8.120}$$

Thus

$$Q_s(t) = \Pr\left\{\bigcup_{j=1}^{m} d_j\right\} \tag{8.121}$$

$$\begin{aligned} &= \sum_{j=1}^{m} \Pr\{d_j\} - \sum_{j=1}^{m-1} \sum_{k=j+1}^{m} \Pr\{d_j \cap d_k\} \\ &+ \cdots + (-1)^{r-1} \sum_{1 \le j_1 < j_2 < \cdots < j_r \le m} \Pr\{d_{j_1} \cap d_{j_2} \cap \cdots \cap d_{j_r}\} \\ &+ \cdots + (-1)^{m-1} \Pr\{d_1 \cap d_2 \cap \cdots \cap d_m\} \end{aligned} \tag{8.122}$$

Equation (8.122) is an expansion of (8.121) obtained by the so-called *inclusion-exclusion formula*. The rth term on the right-hand side of (8.122) implies the contribution to $Q_s(t)$ from r out of m minimal cut sets being simultaneously failed at time t; that is, all the basic events in these r minimal cut sets exist. A very useful property of (8.122) is that the top event probability is given in terms of intersections, which are easier to calculate than the unions in (8.121).

For small systems it is relatively easy to get exact values for $Q_s(t)$, and this is demonstrated by the following example.

Example 11—Two-out-of-three system. Calculate $Q_s(t)$ for the two-out-of-three voting system of Figure 8.8 by assuming the component unavailabilities of (8.68), using (8.122).

Solution: From the three minimal cut sets of the system, we have

$$d_1 = B_1 \cap B_2, \qquad d_2 = B_2 \cap B_3, \qquad d_3 = B_3 \cap B_1 \tag{8.123}$$

The exact expression for $Q_s(t)$ from (8.122) is

$$\begin{aligned} Q_s(t) &= \sum_{j=1}^{3} \Pr\{d_j\} - \sum_{j=1}^{2} \sum_{k=j+1}^{3} \Pr\{d_j \cap d_k\} + \sum_{j=1}^{1} \sum_{k=j+1}^{2} \sum_{l=k+1}^{3} \Pr\{d_j \cap d_k \cap d_l\} \\ &= \Pr\{d_1\} + \Pr\{d_2\} + \Pr\{d_3\} \\ &\quad - [\Pr\{d_1 \cap d_2\} + \Pr\{d_1 \cap d_3\} + \Pr\{d_2 \cap d_3\}] + \Pr\{d_1 \cap d_2 \cap d_3\} \end{aligned} \tag{8.124}$$

$$\begin{aligned} [A] &\equiv [\Pr\{d_1\} + \Pr\{d_2\} + \Pr\{d_3\}] = Q^2 + Q^2 + Q^2 = 1.08 \\ [B] &\equiv [\Pr\{d_1 \cap d_2\} + \Pr\{d_1 \cap d_3\} + \Pr\{d_2 \cap d_3\}] = Q^3 + Q^3 + Q^3 = 0.65 \\ [C] &\equiv \Pr\{d_1 \cap d_2 \cap d_3\} = Q^3 = 0.22 \end{aligned} \tag{8.125}$$

Thus

$$Q_s(t) = [A] - [B] + [C] = 0.65 \tag{8.126}$$

This confirms (8.71). ■

We note here an expression of $Q_s(t)$ in terms of coverage $\alpha(Y)$ of cut sets.

$$\alpha(Y) \equiv \sum_{j=1}^{m} \kappa_j(Y) \tag{8.127}$$

$$Q_s(t) = \sum_{Y,\alpha(Y)\geq 1} \sum_{j=1}^{m} [1/\alpha(Y)]\kappa_j(Y)\Pr\{Y\} \tag{8.128}$$

This is called a *coverage formula* for $Q_s(t)$. Function α denotes how many cut sets exist at state vector Y.

8.6 LOWER AND UPPER BOUNDS FOR SYSTEM UNAVAILABILITY

For a large, complicated fault tree, exact system unavailability calculation by the methods of the preceding sections are time consuming. When computing time becomes a factor, unavailability lower and upper bounds can be calculated by the short-cut methods in this section.

8.6.1 Inclusion-Exclusion Bounds

Equation (8.122) can be bracketed by

$$\sum_{j=1}^{m} \Pr\{d_j\} - \sum_{j=1}^{m-1} \sum_{k=j+1}^{m} \Pr\{d_j \cap d_k\} \leq Q_s(t) \leq \sum_{j=1}^{m} \Pr\{d_j\} \tag{8.129}$$

Example 12—Two-out-of-three system. For Example 11 in the preceding section we have

$$Q_s(t)_{\min} = [A] - [B] = 0.43$$
$$Q_s(t)_{\max} = [A] = 1.08$$

The exact value of $Q_s(t)$ is 0.65, so these lower and upper bounds are approximate. However, the brackets are normally within three significant figures of one another because component unavailabilities are usually much less than 1. ■

Example 13—Two-out-of-three system. Calculate $Q_s(t)$, $Q_s(t)_{\min}$, and $Q_s(t)_{\max}$ by assuming $Q = 0.001$ in Example 12.

Solution: From (8.125)

$$[A] = Q^2 + Q^2 + Q^2 = 3.0 \times 10^{-6}$$
$$[B] = Q^3 + Q^3 + Q^3 = 3.0 \times 10^{-9}$$
$$[C] = Q^3 = 1.0 \times 10^{-9}$$

Thus

$$Q_s(t) = [A] - [B] + [C] = 2.998 \times 10^{-6}$$
$$Q_s(t)_{\min} = [A] - [B] = 2.997 \times 10^{-6}$$
$$Q_s(t)_{\max} = [A] = 3.0 \times 10^{-6}$$

We have tight lower and upper bounds. ■

In general, the formula gives a lower bound when r is even; the formula yields an upper bound when r is odd.

8.6.2 Esary and Proschan Bounds

We now restrict our attention to structure functions that are coherent (monotonic). The engineering interpretation of this is that, in a coherent system, the occurrence of a component failure always results in system degradation. Formally, $\psi(Y)$ is coherent if [3]:

1. $\psi(Y) = 1$ if $Y = (1, 1, \ldots, 1)$
2. $\psi(Y) = 0$ if $Y = (0, 0, \ldots, 0)$
3. $\psi(Y) \geq \psi(X)$ if $Y_i \geq X_i$ for all $i = 1, \ldots, n$
4. each basic event appears in at least one minimal cut set

For a coherent structure function, the right-hand sides of (8.104) and (8.105) give upper and lower bounds for the system unavailability $Q_s(t)$ [4]:

$$\prod_{j=1}^{m(p)} E\{\rho_j(Y)\} \leq Q_s(t) \leq 1 - \prod_{j=1}^{m(c)} [1 - E\{\kappa_j(Y)\}] \tag{8.130}$$

where $m(p)$ and $m(c)$ are total numbers of minimal path sets and cut sets, respectively.

Example 14—Two-out-of-three system. Calculate Esary and Proschan bounds for the problem in Example 13 of the preceding section.

Solution:

$$\begin{aligned} \kappa_1 &= Y_1Y_2, \qquad \kappa_2 = Y_2Y_3, \qquad \kappa_3 = Y_3Y_1 \\ \rho_1 &= Y_1 + Y_2 - Y_1Y_2 \\ \rho_2 &= Y_2 + Y_3 - Y_2Y_3 \\ \rho_3 &= Y_3 + Y_1 - Y_3Y_1 \end{aligned}$$

Because $E\{Y_1\} = E\{Y_2\} = E\{Y_3\} = Q = 0.001$, we have

$$\begin{aligned} Q_s(t)_{\min} &= [Q + Q - Q^2]^3 = 8.0 \times 10^{-9} \\ Q_s(t)_{\max} &= 1 - [1 - Q^2]^3 = 3.0 \times 10^{-6} \end{aligned} \tag{8.131}$$

The upper bound is as good as that obtained by bracketing, while the lower bound is extremely conservative. ■

8.6.3 Partial Minimal Cut Sets and Path Sets

Pick up $m(c)'$ minimal cut sets and $m(p)'$ minimal path sets. Here $m(c)'$ and $m(p)'$ are less than the actual number of minimal cut sets $m(c)$ and path sets $m(p)$, respectively. The structure function $\psi_L(Y)$ with these $m(c)'$ cut sets is

$$\psi_L(Y) = 1 - \prod_{j=1}^{m(c)'} [1 - \kappa_j(Y)] \tag{8.132}$$

where $\kappa_j(Y)$ is the jth minimal cut structure. Similarly, the structure function $\psi_U(Y)$ with the $m(p)'$ path sets is

$$\psi_U(Y) = \prod_{j=1}^{m(p)'} \rho_j(Y) \tag{8.133}$$

Because the structure function $\psi_L(Y)$ has fewer minimal cut sets than $\psi(Y)$, we have

$$\psi_L(Y) \leq \psi(Y) \tag{8.134}$$

Similarly,

$$\psi_U(Y) \geq \psi(Y) \tag{8.135}$$

Thus

$$E\{\psi_L(Y)\} \leq E\{\psi(Y)\} \leq E\{\psi_U(Y)\} \tag{8.136}$$

or

$$Q_s(t)_{\min} \equiv E\{\psi_L(Y)\} \leq Q_s(t) \leq E\{\psi_U(Y)\} \equiv Q_s(t)_{\max} \tag{8.137}$$

Example 15—Tail-gas quench and clean-up system. Calculate $Q_s(t)_{\min}$, $Q_s(t)$, and $Q_s(t)_{\max}$ for the fault tree of Figure 8.13. Assume the component unavailabilities at time t to be 0.001.

Solution: The fault tree has five minimal cut sets,

$$\{A\}, \quad \{D\}, \quad \{G\}, \quad \{B, C\}, \quad \{E, F\} \tag{8.138}$$

and four minimal path sets:

$$\{A, D, G, C, F\}, \quad \{A, D, G, C, E\}, \quad \{A, D, G, B, F\}, \quad \{A, D, G, B, E\} \tag{8.139}$$

Take only the cut sets $\{A\}$, $\{D\}$, and $\{G\}$ (ignore the higher-order ones) and only two path sets $\{A, D, G, C, F\}$ and $\{A, D, G, B, E\}$. Then,

$$\psi(Y) = 1 - [1 - Y_A][1 - Y_D][1 - Y_G][1 - Y_B Y_C][1 - Y_E Y_F] \tag{8.140}$$

$$\psi_L(Y) = 1 - [1 - Y_A][1 - Y_D][1 - Y_G] \tag{8.141}$$

$$\begin{aligned}\psi_U(Y) = {} & [1 - (1 - Y_A)(1 - Y_D)(1 - Y_G)(1 - Y_C)(1 - Y_F)] \\ & \times [1 - (1 - Y_A)(1 - Y_D)(1 - Y_G)(1 - Y_B)(1 - Y_E)]\end{aligned} \tag{8.142}$$

$$\begin{aligned}= {} & 1 - (1 - Y_A)(1 - Y_D)(1 - Y_G)(1 - Y_B)(1 - Y_E) \\ & - (1 - Y_A)(1 - Y_D)(1 - Y_G)(1 - Y_C)(1 - Y_F) \\ & + (1 - Y_A)(1 - Y_D)(1 - Y_G)(1 - Y_B)(1 - Y_E)(1 - Y_C)(1 - Y_F)\end{aligned} \tag{8.143}$$

Thus

$$\begin{aligned}Q_s(t) &= 1 - (0.999)^3(0.999999)^2 = 2.999 \times 10^{-3} \\ Q_s(t)_{\min} &= 1 - (0.999)^3 = 2.997 \times 10^{-3} \\ Q_s(t)_{\max} &= 1 - (0.999)^5 - (0.999)^5 + (0.999)^7 = 3.001 \times 10^{-3}\end{aligned} \tag{8.144}$$

Good upper and lower bounds are obtained. ■

As a first approximation, it is reasonable to include only the one- or two-event minimal cut sets in the $m(c)'$ cut sets. Similarly, we take as the $m(p)'$ path sets, minimal path sets containing the fewest number of basic events. Because fewer cut sets and path sets are involved, the calculation can be simplified. Further simplifications are possible if we pick out nearly disjoint cut sets or path sets because the structure functions $\psi_U(Y)$ and $\psi_L(Y)$ can be expanded into polynomials with fewer terms, each of which consists of independent factors.

8.7 SYSTEM QUANTIFICATION BY KITT

The previous sections covered availability and unavailability quantification methods for relatively simple systems. This section develops the theory and techniques germane to obtaining unavailabilities, availabilities, expected number of failures and repairs, and conditional failure and repair intensities, starting with minimal cut sets or path sets of large and complicated fault trees. We discuss, in some detail, the KITT (kinetic tree theory), and show how system parameters can be guesstimated by approximation techniques based on inclusion-exclusion formulae. To be consistent with previous chapters, we present here a revised version of Vesely's original derivation [5]. A KITT improvement is described in reference [6]. Other computer codes are surveyed in IAEA-TECDOC- 553 [7].

8.7.1 Overview of KITT

The code is an application of kinetic tree theory and will handle independent basic events that are nonrepairable or repairable, provided they have constant failure rates and constant repair rates. However, the exponential failure and/or repair distribution limitation can be circumvented by using the "phased mission" version of the program (KITT-2), which allows for tabular input of time-varying failure and repair rates. KITT also requires as input the minimal cut sets or the minimal path sets. Inhibit gates are permitted.

Exact, time-dependent reliability parameters are determined for each basic event and cut set, but for the system as a whole the parameters are obtained by upper- or lower-bound approximations, or by bracketing. The upper and lower bounds are generally excellent approximations to the exact parameters. In the bracketing procedure the various upper and lower bounds can be obtained as close to each other as desired, and thus exact values for system parameters are obtained if the user so chooses.

The probability characteristics, their definitions, the nomenclature, and the expected (mostly asymptotic) behavior of the variables are summarized in Tables 8.6 and 8.7. A flow sheet of the KITT computation is given as Figure 8.25. The numbers on the flow sheet represent the equations in Table 8.8 used to obtain the parameters.

TABLE 8.6. System Parameters Calculated by KITT

Symbols					
Component	Cut Set	System	KITT Symbol	**Definition**	**Name**
$Q(t)$	$Q^*(t)$	$Q_s(t)$	Q	Probability of a failed state at time t	Unavailability
$w(t)$	$w^*(t)$	$w_s(t)$	W	Expected number of failures per unit time at time t	Unconditional failure intensity
$v(t)$	$v^*(t)$	$v_s(t)$	V	Expected number of repairs per unit time at time t	Unconditional repair intensity
$\lambda(t)$	$\lambda^*(t)$	$\lambda_s(t)$	L	Probability of a failure per unit time at time t, given no failures at time t	Conditional failure intensity
$\mu(t)$	$\mu^*(t)$	$\mu_s(t)$	M	Probability of a repair per unit time at time t, given no repairs at time t	Conditional repair intensity
$W(0, t)$	$W^*(0, t)$	$W_s(0, t)$	$WSUM$	Expected number of failures in time interval $[0, t)$	Expected number of failures
$V(0, t)$	$V^*(0, t)$	$V_s(0, t)$	$VSUM$	Expected number of repairs in time interval $[0, t)$	Expected number of repairs
$F(t)$	$F^*(t)$	$F_s(t)$	Not Available	Probability of one or more failures in time interval $[0, t)$	Unreliability

TABLE 8.7. Behavior of System Parameters with Constant Rates λ and μ

Component Level		
Parameter	Repairable	Nonrepairable
$Q(t)$	Constant $Q(t)$ after $t >$ 3MTTR, $Q(t) << 1$	$Q(t) \to 1$ as $t \to \infty$, $Q(t) = F(t) = W(0, t) = 1 - e^{-\lambda t}$
$w(t)$	Constant $w(t)$ after $t >$ 3MTTR, $w(t) \simeq \lambda$	$w(t)$ decreases with time, $w(t) = f(t) = \lambda e^{-\lambda t}$
$\lambda(t)$	Constant λ. $\lambda \simeq w(t)$ after $t >$ 3 MTTR	Constant λ
$W(0, t)$	$W(0, t) \to \infty$ as $t \to \infty$	$W(0, t) \to 1$ as $t \to \infty$, $W(0, t) = F(t) = Q(t)$
$F(t)$	$F(t) \to 1$ as $t \to \infty$	$F(t) \to 1$ as $t \to \infty$, $F(t) = W(0, t) = Q(t)$

Cut Set Level		
Parameter	Repairable	Nonrepairable
$Q^*(t)$	Constant $Q^*(t)$ after $t >$ 3MTTR, $Q^*(t) << 1$	$Q^*(t) \to 1$ as $t \to \infty$, $Q^*(t) = F^*(t) = W^*(0, t)$
$w^*(t)$	Constant $w^*(t)$ after $t >$ 3MTTR, $w^*(t) \simeq \lambda^*(t)$	$w^*(t)$ increases, then decreases with time, $w^*(t) = f^*(t)$
$\lambda^*(t)$	Constant $\lambda^*(t)$ after $t >$ 3MTTR, $\lambda^*(t) \simeq w^*(t)$	$\lambda^*(t)$ increases with time
$W^*(0, t)$	$W^*(0, t) \to \infty$ as $t \to \infty$	$W^*(0, t) \to 1$ as $t \to \infty$, $W^*(0, t) = F^*(t) = Q^*(t)$
$F^*(t)$	$F^*(t) \to 1$ as $t \to \infty$	$F^*(t) \to 1$ as $t \to \infty$, $F^*(t) = W^*(0, t) = Q^*(t)$

System Level		
Parameter	Repairable	Nonrepairable
$Q_s(t)$	Constant $Q_s(t)$ after $t >$ 3MTTR, $Q_s(t) << 1$	$Q_s(t) \to 1$ as $t \to \infty$, $Q_s(t) = F_s(t) = W_s(0, t)$
$w_s(t)$	Constant $w_s(t)$ after $t >$ 3MTTR, $w_s(t) \simeq \lambda_s(t)$	$w_s(t)$ increases, then decreases with time, $w_s(t) = f_s(t)$
$\lambda_s(t)$	Constant $\lambda_s(t)$ after $t >$ 3MTTR, $\lambda_s(t) \simeq w_s(t)$	$\lambda_s(t)$ increases with time
$W_s(0, t)$	$W_s(0, t) \to \infty$ as $t \to \infty$	$W_s(0, t) \to 1$ as $t \to \infty$, $W_s(0, t) = F_s(t) = Q_s(t)$
$F_s(t)$	$F_s(t) \to 1$ as $t \to \infty$	$F_s(t) \to 1$ as $t \to \infty$, $F_s(t) = W_s(0, t) = Q_s(t)$

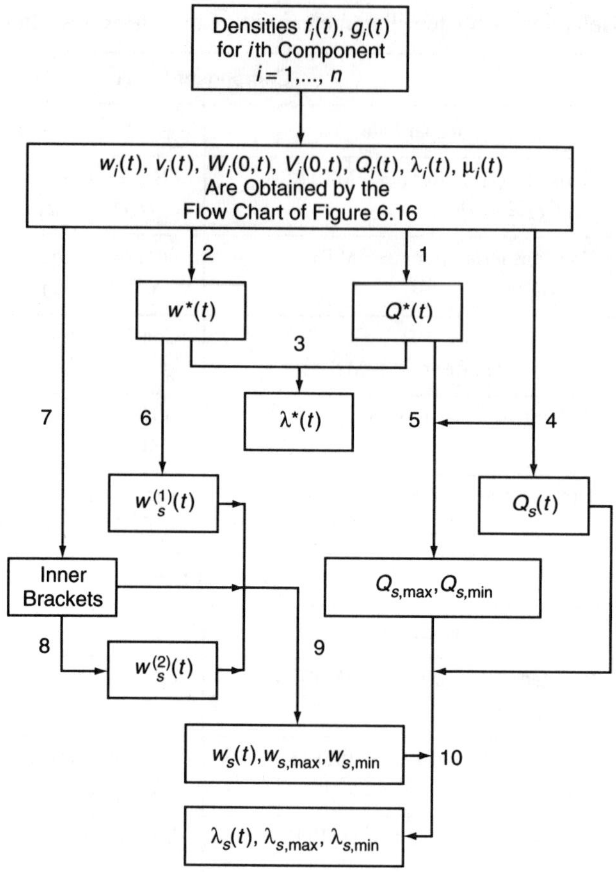

Figure 8.25. Flow sheet of KITT computations.

The program calculates $w(t)$ and $v(t)$ before $Q(t)$, using equation (6.89).

$$w(t) = f(t) + \int_0^t f(t-u)v(u)du \tag{8.145}$$

$$v(t) = \int_0^t g(t-u)w(u)du \tag{8.146}$$

In accordance with the definitions, the first term on the right-hand side of (8.145) is interpreted as the contribution to $w(t)$ from the first occurrence of the basic event, and the second term is the contribution to $w(t)$ from the failure repaired at time u, and then recurring at time t. A similar interpretation can be made for $v(t)$ in (8.146). If a rigorous solution of $w(t)$ and $v(t)$ is required for exponential failure and repair distributions, Laplace transform techniques can be used (Table 6.10). KITT uses a numerical integration.

Before moving on to cut sets and system calculations, we demonstrate the use of these equations by a simple, one-component example. Component reliability parameters are unique and, as a first approximation, independent of the complexity of the system in which they appear. The calculation proceeds according to the flow chart of Figure 6.16.

Example 16—Single-component system. Using Table 6.10, calculate reliability parameters for nonrepairable component 1 with $\lambda_1 = 1.0 \times 10^{-3}$ failures per hour, at $t = 20$,

TABLE 8.8. Equations for KITT Calculations

1	$$Q^*(t) = \Pr\{B_1 \cap B_2 \cap \cdots \cap B_n\} = \prod_{i=1}^{n} Q_i(t)$$
2	$$w^*(t) = \sum_{i=1}^{n} w_i(t) \prod_{l=1, l \neq i}^{n} Q_l(t)$$
3	$$\lambda^*(t) = \frac{w^*(t)}{1 - Q^*(t)}$$
4	$$Q_s(t) = \sum_{j=1}^{m} Q_j^*(t) - \sum_{j=1}^{m-1} \sum_{k=j+1}^{m} \prod_{j,k} Q(t) + + \cdots + (-1)^{r-1} \sum_{1 \leq j_1 < j_2 < \cdots < j_r \leq m} \prod_{j_1 \cdots j_r} Q(t) + \cdots + (-1)^{m-1} \prod_{1 \cdots m} Q(t)$$
5	$$\sum_{j=1}^{m} Q_j^*(t) - \sum_{j=1}^{m-1} \sum_{k=j+1}^{m} \prod_{j,k} Q(t) \leq Q_s(t) \leq \sum_{j=1}^{m} Q_j^*(t)$$
6	$$w_s^{(1)}(t) = \sum_{j=1}^{m} w_j^*(t) - \sum_{j=1}^{m-1} \sum_{k=j+1}^{m} w^*(t; j, k) \prod_{j,k}^{*} Q(t) + \cdots + (-1)^{r-1} \sum_{1 \leq j_1 < j_2 < \cdots < j_r \leq m} w^*(t; j_1, j_2, \ldots, j_r) \prod_{j_1, j_2 \cdots j_r}^{*} Q(t) + \cdots + (-1)^{m-1} w^*(t; 1, \ldots, m) \prod_{1 \cdots m}^{*} Q(t)$$
7	$$\Pr\{e_1 \cap \cdots \cap e_r \cap T\} = \sum_{j=1}^{m} \Pr\{e_1 \cap \cdots \cap e_r \cap d_j\} - \sum_{j=1}^{m-1} \sum_{k=j+1}^{m} \Pr\{e_1 \cap \cdots \cap e_r \cap d_j \cap d_k\} + \cdots + (-1)^{s-1} \sum_{1 \leq j_1 < j_2 < \cdots < j_s \leq m} \Pr\{e_1 \cap \cdots \cap e_r \cap d_{j_1} \cap d_{j_2} \cap \cdots \cap d_{j_s}\} + \cdots + (-1)^{m-1} \Pr\{e_1 \cap \cdots \cap e_r \cap d_1 \cap d_2 \cap \cdots \cap d_m\}$$
8	$$w_s^{(2)}(t)dt = \Pr\left\{ T \bigcup_{j=1}^{m} e_j \right\} = \sum_{j=1}^{m} \Pr\{e_j \cap T\} - \sum_{j=1}^{m-1} \sum_{k=j+1}^{m} \Pr\{e_j \cap e_k \cap T\} + \cdots + (-1)^{r-1} \sum_{1 \leq j_1 < j_2 < \cdots < j_r \leq m} \Pr\{e_{j_1} \cap e_{j_2} \cap \cdots \cap e_{j_r} \cap T\} + \cdots + (-1)^{m-1} \Pr\{e_1 \cap e_2 \cap \cdots \cap e_m \cap T\}$$
9	$$w_s(t) = w_s^{(1)}(t) - w_s^{(2)}(t)$$
10	$$\lambda_s(t) = \frac{w_s(t)}{1 - Q_s(t)}$$

$t = 500$, and $t = 1100$ hr. Repeat the calculations, assuming that the component is repairable with MTTR $= 1/\mu_1 = 10$ hr.

Solution: For the nonrepairable component

$$w(t) = \lambda e^{-\lambda t}, \qquad v(t) = 0 \tag{8.147}$$

$$Q(t) = \int_0^t [w(u) - v(u)]du = 1 - e^{-\lambda t} = F(t) \tag{8.148}$$

$$W(0, t) = \int_0^t w(u)du = 1 - e^{-\lambda t} = F(t) \tag{8.149}$$

$$V(0, t) = \int_0^t v(u)du = 0 \tag{8.150}$$

For the repairable case

$$w(t) = \frac{\lambda\mu}{\lambda + \mu} + \frac{\lambda^2}{\lambda + \mu} e^{-(\lambda+\mu)t} \tag{8.151}$$

$$v(t) = \frac{\lambda\mu}{\lambda + \mu}[1 - e^{-(\lambda+\mu)t}] \tag{8.152}$$

$$Q(t) = \int_0^t [w(u) - v(u)]du = \frac{\lambda}{\lambda + \mu}[1 - e^{-(\lambda+\mu)t}] \tag{8.153}$$

$$W(0, t) = \int_0^t w(u)du = \frac{\lambda\mu}{\lambda + \mu} t + \frac{\lambda^2}{(\lambda + \mu)^2}[1 - e^{-(\lambda+\mu)t}] \tag{8.154}$$

$$V(0, t) = \int_0^t v(u)du = \frac{\lambda\mu}{\lambda + \mu} t - \frac{\lambda\mu}{(\lambda + \mu)^2}[1 - e^{-(\lambda+\mu)t}] \tag{8.155}$$

The values of $Q(t)$, $w(t)$, and $W(0, t)$ are listed in Table 8.9.

TABLE 8.9. Results of Example 16

Nonrepairable Component, MTTR$_1$ = ∞				
t	$w(t)$	$Q(t)$	$W(0, t)$	$V(0, t)$
20	9.80×10^{-4}	1.98×10^{-2}	1.98×10^{-2}	0.0
500	6.06×10^{-4}	3.93×10^{-1}	3.93×10^{-1}	0.0
1100	3.33×10^{-4}	6.32×10^{-1}	6.32×10^{-1}	0.0
Repairable Component, MTTR$_1$ = 10				
t	$w(t)$	$Q(t)$	$W(0, t)$	$V(0, t)$
20	9.91×10^{-4}	8.59×10^{-3}	1.99×10^{-2}	1.13×10^{-2}
500	9.90×10^{-4}	9.90×10^{-3}	4.95×10^{-1}	4.85×10^{-1}
1100	9.90×10^{-4}	9.90×10^{-3}	$1.09 \times 10^{+0}$	$1.08 \times 10^{+0}$

Failure Rate $\lambda_1 = 0.001$

At $t = 1100$, 63.2% of the steady-state unavailability $Q(\infty)$ is attained for the nonrepairable case, which is consistent with a mean time to failure of 1000 hr. Further, parameter $W(0, t)$ coincides with unreliability or unavailability $Q(t)$. For the repairable case, steady state is generally reached in a few multiples of the repair time because λ is usually far smaller than μ, and $(\lambda + \mu)$ is nearly equal to μ. The unreliability $F(t)$ must approach one, but $W(0, t)$ can be greater than one.

For the repairable component, we observe the equalities at steady state.

$$w(\infty) = v(\infty) = \frac{\lambda\mu}{\lambda + \mu} \tag{8.156}$$

$$1/w(\infty) = 1/v(\infty) = \text{MTTF} + \text{MTTR} \tag{8.157}$$

The inverse of $w(\infty)$ or $v(\infty)$ coincides with the mean time between failures, which is intuitively correct. ■

8.7.2 Minimal Cut Set Parameters

A cut set exists if all basic events in the cut set exist. The probability of a cut set existing at time t, $Q^*(t)$, is obtained from the intersections of basic events [see equation (8.10)]

$$Q^*(t) = \Pr\{B_1 \cap B_2 \cap \cdots \cap B_n\} = \prod_{i=1}^{n} Q_i(t) \tag{8.158}$$

where n is the number of cut set members, $Q_i(t)$ the probability of ith basic event existing at time t, and superscript $*$ denotes a cut set parameter.

Examples 17, 18, and 19 demonstrate the procedure for calculating cut set parameters for a series, a parallel, and a two-out-of-three system.

Example 17—Three-component series system. Calculate the cut set reliability parameters for a three-component, repairable and nonrepairable series system at $t = 20$, $t = 500$, and $t = 1100$ hr, where the components have the following parameters.

Component 1		Component 2		Component 3	
$\lambda_1 = 10^{-3}$,	$\mu_1 = 1/10$	$\lambda_2 = 2 \times 10^{-3}$,	$\mu_2 = 1/40$	$\lambda_3 = 3 \times 10^{-3}$,	$\mu_3 = 1/60$

Solution: For this configuration there are three cut sets, each component being a cut set. Thus $Q_1^*(t) = Q_1(t)$, $Q_2^*(t) = Q_2(t)$, $Q_3^*(t) = Q_3(t)$, and so on. The parameters for component 1 were calculated in Example 16. For the three components (cut sets) we have Table 8.10. ■

An n-component parallel system has a cut set of the form $\{B_1, B_2, \ldots, B_n\}$. Thus the calculation of $Q^*(t)$ represents no problem because

$$Q^*(t) = Q_1(t)Q_2(t)\cdots Q_n(t) \tag{8.159}$$

An extension of the theory must be made, however, before $w^*(t)$ and $\lambda^*(t)$ can be obtained. Let us first examine $\lambda^*(t)$, which is defined by the probability of the occurrence of a cut set per unit time at time t, given no cut set failure at time t. Thus $\lambda^*(t)dt$ is the probability that the cut set occurs during time interval $[t, t + dt)$, given that it is not active at time t:

$$\lambda^*(t)dt = \Pr\{C^*(t, t + dt)|\overline{C}^*(t)\} \tag{8.160}$$

$$= \frac{\Pr\{C^*(t, t + dt) \cap \overline{C}^*(t)\}}{\Pr\{\overline{C}^*(t)\}} \tag{8.161}$$

$$= \frac{\Pr\{C^*(t, t + dt)\}}{\Pr\{\overline{C}^*(t)\}} \tag{8.162}$$

TABLE 8.10. Results of Example 17 (Series System)

Nonrepairable Single-Event Cut {1}, $MTTR_1 = \infty$			
t	$w^*(t)$	$Q^*(t)$	$W^*(0, t)$
20	9.80×10^{-4}	1.98×10^{-2}	1.98×10^{-2}
500	6.06×10^{-4}	3.93×10^{-1}	3.93×10^{-1}
1100	3.33×10^{-4}	6.32×10^{-1}	6.32×10^{-1}
Repairable Single-Event Cut {1}, $MTTR_1 = 10$			
t	$w^*(t)$	$Q^*(t)$	$W^*(0, t)$
20	9.91×10^{-4}	8.59×10^{-3}	1.99×10^{-2}
500	9.90×10^{-4}	9.90×10^{-3}	4.95×10^{-1}
1100	9.90×10^{-4}	9.90×10^{-3}	$1.09 \times 10^{+0}$
Nonepairable Single-Event Cut {2}, $MTTR_2 = \infty$			
t	$w^*(t)$	$Q^*(t)$	$W^*(0, t)$
20	1.92×10^{-3}	3.92×10^{-2}	3.92×10^{-2}
500	7.36×10^{-4}	6.32×10^{-1}	6.32×10^{-1}
1100	2.22×10^{-4}	8.89×10^{-1}	8.89×10^{-1}
Repairable Single-Event Cut {2}, $MTTR_2 = 40$			
t	$w^*(t)$	$Q^*(t)$	$W^*(0, t)$
20	1.94×10^{-3}	3.09×10^{-2}	3.93×10^{-2}
500	1.85×10^{-3}	7.41×10^{-2}	9.31×10^{-1}
1100	1.85×10^{-3}	7.41×10^{-2}	$2.04 \times 10^{+0}$
Nonrepairable Single-Event Cut {3}, $MTTR_3 = \infty$			
t	$w^*(t)$	$Q^*(t)$	$W^*(0, t)$
20	2.83×10^{-3}	5.82×10^{-2}	5.82×10^{-2}
500	6.69×10^{-4}	7.77×10^{-1}	7.77×10^{-1}
1100	1.11×10^{-4}	9.63×10^{-1}	9.63×10^{-1}
Repairable Single-Event Cut {3}, $MTTR_3 = 60$			
t	$w^*(t)$	$Q^*(t)$	$W^*(0, t)$
20	2.85×10^{-3}	4.96×10^{-2}	5.84×10^{-2}
500	2.54×10^{-3}	1.53×10^{-1}	$1.29 \times 10^{+0}$
1100	2.54×10^{-3}	1.53×10^{-1}	$2.81 \times 10^{+0}$

Failure Rate $\lambda_1 = 0.001$; Failure Rate $\lambda_2 = 0.002$;
Failure Rate $\lambda_3 = 0.003$

where $C^*(t, t + dt)$ is the event occurrence of the cut set during $[t, t + dt)$, and $\overline{C}^*(t)$ is the event nonexistence of the cut set failure at time t. The denominator is given by

$$\Pr\{\overline{C}^*(t)\} = 1 - Q^*(t) \tag{8.163}$$

Consider the numerator of (8.162). The cut set failure occurs if and only if one of the basic events in the cut set does not exist at t and then occurs during $[t, t+dt)$, and all other basic events exist at t. Thus

$$\Pr\{C^*(t, t+dt)\} = \sum_{i=1}^{n} \Pr\{\text{event } i \text{ occurs during } [t, t+dt), \text{ and the other events exist at } t\} \tag{8.164}$$

Because the basic events are mutually independent,

$$\Pr\{C^*(t, t+dt)\} = \sum_{i=1}^{n} \Pr\{\text{event } i \text{ occurs during } [t, t+dt)\} \times \Pr\{\text{the other events exist at } t\} \tag{8.165}$$

$$= \sum_{i=1}^{n} w_i(t)dt \prod_{l=1, l\neq i}^{n} Q_l(t) \tag{8.166}$$

Consequently, (8.162) can be written

$$\lambda^*(t)dt = \frac{\sum_{i=1}^{n} w_i(t)dt \prod_{l=1, l\neq i}^{n} Q_l(t)}{1 - Q^*(t)} \tag{8.167}$$

The denominator on the right-hand side of (8.167) represents the probability of the nonexistence of the cut set failure at time t. Each term of the summation is the probability of the ith basic event during $[t, t+dt)$ with the remaining basic events already existing at time t. At most, one basic event occurs during the small time interval $[t, t+dt)$, and the terms describing the probability of two or more basic events can be neglected.

The expected number of times the cut set occurs per unit time at time t, that is, $w^*(t)$, is equal to the numerator of (8.167) divided by dt, and given by

$$w^*(t) = \sum_{i=1}^{n} w_i(t) \prod_{l=1, l\neq i}^{n} Q_l(t) \tag{8.168}$$

Thus $\lambda^*(t)$ in (8.167) is calculated from $w^*(t)$ and $Q^*(t)$:

$$\lambda^*(t) = \frac{w^*(t)}{1 - Q^*(t)} \tag{8.169}$$

Similar equations hold for $\mu^*(t)$ and $v^*(t)$, that is, $v^*(t)$ can be calculated by

$$v^*(t) = \sum_{i=1}^{n} v_i(t) \prod_{l=1, l\neq i}^{n} Q_l(t) \tag{8.170}$$

and $\mu^*(t)$ is given by

$$\mu^*(t) = \frac{v^*(t)}{Q^*(t)} \tag{8.171}$$

The integral values $W^*(0, t)$ and $V^*(0, t)$ are, as before, obtained from the differentials $w^*(t)$ and $v^*(t)$:

$$W^*(0, t) = \int_0^t w^*(u)du \tag{8.172}$$

$$V^*(0, t) = \int_0^t v^*(u)du \tag{8.173}$$

These equations are applied in Example 18 to a simple parallel system, and in Example 19 to a two-out-of-three voting configuration.

Example 18—Two-component parallel system. Calculate the cut set parameters for a repairable and nonrepairable parallel system consisting of components 1 and 2 of Example 17 at $t = 20$, 500, and 1100.

Solution: Applying (8.158) to the two-component cut set {1, 2} we have

$$Q^*(t) = Q_1(t)Q_2(t) \tag{8.174}$$

For the repairable case, at 20 hr

$$Q^*(t) = (8.59 \times 10^{-3})(3.09 \times 10^{-2}) = 2.65 \times 10^{-4} \tag{8.175}$$

From (8.168), $w^*(t) = w_1(t)Q_2(t) + w_2(t)Q_1(t)$; thus for the repairable case, at 20 hr,

$$\begin{aligned} w^*(t) &= (9.91 \times 10^{-4})(3.09 \times 10^{-2}) + (1.94 \times 10^{-3})(8.59 \times 10^{-3}) \\ &= 4.73 \times 10^{-5} \end{aligned} \tag{8.176}$$

From (8.169), $\lambda^*(t) = w^*(t)/[1 - Q^*(t)]$. At 20 hr, for the repairable case,

$$\lambda^*(t) = \frac{4.73 \times 10^{-5}}{1 - 2.65 \times 10^{-4}} = 4.73 \times 10^{-5} \tag{8.177}$$

Other differentials $v^*(t)$ and $\mu^*(t)$ are calculated by (8.170) and (8.171). The integral parameters $W^*(0, t)$ and $V^*(0, t)$ are readily obtained by equations (8.172) and (8.173). Part of the final results are listed in Table 8.11.

TABLE 8.11. Results of Example 18

Nonrepairable System				
t	$w^*(t)$	$Q^*(t)$	$W^*(0, t)$	$\lambda^*(t)$
20	7.65×10^{-5}	7.76×10^{-4}	7.73×10^{-4}	7.65×10^{-5}
500	6.73×10^{-4}	2.49×10^{-1}	2.49×10^{-1}	8.96×10^{-4}
1100	4.44×10^{-4}	5.93×10^{-1}	5.93×10^{-1}	1.09×10^{-3}
Repairable System				
t	$w^*(t)$	$Q^*(t)$	$W^*(0, t)$	$\lambda^*(t)$
20	4.73×10^{-5}	2.65×10^{-4}	5.78×10^{-4}	4.73×10^{-5}
500	9.17×10^{-5}	7.33×10^{-4}	4.30×10^{-2}	9.17×10^{-5}
1100	9.17×10^{-5}	7.33×10^{-4}	9.80×10^{-2}	9.17×10^{-5}

As expected, the parallel (redundant) configuration is more reliable than the single-component system of Example 16. For the nonrepairable case, $Q^*(t)$ equals $W^*(0, t)$ and, for the repairable case, $\lambda^*(t) \simeq w^*(t)$ because $Q^*(t) << 1$. ■

Example 19—Two-out-of-three system. Calculate the cut set parameters for a repairable and nonrepairable two-out-of-three voting system consisting of the three components of Example 17 at $t = 20$, 500, and 1100 hr.

Solution: The fault tree for this system is given in Figure 8.8, and the cut sets are easily identified as $K_1 = \{1, 2\}$, $K_2 = \{2, 3\}$, $K_3 = \{3, 1\}$. Reliability parameters for K_1 are obtained in Example 18. Parameters for the three cut sets are listed in Table 8.12.

TABLE 8.12. Results of Example 19 (Two-out-of-Three System)

Nonrepairable System $K_1(1, 2)$

t	$w^*(t)$	$Q^*(t)$	$W^*(0, t)$	$\lambda^*(t)$
20	7.65×10^{-5}	7.76×10^{-4}	7.73×10^{-4}	7.65×10^{-5}
500	6.73×10^{-4}	2.49×10^{-1}	2.49×10^{-1}	8.96×10^{-4}
1100	4.44×10^{-4}	5.93×10^{-1}	5.93×10^{-1}	1.09×10^{-3}

Repairable System $K_1(1, 2)$

t	$w^*(t)$	$Q^*(t)$	$W^*(0, t)$	$\lambda^*(t)$
20	4.73×10^{-5}	2.65×10^{-4}	5.78×10^{-4}	4.73×10^{-5}
500	9.17×10^{-5}	7.33×10^{-4}	4.30×10^{-2}	9.17×10^{-5}
1100	9.17×10^{-5}	7.33×10^{-4}	9.80×10^{-2}	9.17×10^{-5}

Nonrepairable System $K_2(2, 3)$

t	$w^*(t)$	$Q^*(t)$	$W^*(0, t)$	$\lambda^*(t)$
20	2.23×10^{-4}	2.28×10^{-3}	2.27×10^{-3}	2.23×10^{-4}
500	9.95×10^{-4}	4.91×10^{-1}	4.91×10^{-1}	1.95×10^{-3}
1100	3.12×10^{-4}	8.56×10^{-1}	8.56×10^{-1}	2.17×10^{-3}

Repairable System $K_2(2, 3)$

t	$w^*(t)$	$Q^*(t)$	$W^*(0, t)$	$\lambda^*(t)$
20	1.84×10^{-4}	1.53×10^{-3}	1.97×10^{-3}	1.85×10^{-4}
500	4.71×10^{-4}	1.13×10^{-2}	2.15×10^{-1}	4.76×10^{-4}
1100	4.71×10^{-4}	1.13×10^{-2}	4.98×10^{-1}	4.76×10^{-4}

Nonrepairable System $K_3(3, 1)$

t	$w^*(t)$	$Q^*(t)$	$W^*(0, t)$	$\lambda^*(t)$
20	1.13×10^{-4}	1.15×10^{-3}	1.48×10^{-3}	1.13×10^{-4}
500	7.35×10^{-4}	3.06×10^{-1}	3.06×10^{-1}	1.06×10^{-3}
1100	3.94×10^{-4}	6.43×10^{-1}	6.42×10^{-1}	1.10×10^{-3}

Repairable System $K_3(3, 1)$

t	$w^*(t)$	$Q^*(t)$	$W^*(0, t)$	$\lambda^*(t)$
20	7.37×10^{-5}	4.26×10^{-4}	8.23×10^{-4}	7.37×10^{-5}
500	1.76×10^{-4}	1.51×10^{-3}	8.03×10^{-2}	1.76×10^{-4}
1100	1.76×10^{-4}	1.51×10^{-3}	1.86×10^{-1}	1.76×10^{-4}

These results contain no surprises. The mean time to failure for the components is $\text{MTTF}_3 < \text{MTTF}_2 < \text{MTTF}_1$; thus we would expect $Q_1^*(t) < Q_3^*(t) < Q_2^*(t)$ for the nonrepairable case, and that result is confirmed at 1100 hr:* $0.593 < 0.643 < 0.856$. For the repairable case, we also see that

*Suffix j attached to the cut set parameters refers to the jth cut set. Cut set 1 = {1, 2}, cut set 2 = {2, 3}, cut set 3 = {3, 1}.

$Q_1^*(t) < Q_3^*(t) < Q_2^*(t)$; $7.33 \times 10^{-4} < 1.51 \times 10^{-3} < 1.13 \times 10^{-2}$ because of the shorter repair times for the more reliable components.

Another point to note is that a system composed of components having constant failure rates or constant conditional failure intensities λ will not necessarily have a constant conditional failure intensity λ^* on a cut set level. We see also that, unlike for a nonrepairable component where $w(t)$ decreases with time, $w^*(t)$ increases briefly, and then decreases. ■

The KITT program accepts as input path sets as well as cut sets, the calculations being done in much the same way. We do not discuss this option.

8.7.3 System Unavailability $Q_s(t)$

As in Section 8.5.4, we define event d_j as

$$\begin{aligned} d_j &= \text{all basic events exist in the } j\text{th minimal cut set at time } t \\ &= \text{the } j\text{th minimal cut set failure exists at time } t. \end{aligned}$$

The expansion (8.122) in Section 8.5.4 was obtained by the inclusion-exclusion formula. The rth term on the right-hand side of (8.122) is the contribution to $Q_s(t)$ from r minimal cut set failures existing simultaneously at time t. Thus (8.122) can be rewritten as

$$\begin{aligned} Q_s(t) = &\sum_{j=1}^{m} Q_j^*(t) - \sum_{j=1}^{m-1} \sum_{k=j+1}^{m} \prod_{j,k} Q(t) \\ &+ \cdots + (-1)^{r-1} \sum_{1 \le j_1 < j_2 < \cdots < j_r \le m} \prod_{j_1 \cdots j_r} Q(t) \\ &+ \cdots + (-1)^{m-1} \prod_{1 \cdots m} Q(t) \end{aligned} \tag{8.178}$$

where $\prod_{j_1 \cdots j_r}$ is the product of $Q(t)$'s for the basic events in cut set j_1, or $j_2, \ldots,$ or j_r.

The lower and upper bounds of (8.129) can be rewritten as

$$\sum_{j=1}^{m} Q_j^*(t) - \sum_{j=1}^{m-1} \sum_{k=j+1}^{m} \prod_{j,k} Q(t) \le Q_s(t) \le \sum_{j=1}^{m} Q_j^*(t) \tag{8.179}$$

where $\prod_{j,k}$ is the product of $Q(t)$'s for the basic event that is a member of cut set j or k. Because $Q(t)$ is usually much less than one, the brackets are within three significant figures of one another.

The Esary and Proschan upper bound of (8.130) can be written as

True Value	Upper Bound	
$Q_s(t)$	$\le 1 - \prod_{j=1}^{m} [1 - Q_j^*(t)]$	(8.180)

This is exact when the cut sets are disjoint sets of basic events.

Example 20—Two-component series system. Find the upper and lower brackets for $Q_s(t)$ at $t = 20$ hr for a two-component, series, repairable system. The components are 1 and 2 of Example 17.

Solution: From Table 8.10, the cut set and component values at 20 hr are

$$Q_1^*(t) = Q_1(t) = 8.59 \times 10^{-3}$$
$$Q_2^*(t) = Q_2(t) = 3.09 \times 10^{-2}$$

From (8.179),

$$\begin{aligned} Q_s(t)_{\max} &= Q_1^*(t) + Q_2^*(t) \\ &= 8.59 \times 10^{-3} + 3.09 \times 10^{-2} \\ &= 3.95 \times 10^{-2} \\ Q_s(t)_{\min} &= Q_1^*(t) + Q_2^*(t) - Q_1(t)Q_2(t) \\ &= 3.92 \times 10^{-2} \end{aligned}$$

The lower bound, the last bracket, is the best. It coincides with the exact system unavailability $Q_s(t)$ because all terms in the expansion are included. ■

Example 21—Two-component parallel system. Obtain the upper and lower brackets of $Q_s(t)$ for the parallel, two-component system of Example 18.

Solution: Here we have only one cut set, and so $Q_s(t)$ is exactly equal to $Q^*(t)$ and the upper and lower bounds are identical. ■

Example 22—Two-out-of-three system. Find the upper and lower brackets for $Q_s(t)$ at 500 hr for the two-out-of-three system of Example 19 (nonrepairable case), and compare the values with $Q_s(t)$ upper bound obtained from equation (8.180).

Solution: From Table 8.10, at $t = 500$ hr,

$$Q_1(t) = 3.93 \times 10^{-1}, \qquad Q_2(t) = 6.32 \times 10^{-1}, \qquad Q_3(t) = 7.77 \times 10^{-1}$$

From Table 8.12,

$$Q_1^*(t) = 2.49 \times 10^{-1}, \qquad Q_2^*(t) = 4.91 \times 10^{-1}, \qquad Q_3^*(t) = 3.06 \times 10^{-1} \tag{8.181}$$

The exact expression for $Q_s(t)$ from equation (8.178) or Example 11 is

$$\begin{aligned} Q_s(t) &= \sum_{j=1}^{3} \Pr\{d_j\} - \sum_{j=1}^{2}\sum_{k=j+1}^{3} \Pr\{d_j \cap d_k\} + \sum_{j=1}^{1}\sum_{k=j+1}^{2}\sum_{l=k+1}^{3} \Pr\{d_j \cap d_k \cap d_l\} \\ &= \Pr\{d_1\} + \Pr\{d_2\} + \Pr\{d_3\} - [\Pr\{d_1 \cap d_2\} + \Pr\{d_1 \cap d_3\} \\ &\quad + \Pr\{d_2 \cap d_3\}] + \Pr\{d_1 \cap d_2 \cap d_3\} \end{aligned} \tag{8.182}$$

where

$$[A] \equiv [\Pr\{d_1\} + \Pr\{d_2\} + \Pr\{d_3\}] = Q_1^*(t) + Q_2^*(t) + Q_3^*(t) = 1.05$$

$$\begin{aligned} [B] &\equiv [\Pr\{d_1 \cap d_2\} + \Pr\{d_1 \cap d_3\} + \Pr\{d_2 \cap d_3\}] = \prod_{1,2} Q(t) + \prod_{1,3} Q(t) + \prod_{2,3} Q(t) \\ &= Q_1(t)Q_2(t)Q_3(t) + Q_1(t)Q_2(t)Q_3(t) + Q_1(t)Q_2(t)Q_3(t) = 5.79 \times 10^{-1} \end{aligned}$$

$$[C] \equiv \Pr\{d_1 \cap d_2 \cap d_3\} = \prod_{1,2,3} Q(t) = Q_1(t)Q_2(t)Q_3(t) = 1.93 \times 10^{-1}$$

Thus

$$\begin{aligned} Q_s(t)_{\max} &= [A] = 1.05 \\ Q_s(t)_{\min} &= [A] - [B] = 4.66 \times 10^{-1} \\ Q_s(t)_{\max} &= [A] - [B] + [C] = 6.59 \times 10^{-1} \end{aligned}$$

In this case, the second $Q_s(t)_{\max}$ is the exact value and is the last bracket. As in the last example, all terms are included.

The upper bound obtained by (8.180) is

$$\begin{aligned} Q_s(t)\text{upper} &= 1 - [1 - 2.49 \times 10^{-1}][1 - 4.91 \times 10^{-1}][1 - 3.06 \times 10^{-1}] \\ &= 7.35 \times 10^{-1} \end{aligned} \tag{8.183}$$

We see that this upper bound is a conservative estimate compared to the second $Q_s(t)_{\max}$. ■

8.7.4 System Parameter $w_s(t)$

The parameter $w_s(t)$ is the expected number of times the top event occurs at time t, per unit time; thus $w_s(t)dt$ is the expected number of times the top event occurs during $[t, t + dt)$. We now let

e_j = the event that the jth cut set failure occurs during $[t, t + dt)$; that is, $\Pr\{e_j\} = w_j^*(t)dt$

For the top event to occur in the interval $[t, t + dt)$, none of the cut set failures can exist at time t, and then one (or more) of them must fail in time t to $t + dt$. Hence

$$w_s(t)dt = \Pr\left\{\overline{T} \cap \left[\bigcup_{j=1}^{m} e_j\right]\right\} = \Pr\left\{\bigcup_{j=1}^{m} e_j\right\} - \Pr\left\{T \left[\bigcup_{j=1}^{m} e_j\right]\right\} \tag{8.184}$$

$$T \equiv \bigcup_{j=1}^{m} d_j \tag{8.185}$$

or, equivalently,

$$w_s(t) = w_s^{(1)}(t) - w_s^{(2)}(t) \tag{8.186}$$

The first right-hand term is the contribution from the event that one or more cut sets fail during $[t, t + dt)$. The second accounts for those cases in which one or more cut sets fail during $[t, t + dt)$ while other cut sets, already failed to time t, have not been repaired. It is a second-order correction term; hence we label it $w_s^{(2)}(t)$. The first term $w_s^{(1)}(t)$ gives an upper bound for $w_s(t)$.

8.7.4.1 *First term* $w_s^{(1)}(t)$.

Expanding $w_s^{(1)}(t)$ in the same manner as (8.122) yields

$$\begin{aligned} w_s^{(1)}(t)dt &= \Pr\left\{\bigcup_{j=1}^{m} e_j\right\} \\ &= \sum_{j=1}^{m} w_j^*(t)dt - \sum_{j=1}^{m-1} \sum_{k=j+1}^{m} \Pr\{e_j \cap e_k\} \\ &\quad + \cdots + (-1)^{r-1} \sum_{1 \le j_1 < j_2 < \cdots < j_r \le m} \Pr\{e_{j_1} \cap e_{j_2} \cap \cdots \cap e_{j_r}\} \\ &\quad + \cdots + (-1)^{m-1} \Pr\{e_1 \cap e_2 \cap \cdots \cap e_m\} \end{aligned} \tag{8.187}$$

The first summation, as in equation (8.122), is simply the contribution from cut set failures, whereas the second and following terms involve the simultaneous occurrence of two or more failures. The cut set failures considered in the particular combinations must not exist at time t and then must all simultaneously occur in t to $t + dt$.

The foregoing equations are adequate to obtain upper estimates $w_s^{(1)}(t)$ of $w_s(t)$ for simple series systems: The expansion terms $\Pr\{e_j \cap e_k\}$ are zero because the cut sets do not have any common component. For parallel systems, $w_s = w^*$, there being only one cut set.

Example 23—Two-component series system. Calculate $w_s^{(1)}(t)$ at 20 hr for a two-component ($\lambda_1 = 10^{-3}, \lambda_2 = 2 \times 10^{-3}$), repairable ($\mu_1 = 1/10, \mu_2 = 1/40$), series system at 20 hr.

Solution: From Table 8.10,

$$w_1^*(20) = 9.91 \times 10^{-4}, \qquad w_2^*(20) = 1.94 \times 10^{-3} \tag{8.188}$$

Noting that the second and the following terms on the right-hand side of (8.187) are equal to zero,

$$\begin{aligned} w_s^{(1)}(20) &= \sum_{j=1}^{m} w_j^*(20) = w_1^*(20) + w_2^*(20) \\ &= 9.91 \times 10^{-4} + 1.94 \times 10^{-3} \\ &= 2.93 \times 10^{-3} \end{aligned}$$

This is maximum w_s, with $w_s^{(2)} = 0$ in (8.186). A nonrepairable system would be treated in exactly the same way. ■

The simultaneous occurrence of two or more cut sets can only be caused by one basic event occurring and, moreover, this basic event must be a common member of all those cut sets that must occur simultaneously.* Consider the general event $e_1 \cap e_2 \cap \cdots \cap e_r$, that is, the simultaneous occurrence of the r cut sets. Let there be α unique basic events that are common members to all of the r cut sets: Each of these basic events must be a member of every one of the cut sets $1, \ldots, r$. If α is zero, then the event $e_1 \cap e_2 \cap \cdots \cap e_r$ cannot occur, and its associated probability is zero. Assume, therefore, that α is greater than zero.

If one of these α basic events does not exist at t and then occurs in t to $t + dt$, and all the other basic events of the r cut sets exist at t (including the $\alpha - 1$ common basic events), then the event $e_1 \cap e_2 \cap \cdots \cap e_r$ will occur. The probability of the event $e_1 \cap e_2 \cap \cdots \cap e_r$ is

$$\Pr\{e_1 \cap e_2 \cap \cdots \cap e_r\} = w^*(t; 1, \ldots, r)dt \prod_{1 \cdots r}^{*} Q(t) \tag{8.189}$$

The product symbol in equation (8.189) is defined such that

$\prod_{1 \cdots r}^{*} Q(t)$ = the product of $Q(t)$ for the basic event that is a member of at least one of the cut sets $1, \ldots, r$ but is not a common member of all of them.

The product in equation (8.189) is, therefore, the product of the existence probabilities of those basic events other than the α common basic events. Also, a basic event existence probability $Q(t)$ appears only once in the product even though it is a member of two or more cut sets (it cannot be a member of all r cut sets because these are the α common basic events).

The quantity $w^*(t; 1, \ldots, r)dt$ accounts for the α common basic events and is defined such that

---

*The next few pages of this discussion closely follow Vesely's original derivation.

$w^*(t; 1 \cdots r)dt =$ the unconditional failure intensity for a cut set that has as its basic events the basic events that are common members to all the cut sets $1, \ldots, r$.

If the r cut sets have no basic events common to all of them, then $w^*(t; 1, \ldots, r)$ is defined to be identically zero:

$$w^*(t; 1, \ldots, r)dt = 0, \quad \text{no basic events common to all } r \text{ cut sets.} \tag{8.190}$$

The expression for a cut set failure intensity $w^*(t)$, equation (8.168), shows that the intensity consists of one basic event occurring and the other basic events already existing. This is precisely what is needed for the α common basic events. Computation of $w^*(t; 1, \ldots, r)dt$ therefore consists of considering the α common basic events as being members of a cut set, and using equation (8.168) to calculate $w^*(t; 1, \ldots, r)dt$, the unconditional failure intensity for a cut set.

Computation of the probability of r cut sets simultaneously occurring by equation (8.189) is therefore quite direct. The unique basic events that are members of any of the r cut sets are first separated into two groups: those that are common to all r cut sets and those that are not common to all the cut sets. The common group is considered as a cut set in itself, and $w^*(t; 1, \ldots, r)dt$ is computed for this group directly from equation (8.168). If there are no basic events in this common group, then $w^*(t; 1, \ldots, r)dt$ is identically zero and computation need proceed no further, such as $\Pr\{e_1 \cap \cdots \cap e_r\} = 0$. For the uncommon group, the product of the existence probabilities $Q(t)$ for the member basic events is computed. This product and $w^*(t; 1, \ldots, r)dt$ are multiplied and $\Pr\{e_1 \cap \cdots \cap e_r\}$ is obtained. The factor dt will cancel out in the final expression for $w_s^{(1)}(t)$.

With the general term $\Pr\{e_1 \cap \cdots \cap e_r\}$ being determined, equation (8.187), which gives the first term of $w_s(t)dt$, is subsequently evaluated.

$$\begin{aligned} w_s^{(1)}(t) &= \sum_{j=1}^{m} w_j^*(t) - \sum_{j=1}^{m-1} \sum_{k=j+1}^{m} w^*(t; j, k) \prod_{j,k}^{*} Q(t) \\ &+ \cdots + (-1)^{r-1} \sum_{1 \le j_1 < j_2 < \cdots < j_r \le m} w^*(t; j_1, j_2, \ldots, j_r) \prod_{j_1, j_2 \cdots j_r}^{*} Q(t) \\ &+ \cdots + (-1)^{m-1} w^*(t; 1, \ldots, m) \prod_{1 \cdots m}^{*} Q(t) \end{aligned} \tag{8.191}$$

The first term on the right-hand side of this equation is simply the sum of the unconditional failure intensities of the individual cut sets. Each product in the remaining terms consists of separating the common and uncommon basic events for the particular combination of cut sets and then performing the operations described in the preceding paragraphs. Moreover, each succeeding term on the right-hand side of equation (8.191) consists of combinations of a larger number of products of $Q(t)$. Therefore, each succeeding term rapidly decreases in value and the bracketing procedure is extremely efficient when applied to equation (8.191).

8.7.4.2 Second correction term $\mathbf{w_s^{(2)}(t)}$

Outer brackets. Equation (8.191) consequently determines the first term for $w_s(t)$ of (8.186), and the second term $w_s^{(2)}$ must now be determined. Expanding this second term yields

$$
\begin{aligned}
w_s^{(2)}(t)dt &= \Pr\left\{T \bigcup_{j=1}^{m} e_j\right\} \\
&= \sum_{j=1}^{m} \Pr\{e_j \cap T\} - \sum_{j=1}^{m-1}\sum_{k=j+1}^{m} \Pr\{e_j \cap e_k \cap T\} \\
&\quad + \cdots + (-1)^{r-1} \sum_{1\le j_1<j_2<\cdots<j_r\le m} \Pr\{e_{j_1} \cap e_{j_2} \cap \cdots \cap e_{j_r} \cap T\} \\
&\quad + \cdots + (-1)^{m-1}\Pr\{e_1 \cap e_2 \cap \cdots \cap e_m \cap T\}
\end{aligned}
\tag{8.192}
$$

Consider a general term in this expression $\Pr\{e_1 \cap \cdots \cap e_r \cap T\}$. This term is the probability of the r cut sets simultaneously occurring in t to $t + dt$ with one or more of the other cut sets already existing at time t (event T).

Inner brackets. Because event T involves a union, the general term may be expanded:

$$
\begin{aligned}
\Pr\{e_1 \cap \cdots \cap e_r \cap T\} &= \sum_{j=1}^{m} \Pr\{e_1 \cap \cdots \cap e_r \cap d_j\} \\
&\quad - \sum_{j=1}^{m-1}\sum_{k=j+1}^{m} \Pr\{e_1 \cap \cdots \cap e_r \cap d_j \cap d_k\} \\
&\quad + \cdots + (-1)^{s-1} \sum_{1\le j_1<j_2<\cdots<j_s\le m} \\
&\quad \times \Pr\{e_1 \cap \cdots \cap e_r \cap d_{j_1} \cap d_{j_2} \cap \cdots \cap d_{j_s}\} \\
&\quad + \cdots + (-1)^{m-1}\Pr\{e_1 \cap \cdots \cap e_r \cap d_1 \cap d_2 \cap \cdots \cap d_m\}
\end{aligned}
\tag{8.193}
$$

where d_j is the event of the jth cut set failure existing at time t. Consider now a general term in this expansion, $\Pr\{e_1 \cap \cdots \cap e_r \cap d_1 \cap \cdots d_s\}$. If this term is evaluated then $\Pr\{e_1 \cap \cdots \cap e_r \cap T\}$ will be determined and, hence, $w_s^{(2)}(t)dt$.

The event $\Pr\{e_1 \cap \cdots \cap e_r \cap d_1 \cap \cdots d_s\}$ is similar to the event $\Pr\{e_1 \cap \cdots \cap e_r\}$ with the exception that now the cut sets $1, \ldots, s$ must also exist at time t. If a cut set exists at time t, all its basic events must exist at time t, and these basic events cannot occur in t to $t + dt$ because an occurrence calls for a nonexistence at t and then an existence at $t + dt$. The expression for $\Pr\{e_1 \cap \cdots \cap e_r \cap d_1 \cap \cdots d_s\}$ is, therefore, analogous to the previous expression for $\Pr\{e_1 \cap \cdots \cap e_r\}$ [eq. (8.189)] with one alteration. Those basic events common to all the r cut sets $1, \ldots, r$, which are also in any of the s cut sets $1, \ldots, s$, cannot contribute to $\Pr\{e_1 \cap \cdots \cap e_r \cap d_1 \cap \cdots d_s\}$ because they must already exist at time t (for the event $d_1 \cap \cdots \cap d_s$). Hence these basic events, common to all r cut sets and also in any of the s cut sets, must be deleted from $w^*(t; 1, \ldots, r)$ and must be incorporated in the product of basic event existence probabilities appearing in equation (8.189).

8.7.4.3 Bracketing procedure. For fault trees with a large number of cut sets, the bracketing procedure is an extremely efficient method of obtaining as tight an envelope as desired for $w_s(t)$. In equations (8.191), (8.192), and (8.193), an upper bound can be obtained for $w_s^{(1)}(t)$, $w_s^{(2)}(t)$, or $\Pr\{e_1 \cap \cdots \cap e_r \cap T\}$ by considering just the first terms in the respective right-hand expressions. Lower bounds can be obtained by considering the first two terms and so forth. Various combinations of these successive upper and lower bounds will give successive upper and lower bounds for $w_s(t)$.

As an example of the application of the bracketing procedure, a first (and simple) upper bound for $w_s(t)$, $w_s(t)_{\max}$ is given by the relations

$$w_s(t)_{\max} = w_s^{(1)}(t)_{\max} \tag{8.194}$$

where

$$w_s^{(1)}(t)_{\max} = \sum_{j=1}^{m} w_j^*(t) \tag{8.195}$$

This was done in Example 23.

The computer code based on these equations allows the user the luxury of determining how many terms are used in equations (8.191), (8.192), and (8.193). This introduces a number of complications because the terms are alternatively plus and minus. If one chooses, for example, to use two terms in equation (8.191), then $w_s^{(1)}(t)$ is a lower bound with respect to the first term, and the best solution is the lower bound. If three terms are considered, then the best solution is the upper bound. The same consideration applies to $w_s^{(2)}(t)$, so the final $w_s(t)$ brackets must be interpreted cautiously.

The overall system bounds are

$$w_s(t)_{\min} \le w_s(t) \le w_s(t)_{\max}$$

$$w_s(t)_{\min} \equiv w_s^{(1)}(t)_{\min} - w_s^{(2)}(t)_{\max}$$

$$w_s(t)_{\max} \equiv w_s^{(1)}(t)_{\max} - w_s^{(2)}(t)_{\min}$$

Example 24 will hopefully clarify the theory and equations.

Example 24—Two-out-of-three system. Calculate w_s and the associated brackets for the two-out-of-three nonrepairable voting system of Example 22 at 500 hr.

Solution: The system parameters at 500 hr (see Tables 8.10 and 8.12) were:

$$w_1^*(1,2) = 6.73 \times 10^{-4} \qquad w_2^*(2,3) = 9.95 \times 10^{-4} \qquad w_3^*(1,3) = 7.35 \times 10^{-4}$$

$$Q_1 = 3.93 \times 10^{-1} \qquad Q_2 = 6.32 \times 10^{-1} \qquad Q_3 = 7.77 \times 10^{-1}$$

$$w_1 = 6.06 \times 10^{-4} \qquad w_2 = 7.36 \times 10^{-4} \qquad w_3 = 6.69 \times 10^{-4}$$

We proceed with a term-by-term evaluation of $w_s^{(1)}$, using equation (8.191).

1. First term, A:

$$\sum_{j=1}^{3} w_j^*(t) = w_1^*(t) + w_2^*(t) + w_3^*(t) = 2.40 \times 10^{-3} \tag{8.196}$$

2. Second term, B:

$$\sum_{j=1}^{2}\sum_{k=j+1}^{3} w^*(t;j,k)\prod_{j,k}^{*} Q(t) = w^*(t;1,2)\prod_{1,2}^{*} Q(t) + w^*(t;1,3)\prod_{1,3}^{*} Q(t)$$

$$+\, w^*(t;2,3)\prod_{2,3}^{*} Q(t)$$

$$= w_2Q_1Q_3 + w_1Q_2Q_3 + w_3Q_1Q_2 = 6.89 \times 10^{-4}$$

3. Third term, C:

$$\sum_{j=1}^{1}\sum_{k=j+1}^{2}\sum_{l=k+1}^{3} w^*(t;j,k,l)\prod_{j,k,l}^{*} Q(t) = w^*(t;1,2,3)\prod_{1,2,3} Q(t) = 0\cdot Q_1Q_2Q_3 = 0$$

The calculation of $w_s^{(2)}(t)$ is done by using equations (8.192) and (8.193).

4. First term, D:

$$\sum_{j=1}^{3}\Pr\{e_j\cap T\} = \sum_{j=1}^{3}\left[\sum_{k=1}^{3}\Pr\{e_j\cap d_k\} - \sum_{k=1}^{2}\sum_{l=k+1}^{3}\Pr\{e_j\cap d_k\cap d_l\} + \sum_{k=1}^{1}\sum_{l=k+1}^{2}\sum_{q=l+1}^{3}\Pr\{e_j\cap d_k\cap d_l\cap d_q\}\right]$$

Recall now that e_j is the event of the jth cut set failure occurring in t to $t+dt$, and d_j is the event of the jth cut set failure existing at t. The first term in the inner bracket is

$$j=1;\ \Pr\{e_1\cap d_1\}+\Pr\{e_1\cap d_2\}+\Pr\{e_1\cap d_3\} = 0 + w_1Q_2Q_3 + w_2Q_1Q_3$$

If, for example, d_1 exists at time t, components 1 and 2 have failed, and $\Pr\{e_1\} = 0$ (term 1). If d_2 exists, components 2 and 3 have failed, and only component 1 can fail, and so on. The second term in the inner bracket is zero because if two cut sets have failed, all components have failed. This is true of term 3 also.

$$j = 2;\ \Pr\{e_2\cap d_1\}+\Pr\{e_2\cap d_2\}+\Pr\{e_2\cap d_3\} = w_3Q_1Q_2 + 0 + w_2Q_1Q_3$$
$$j = 3;\ \Pr\{e_3\cap d_1\}+\Pr\{e_3\cap d_2\}+\Pr\{e_3\cap d_3\} = w_3Q_1Q_2 + w_1Q_2Q_3 + 0$$

$$\sum_{j=1}^{3}\Pr\{e_j\cap T\} = 2[w_3Q_1Q_2 + w_1Q_2Q_3 + w_2Q_1Q_3] = 1.38\times10^{-3}$$

5. Second term, E:

(a) $\sum_{j=1}^{2}\sum_{k=j+1}^{3}\Pr\{e_j\cap e_k\cap T\} = \sum_{j=1}^{2}\sum_{k=j+1}^{3}\Big[\sum_{l=1}^{3}\Pr\{e_j\cap e_k\cap d_l\} - \sum_{l=1}^{2}\sum_{q=l+1}^{3}$ $\times\Pr\{e_j\cap e_k\cap d_l\cap d_q\} + \sum_{l=1}^{1}\sum_{q=l+1}^{2}\sum_{r=q+1}^{3}\Pr\{e_j\cap e_k\cap d_l\cap d_q\cap d_r\}\Big]$

(b) $j=1, k=2;\ \Pr\{e_1\cap e_2\cap d_1\}+\Pr\{e_1\cap e_2\cap d_2\}+\Pr\{e_1\cap e_2\cap d_3\}$ $-\Pr\{e_1\cap e_2\cap d_1\cap d_2\}-\Pr\{e_1\cap e_2\cap d_1\cap d_3\}-\Pr\{e_1\cap e_2\cap d_2\cap d_3\}+$higher order terms (all zero) $= 0+0+w_2Q_1Q_3-0-0-0+0$

(c) $j=1, k=3;\ \Pr\{e_1\cap e_3\cap d_1\}+\Pr\{e_1\cap e_3\cap d_2\}+\Pr\{e_1\cap e_3\cap d_3\}$ $-\Pr\{e_1\cap e_3\cap d_1\cap d_2\}-\Pr\{e_1\cap e_3\cap d_1\cap d_3\}-\Pr\{e_1\cap e_3\cap d_2\cap d_3\}+$higher order terms (all zero) $= 0+w_1Q_2Q_3+0-0-0-0+0$

(d) $j=2, k=3;\ \Pr\{e_2\cap e_3\cap d_1\}+\Pr\{e_2\cap e_3\cap d_2\}+\Pr\{e_2\cap e_3\cap d_3\}$ $-\Pr\{e_2\cap e_3\cap d_1\cap d_2\}-\Pr\{e_2\cap e_3\cap d_1\cap d_3\}-\Pr\{e_2\cap e_3\cap d_2\cap d_3\}+$higher order terms (all zero) $= w_3Q_1Q_2+0+0-0-0-0+0$

(e) $\sum_{j=1}^{2}\sum_{k=j+1}^{3}\Pr\{e_j\cap e_k\cap T\} = w_2Q_1Q_3 + w_1Q_2Q_3 + w_3Q_1Q_2 = 0.5\times[D]$

(f) $w_s = w_s^{(1)} - w_s^{(2)} = [A-B+C]-[D-E] = 1.71\times10^{-3} - 6.9\times10^{-4} = 1.02\times10^{-3}$

■

It appears that there is an error in the original KITT code subroutine that produces $w_s^{(2)}$.

8.7.5 Other System Parameters

Once Q_s and w_s have been computed, it is comparatively easy to obtain the other system parameters, λ_s and W_s. As with $\lambda^*(t)dt$, its cut set analog, the probability that the top event occurs in time t to $t + dt$, given there is no top event failure at t, is related to $w_s(t)dt$ and $Q_s(t)$ by

$$\lambda_s(t) = \frac{w_s(t)}{1 - Q_s(t)} \tag{8.197}$$

This is identical to equation (8.169), the cut set analog. For the failure to occur in t to $t+dt$, $(w_s(t)dt)$, it must not exist at time t, $(1 - Q_s(t))$, and must occur in time t to $t+dt$, $(\lambda_s(t)dt)$.

The integral value $W_s(0, t)$ is, as before, obtained from the differential $w_s(t)$ by

$$W_s(0, t) = \int_0^t w_s(u)du \tag{8.198}$$

Example 25—Two-out-of-three system. Calculate $\lambda_s(t)$ at 500 hr for the two-out-of-three nonrepairable voting system of Example 22, using Q_s and w_s values from Examples 22 and 24.

Solution: Using the KITT w_s value from Example 24 and Q_s from Example 22:

$$\lambda_s(500) = \frac{w_s}{1 - Q_s} = \frac{1.02 \times 10^{-3}}{1 - 6.59 \times 10^{-1}} = 2.99 \times 10^{-3}$$

■

8.7.6 Short-Cut Calculation Methods

Back-of-the-envelope guesstimates have a time-honored role in engineering and will always be with us, computers notwithstanding. In this section we develop a modified version of a calculation technique originated by Fussell [8]. It requires as input failure and repair rates for each component and minimal cut sets. It assumes exponential distributions with rates λ and μ and independence of component failures. We begin the derivation by restating a few equations presented earlier in this chapter and Table 6.10. We use Q_i as the symbol for component unavailability. Suffix i refers to a component; suffix j to a cut set. As shown in Figure 8.26, for nonrepairable component i,

$$Q_i = 1 - e^{-\lambda_i t} \simeq \lambda_i t \tag{8.199}$$

If the component is repairable,

$$Q_i = \frac{\lambda_i}{\lambda_i + \mu_i}\left[1 - e^{-(\lambda_i + \mu_i)t}\right] \tag{8.200}$$

As t becomes large and if $\lambda_i/\mu_i << 1$,

$$Q_i \simeq \frac{\lambda_i}{\lambda_i + \mu_i} \simeq \frac{\lambda_i}{\mu_i} \tag{8.201}$$

Figure 8.27 shows an approximation for $\lambda = 0.003$ and $\mu = 1/60$. These approximations for nonrepairable and repairable cases overpredict Q_i, in general.

To obtain the cut set reliability parameters, we write the familiar

$$Q_j^* = \prod_{i=1}^{n} Q_i \tag{8.202}$$

Equation (8.202), coupled with equation (8.201), gives the steady-state value for Q_j^* directly. To calculate the other cut set parameters, further approximations need to be made.

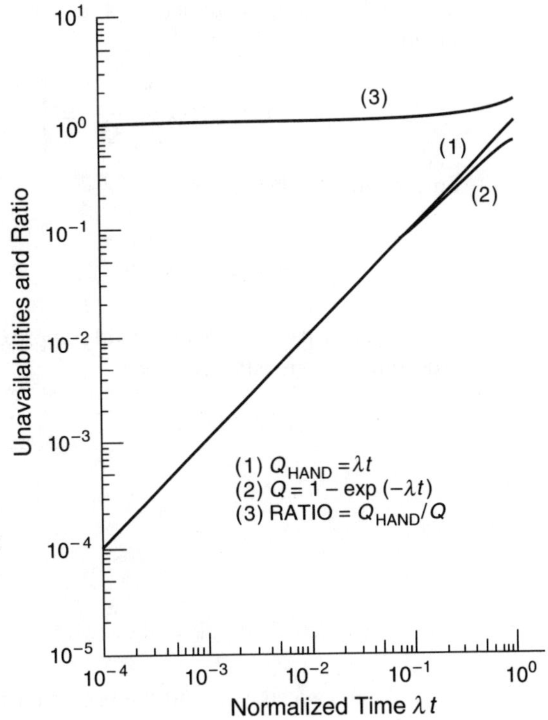

Figure 8.26. Approximation of non-repairable component unavailability.

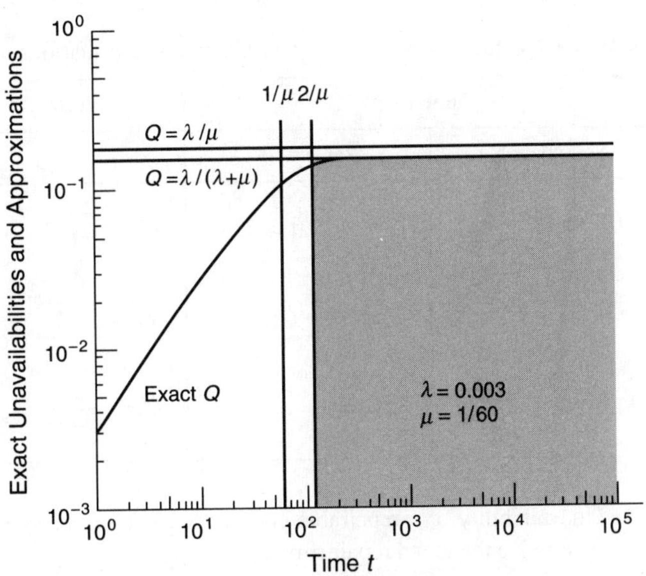

Figure 8.27. Approximation of repairable component unavailability.

We start by combining equations (8.168) with (6.105) to get

$$w_j^*(t) = \sum_{i=1}^{n} [1 - Q_i(t)]\lambda_i(t) \prod_{l=1, l \neq i}^{n} Q_l(t) \tag{8.203}$$

Substituting equation (8.202) and making the approximation that $[1 - Q_i(t)] = 1$ we obtain

$$w_j^*(t) \simeq Q_j^*(t) \sum_{i=1}^{n} \frac{\lambda_i}{Q_i} = \begin{cases} Q_j^*(t) \cdot (n/t), & \text{nonrepairable} \\ Q_j^*(t) \cdot \sum_{i=1}^{n} \mu_i, & \text{repairable} \end{cases} \tag{8.204}$$

Furthermore we have, for λ_j^*,

$$\lambda_j^* = \frac{w_j^*}{1 - Q_j^*} \tag{8.205}$$

System parameters are readily approximated from cut set parameters by bounding procedures previously developed.

$$Q_s \simeq \sum_{j=1}^{m} Q_j^* \tag{8.206}$$

$$\lambda_s \simeq \sum_{j=1}^{m} \lambda_j^* \tag{8.207}$$

$$w_s \simeq \sum_{j=1}^{m} w_j^* \tag{8.208}$$

Some caveats apply to the use of these equations, which are summarized in Table 8.13. In general, the overprediction can become significant in the following cases.

TABLE 8.13. Summary of Short-Cut Calculation Equations

Component		Cut Set	System
Nonrepairable	Repairable		
$Q = \lambda t$, $(\lambda t < 0.1)$	$Q = \lambda/\mu$, $(t > 2/\mu)$	$Q^* = \prod_{i=1}^{n} Q_i$	$Q_s = \sum_{j=1}^{m} Q_j^*$
$w = \lambda[1 - Q]$	$w = \lambda[1 - Q]$	$w_* = Q^* \sum_{i=1}^{n} \frac{\lambda_i}{Q_i}$	$w_s = \sum_{j=1}^{m} w_j^*$
λ: Given	λ: Given	$\lambda^* = \frac{w^*}{1 - Q^*}$	$\lambda_s = \sum_{j=1}^{m} \lambda_j^*$

1. Unavailability of a repairable component, cut set, or system is evaluated at less than twice the mean repair time $1/\mu_i$.
2. Unavailability of a nonrepairable component, system, or cut set is evaluated at more than one-tenth the MTTF = $1/\lambda_i$.
3. When component, cut set, or system unavailabilities are greater than 0.1.

We now test these equations by using them to calculate the reliability parameters for the two-out-of-three system at 100 hr. The input information is, as before:

Component	$\lambda(\text{hr}^{-1})$	$\mu(\text{hr}^{-1})$
1	10^{-3}	1/10
2	2×10^{-3}	1/40
3	3×10^{-3}	1/60

Cut sets are {1, 2}, {2, 3}, {1, 3}.

The calculations are summarized in Table 8.14. The test example is a particularly severe one because, at 100 hr, we are below the minimum time required by component 3 to come to steady state ($t = 100 = 1.67 \times 60 = 1.67 \times (1/\mu_3)$). As shown in Table 8.14, we see that Q_s has been calculated conservatively to an accuracy of 30%.

TABLE 8.14. Repairable and Nonrepairable Cases for Short-Cut Calculations

Parameter	Approximation	Numerical Result (Short-Cut)	Exact Value (Computer)	Time Bounds to Ensure Small Overprediction	
				Minimum	Maximum
		Nonrepairable Case			
Q_1	$\lambda_1 t$	10^{-1}	0.95×10^{-1}	0	100
Q_2	$\lambda_2 t$	2×10^{-1}	1.8×10^{-1}	0	50
Q_3	$\lambda_3 t$	3×10^{-1}	2.6×10^{-1}	0	33
Q_1^*	$Q_1 Q_2$	2×10^{-2}	1.8×10^{-2}		
Q_2^*	$Q_2 Q_3$	6×10^{-2}	4.7×10^{-2}		
Q_3^*	$Q_1 Q_3$	3×10^{-2}	2.5×10^{-2}		
w_1^*	$Q_1^* \sum (\lambda_i / Q_i)$	4×10^{-4}	3.2×10^{-4}		
w_2^*	$Q_2^* \sum (\lambda_i / Q_i)$	12×10^{-4}	8.3×10^{-4}		
w_3^*	$Q_3^* \sum (\lambda_i / Q_i)$	6×10^{-4}	4.5×10^{-4}		
Q_s	$\sum Q_j^*$	11×10^{-2}	9×10^{-2}		
w_s	$\sum w_j^*$	2.2×10^{-3}	1.5×10^{-3}		
		Repairable Case			
Q_1	λ_1 / μ_1	10×10^{-3}	9.9×10^{-3}	20	∞
Q_2	λ_2 / μ_2	80×10^{-3}	74×10^{-3}	80	∞
Q_3	λ_3 / μ_3	180×10^{-3}	152×10^{-3}	120	∞
Q_1^*	$Q_1 Q_2$	8×10^{-4}	7.3×10^{-4}		
Q_2^*	$Q_2 Q_3$	14.4×10^{-3}	11×10^{-3}		
Q_3^*	$Q_1 Q_3$	1.8×10^{-3}	1.5×10^{-3}		
w_1^*	$Q_1^* \sum (\lambda_i / Q_i)$	10×10^{-5}	9.2×10^{-5}		
w_2^*	$Q_2^* \sum (\lambda_i / Q_i)$	6×10^{-4}	4.2×10^{-4}		
w_3^*	$Q_3^* \sum (\lambda_i / Q_i)$	2.1×10^{-4}	1.8×10^{-4}		
Q_s	$\sum Q_j^*$	17×10^{-3}	13×10^{-3}		
w_s	$\sum w_j^*$	9.1×10^{-4}	7×10^{-4}		

8.7.7 The Inhibit Gate

An inhibit gate, Figure 8.28, represents an event that occurs with some fixed probability of occurrence.* It produces the output event only if its input event exists and the inhibit condition has occurred.

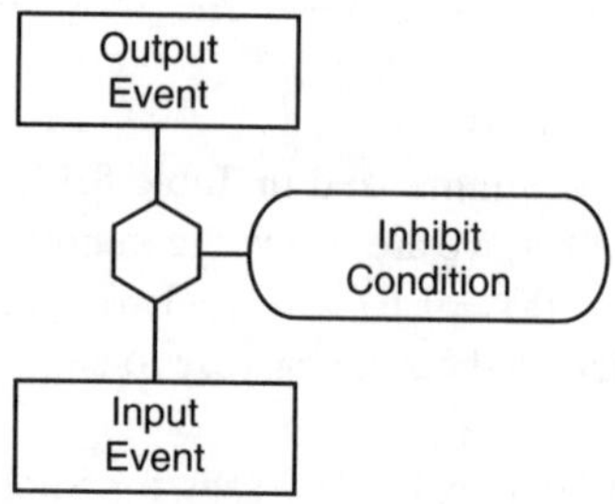

Figure 8.28. Inhibit gate.

An example of a section of a fault tree containing an inhibit gate is shown in Figure 8.29. The event "fuse cut" occurs if a primary or secondary fuse failure occurs. Secondary fuse failure can occur if an excessive current in the circuit occurs because an excessive current can cause a fuse to open.

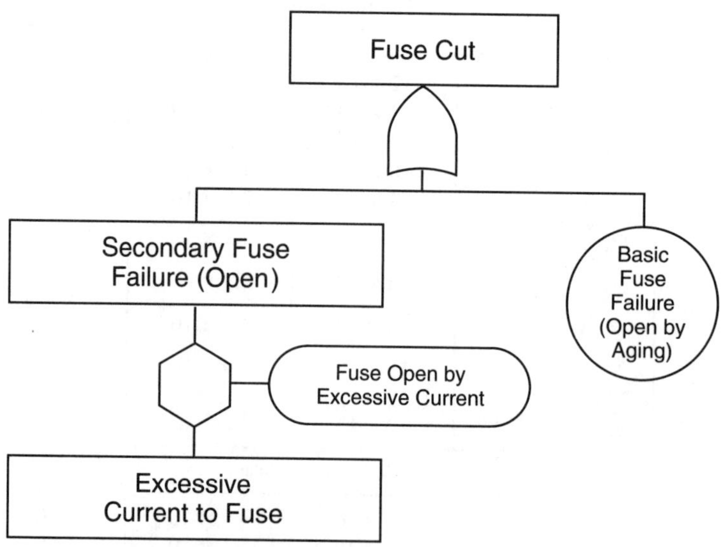

Figure 8.29. Fault tree for fuse.

The fuse does not open, however, every time an excessive current is present in the circuit because there may not be sufficient overcurrent to open the fuse. The inhibit condition is then used as a weighting factor applied to all the failure events in the domain of the inhibit gate. Because the inhibit condition is treated as an AND logic gate in a probabilistic analysis, it is a probabilistic weighting factor. The inhibit condition has many uses in fault-tree analysis, but in all cases it represents a probabilistic weighting factor. A human operator, for example, is simulated by an inhibit gate when his reliability or availability is a time-independent constant.

---

*See also row 3, Table 4.1.

If, in the input to KITT, an event is identified as an inhibit condition, the cut set parameters Q^* and w^* are multiplied by the inhibit value. In the two-component parallel system of Figure 8.30, a value of 0.1 is assigned to the inhibit condition, $Q_2 = 0.1$. The results of the computations are summarized in Table 8.15. We see that the effect of the inhibit gate in Figure 8.30 is to yield $Q^* = Q_1 Q_2 = Q_1 \times 0.1$ and $w^* = w_1 \times 0.1$, with Q_2 independent of time.

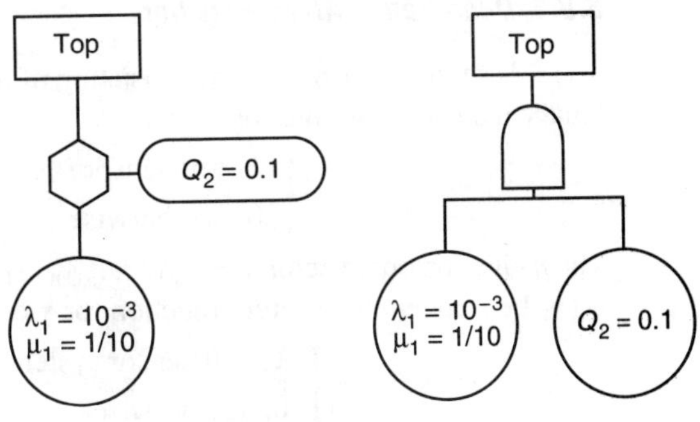

Figure 8.30. Example system with inhibit gate.

TABLE 8.15. Computation for Inhibit Gate

Time	Q_1	w_1	Q_s	w_s
20	8.59×10^{-3}	9.91×10^{-4}	8.59×10^{-4}	9.91×10^{-5}
500	9.90×10^{-3}	9.90×10^{-4}	9.90×10^{-4}	9.90×10^{-5}

8.7.8 Remarks on Quantification Methods

8.7.8.1 Component unavailability for age-dependent failure rate. Assume a component has an age-dependent failure rate $r(s)$, where s denotes age. The equation

$$r(t) = \frac{w(t)}{1 - Q(t)} \tag{8.209}$$

incorrectly quantifies unavailability $Q(t)$ at time t, for a given $r(t)$ and $w(t)$. This equation is correct if $r(t)$ is replaced by $\lambda(t)$, the conditional failure intensity of the component:

$$\lambda(t) = \frac{w(t)}{1 - Q(t)} \tag{8.210}$$

It is difficult to use this equation for the quantification of $Q(t)$, however, because $\lambda(t)$ itself is an unknown parameter. One feasible approach is to use (6.96) to quantify $Q(t)$.

8.7.8.2 Cut set or system reliability

$$R(t) = \exp\left[-\int_0^t \lambda(u)du\right] \tag{8.211}$$

This equation is not generally true. The correct equation is (6.67),

$$R(t) = \exp\left[-\int_0^t r(u)du\right] \tag{8.212}$$

Equation (8.211) is correct only in the case where failure rate $r(t)$ is constant and hence coincides with the (constant) conditional failure intensity $\lambda(t) = \lambda$. For cut sets or systems, the conditional failure intensity is not constant, so we cannot use (8.211). In Chapter 9, we develop Markov transition methods whereby system reliability can be obtained.

8.8 ALARM FUNCTION AND TWO TYPES OF FAILURE

8.8.1 Definition of Alarm Function

Assume a sensor system consisting of n sensors, not necessarily identical. Define a binary indicator variable for sensor i:

$$y_i = \begin{cases} 1, & \text{if sensor } i \text{ is generating its sensor alarm} \\ 0, & \text{otherwise} \end{cases} \tag{8.213}$$

The n-dimensional vector $y = (y_1, \ldots, y_n)$ specifies an overall state for the n sensors. Let $\psi(y)$ be a coherent structure function for y defined by

$$\psi(y) = \begin{cases} 1, & \text{if sensor system is generating its system alarm} \\ 0, & \text{otherwise} \end{cases} \tag{8.214}$$

The function $\psi(y)$ is an alarm function because it tells us how the sensor system generates a system alarm, based on state y of the sensors.

1. Series system:

$$\psi(y_1, y_2) = y_1 y_2 \tag{8.215}$$

2. Parallel system:

$$\psi(y_1, y_2) = 1 - (1 - y_1)(1 - y_2) \tag{8.216}$$

3. Two-out-of-three system:

$$\psi(y_1, y_2, y_3) = 1 - (1 - y_1 y_2)(1 - y_2 y_3)(1 - y_1 y_3) \tag{8.217}$$

Figure 8.31 enumerates the coherent logic for three-sensor systems.

8.8.2 Failed-Safe and Failed-Dangerous Failures

A sensor or a sensor system is failed-safe (FS) if it generates a spurious alarm in a safe environment. On the other hand, a sensor or a sensor system is failed-dangerous (FD) if it does not generate an alarm in an unsafe environment.

8.8.2.1 Failed-safe failure. Assume that the sensor system is in a safe environment. Sensor-state vector y is now conditioned by the environment, and the FS function $\psi_{FS}(y)$ of the sensor system is defined by

$$\psi_{FS}(y) = \begin{cases} 1, & \text{if sensor system is FS} \\ 0, & \text{otherwise} \end{cases} \tag{8.218}$$

where

$$y_i = \begin{cases} 1, & \text{if sensor } i \text{ is FS} \\ 0, & \text{otherwise} \end{cases} \tag{8.219}$$

The sensor system is FS if and only if FS sensors generates the system alarm through alarm function $\psi(y)$. Thus the FS function coincides with alarm function $\psi(y)$, where state vector y is now conditioned by the safe environment.

$$\psi_{FS}(y) = \psi(y) \tag{8.220}$$

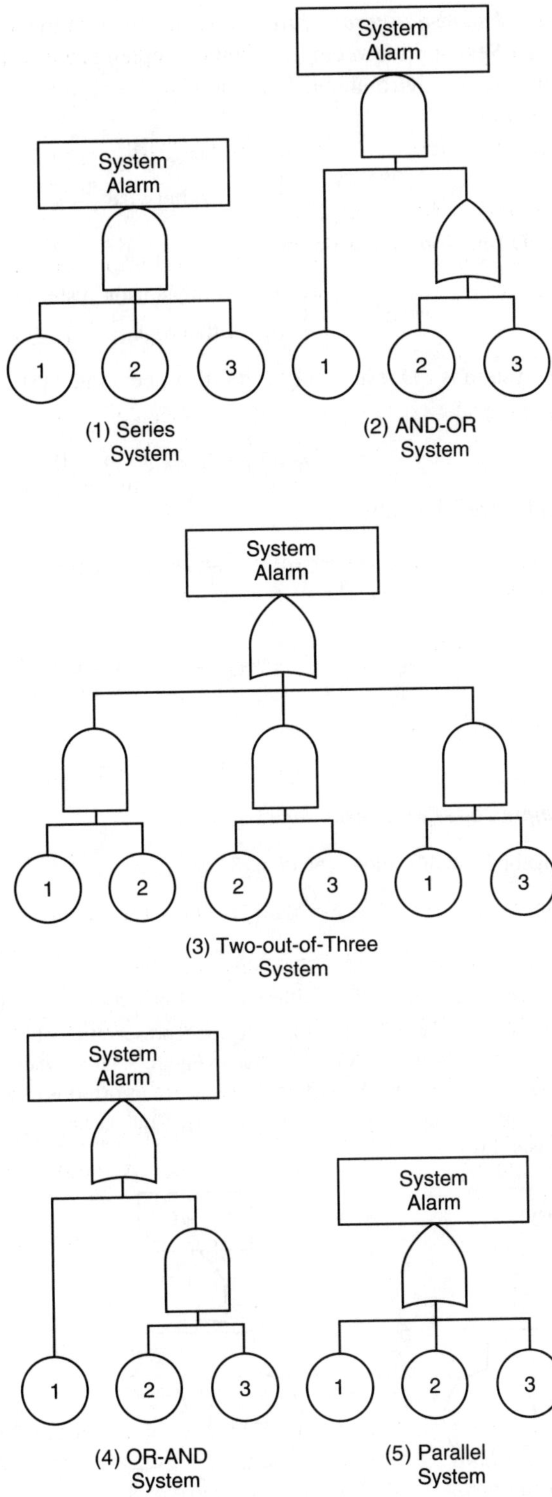

Figure 8.31. Coherent alarm-generation logic for three-sensor system.

8.8.2.2 Failed-dangerous failure. Assume that the sensor system is in an unsafe environment. Sensor-state vector y and its complement $\overline{y} = (\overline{y_1}, \ldots, \overline{y_n})$ are now conditioned by the unsafe environment. Variable $\overline{y_i} = 1 - y_i$, the complement of y_i, tells whether sensor i is FD or not:

$$\overline{y}_i = \begin{cases} 1, & \text{if sensor } i \text{ is FD} \\ 0, & \text{otherwise} \end{cases} \tag{8.221}$$

The FD function of $\overline{y}$ is defined by

$$\psi_{\text{FD}}(\overline{y}) = \begin{cases} 1, & \text{if the sensor system is FD} \\ 0, & \text{otherwise} \end{cases} \tag{8.222}$$

The sensor system is FD if and only if it fails to generate system alarms in unsafe environments:

$$\psi_{\text{FD}}(\overline{y}) = 1 \Leftrightarrow \psi(y) = 0 \tag{8.223}$$

where $\overline{y}$ and y are related by

$$\overline{y} = 1 - y \tag{8.224}$$

Therefore,

$$\psi_{\text{FD}}(\overline{y}) = 1 - \psi(y) = \text{ complement of } \psi(y) \tag{8.225}$$

or

$$\psi_{\text{FD}}(\overline{y}) = 1 - \psi(1 - \overline{y}) \tag{8.226}$$

Example 26—Two-sensor series system

1. Algebraic modification: equation (8.226) yields

$$\psi_{\text{FD}}(\overline{y}) = 1 - y_1 y_2 \tag{8.227}$$

$$= 1 - (1 - \overline{y}_1)(1 - \overline{y}_2) \tag{8.228}$$

The sensor system is FD if either sensor 1 or sensor 2 is FD (i.e., $\overline{y}_1 = 1$ or $\overline{y}_2 = 1$).

2. Fault trees: Figure 8.32(a) is a fault-tree representation of the alarm function $\psi(y) = y_1 y_2$. The complement of $\psi(y)$ is depicted in Figure 8.32(b), where the basic events are expressed in terms of y_1 and y_2. Rewriting the basic events in terms of $\overline{y}_1$ and $\overline{y}_2$ yields Figure 8.32(c), the representation of the FD function $\psi_{\text{FD}}(\overline{y})$; the sensor system is FD if either sensor 1 or sensor 2 is FD. ■

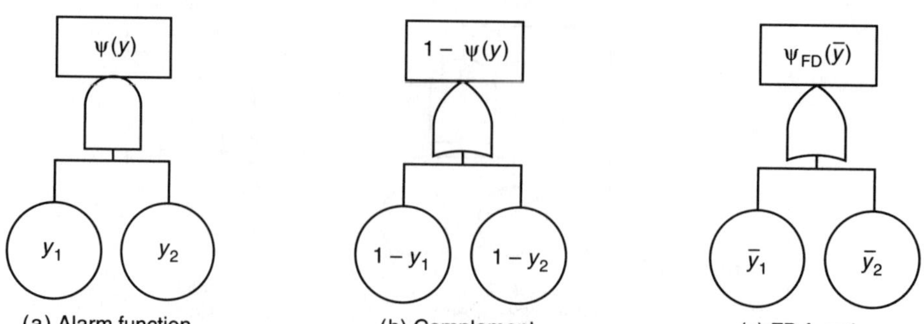

Figure 8.32. FD function for series system.

8.8.3 Probabilistic Parameters

8.8.3.1 Demand probability. Let x be an indicator variable for the environment monitored by the sensor system. It is either safe or unsafe:

$$x = \begin{cases} 1, & \text{if the environment is unsafe} \\ 0, & \text{otherwise} \end{cases} \tag{8.229}$$

The demand probability p is expressed as

$$p = \Pr\{x = 1\} \tag{8.230}$$

8.8.3.2 Sensor. Assume that sensor i monitors the environment. Sensor i is FS if and only if it generates a sensor alarm in a safe environment. Thus the conditional FS probability a_i of sensor i is

$$a_i = \Pr\{y_i = 1 | x = 0\} \tag{8.231}$$

Sensor i is FD if and only if it fails to generate a sensor alarm in the unsafe environment. The conditional FD probability b_i of sensor i is

$$b_i = \Pr\{y_i = 0 | x = 1\} \tag{8.232}$$

8.8.3.3 Sensor system. The conditional FS probability a_s for a sensor system is

$$a_s = \Pr\{\psi_{\text{FS}}(y) = 1 | x = 0\} = E\{\psi_{\text{FS}}(y) | x = 0\} \tag{8.233}$$

$$= \sum_y \psi(y) \Pr\{y | x = 0\} \tag{8.234}$$

Let $h(y)$ be a sum-of- products (sop) expression for alarm function $\psi(y)$. As described in previous sections, two methods are customarily used to obtain $h(y)$:

1. Truth-table approach: Function $h(y)$ is obtained by picking, from a truth table, exclusive combinations of sensor states yielding $\psi(y) = 1$ [see (8.79)]:

$$h(y) = \sum_u \psi(u) \left[\prod_{i=1}^{n} y_i^{u_i} (1 - y_i)^{u_i} \right] \tag{8.235}$$

2. Expansion approach: Function $h(y)$ is obtained by expanding the minimal cut representation or the minimal path representation or any other form of $\psi(y)$.

If the sensors are statistically independent in the safe environment, we have

$$a_s = h(a), \qquad a \equiv (a_1, \ldots, a_n) \tag{8.236}$$

The sensor system is FD if and only if it fails to generate the system alarm in an unsafe environment. The conditional FD probability b_s is

$$b_s = \Pr\{\psi_{\text{FD}}(\overline{y}) = 1 | x = 1\} = E\{1 - \psi(y) | x = 1\} \tag{8.237}$$

$$= E\{1 - h(y) | x = 1\} \tag{8.238}$$

If the sensors are statistically independent in the unsafe environment, we have

$$b_s = 1 - h(1 - b), \qquad b \equiv (b_1, \ldots, b_n) \tag{8.239}$$

Example 27—Two-sensor system. For a two-sensor series system, $h(y) = y_1 y_2$. Thus

$$a_s = a_1 a_2 \tag{8.240}$$

$$b_s = 1 - (1 - b_1)(1 - b_2) = b_1 + b_2 - b_1 b_2 \tag{8.241}$$

For a two-sensor parallel system, $h(y) = y_1 + y_2 - y_1 y_2$. Thus

$$a_s = a_1 + a_2 - a_1 a_2 \tag{8.242}$$

$$\begin{aligned} b_s &= 1 - (1 - b_1) - (1 - b_2) + (1 - b_1)(1 - b_2) \\ &= b_1 b_2 \end{aligned} \tag{8.243}$$

It can be shown that a series system consisting of identical sensors has fewer FS failures than a parallel system; the parallel system is less susceptible to FD failures than the series system. ■

Probabilistic parameters for three-sensor systems are summarized in Table 8.16. Let us now compare alarm-generating logic, assuming identical sensors ($a_i = a, b_i = b$). It can be shown easily that

$$a_s^{(1)} \le a_s^{(2)} \le a_s^{(3)} \le a_s^{(4)} \le a_s^{(5)} \tag{8.244}$$

$$b_s^{(1)} \ge b_s^{(2)} \ge b_s^{(3)} \ge b_s^{(4)} \ge b_s^{(5)} \tag{8.245}$$

where superscripts have the following meanings: (1) = series system (i.e., three-out-of-three system), (2) = AND-OR system, (3) = two-out-of-three system, (4) = OR-AND system, (5) = parallel system (i.e., one-out-of-three system).

TABLE 8.16. Probabilistic Parameters for Three-Sensor Systems

Parameter	(1) Series	(2) AND-OR	(3) Two-out-of-Three	(4) OR-AND	(5) Parallel
General Components					
a_s	$a_1 a_2 a_3$	$a_1 a_2 + a_1 a_3 - a_1 a_2 a_3$	$a_1 a_2 + a_1 a_3 + a_2 a_3 - 2a_1 a_2 a_3$	$a_1 + a_2 a_3 - a_1 a_2 a_3$	$a_1 + a_2 + a_3 - a_1 a_2 - a_1 a_3 - a_2 a_3 + a_1 a_2 a_3$
b_s	$b_1 + b_2 + b_3 - b_1 b_2 - b_1 b_3 - b_2 b_3 + b_1 b_2 b_3$	$b_1 + b_2 b_3 - b_1 b_2 b_3$	$b_1 b_2 + b_1 b_3 + b_2 b_3 - 2b_1 b_2 b_3$	$b_1 b_2 + b_1 b_3 - b_1 b_2 b_3$	$b_1 b_2 b_3$
Identical Components					
a_s	a^3	$2a^2 - a^3$	$3a^2 - 2a^3$	$a + a^2 - a^3$	$3a - 3a^2 + a^3$
b_s	$3b - 3b^2 + b^3$	$b + b^2 - b^3$	$3b^2 - 2b^3$	$2b^2 - b^3$	b^3

REFERENCES

[1] Vesely, W. E. "A time-dependent methodology for fault tree evaluation," *Nuclear Engineering and Design*, vol. 13, no. 2, pp. 337–360, 1970.

[2] Caceres, S., and E. J. Henley. "Process analysis by block diagrams and fault trees," *Industrial Engineering Chemistry: Fundamentals*, vol. 15, no. 2, pp. 128–133, 1976.

[3] Esary, J. D., and F. Proschan. "Coherent structures with non-identical components," *Technometrics*, vol. 5, pp. 191–209, 1963.

[4] Esary, J. D., and F. Proschan. "A reliability bound for systems of maintained and independent components," *J. of the American Statistical Assoc.*, vol. 65, pp. 329–338, 1970.

[5] Vesely, W. E., and R. E. Narum. "PREP and KITT: Computer codes for automatic evaluation of fault trees," Idaho Nuclear Corp., IN1349, 1970.

[6] Jingcheng, L., and P. Zhijie. "An improved algorithm of kinetic tree theory," *Reliability Engineering and System Safety*, vol. 23, pp. 167–175, 1988.

[7] IAEA. "Computer codes for level 1 probabilistic safety assessment," IAEA, IAEA-TECDOC-553, June 1990.

[8] Fussell, J. "How to hand-calculate system reliability and safety characteristics," *IEEE Trans. on Reliability*, vol. 24, no. 3, pp. 169–174, 1975.

PROBLEMS

8.1. Calculate unavailability $Q_s(t)$ for the three-out-of-six voting system, assuming component unavailabilities of 0.1 at time t.

8.2. Calculate unavailability $Q_s(t)$ of the tail-gas quench and clean-up system of Figure 8.12, using as data

$$\Pr\{A\} = \Pr\{D\} = \Pr\{G\} = 0.01$$
$$\Pr\{B\} = \Pr\{C\} = \Pr\{E\} = \Pr\{F\} = 0.1$$

8.3. Calculate availability $A_s(t)$ of the tail-gas quench and clean-up system, using the data in Problem 8.2 and the success tree of Figure 8.15. Confirm that

$$A_s(t) + Q_s(t) = 1$$

8.4. A safety system consists of three monitors. A plant abnormal state requiring shutdown occurs with probability of 0.2. If the safety system fails to shut down, $10,000 is lost. Each spurious shutdown costs $4000. Determine the optimal m-out-of-three safety system, using as data

$$\Pr\{\text{monitor shutdown failure}|\text{abnormal plant}\} = 0.01$$
$$\Pr\{\text{monitor spurious signal}|\text{normal plant}\} = 0.05$$

Assume statistically independent failures. Use the truth-table method.

8.5. **(a)** Obtain the structure functions ψ_1, ψ_2, ψ_3, and ψ for the reliability lock diagram of Figure P8.5.

(b) Calculate the system unavailability, using the component unavailabilities:

$$Q_1 = 0.01, \qquad Q_2 = 0.1, \qquad Q_3 = 0.05$$

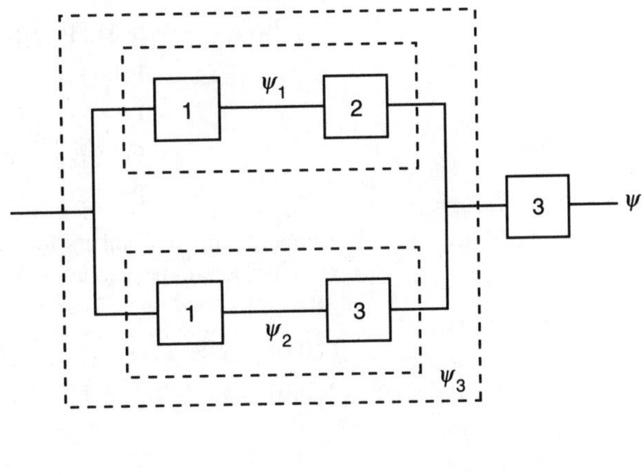

Figure P8.5. A reliability block diagram.

8.6. Consider the reliability block diagram of Figure P8.6. Assume stationary unavailabilities:

$$Q_1 = Q_2 = Q_3 = Q_4 = 0.05, \qquad Q_5 = 0.01$$

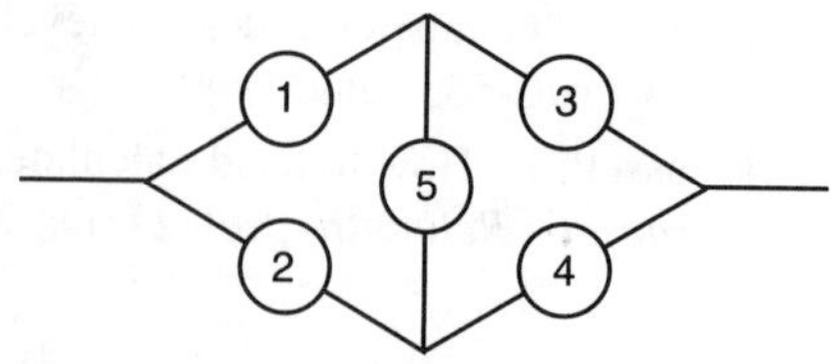

Figure P8.6. A bridge circuit.

(a) Obtain minimal cuts and minimal paths by inspection.
(b) Determine the minimal cut and minimal path representation of the structure function.
(c) Calculate the system unavailability by expanding the two structure functions.
(d) Obtain the system unavailability by the partial pivotal decomposition of the minimal cut representation.
(e) Calculate each bracket of the inclusion-exclusion principle. Obtain the successive lower and upper bounds. Obtain the Esary and Proschan lower and upper bound as well.
(f) Obtain lower and upper bounds using two-event minimal cut sets and minimal path sets.
(g) Assume constant failure rates (conditional failure intensities), $\lambda_1 = \lambda_2 = \lambda_3 = \lambda_4 = \lambda_5 = 0.01$. Obtain constant repair rates (conditional repair intensities), $\mu_1, \ldots, \mu_5$.

8.7. Assume the following rates for the bridge circuit of Figure P8.6.

$$\lambda_1 = \lambda_2 = \lambda_3 = \lambda_4 = \lambda_5 = 0.001 = \lambda$$
$$\mu_1 = \mu_2 = \mu_3 = \mu_4 = \mu_5 = 0.01 = \mu$$

(a) Obtain component parameters Q_i, w_i, and v_i at $t = 100$.
(b) The bridge circuit has four minimal cut sets: $K_1 = \{1, 2\}$, $K_2 = \{3, 4\}$, $K_3 = \{1, 4, 5\}$, and $K_4 = \{2, 3, 5\}$. Calculate cut set parameters Q_i^*, w_i^*, λ_i^*, v_i^*, and μ_i^* at $t = 100$.
(c) Define by

$$e_1 : \text{cut set } \{1, 2\} \text{ occurs at time } t$$
$$e_2 : \text{cut set } \{3, 4\} \text{ occurs at time } t$$
$$e_3 : \text{cut set } \{1, 4, 5\} \text{ occurs at time } t$$
$$e_4 : \text{cut set } \{2, 3, 5\} \text{ occurs at time } t$$

Show that $w_s^{(1)}(t)dt$ of (8.187) becomes

$$\begin{aligned} w_s^{(1)}(t)dt = \; & \Pr\{e_1\} + \Pr\{e_2\} + \Pr\{e_3\} + \Pr\{e_4\} \\ & - \Pr\{e_1 \cap e_2\} - \Pr\{e_1 \cap e_3\} - \Pr\{e_1 \cap e_4\} \\ & - \Pr\{e_2 \cap e_3\} - \Pr\{e_2 \cap e_4\} - \Pr\{e_3 \cap e_4\} \\ & + \Pr\{e_1 \cap e_2 \cap e_3\} + \Pr\{e_1 \cap e_2 \cap e_4\} + \Pr\{e_1 \cap e_3 \cap e_4\} \\ & + \Pr\{e_2 \cap e_3 \cap e_4\} - \Pr\{e_1 \cap e_2 \cap e_3 \cap e_4\} \end{aligned}$$

(d) Determine common members for each term on the right-hand side of the above expression. Determine also $w^*(t; 1, \ldots, r)$ and $\prod_{1\cdots r}^{*} Q(t)$ of (8.189).
(e) Calculate lower and upper bounds for $w_s^{(1)}(100)$, using as data:

$$Q_i(100) = 6.06 \times 10^{-2}, \qquad w_i(100) = 9.39 \times 10^{-4}, \qquad i = 1, \ldots, 5$$
$$w_1^*(100) = w_2^*(100) = 1.14 \times 10^{-4}, \qquad w_3^*(100) = w_4^*(100) = 1.04 \times 10^{-5}$$

8.8. **(a)** If cut sets $K_{j_1}, \ldots, K_{j_r}$ have no common members, then $\Pr\{e_{j_1} \cap \cdots \cap e_{j_r} \cap T\}$ in (8.192) is zero. Noting this, show for the bridge circuit of Figure P8.6 that

$$
\begin{aligned}
w_s^{(2)}(t) &= \Pr\{e_1 \cap T\} + \Pr\{e_2 \cap T\} + \Pr\{e_3 \cap T\} + \Pr\{e_4 \cap T\} \\
&\quad - \Pr\{e_1 \cap e_3 \cap T\} - \Pr\{e_1 \cap e_4 \cap T\} - \Pr\{e_2 \cap e_3 \cap T\} \\
&\quad - \Pr\{e_2 \cap e_4 \cap T\} - \Pr\{e_3 \cap e_4 \cap T\}
\end{aligned}
$$

(b) Expand each term in the above equation, and simplify the results.

(c) Obtain lower and upper bounds for $w_s^{(2)}(100)$ using Q_i, w_i, and w_j^* from Problem 8.7.

8.9. **(a)** Obtain successive lower and upper bounds of $w_s(100)$ using the successive bounds:

$$
\begin{aligned}
w_s^{(1)}(100)_{\max,1} &= 2.49 \times 10^{-4} \\
w_s^{(1)}(100)_{\min,1} &= 2.48 \times 10^{-4} \\
w_s^{(1)}(100)_{\max,2} &= 2.48 \times 10^{-4} = w_s^{(1)}(100)_{\min,2} = \text{last bracket} \\
w_s^{(2)}(100)_{\max,1} &= 3.28 \times 10^{-6} \\
w_s^{(2)}(100)_{\min,1} &= 3.21 \times 10^{-6} \\
w_s^{(2)}(100)_{\max,2} &= 3.21 \times 10^{-6} = w_s^{(2)}(100)_{\min,2} = \text{last bracket}
\end{aligned}
$$

(b) Obtain an upper bound of $\lambda_s(100)$, using $Q_s(100)_{\max} = 7.80 \times 10^{-3}$.

8.10. Apply the short-cut calculation of the reliability parameters for the bridge circuit of Figure P8.6 at $t = 500$, assuming the rates

$$
\begin{aligned}
\lambda_1 &= \lambda_2 = \lambda_3 = \lambda_4 = \lambda_5 = 0.001 = \lambda \\
\mu_1 &= \mu_2 = \mu_3 = \mu_4 = \mu_5 = 0.01 = \mu
\end{aligned}
$$

9

System Quantification for Dependent Events

9.1 DEPENDENT FAILURES

Dependent failures are classified as functional and common-unit interdependencies of components or systems, common-cause failures, and subtle dependencies.

9.1.1 Functional and Common-Unit Dependency

Functional and common-unit dependencies are called *cascade failures*, *propagating failures*, or *command failures*. They exist when a system or a component is unavailable because of the lack of required input from support systems. Functional and common-unit dependencies are caused by functional coupling and common-unit coupling, described in Chapter 2. Most PRAs explicitly represent functional and common-unit dependencies by event trees, fault trees, reliability block diagrams, or Boolean expressions. These representations are *explicit models* because cause-effect relationships are modeled explicitly by the logic models. There are two types of functional and common-unit dependencies: intrasystem (i.e., within a system) and intersystem (i.e., between or among systems) [1].

1. Intrasystem dependencies: These are incorporated directly into the logic model. For example, the fact that a valve cannot supply water to a steam generator unless a pump functions properly is expressed by the feedwater-system fault tree or reliability block diagram.
2. Intersystem dependencies: For this type of dependency (e.g., the dependence of a motor-operated pump in a feedwater system on the supply of electric power), there are two approaches. If a small-event-tree approach is followed, a relatively large fault tree for the feedwater system can be constructed to explicitly include the power supply failure as a cause of motor-operated pump failure. If a large-event-tree approach is used, the intersystem dependencies can be incorporated into

the event-tree headings so that a relatively small fault tree is constructed for the feedwater system for each different power supply state in the event tree.

9.1.2 Common-Cause Failure

Common-cause failure is defined as the simultaneous failure or unavailability of more than one component due to shared causes other than the functional and common-unit dependencies already modeled in the logic model. The occurrence of common-cause failures is affected by factors such as similarity or diversity of components, physical proximity or separation of redundant components, or susceptibilities of components to environmental stresses. An extremely important consideration is the potential for shared human error in design, manufacture, construction, management, and operation of redundant elements.

Models are available for implicitly representing common-cause effects by model parameters. This type of representation is called parametric modeling.

9.1.3 Subtle Dependency

Subtle dependency includes standby redundancies, common loads, and exclusive basic events.

1. Standby redundancy: Standby redundancy is used to improve system availability and reliability. When an operating component fails, a standby component is put into operation, and the system continues to function. Failure of an operating component causes a standby component to be more susceptible to failure because it is now under load. This means that failure of one component affects the failure characteristics of other components, thus component failures are not statistically independent. Typically, Markov models are used to represent dependency due to standby redundancy.
2. Common loads: Assume that a set of components supports loads such as stresses or currents. Failure of one component increases the load carried by the other components. Consequently, the remaining components are more likely to fail, so we cannot assume statistical independence. The dependency among components can be expressed by Markov models.
3. Mutually exclusive events. Consider the basic events, "switch fails to close" and "switch fails to open." These two basic events are mutually exclusive, that is, occurrence of one basic event precludes the other. Thus we encounter dependent basic events when a fault tree involves mutually exclusive basic events. This dependency can be accounted for when minimal cut sets are obtained.

9.1.4 System-Quantification Process

The inclusion-exclusion principle, when coupled with appropriate models, enables us to quantify systems that include dependent basic events. A general procedure for system quantification involving dependent failures is as follows.

1. Represent system parameters by the inclusion-exclusion principle. For each term in the representation, examine whether it involves dependent basic events or not. If a term consists of independent events, quantify it by the methods in Chapter 8. Otherwise, proceed as follows.

2. Model dependent events by an appropriate model.
3. Quantify terms involving dependent events by solving the model.
4. Determine the first bracket to obtain upper bounds for the system parameter. If possible, calculate the second bracket for the lower bound or compute a complete expansion of the system parameter for the exact solution.

This chapter deals with dependencies due to standby redundancies and common causes.

9.2 MARKOV MODEL FOR STANDBY REDUNDANCY

9.2.1 Hot, Cold, and Warm Standby

Consider the tail-gas quench and clean-up system of Figure 8.12. The corresponding fault tree is Figure 8.13. There are two quench pumps, A and B; one is in standby and the other—the principal pump—is in operation.

Assume that pump A is principal at a given time t, whereas pump B is in standby. If pump A fails, standby pump B takes the place of A, and pumping continues. The failed pump A is repaired and then put into standby when the repair is completed. Repaired standby pump A will replace principal pump B when it fails. The redundancy increases system or subsystem reliability. The system has another standby redundancy consisting of the two circulation pumps E and F.

Each component in standby redundancy has three phases: standby, operation, and repair. Components fail only when they are in operation (failure to run) or in standby (failure to start). Depending on component-failure characteristics during these phases, standby redundancy is classified into the following types.

1. Hot Standby: Each component has the same failure rate regardless of whether it is in standby or operation. Hot standby redundancy involves statistically independent components because the failure rate of one component is unique, and not affected by the other components.
2. Cold Standby: Components do not fail when they are in cold standby. Failure of a principal component forces a standby component to start operating and to have a nonzero failure rate. Thus failure characteristics of one component are affected by the other, and cold standby redundancy results in mutually dependent basic events (component failures).
3. Warm Standby: A standby component can fail, but it has a smaller failure rate than a principal component. Failure characteristics of one component are affected by the other, and warm standby induces dependent basic events.

9.2.2 Inclusion-Exclusion Formula

The fault tree in Figure 8.13 has five minimal cut sets:

$$d_1 = \{A\}, \qquad d_2 = \{D\}, \qquad d_3 = \{G\}, \qquad d_4 = \{B, C\}, \qquad d_5 = \{E, F\} \tag{9.1}$$

The inclusion exclusion principle (8.122) gives the following lower and upper bounds for system unavailability $Q_s(t)$.

$$
\begin{aligned}
Q_s(t)_{\max} &= \text{first bracket} \\
&= \Pr\{A\} + \Pr\{D\} + \Pr\{G\} + \Pr\{B \cap C\} + \Pr\{E \cap F\} &\quad (9.2)\\
Q_s(t)_{\min} &= Q_s(t)_{\max} - \text{second bracket} &\quad (9.3)\\
&= Q_s(t)_{\max} - \Pr\{A \cap D\} - \Pr\{A \cap G\} - \Pr\{A \cap B \cap C\} \\
&\quad - \Pr\{A \cap E \cap F\} - \Pr\{D \cap G\} - \Pr\{D \cap B \cap C\} \\
&\quad - \Pr\{D \cap E \cap F\} - \Pr\{G \cap B \cap C\} - \Pr\{G \cap E \cap F\} &\quad (9.4)\\
&\quad - \Pr\{B \cap C \cap E \cap F\}
\end{aligned}
$$

Events A, D, G, $B \cap C$, and $E \cap F$ are mutually independent by assumption, thus (9.4) can be written as

$$
\begin{aligned}
Q_s(t)_{\min} = Q_s(t)_{\max} &- \Pr\{A\}\Pr\{D\} - \Pr\{A\}\Pr\{G\} - \Pr\{A\}\Pr\{B \cap C\} \\
&- \Pr\{A\}\Pr\{E \cap F\} - \Pr\{D\}\Pr\{G\} - \Pr\{D\}\Pr\{B \cap C\} \\
&- \Pr\{D\}\Pr\{E \cap F\} - \Pr\{G\}\Pr\{B \cap C\} \\
&- \Pr\{G\}\Pr\{E \cap F\} - \Pr\{B \cap C\}\Pr\{E \cap F\}
\end{aligned}
\quad (9.5)
$$

Note that the equalities

$$
\left.
\begin{aligned}
\Pr\{B \cap C\} &= \Pr\{B\}\Pr\{C\} \\
\Pr\{E \cap F\} &= \Pr\{E\}\Pr\{F\}
\end{aligned}
\right\}
\quad (9.6)
$$

hold only for hot standby redundancy. Cold or warm standby does not satisfy these equalities.

Probabilities $\Pr\{A\}$, $\Pr\{D\}$, and $\Pr\{G\}$ are component unavailabilities computable by methods in Chapter 6. Probabilities $\Pr\{B \cap C\}$ and $\Pr\{E \cap F\}$ are denoted by $Q_r(t)$, which is the unavailability in standby redundancy calculated by the methods explained in the following sections. In all cases we assume perfect switching, although switching failures could also be expressed by Markov transition models.

9.2.3 Time-Dependent Unavailability

9.2.3.1 Two-component redundancy. Figure 9.1 summarizes the behavior of a standby-redundancy system consisting of components A and B. Each rectangle represents a redundancy state. The extreme left box in a rectangle is a standby component, the middle box is a principal component, and the extreme right box is for components under repair. Thus rectangle 1 represents a state where component B is in standby and component A is operating. Similarly, rectangle 4 expresses the event that component B is operating and component A is under repair. Possible state transitions are shown in the same figure. The warm or hot standby has transitions from state 1 to 3, or state 2 to 4, whereas the cold standby does not. For the warm or hot standby, the standby component fails with constant failure rate $\bar{\lambda}$. For hot standby, $\bar{\lambda}$ is equal to λ, the failure rate for principal components. For cold standby, $\bar{\lambda}$ is zero. The warm standby $(0 \le \bar{\lambda} \le \lambda)$ has as its special cases the hot standby $(\bar{\lambda} = \lambda)$ and the cold standby $(\bar{\lambda} = 0)$. Two or less components can be repaired at a time, and each component has a constant repair rate μ. In all cases, the system fails when it enters state 5.

Denote by $P_i(t)$ the probability that the redundant system is in state i at time t. The derivative $\dot{P}_i(t)$ is given by

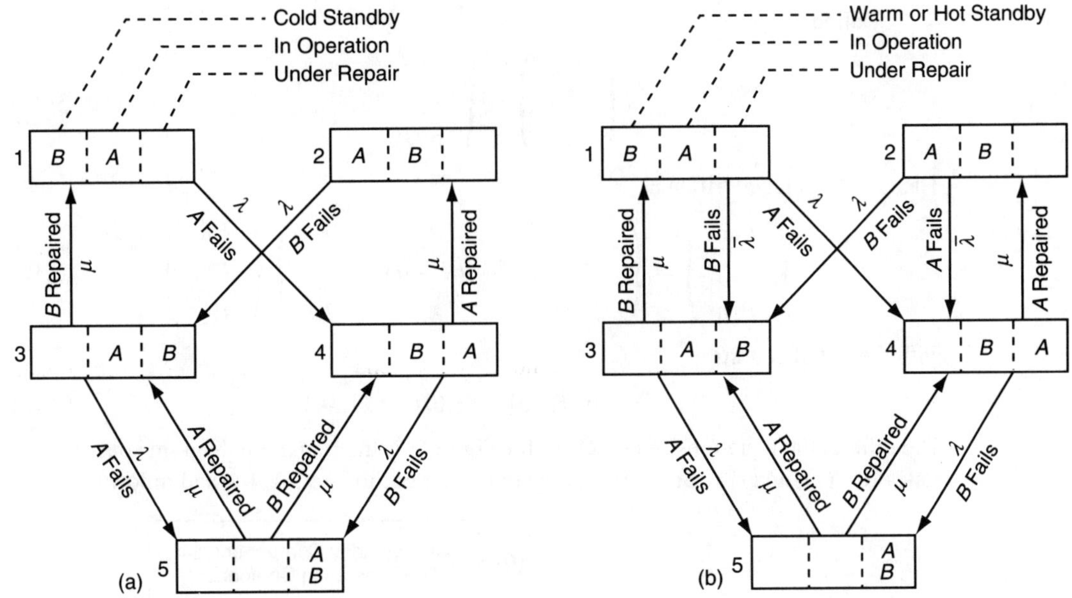

Figure 9.1. Transition diagram for cold, warm, or hot standby. (a) Diagram for cold standby; (b) Diagram for warm or hot standby.

$$
\begin{aligned}
\dot{P}_i(t) &= (\text{inflow to state } i) - (\text{outflow from state } i) \\
&= \sum_{j \neq i} [\text{rate of transition to state } i \text{ from state } j] \times [\text{probability of state } j] \\
&\quad - \sum_{j \neq i} [\text{rate of transition from state } i \text{ to state } j] \times [\text{probability of state } i]
\end{aligned}
\tag{9.7}
$$

Notice that each transition rate is weighted by the corresponding source state probability. The above formula results in a set of differential equations

$$
\begin{pmatrix} \dot{P}_1 \\ \dot{P}_2 \\ \dot{P}_3 \\ \dot{P}_4 \\ \dot{P}_5 \end{pmatrix} = \begin{pmatrix} -(\lambda + \bar{\lambda}) & 0 & \mu & 0 & 0 \\ 0 & -(\lambda + \bar{\lambda}) & 0 & \mu & 0 \\ \bar{\lambda} & \lambda & -(\lambda + \mu) & 0 & \mu \\ \lambda & \bar{\lambda} & 0 & -(\lambda + \mu) & \mu \\ 0 & 0 & \lambda & \lambda & -2\mu \end{pmatrix} \begin{pmatrix} P_1 \\ P_2 \\ P_3 \\ P_4 \\ P_5 \end{pmatrix} \tag{9.8}
$$

The first equation in (9.8) is obtained by noting that state 1 has inflow rate μ from state 3 and two outflow rates, λ and $\bar{\lambda}$. Other equations are obtained in a similar way. Assume that the redundant system is in state 1 at time zero. Then the initial condition for (9.8) is

$$
[P_1(0), P_2(0), \ldots, P_5(0)] = (1, 0, \ldots, 0) \tag{9.9}
$$

Add the first equation of (9.8) to the second, and the third equation to the fourth, respectively. Then

$$
\begin{pmatrix} d[P_1 + P_2]/dt \\ d[P_3 + P_4]/dt \\ dP_5/dt \end{pmatrix} = \begin{pmatrix} -(\lambda + \bar{\lambda}) & \mu & 0 \\ \lambda + \bar{\lambda} & -(\lambda + \mu) & 2\mu \\ 0 & \lambda & -2\mu \end{pmatrix} \begin{pmatrix} P_1 + P_2 \\ P_3 + P_4 \\ P_5 \end{pmatrix} \tag{9.10}
$$

Define

$$\begin{pmatrix} P_{(0)} \\ P_{(1)} \\ P_{(2)} \end{pmatrix} = \begin{pmatrix} P_1 + P_2 \\ P_3 + P_4 \\ P_5 \end{pmatrix} \tag{9.11}$$

Then (9.10) can be written as

$$\begin{pmatrix} \dot{P}_{(0)} \\ \dot{P}_{(1)} \\ \dot{P}_{(2)} \end{pmatrix} = \begin{pmatrix} -(\lambda + \bar{\lambda}) & \mu & 0 \\ \lambda + \bar{\lambda} & -(\lambda + \mu) & 2\mu \\ 0 & \lambda & -2\mu \end{pmatrix} \begin{pmatrix} P_{(0)} \\ P_{(1)} \\ P_{(2)} \end{pmatrix} \tag{9.12}$$

with the initial condition

$$[P_{(0)}(0), P_{(1)}(0), P_{(2)}(0)] = (1, 0, 0) \tag{9.13}$$

The differential equations of (9.12) are for Figure 9.2, the transition diagram consisting of states (0), (1), and (2). State (0), for example, has outflow rate $\lambda + \bar{\lambda}$ and inflow rate μ.

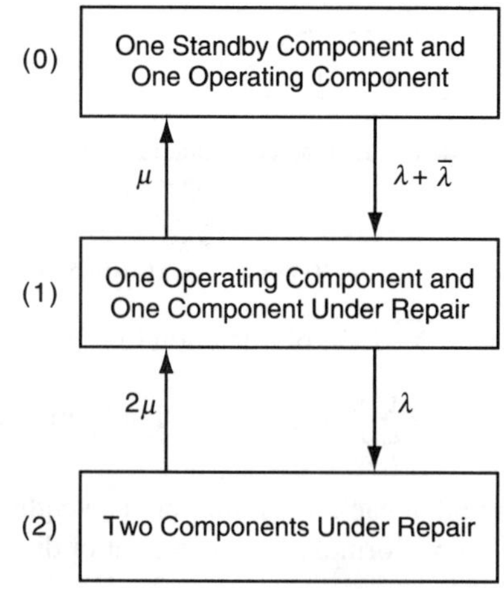

Figure 9.2. Simplified Markov transition diagram: redundant configuration.

Equation (9.12) can be integrated numerically or, if an analytical solution for $P_{(i)}$ is required, Laplace transforms may be used. The Markov differential equations represent dependent failures by introducing state-dependent transition rates; interconnected components do not necessarily operate independently, nor are repairs of failed components necessarily made independently. For more information on Markov models, analytical solutions, numerical calculations, and reliability applications, the reader can consult the articles and textbooks cited in reference [2].

The parameter $Q_r(t) = \Pr\{A \cap B\}$ is the unavailability of the standby redundancy $\{A, B\}$ and equals the probability that both components A and B are under repair at time t. Thus

$$Q_r(t) = P_{(2)}(t) \tag{9.14}$$

Example 1—Warm standby. Consider the redundant quench pumps B and C of Figure 8.12. Assume the following failure and repair rates for each pump.

$$\lambda = 10^{-3}(\text{hr}^{-1}), \qquad \bar{\lambda} = 0.5 \times 10^{-3}\ (\text{hr}^{-1}), \qquad \mu = 10^{-2}\ (\text{hr}^{-1}) \tag{9.15}$$

Calculate parameter $Q_r(t)$ at $t = 100$, 500, and 1000 hr.

Solution: Substitute $P_{(2)} = 1 - P_{(0)} - P_{(1)}$ into the second equation of (9.12). Then,

$$\begin{pmatrix} \dot{P}_{(0)} \\ \dot{P}_{(1)} \end{pmatrix} = \begin{pmatrix} -(\lambda+\bar{\lambda}), & \mu \\ \lambda+\bar{\lambda}-2\mu, & -(\lambda+3\mu) \end{pmatrix} \begin{pmatrix} P_{(0)} \\ P_{(1)} \end{pmatrix} + \begin{pmatrix} 0 \\ 2\mu \end{pmatrix} \tag{9.16}$$

The Laplace transform of $\dot{P}_{(i)}$ is related to $L[P_{(i)}]$ and $P_{(i)}(0)$ by

$$L[\dot{P}_{(i)}] = \int_0^\infty \dot{P}_{(i)}(t)e^{-st}dt = sL[P_{(i)}] - P_{(i)}(0) \tag{9.17}$$

and the Laplace transform of the constant 2μ is

$$L[2\mu] = \int_0^\infty 2\mu e^{-st}dt = 2\mu/s \tag{9.18}$$

Thus transformation of both sides of (9.16) yields

$$\begin{pmatrix} sL[P_{(0)}]-1 \\ sL[P_{(1)}]-0 \end{pmatrix} = \begin{pmatrix} -(\lambda+\bar{\lambda}), & \mu \\ \lambda+\bar{\lambda}-2\mu, & -(\lambda+3\mu) \end{pmatrix} \begin{pmatrix} L[P_{(0)}] \\ L[P_{(1)}] \end{pmatrix} + \begin{pmatrix} 0 \\ 2\mu/s \end{pmatrix} \tag{9.19}$$

or

$$\begin{pmatrix} \lambda+\bar{\lambda}+s, & -\mu \\ -\lambda-\bar{\lambda}+2\mu, & \lambda+3\mu+s \end{pmatrix} \begin{pmatrix} L[P_{(0)}] \\ L[P_{(1)}] \end{pmatrix} = \begin{pmatrix} 1 \\ 2\mu/s \end{pmatrix} \tag{9.20}$$

Substituting failure and repair rates into (9.20):

$$\begin{pmatrix} s+1.5\times10^{-3}, & -10^{-2} \\ 1.85\times10^{-2}, & s+3.1\times10^{-2} \end{pmatrix} \begin{pmatrix} L[P_{(0)}] \\ L[P_{(1)}] \end{pmatrix} = \begin{pmatrix} 1 \\ 2\times10^{-2}/s \end{pmatrix} \tag{9.21}$$

These are linear simultaneous equations for $L[P_{(0)}]$ and $L[P_{(1)}]$ and can be solved:

$$\begin{pmatrix} L[P_{(0)}] \\ L[P_{(1)}] \end{pmatrix} = \begin{pmatrix} s+1.5\times10^{-3}, & -10^{-2} \\ 1.85\times10^{-2}, & s+3.1\times10^{-2} \end{pmatrix}^{-1} \begin{pmatrix} 1 \\ 2\times10^{-2}/s \end{pmatrix} \tag{9.22}$$

or

$$L[P_{(0)}] = \frac{s+3.1\times10^{-2}}{(s+a)(s+b)} + \frac{2\times10^{-4}}{s(s+a)(s+b)} \tag{9.23}$$

$$L[P_{(1)}] = \frac{1.5\times10^{-3}}{(s+a)(s+b)} + \frac{3\times10^{-5}}{s(s+a)(s+b)} \tag{9.24}$$

where $a = 1.05\times10^{-2}$ and $b = 2.20\times10^{-2}$.

From standard tables of inverse Laplace transforms,

$$L^{-1}\left(\frac{K}{(s+a)(s+b)}\right) = \frac{K}{b-a}(e^{-at} - e^{-bt}) \tag{9.25}$$

$$L^{-1}\left(\frac{K(s+z)}{(s+a)(s+b)}\right) = \frac{K}{b-a}[(z-a)e^{-at} - (z-b)e^{-bt}] \tag{9.26}$$

$$L^{-1}\left(\frac{K}{s(s+a)(s+b)}\right) = \frac{K}{ab}\left(1 - \frac{be^{-at}}{b-a} + \frac{ae^{-bt}}{b-a}\right) \tag{9.27}$$

These inverse transforms give

$$P_{(0)} = 0.8639 + 0.1303e^{-at} + 0.0057e^{-bt} \tag{9.28}$$

$$P_{(1)} = 0.1296 - 0.1179e^{-at} - 0.0117e^{-bt} \tag{9.29}$$

and, at the steady state,

$$P_{(0)}(\infty) = 0.8639 \tag{9.30}$$
$$P_{(1)}(\infty) = 0.1296 \tag{9.31}$$

Thus the cut set parameter $Q_s(t)$ is

$$Q_r(t) = 1 - P_{(0)} - P_{(1)} \tag{9.32}$$
$$= 0.0065 - 0.0124e^{-0.0105t} + 0.0060e^{-0.022t} \tag{9.33}$$

yielding

t	$Q_r(t)$
100	0.0028
500	0.0064
1000	0.0065

A steady state $Q_r(\infty) = 0.0065$ is reached at $t = 1000$. ■

Example 2—Cold standby. Assume the following failure and repair rates for quench pumps B and C.

$$\lambda = 10^{-3}\ (\text{hr}^{-1}), \qquad \bar{\lambda} = 0\ (\text{hr}^{-1}), \qquad \mu = 10^{-2}\ (\text{hr}^{-1}) \tag{9.34}$$

Calculate parameter $Q_r(t)$ at $t = 100$, 500, and 1000 hr.

Solution: Substitute the failure and repair rates into (9.20).

$$\begin{pmatrix} s+0.001, & -0.01 \\ 0.019, & s+0.031 \end{pmatrix} \begin{pmatrix} L[P_{(0)}] \\ L[P_{(1)}] \end{pmatrix} = \begin{pmatrix} 1 \\ 0.02/s \end{pmatrix} \tag{9.35}$$

$$L[P_{(0)}] = \frac{s+0.031}{(s+a)(s+b)} + \frac{0.0002}{s(s+a)(s+b)} \tag{9.36}$$

$$L[P_{(1)}] = \frac{0.001}{(s+a)(s+b)} + \frac{0.00002}{s(s+a)(s+b)} \tag{9.37}$$

where $a = 0.010$ and $b = 0.022$.

The inverse transformations (9.25) to (9.27) give

$$P_{(0)} = 0.9050 + 0.0915e^{-at} + 0.0035e^{-bt} \tag{9.38}$$
$$P_{(1)} = 0.0905 - 0.0831e^{-at} - 0.0074e^{-bt} \tag{9.39}$$
$$Q_r(t) = 1 - P_{(0)} - P_{(1)} \tag{9.40}$$
$$= 0.0045 - 0.0084e^{-0.010t} + 0.0039e^{-0.022t} \tag{9.41}$$

yielding

t	$Q_r(t)$
100	0.0019
500	0.0045
1000	0.0045

■

Example 3—Hot standby. Let quench pumps A and B have the failure and the repair rates

$$\lambda = \bar{\lambda} = 10^{-3} \text{ (hr}^{-1}), \qquad \mu = 10^{-2} \text{ (hr}^{-1}) \tag{9.42}$$

Calculate $Q_r(t)$ at $t = 100$, 500, and 1000 hr.

Solution: In this case, pumps B and C are statistically independent and we calculate $Q_r(t)$ without solving differential equation (9.16).

From Table 6.10,

$$\begin{aligned} Q(t) &= \text{unavailability of pump } B \\ &= \text{unavailability of pump } C \\ &= \frac{\lambda}{\lambda + \mu}(1 - e^{-(\lambda+\mu)t}) \end{aligned} \tag{9.43}$$

Thus

$$Q_r(t) = Q(t)^2 = \left(\frac{\lambda}{\lambda+\mu}\right)^2 \left[1 - e^{-(\lambda+\mu)t}\right]^2 \tag{9.44}$$

$$= \left(\frac{\lambda}{\lambda+\mu}\right)^2 - 2\left(\frac{\lambda}{\lambda+\mu}\right)^2 e^{-(\lambda+\mu)t} + \left(\frac{\lambda}{\lambda+\mu}\right)^2 e^{-2(\lambda+\mu)t} \tag{9.45}$$

$$= 0.0083 - 0.0165e^{-0.011t} + 0.0083e^{-0.022t} \tag{9.46}$$

Therefore

t	$Q_r(t)$
100	0.0037
500	0.0082
1000	0.0083

Table 9.1 summarizes the results of Examples 1 to 3. As expected,

$$\begin{aligned} &\text{unavailability of hot standby} > \text{unavailability of warm standby} \\ &\qquad > \text{unavailability of cold standby} \end{aligned} \tag{9.47}$$

TABLE 9.1. Summary of Examples 1 to 3

	Example 1 Warm	Example 2 Cold	Example 3 Hot
$Q_r(100)$	0.0028	0.0019	0.0037
$Q_r(500)$	0.0064	0.0045	0.0082
$Q_r(1000)$	0.0065	0.0045	0.0083
λ	0.001	0.001	0.001
$\bar{\lambda}$	0.0005	0	0.001
μ	0.01	0.01	0.01

■

Example 4—Tail-gas system unavailability. Consider the tail-gas quench clean-up system of Figure 8.12. Assume the failure and repair rates in Example 1 for the quench pumps (warm standby); the rates in Example 2 for the circulation pumps (cold standby); and the following rates for booster fan A, feed pump D, and filter G:

$$\lambda^* = 10^{-4}, \qquad \mu^* = 10^{-2} \tag{9.48}$$

Evaluate the system unavailability $Q_s(t)$ at $t = 100$, 500, and 1000 hr.

Solution: From Examples 1 and 2, we have

t	$Q'_r(t) = \Pr\{B \cap C\}$	$Q''_r(t) = \Pr\{E \cap F\}$
100	0.0028	0.0019
500	0.0064	0.0045
1000	0.0065	0.0045

and,

$$\begin{aligned} Q^*(t) &= \Pr\{A\} = \Pr\{D\} = \Pr\{G\} \\ &= \frac{\lambda^*}{\lambda^* + \mu^*}(1 - e^{-(\lambda^*+\mu^*)t}) \\ &= 0.0099[1 - e^{-0.0101t}] \end{aligned} \tag{9.49}$$

Thus

t	$Q^*(t)$
100	0.0063
500	0.0098
1000	0.0099

Equations (9.2) and (9.4) become

$$\begin{aligned} Q_s(t)_{\max} &= 3Q^*(t) + Q'_r(t) + Q''_r(t) \\ Q_s(t)_{\min} &= Q_s(t)_{\max} - 3Q^*(t)^2 - 3Q^*(t)Q'_r(t) - 3Q^*(t)Q''_r(t) - Q'_r(t)Q''_r(t) \end{aligned} \tag{9.50}$$

yielding

t	$Q_s(t)_{\max}$	$Q_s(t)_{\min}$
100	0.025	0.025
500	0.040	0.040
1000	0.041	0.040

■

9.2.3.2 Three-component redundancy. So far we have treated standby redundancy with two components. Let us now consider the tail-gas quench and clean-up system of Figure 9.3, which has a two-out-of-three quench-pump system. Assume that each pump has failure rate λ when it is operating and failure rate $\bar{\lambda}$ when it is in standby, and that only one pump at a time can be repaired. Note that two or less pumps are repaired at a time in Figure 9.1. Possible state transitions are shown in Figure 9.4. State 1 means that pump A is in standby and pumps D and B are principal (working). State 13 shows that pumps A, D, and B are under repair, but only pump A is currently being repaired. Transition from state 7 to 13 occurs when pump B fails; it is assumed that pump B is still operating in state 7 and rate λ is used, although the two-out-of-three system is failed in this state;

if the pump stops operating at state 7, rate $\overline{\lambda}$ is used. Pump B is in the last place in the repair queue in state 13, and transition from state 13 to 12 happens when repair of pump A is complete. Pump D is being repaired in state 12. The other transitions have similar explanations.

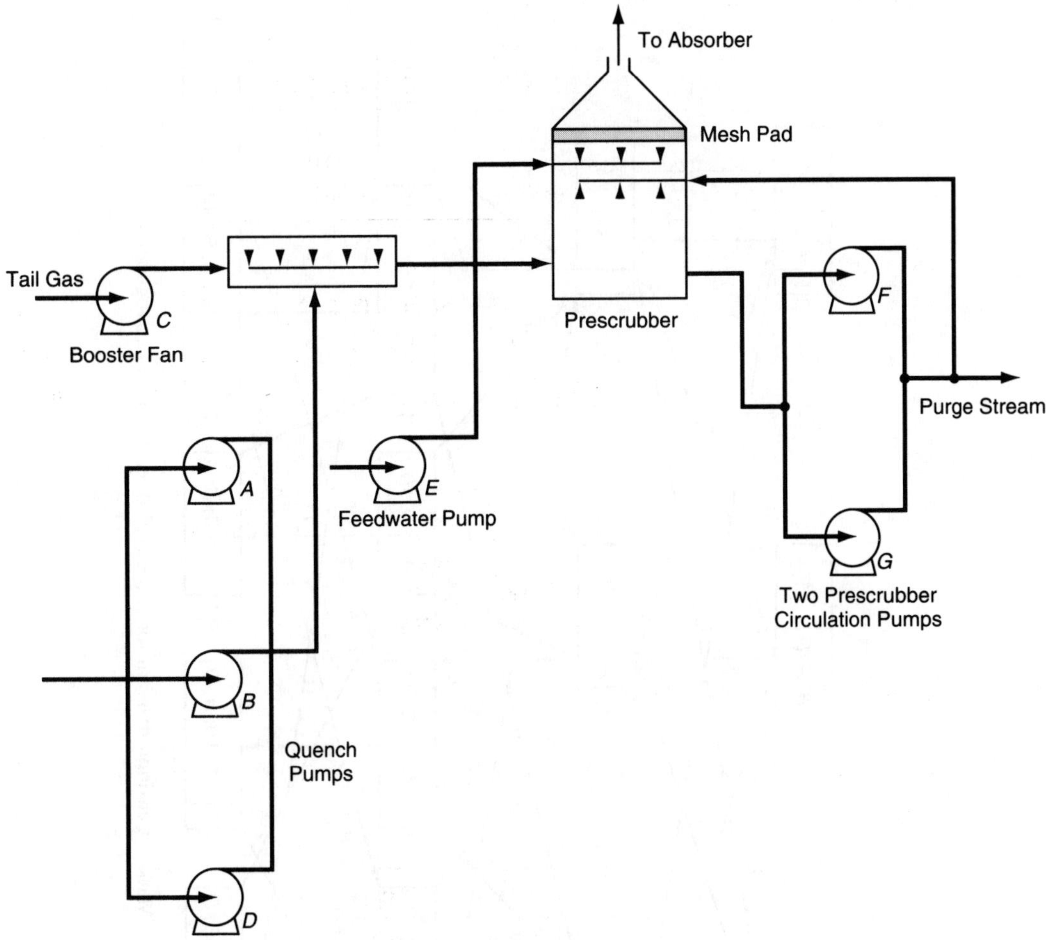

Figure 9.3. Tail-gas quench and clean-up system with 2/3 quench pumps.

The states in Figure 9.4 can be aggregated as shown in Figure 9.5. The states in the first row of Figure 9.4 are substates of state (0) of Figure 9.5. State (0) implies one standby pump and two operating pumps, and the states in the second row of Figure 9.4 are substates of state (1), which has two principal pumps and one pump under repair.

State (0) has substates 1, 2, and 3. Each substate goes into state (1) at the rate $2\lambda + \overline{\lambda}$. Thus the inflow from state (0) to state (1) is

$$\begin{aligned}(2\lambda + \overline{\lambda})P_1 + (2\lambda + \overline{\lambda})P_2 + (2\lambda + \overline{\lambda})P_3 &= (2\lambda + \overline{\lambda})(P_1 + P_2 + P_3) \\ &= (2\lambda + \overline{\lambda})P_{(0)}\end{aligned} \tag{9.51}$$

This means that the rate of transition from state (0) to state (1) is $(2\lambda + \overline{\lambda})$ as shown in Figure 9.5. Rates of the other transitions are obtained in a similar manner.

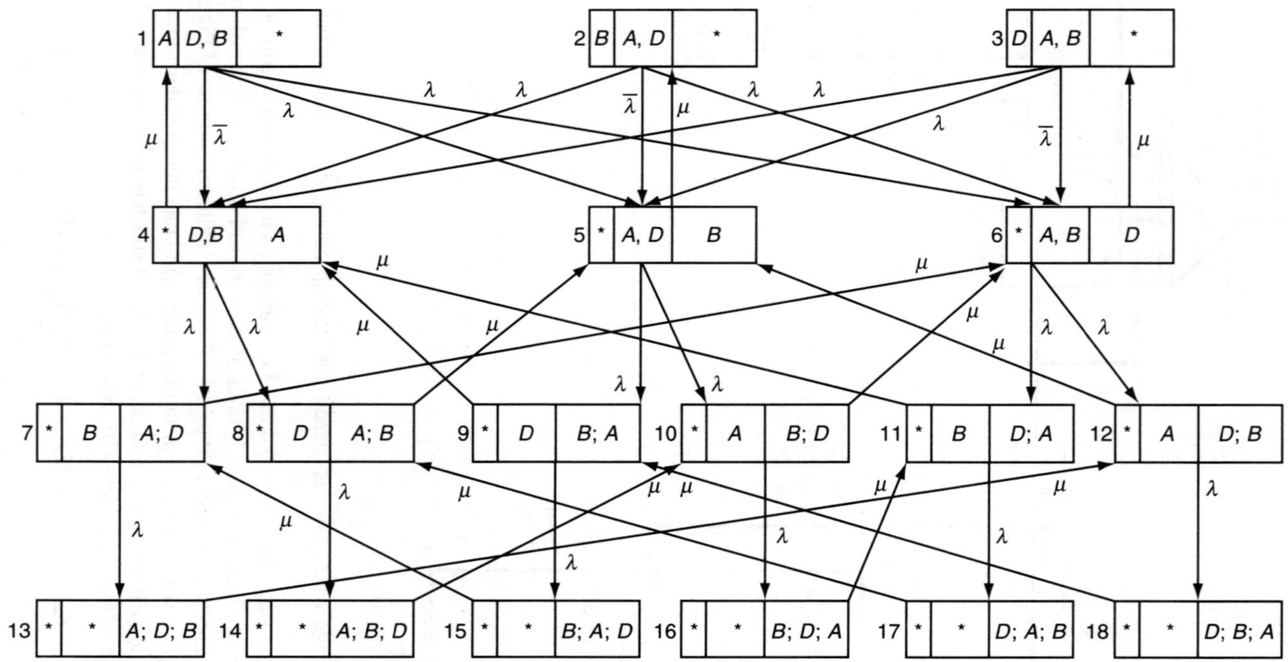

Figure 9.4. Markov transition diagram for two-out-of-three redundant configuration.

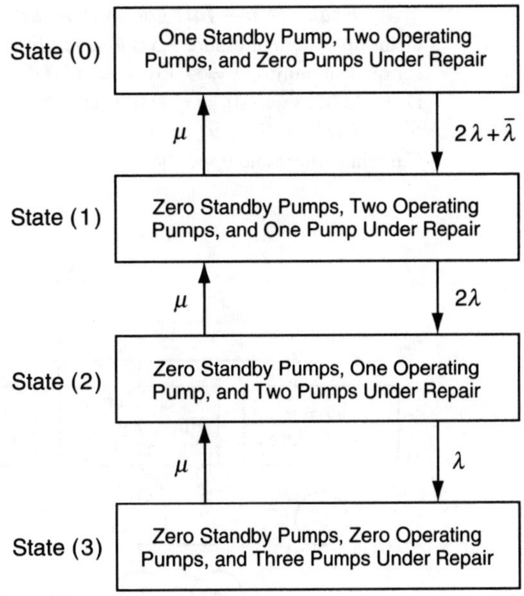

Figure 9.5. Simplified transition diagram for two-out-of-three redundant configuration.

The transition diagram of Figure 9.5 gives the following differential equation.

$$\begin{pmatrix} \dot{P}_{(0)} \\ \dot{P}_{(1)} \\ \dot{P}_{(2)} \\ \dot{P}_{(3)} \end{pmatrix} = \begin{pmatrix} -(2\lambda+\bar{\lambda}) & \mu & 0 & 0 \\ 2\lambda+\bar{\lambda} & -(2\lambda+\mu) & \mu & 0 \\ 0 & 2\lambda & -(\lambda+\mu) & \mu \\ 0 & 0 & \lambda & -\mu \end{pmatrix} \begin{pmatrix} P_{(0)} \\ P_{(1)} \\ P_{(2)} \\ P_{(3)} \end{pmatrix} \tag{9.52}$$

with the initial condition

$$(P_{(0)}, P_{(1)}, P_{(2)}, P_{(3)}) = (1, 0, 0, 0) \tag{9.53}$$

This can be integrated numerically to obtain probabilities $P_{(i)}$.

Two pumps must operate for the quench-pump system of Figure 9.3 to function. Thus the redundancy parameter $Q_r(t)$ for the event "less than two pumps operating" is given by

$$Q_r(t) = P_{(2)}(t) + P_{(3)}(t) \tag{9.54}$$

Example 5—Three-pump standby redundancy. Assume the failure and repair rates (hr^{-1}),

$$\lambda = 10^{-3}, \qquad \bar{\lambda} = 0.5 \times 10^{-3}, \qquad \mu = 10^{-2} \tag{9.55}$$

Calculate $Q_r(t)$ at t = 100, 500, and 1000 hour.

Solution: Substitute the failure and repair rates into (9.52). The resulting differential equations are integrated numerically, yielding

t	$P_{(2)}(t)$	$P_{(3)}(t)$	$Q_r(t)$
100	0.011	0.003	0.014
500	0.036	0.004	0.040
1000	0.038	0.004	0.042

■

Example 6—Tail-gas system unavailability. A fault tree for the tail-gas quench and clean-up system of Figure 9.3 is given as Figure 9.6. Assume the failure and repair rates in Example 1 for quench pumps ($\lambda = 0.001, \bar{\lambda} = 0.0005, \mu = 0.01$); the rates in Example 2 for circulation pumps ($\lambda = 0.001, \bar{\lambda} = 0.0, \mu = 0.01$); and the rates in Example 4 for booster fan C, feed pump E, and filter H ($\lambda^* = 10^{-4}, \mu^* = 10^{-2}$). The results of Examples 4 and 5 are summarized in Table 9.2. Calculate lower and upper bounds for the system unavailability $Q_s(t)$ at $t = 1000$ hr.

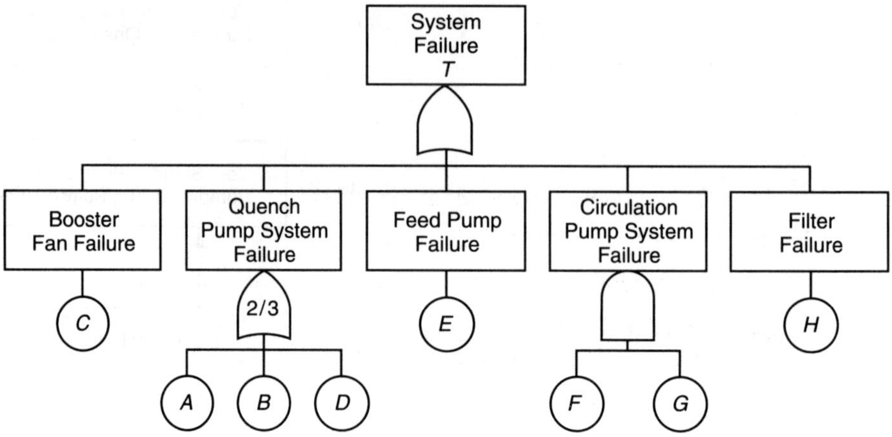

Figure 9.6. Fault tree for tail-gas quench and clean-up system.

TABLE 9.2. Summary of Examples 4 and 5

Example 4	Example 4	Example 5
$Q_r''(1000)$	$Q^*(1000)$	$Q_r(1000)$
0.0045	0.0099	0.042

Solution: The fault tree has minimal cut sets

$$\{C\}, \{E\}, \{H\}, \{A, B\}, \{B, D\}, \{D, A\}, \{F, G\} \tag{9.56}$$

The inclusion-exclusion principle (8.122) gives the following upper and lower bounds for

$$Q_s(t) = \Pr\{C \cup E \cup H \cup [(A \cap B) \cup (B \cap D) \cup (D \cap A)] \cup [F \cap G]\} \tag{9.57}$$

$$\begin{aligned} \text{First bracket} &= Q_s(t)_{\max} = \Pr\{C\} + \Pr\{E\} + \Pr\{H\} \\ &\quad + \Pr\{(A \cap B) \cup (B \cap D) \cup (D \cap A)\} + \Pr\{F \cap G\} \end{aligned} \tag{9.58}$$

$$\begin{aligned} \text{Second bracket} &= Q_s(t)_{\max} - \Pr\{C\}\Pr\{E\} - \Pr\{C\}\Pr\{H\} - \Pr\{E\}\Pr\{H\} \\ &\quad - \Pr\{C\}\Pr\{(A \cap B) \cup (B \cap D) \cup (D \cap A)\} - \Pr\{C\}\Pr\{F \cap G\} \\ &\quad - \Pr\{E\}\Pr\{(A \cap B) \cup (B \cap D) \cup (D \cap A)\} - \Pr\{E\}\Pr\{F \cap G\} \\ &\quad - \Pr\{H\}\Pr\{(A \cap B) \cup (B \cap D) \cup (D \cap A)\} - \Pr\{H\}\Pr\{F \cap G\} \\ &\quad - \Pr\{(A \cap B) \cup (B \cap D) \cup (D \cap A)\}\Pr\{F \cap G\} \end{aligned} \tag{9.59}$$

The probability $\Pr\{(A \cap B) \cup (B \cap D) \cup (D \cap A)\}$ is given by $Q_r(t)$ in Example 5, $\Pr\{C\} = \Pr\{E\} = \Pr\{H\}$ is calculated as $Q^*(t)$ in Example 4, and $\Pr\{F \cap G\}$ is equal to $Q_r''(t)$ in Example 4.

Thus

$$
\begin{aligned}
Q_s(t)_{\max} &= 3Q^*(t) + Q_r(t) + Q_r''(t) \\
&= 3 \times 0.0099 + 0.042 + 0.0045 = 0.076 \\
Q_s(t)_{\min} &= 0.076 - 3Q^*(t)^2 - 3Q^*(t)Q_r(t) - 3Q^*(t)Q_r''(t) - Q_r(t)Q_r''(t) \\
&= 0.076 - 0.0003 - 0.0013 - 0.0001 - 0.0002 \\
&= 0.074
\end{aligned}
\tag{9.60}
$$

and the system unavailability is bracketed by

$$
0.074 \le Q_s(t) \le 0.076 \tag{9.61}
$$

■

9.2.3.3* n-*Component redundancy. As a general case, consider standby redundancies satisfying the following requirements.

1. The standby redundancy consists of n identical components.
2. The redundant configuration has m $(\le n)$ principal components.
3. At most, r (≥ 1) components can be repaired at a time.

An aggregated transition diagram is shown in Figure 9.7, and we have the differential equations

$$
\left.
\begin{aligned}
\dot{P}_{(0)} &= -\lambda_0 P_{(0)} + \mu_1 P_{(1)} \\
&\vdots \\
\dot{P}_{(k)} &= \lambda_{k-1} P_{(k-1)} - (\lambda_k + \mu_k) P_{(k)} + \mu_{k+1} P_{(k+1)} \\
&\vdots \\
\dot{P}_{(n)} &= \lambda_{n-1} P_{(n-1)} - \mu_n P_{(n)}
\end{aligned}
\right\}
\tag{9.62}
$$

where

$$
\left.
\begin{aligned}
k &\equiv \text{number of components under repair} \\
\lambda_k &\equiv m\lambda + (n - m - k)\bar{\lambda}, \quad \text{for } k = 0, \ldots, n - m \\
\lambda_k &\equiv (n - k)\lambda, \quad \text{for } k = n - m + 1, \ldots, n - 1 \\
\mu_k &\equiv \min\{r, k\} \times \mu, \quad \text{for } k = 1, \ldots, n
\end{aligned}
\right\}
\tag{9.63}
$$

The parameter $Q_r(t)$ is given by

$$
Q_r(t) = P_{(n-m+1)}(t) + \cdots + P_{(n)}(t) \tag{9.64}
$$

Equation (9.12) is a special case of (9.62), where $n = 2, m = 1$, and $r = 2$. Similarly, equation (9.52) is obtained from (9.62) by setting $n = 3, m = 2$, and $r = 1$.

9.2.4 Steady-State Unavailability

The steady-state solution of (9.62) satisfies

$$
\left.
\begin{aligned}
0 &= -\lambda_0 P_{(0)} + \mu_1 P_{(1)} \\
&\vdots \\
0 &= \lambda_{k-1} P_{(k-1)} - (\lambda_k + \mu_k) P_{(k)} + \mu_{k+1} P_{(k+1)} \\
&\vdots \\
0 &= \lambda_{n-1} P_{(n-1)} - \mu_n P_{(n)}
\end{aligned}
\right\}
\tag{9.65}
$$

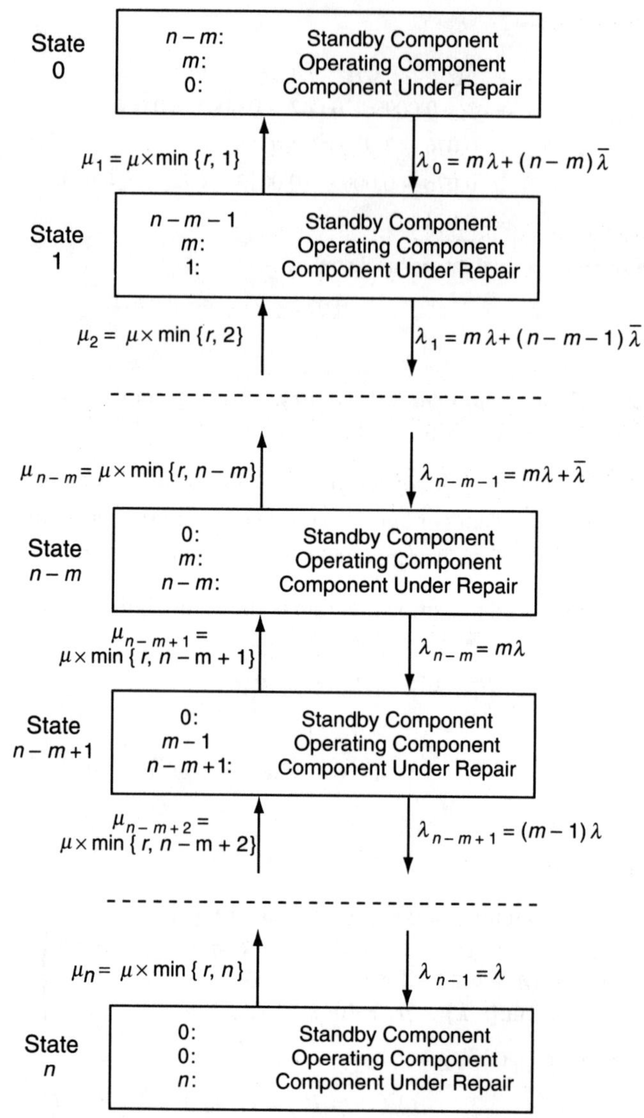

Figure 9.7. Transition diagram for m-out-of-n redundant configuration.

Define

$$\pi_k = \lambda_k P_{(k)} - \mu_{k+1} P_{(k+1)}, \qquad k = 0, \ldots, n-1 \tag{9.66}$$

Then (9.65) can be written as

$$\left.\begin{aligned} \pi_0 &= 0 \\ &\vdots \\ \pi_k - \pi_{k-1} &= 0, \qquad k = 1, \ldots, n-1 \\ &\vdots \\ \pi_{n-1} &= 0 \end{aligned}\right\} \tag{9.67}$$

In other words,

$$\pi_0 = \pi_1 = \cdots = \pi_{n-1} = 0 \tag{9.68}$$

Because $\mu_k \neq 0$ for $k = 1, \ldots, n$, we have from $\pi_{k-1} = 0$,

$$P_{(k)} = \frac{\lambda_{k-1}}{\mu_k} P_{(k-1)} = \frac{\lambda_0 \lambda_1 \ldots \lambda_{k-1}}{\mu_1 \mu_2 \ldots \mu_k} P_{(0)} \equiv \theta_k P_{(0)}, \qquad k = 1, \ldots, n \tag{9.69}$$

Because the sum of all probabilities is equal to unity,

$$P_{(k)} = \theta_k / (\theta_0 + \theta_1 + \cdots + \theta_n) \tag{9.70}$$

where

$$\theta_0 \equiv 1, \qquad \theta_j \equiv \lambda_0 \lambda_1 \cdots \lambda_{j-1} / (\mu_1 \mu_2 \cdots \mu_j), \qquad j = 1, \ldots, n \tag{9.71}$$

The steady state $Q_r(\infty)$ can readily be obtained from (9.70).

Example 7—Two-pump standby redundancy. Calculate the steady-state unavailability $Q_r(\infty)$ for the pump system of Examples 1, 2, and 3.

Solution: Note that $n = 2$, $m = 1$, and $r = 2$. Equation (9.63) or Figure 9.2 gives as values for λ_0, λ_1, μ_1, and μ_2:

	Warm Standby	Cold Standby	Hot Standby
$\lambda_0 = \lambda + \bar{\lambda}$	0.0015	0.001	0.020
$\lambda_1 = \lambda$	0.001	0.001	0.001
$\mu_1 = \mu$	0.01	0.01	0.01
$\mu_2 = 2\mu$	0.02	0.02	0.02

The values for θ_0, θ_1, and θ_2 are

	Warm Standby	Cold Standby	Hot Standby
$\theta_0 = 1$	1	1	1
$\theta_1 = \lambda_0/\mu_1$	0.15	0.1	0.2
$\theta_2 = \lambda_0\lambda_1/(\mu_1\mu_2)$	0.0075	0.005	0.01

Therefore, the probabilities $P_{(k)}$ and $Q_r(\infty)$ are

	Warm Standby	Cold Standby	Hot Standby
$\sum \theta$	1.1575	1.105	1.21
$P_{(0)} = \theta_0 / \sum \theta$	0.864	0.905	0.826
$P_{(1)} = \theta_1 / \sum \theta$	0.130	0.090	0.165
$P_{(2)} = \theta_2 / \sum \theta$	0.006	0.005	0.008
$Q_r(\infty) = P_{(2)}$	0.006	0.005	0.008

We observe from Examples 1, 2, and 3 that the steady-state values of $Q_r(t)$ are attained at $t = 1000$ within round-off error accuracy. ■

Example 8—Three-pump standby redundancy. Consider the pumping system of Example 5. Calculate the steady-state $Q_r(\infty)$ for the event "less than two pumps operating."

Solution: We note that $n = 3$, $m = 2$, and $r = 1$. Equation (9.52) or Figure 9.5 gives

$$\begin{array}{ll} \lambda_0 = 2\lambda + \bar{\lambda} = 0.0025, & \mu_1 = \mu = 0.01 \\ \lambda_1 = 2\lambda = 0.002, & \mu_2 = \mu = 0.01 \\ \lambda_2 = \lambda = 0.001, & \mu_3 = \mu = 0.01 \end{array} \tag{9.72}$$

Values of θ_k are

$$\begin{aligned} \theta_0 &= 1 \\ \theta_1 &= \lambda_0/\mu_1 = 0.25 \\ \theta_2 &= \lambda_0\lambda_1/(\mu_1\mu_2) = 0.05 \\ \theta_3 &= \lambda_0\lambda_1\lambda_2/(\mu_1\mu_2\mu_3) = 0.005 \end{aligned}$$

Equation (9.70) gives

$\sum\theta$	$P_{(0)} = \theta_0/\sum\theta$	$P_{(1)} = \theta_1/\sum\theta$	$P_{(2)} = \theta_2/\sum\theta$	$P_{(3)} = \theta_3/\sum\theta$
1.305	0.766	0.192	0.038	0.004

(9.73)

Hence from (9.54)

$$Q_r(\infty) = 0.038 + 0.004 = 0.042 \tag{9.74}$$

This steady-state value confirms $Q_r(t)$ at $t = 1000$, as in Example 5. ■

9.2.5 Failures per Unit Time

9.2.5.1 Two-component redundancy. The parameter $w_s(t)$ is important in that its integration over a time interval is the expected number of system failures during the interval. As shown by (8.194) and (8.195), an upper bound for $w_s(t)$ is

$$w_s(t)_{\max} = \sum_{i=1}^{m} w_i^*(t) \tag{9.75}$$

Consider the fault tree of Figure 8.13 that has five minimal cut sets:

$$d_1 = \{A\} \qquad d_2 = \{D\} \qquad d_3 = \{G\} \qquad d_4 = \{B, C\} \qquad d_5 = \{E, F\} \tag{9.76}$$

Equation (9.75) becomes

$$w_s(t)_{\max} = w_1^*(t) + w_2^*(t) + w_3^*(t) + w_4^*(t) + w_5^*(t) \tag{9.77}$$

For cut set $\{B, C\}$ to fail, either one of B and C should fail in t to $t + dt$ with the other remaining basic event already existing at time t. Thus $w_4^*(t)dt$ is

$$\begin{aligned} w_4^*(t)dt = {} & \Pr\{B \text{ fails during } [t, t+dt) | \overline{B} \cap C \text{ at time } t\} \Pr\{\overline{B} \cap C \text{ at time } t\} \\ & + \Pr\{C \text{ fails during } [t, t+dt) | B \cap \overline{C} \text{ at time } t\} \Pr\{B \cap \overline{C} \text{ at time } t\} \end{aligned} \tag{9.78}$$

Assume failure rate λ' for pumps B and C. Then

$$\begin{aligned} w_4^*(t)dt &= \lambda' dt \times [\Pr\{\overline{B} \cap C \text{ at time } t\} + \Pr\{B \cap \overline{C} \text{ at time } t\}] \\ &= \lambda' dt \cdot P'_{(1)}(t) \end{aligned} \tag{9.79}$$

where $P'_{(1)}(t)$ is the probability of one failed pump existing at time t, and is given by the solution of (9.12). Similarly,

$$w_5^*(t)dt = \lambda'' dt \cdot P''_{(1)}(t) \tag{9.80}$$

where λ'' = failure rate for pumps E and F,
$P''_{(1)}(t)$ = probability of either pump E or F, but not both, being failed at time t

Thus the upper bound $w_s(t)$ can be calculated by

$$\begin{aligned} w_s(t)_{\max} = &\lambda_1[1 - Q_1(t)] + \lambda_2[1 - Q_2(t)] + \lambda_3[1 - Q_3(t)] \\ &+ \lambda' P'_{(1)}(t) + \lambda'' P'_{(2)}(t) \end{aligned} \tag{9.81}$$

Example 9—Tail-gas system configuration 1. Calculate $w_s(1000)_{\max}$ for Figure 8.12 using the failure and repair rates of Example 4.

Solution: We have, from Example 4,

$$\lambda_1 = \lambda_2 = \lambda_3 = \lambda^* = 10^{-4} \tag{9.82}$$

$$\mu_1 = \mu_2 = \mu_3 = \mu^* = 10^{-3} \tag{9.83}$$

$$\begin{aligned} Q_1(t) &= Q_2(t) = Q_3(t) = \frac{\lambda^*}{\lambda^* + \mu^*}\left[1 - e^{-(\lambda^*+\mu^*)t}\right] \\ &= 0.0099 \quad \text{at} \quad t = 1000 \end{aligned} \tag{9.84}$$

$$\lambda' = \lambda'' = \lambda = 10^{-3} \tag{9.85}$$

Using (9.29) and (9.39),

$$\begin{aligned} P'_{(1)} &= 0.1296 - 0.1179e^{-at} - 0.0117e^{-bt} \\ &= 0.130 \quad \text{at} \quad t = 1000, \text{ warm standby} \end{aligned} \tag{9.86}$$

$$\begin{aligned} P''_{(1)} &= 0.0905 - 0.0831e^{-at} - 0.0074e^{-bt} \\ &= 0.090 \quad \text{at} \quad t = 1000, \text{ cold standby} \end{aligned} \tag{9.87}$$

Substituting these values into (9.81),

$$\begin{aligned} w_s(1000)_{\max} &= 3 \times 10^{-4} \times [1 - 0.0099] + 10^{-3} \times 0.130 + 10^{-3} \times 0.090 \\ &= 0.00052 \text{ times/hr} \end{aligned} \tag{9.88}$$

The MTBF is approximated by

$$\text{MTBF} = 1/0.00052 \text{ hr} = 80 \text{ days} \tag{9.89}$$

■

9.2.5.2 Three-component redundancy. Next consider the fault tree of Figure 9.6 that has seven minimal cut sets:

$$\begin{aligned} &d_1 = \{C\}, \quad d_2 = \{E\}, \quad d_3 = \{H\}, \quad d_4 = \{A, B\} \\ &d_5 = \{B, D\}, \quad d_6 = \{D, A\}, \quad d_7 = \{F, G\} \end{aligned} \tag{9.90}$$

Denote by $w_r(t)$ the expected number of times that the quench-pump system fails per unit time at time t. Then, similarly to (9.75), we have as an upper bound

$$w_s(t)_{\max} = w_1^* + w_2^* + w_3^* + w_r + w_7^* \tag{9.91}$$

For the redundant system to fail in time t to $t + dt$, one pump must fail during $[t, t + dt)$ with the redundant system already in state (1) of Figure 9.5. The rate of transition from state (1) to (2) is 2λ. Thus

$$w_r(t) = 2\lambda \cdot P_{(1)}(t) \tag{9.92}$$

where $P_{(1)}(t)$ is the probability that the redundant system has one failed pump at time t, as given by (9.52).

Example 10—Tail-gas system configuration 2. Calculate $w_s(t)_{\max}$ at $t = 1000$ using the failure and repair rates of Example 6.

Solution: Parameter $w_r(t)$ is given by

$$w_r(t) = 2 \times 10^{-3} \times P_{(1)}(1000) = 2 \times 10^{-3} \times 0.19 = 0.00038 \tag{9.93}$$

because numerical integration of (9.52) yields

$$P_{(1)}(1000) = 0.19 \tag{9.94}$$

From the results of Example 9 for $w_1^*(t) = w_2^*(t) = w_3^*(t)$ and $w_7^*(t)$,

$$\begin{aligned} w_s(t)_{\max} &= 3 \times 10^{-4} \times [1 - 0.0099] + 0.00038 + 10^{-3} \times 0.090 \\ &= 0.00077 \end{aligned} \tag{9.95}$$

The MTBF is approximated by

$$\text{MTBF} = 1/0.00077 \text{ hr} = 54 \text{ days} \tag{9.96}$$

■

9.2.5.3 **n-*Component redundancy.*** As a general case, consider an m-out-of-n redundant configuration with r repair crews. Let a fault tree have cut sets that include component failures in the redundancy. The calculation of $w_s(t)_{\max}$ is reduced to evaluating $w_r(t)$, defined as

$$\begin{aligned} w_r(t) &= \text{the expected number of times that the redundant configuration fails per unit time at time } t \\ &= m\lambda P_{(n-m)}(t) \end{aligned}$$

where

$$\begin{aligned} P_{(n-m)}(t) &= \text{the probability of } (n-m) \text{ components being failed at time } t \\ &= \text{the probability of state } (n-m) \text{ in Figure 9.7} \\ m\lambda &= \text{the rate of transition from state } (n-m) \text{ to } (n-m+1) \end{aligned}$$

9.2.6 Reliability and Repairability

As a first step, we partition the set of all states into operational states (U: up) and failed states (D: down). For the m-out-of-n configuration of Figure 9.7, states $0, \ldots, n-m$ are operational and states $n-m+1, \ldots, n$ are failed. For each state S, we write $S \in U$ when the system is operational and $S \in D$ when the system is failed. System reliability $R(t)$, availability $A(t)$, and repairability $M(t)$ are defined by [2]

$$R(t) \equiv \Pr\{S \in U \text{ during } (0, t] | S(\in U) \text{ at time } 0\} \tag{9.97}$$

$$A(t) \equiv \Pr\{S \in U \text{ at time } t | S(\in U \cup D) \text{ at time } 0\} \tag{9.98}$$

$$M(t) \equiv 1 - \Pr\{S \in D \text{ during } (0, t] | S(\in D) \text{ at time } 0\} \tag{9.99}$$

The system availability is calculated by solving differential equations such as (9.62). To calculate the system reliability, the transition diagram of Figure 9.7 is modified in the following way.

1. Remove transitions from failed states to operational states.
2. Remove transitions among failed states.
3. Remove failed states.

The resulting diagram is shown in Figure 9.8(a), and the corresponding differential equations are

$$\left.\begin{aligned} \dot{P}_{(0)} &= -\lambda_0 P_{(0)} + \mu_1 P_{(1)} \\ &\vdots \\ \dot{P}_{(k)} &= \lambda_{k-1} P_{(k-1)} - (\lambda_k + \mu_k) P_{(k)} + \mu_{k+1} P_{(k+1)} \\ &\vdots \\ \dot{P}_{(n-m)} &= \lambda_{n-m-1} P_{(n-m-1)} - (\lambda_{n-m} + \mu_{n-m}) P_{(n-m)} \end{aligned}\right\} \qquad (9.100)$$

The system reliability is then calculated as

$$R = P_{(0)} + \cdots + P_{(n-m)} \qquad (9.101)$$

The repairability transition diagram is obtained as follows.

1. Remove transitions from operational states to failed states.
2. Remove transitions among operational states.
3. Remove operational states.

The resulting diagram is Figure 9.8(b). The repairability is calculated as

$$M = 1 - P_{(n-m+1)} - \cdots - P_{(n)} \qquad (9.102)$$

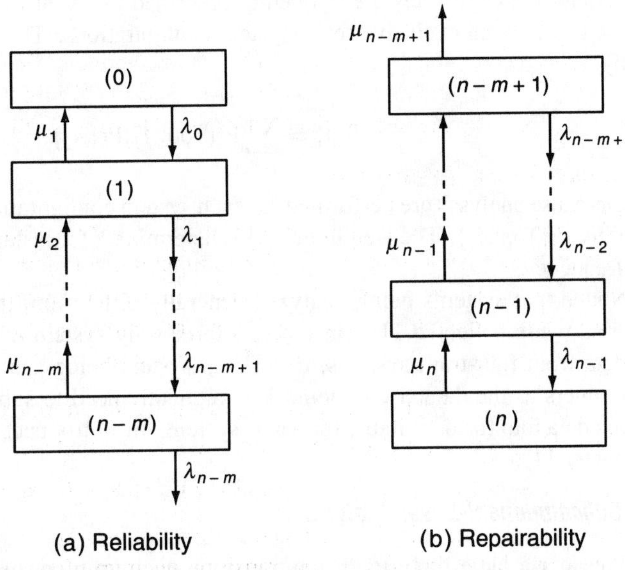

Figure 9.8. Transition diagram for reliability and repairability calculation.

9.3 COMMON-CAUSE FAILURE ANALYSIS

The tail-gas quench and clean-up system of Figure 8.12 has two redundant configurations. Redundancy improves system reliability. The configurations, however, do not necessarily lead to substantial improvement if common-cause failures exist.

There are several models for quantifying systems subject to common-cause failure [1]. The beta-factor (BF) model is the most basic [3]. A generalization of the beta-factor model is the multiple Greek letter (MGL) model [4]. A subset of the Marshall-Olkin model [5] is the basic-parameter (BP) model [6]. The MGL model is mathematically equivalent to the BP model, which was originally used to help establish the MGL model. A binomial failure-rate (BFR) model [7,8] includes, as a special case, the beta-factor model. The BFR model is also called a *shock model*. In this book, we present these models in the manner of reference [1]. The BF, BP, MGL, and BFR models are examples of parametric or implicit modeling because cause-effect relationships are considered by model parameters implicitly. Common-cause analyses are important for evaluating redundancy and diversity as a means of improving system performance.

In the following description, we assume that functional and common-unit dependencies are modeled explicitly by logic models such as fault and event trees, and that component-level minimal cut sets are available.

In the common-cause models, a component failure is classified as either of the following.

1. Failure on demand: A component fails to start operating due to latent or random defects.
2. Failure during operation, that is, failure to continue running.

Likelihoods of these failures depend on system configurations: normal, test, maintenance, and abnormal conditions, such as lack of power. For instance, in maintenance, some components may be out of service, so fewer additional failures would cause the top event. Abnormal conditions are frequently described by event-tree headings. Denote by $A_j,\ j = 1, \dots, N$ an exclusive set of system configurations. The top-event probability is given by

$$\Pr\{\text{Top}\} = \sum_{j=1}^{N} \Pr\{\text{Top}|A_j\}\Pr\{A_j\} \tag{9.103}$$

Common-cause analyses are performed for each system configuration to obtain conditional probability $\Pr\{\text{Top}|A_j\}$. The weight $\Pr\{A_j\}$ is determined, for instance, by test and maintenance frequency.

Notice that systems being analyzed generally differ from the systems from which failure data were collected. For instance, a three-train system may have to be analyzed using data from four-train systems; or a pump system being analyzed may not have the same strainers as the database system. We frequently need to subjectively transform old operating data into forms suitable for a new system; this introduces a source of uncertainty (see Chapter 11).

9.3.1 Subcomponent-Level Analysis

Consider a large three-train pump system, each train consisting of a pump and its drive (Figure 9.9). The three pumps are identical, but the pump drives are different; train

1 pump is turbine-driven, while in trains 2 and 3 pumps are motor-driven. Consider first a one-out-of-three parallel configuration where a fault-tree analysis yields the top-event expression:

$$\text{Top} = (P1 \vee T1) \wedge (P2 \vee M2) \wedge (P3 \vee M3) \tag{9.104}$$

where $P1$ denotes the pump failure of train 1, $T1$ is the turbine-drive failure of train 1, $M2$ denotes the motor-drive failure of train 2, and so on.

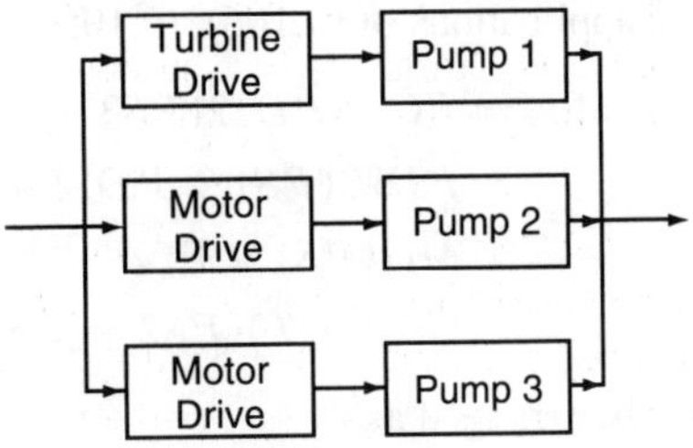

Figure 9.9. One-out-of-three pump system with diverse pump drives.

The following subcomponent-level causes are enumerated for the three pump failures.

1. $PS1$: This causes a single failure of the train 1 pump. The P stands for pump, the S for single, and the 1 refers to the first pump.
2. $PD12$: This causes a simultaneous failure of the two pumps in trains 1 and 2. The D stands for double. Causes $PD13$ and $PD23$ are defined similarly.
3. PG: This causes a simultaneous failure of the three pumps in trains 1, 2, and 3. The character G denotes a global failure of the three pumps.

Subcomponent-level causes for the two motor drives in trains 2 and 3 are $MS2$, $MS3$, and MG; $MS2$ and $MS3$ cause single-drive failures in trains 2 and 3, respectively; MG causes a simultaneous failure of the two motor drives. For the single turbine-drive, only one cause T is considered; this includes single-failure cause $TS1$ and global cause TG. The Boolean top-event expression is

$$\begin{aligned}\text{Top} = {} & (PS1 \vee PD12 \vee PD13 \vee PG \vee T) \wedge \\ & (PS2 \vee PD12 \vee PD23 \vee PG \vee MS2 \vee MG) \wedge \\ & (PS3 \vee PD13 \vee PD23 \vee PG \vee MS3 \vee MG)\end{aligned} \tag{9.105}$$

Only common causes affecting the same type of components are considered in the above example:

Group 1: Three pumps
Group 2: Two motor drives

This grouping, which depends on the analyst's judgment, is a common-cause group.

Theoretically, a large number of dependent relationships must be considered, including cross-component dependencies as in those between the pumps and their drives. In practice, these cross-component failures can generally be neglected, thus keeping the combinations at a manageable level.

The subcomponent-level analysis increases the cut sets that have common causes; equation (9.104) has 8 component-level cut sets, while (9.108) has 22 subcomponent-level cut sets. In the probability expression (9.109), these 22 cut sets are reduced to nine terms by symmetry assumptions.

Consider a consensus operation, described in Chapter 5. The operation with respect to biform variable Y_i in (8.107) yields the consensus $\psi(1_i, Y) \wedge \psi(0_i, Y)$. Because function $\psi(Y)$ is monotonically increasing, this consensus simplifies to $\psi(0_i, Y)$, and the following expansion holds.

$$\psi(Y) = Y_i \psi(1_i, Y) \vee \psi(0_i, Y) \tag{9.106}$$

Consider a sequence of biform variables PG, $PD12$, $PD23$, $PD13$, and MG. By repeated applications of (9.106), (9.105) can be expanded in the following way:

$$\begin{aligned} \text{Top} = {} & PG \vee PD12(PS3 \vee PD13 \vee PD23 \vee MS3 \vee MG) \vee \\ & PD23(PS1 \vee PD13 \vee T) \vee PD13(PS2 \vee MS2 \vee MG) \vee \\ & MG(PS1 \vee T) \vee \\ & (PS1 + T)(PS2 + MS2)(PS3 + MS3) \end{aligned} \tag{9.107}$$

This can be arranged as

$$\begin{aligned} \text{Top} = {} & PG \vee (PD12PD13 \vee PD12PD23 \vee PD13PD23) \vee \\ & (PD12PS3 \vee PD23PS1 \vee PD13PS2) \vee (PD12MG \vee PD13MG) \vee \\ & (PD12MS3 \vee PD13MS2) \vee PD23T \vee MGT \vee MGPS1 \vee \\ & (PS1 + T)(PS2 + MS2)(PS3 + MS3) \end{aligned} \tag{9.108}$$

The last term represents the pure single-failure contribution.

All subcomponent-level causes are mutually independent. Because of the symmetry within a common-cause group of components (i.e., a group of pumps or a group of motor drives), we have the probability expression

$$\begin{aligned} \Pr\{\text{Top}\} \simeq {} & P_3 + 3P_2^2 + 3P_2P_1 + 2P_2M_2 + 2P_2M_1 + P_2T + M_2T \\ & + M_2P_1 + (P_1 + T)(P_1 + M_1)^2 \end{aligned} \tag{9.109}$$

P_3 denotes the triple-failure probability of three pumps at the same time, P_2 the double-failure probability of pumps 1 and 2 (with pump 3 normal), and so on. Note that P_2 is also a failure probability of pumps 1 and 3 (or pumps 2 and 3). In other words, P_j is the simultaneous-failure probability within a particular group of j pumps, while the pumps outside the group are normal.

To obtain the top-event probability, we first calculate the following quantities using the models described in the following sections.

$$P_3, P_2, P_1: \quad \text{for the 3 pumps} \tag{9.110}$$

$$M_2, M_1: \quad \text{for the 2 motor-drives} \tag{9.111}$$

$$T: \quad \text{for the single turbine drive} \tag{9.112}$$

It is noted that, prior to the application of common-cause models, top-event expressions are obtained in terms of the following.

1. Component failures by component-level fault trees, reliability block diagrams, Boolean expressions, and so forth. Equation (9.104) is an example.
2. Subcomponent level of causes [eq. (9.105)].
3. Boolean reduction of subcomponent-level expression [eq. (9.108)].
4. Top-event probability expression in terms of combinations of simultaneous failures [eq. (9.109)].

9.3.2 Beta-Factor Model

9.3.2.1 Demand-failure model parameters. Consider a system or a group consisting of m identical or similar components in standby. The beta-factor model assumes that all m components fail when a common cause occurs. Only one component fails by an independent cause among the m components. Multiple independent failures are neglected. Thus double-pump failure probability P_2 and independent terms in (9.109) are zero in the beta-factor model.

$$\Pr\{\text{Top}\} = P_3 + M_2 T + M_2 P_1 \tag{9.113}$$

Figure 9.10 shows possible state transitions of a three-component system prior to a demand; component failures to start on demand are enumerated in Table 9.3, where the following *exclusive* cases occur.

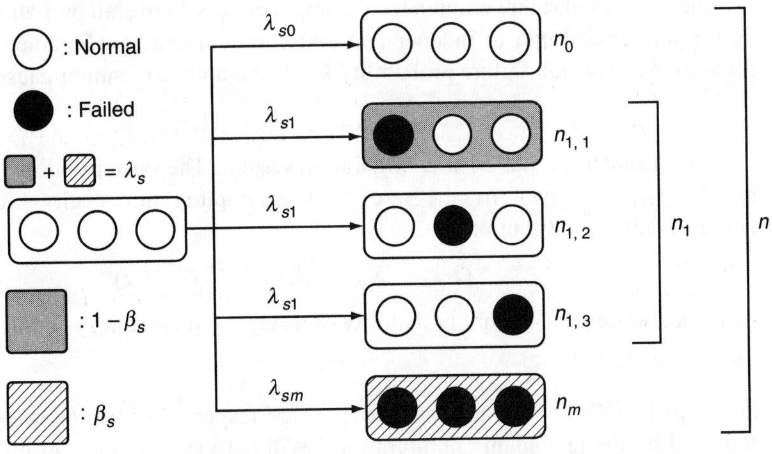

Figure 9.10. Beta-factor state transition model prior to a demand.

TABLE 9.3. Exclusive Component Failures on Demand (β-Factor Model)

Cases	Components			Probabilities	
	C1	C2	C3	Probability	C1 Failures
All Success	S	S	S	λ_{s0}	
Single Failure	F	S	S	λ_{s1}	$\lambda_{s1} = (1-\beta_s)\lambda_s$
	S	F	S	λ_{s1}	
	S	S	F	λ_{s1}	
All Failure	F	F	F	λ_{sm}	$\lambda_{sm} = \beta_s \lambda_s$
			Total	1	$\lambda_s = \lambda_{s1} + \lambda_{sm}$

S: success, F: failure

1. Only one component fails by an independent cause. By convention, this probability is denoted by λ_{s1}, where subscript 1 stands for a single failure by an independent cause, and subscript s denotes a "failure to start." For components that are identical or similar, probability λ_{s1} is the same.

2. All components fail simultaneously by a common cause. This probability is denoted by λ_{sm}, where subscript m stands for simultaneous failure of m components by a common cause, and subscript s, as before, denotes a failure to start.

Two or more components may fail simultaneously due to independent causes; however, these cases are excluded from Table 9.3 by the rare-event assumption.

Consider a component that fails either by an independent or common cause. From Table 9.3, the conditional probability β_s of the common-cause failure, given an independent- (single-) or simultaneous-component failure, is

$$\beta_s = \frac{\lambda_{sm}}{\lambda_{sm} + \lambda_{s1}} = \frac{\lambda_{sm}}{\lambda_s} \tag{9.114}$$

$$\lambda_s \equiv \lambda_{sm} + \lambda_{s1} \tag{9.115}$$

Parameter λ_s, a constant common to all components, is an overall probability of component failure on demand due to independent and common causes. Parameter β_s denotes the fraction of the overall failure probability λ_s attributable to common-cause failures. Thus

$$\lambda_{sm} = \beta_s \lambda_s, \qquad \lambda_{s1} = (1 - \beta_s)\lambda_s \tag{9.116}$$

Consider a one-out-of-m configuration system. The system-failure probability on demand, $Q_{1/m}$, is given by the rare-event assumption that neglects the independent- (single-) failure contribution.

$$Q_{1/m} \sim \lambda_{sm} = \beta_s \lambda_s, \qquad (m \geq 2) \tag{9.117}$$

Note that the demand-failure probability of a single-component system is

$$Q_{1/1} = \lambda_s \tag{9.118}$$

Equation (9.117) shows that parameter β_s corresponds to the unavailability reduction achieved by the redundant configuration. Without the common cause ($\beta_s = 0$), probability $Q_{1/m}$ is underestimated because

$$Q_{1/m} = \lambda_s^m, \quad \text{for independent case} \tag{9.119}$$

9.3.2.2 Data required. For a complete analysis, the following data are required (see Figure 9.10):

1. $n \equiv$ number of demands on a system level.
2. $n_{1,i} \equiv$ number of independent demand failures for component i.
3. $n_1 \equiv$ number of independent failures for all components, such as

$$n_1 = \sum_{i=1}^{m} n_{1,i} \tag{9.120}$$

4. $n_m \equiv$ number of common-cause failures where all m components fail simultaneously, and
5. $n_0 \equiv$ number of successful responses to demands where all m components operate normally.

9.3.2.3 Parameter estimation. The following equations hold:

$$n = n_0 + n_m + \sum_{i=1}^{m} n_{1,i} \tag{9.121}$$

$$= n_0 + n_m + n_1 \tag{9.122}$$

Denote by λ_{s0} the component-success probability on demand. Because the events in Table 9.3 are exclusive and there are $m = 3$ cases of single-component failures,

$$1 = \lambda_{s0} + \lambda_{sm} + m\lambda_{s1} \tag{9.123}$$

For each demand, one case in Table 9.3 applies; all components normal, one component fails, or all components fail. When probabilities λ_{s0}, λ_{sm}, and λ_{s1} are given, the probability Λ of obtaining n_0, n_m, and n_1 is

$$\Lambda = \lambda_{s0}^{n_0}\lambda_{sm}^{n_m}\prod_{i=1}^{m}\lambda_{s1}^{n_{1,i}} \tag{9.124}$$

$$= \lambda_{s0}^{n_0}\lambda_{sm}^{n_m}\lambda_{s1}^{n_1} \tag{9.125}$$

Maximum-likelihood estimators for λ_{s0}, λ_{sm}, and λ_{s1} are obtained by maximizing probability Λ under the constraint of (9.123). A Lagrange multiplier method with the constraint (9.123) yields a maximization problem (v: Lagrange multiplier).

$$\text{Maximize } L = \Lambda + v(1 - \lambda_{s0} - \lambda_{sm} - m\lambda_{s1}) \tag{9.126}$$

Intermediate results are

$$\hat{\lambda}_{sm} = \lambda_{s0}n_m/n_0, \qquad \hat{\lambda}_{s1} = \lambda_{s0}n_1/(mn_0) \tag{9.127}$$

Substituting $\hat{\lambda}_{sm}$ and $\hat{\lambda}_{s1}$ into constraint (9.123) and using the relation (9.122), we have

$$\hat{\lambda}_{sm} = n_m/n, \qquad \hat{\lambda}_{s1} = n_1/(mn) \tag{9.128}$$

Parameter β_s in (9.114) is now

$$\hat{\beta}_s = \frac{n_m}{n_m + (n_1/m)} \tag{9.129}$$

The overall component-failure probability (9.115) is

$$\hat{\lambda}_s = \frac{n_m + (n_1/m)}{n} \tag{9.130}$$

Determination of β_s does not require the total number n of system-level demands; it is a ratio of n_m to $n_m + (n_1/m)$, the total number of failures of a component.

9.3.2.4 Run failure. So far we have considered failures to start on demand. Another type of failure—failures during operation after a successful start can be dealt with in a similar way if the number n of demands is replaced by the total system run time T; a common mission time ($t \leq T$) is assumed for all systems tested. In this case, parameters such as λ_{rm} and λ_{r1} become failure rates rather than probabilities, and subscript r stands for a "run failure." Corresponding failure probabilities during mission time t of the system being analyzed are given by $\lambda_{rm}t$ and $\lambda_{r1}t$, respectively. These probabilities are a first-order approximation for exponential failure distributions.

$$1 - \exp(-at) \simeq at, \qquad 0 < at << 1 \tag{9.131}$$

Denote by λ_r the overall failure rate for an operating component due to independent and common causes. The failure probability, $Q_{1/m}$, for one-out-of-m system ($m \geq 2$) is given by the rare-event approximation.

$$Q_{1/m} = \beta_r(\lambda_r t), \qquad (m \geq 2) \tag{9.132}$$

9.3.2.5 Diverse components. For dissimilar or diverse components, parameter β_s or (β_r) varies from component to component, and its maximum-likelihood estimator is

$$\hat{\beta}_{s,i} = \frac{n_m}{n_m + n_{1,i}} \tag{9.133}$$

In the beta-factor estimators of (9.129) and (9.133), susceptibilities of dissimilar or diverse components to common-cause failures are reflected in the number n_m of common-cause events resulting in total system failures; if diverse components are impervious to common causes, they yield no common-cause events. The use of different $\beta_{s,i}$ values for dissimilar components implies a number $n_{1,i}$ of independent failures specific to the component. However, the component-dependent beta-factor in (9.133) for diverse components offers little improvement over the component-independent beta-factor model. This is shown when we consider diverse components that are similar in independent-failure characteristics ($n_{1,1} \simeq n_{1,2} \simeq n_{1,3}$); common-cause susceptibilities are reflected by n_m in the expression for β_s.

9.3.2.6 Number of demands and system run time. Notice that n, the number of demands, is frequently unavailable. In this case, λ_s is replaced by a generic database estimate $\hat{\lambda}_s$. Given $\hat{\lambda}_s$, the independent failure rate λ_{s1} can be calculated from

$$\hat{\lambda}_{s1} = (1 - \beta_s)\hat{\lambda}_s \tag{9.134}$$

The number n of demands is estimated by solving the equation

$$\hat{\lambda}_{s1} = n_1/(mn), \text{ i.e.,} \qquad n = n_1/(m\hat{\lambda}_{s1}) \tag{9.135}$$

When redundant configurations with different sizes are involved, average number $\overline{m}$ of components is used to replace m. Equation (9.135) cannot be used when we have no single failures, $n_1 = 0$. In such a case, the following Bayes estimate is used.

Assume for λ_{s1} a beta prior distribution with parameter a and b:

$$p\{\lambda_{s1}\} = \frac{\lambda_{s1}^a(1 - \lambda_{s1})^b}{\text{const.}} \tag{9.136}$$

The likelihood of obtaining n_1 component failures for nm demand is

$$p\{n_1|\lambda_{s1}\} = \frac{\lambda_{s1}^{n_1}(1 - \lambda_{s1})^{nm-n_1}}{\text{const.}} \tag{9.137}$$

From Bayes theorem in the appendix of Chapter 3, a posterior distribution of λ_{s1} is

$$p\{\lambda_{s1}|n_1\} = \frac{\lambda_{s1}^{a+n_1}(1 - \lambda_{s1})^{b+nm-n_1}}{\text{const.}} \tag{9.138}$$

Therefore, the posterior mean of λ_{s1} is

$$\hat{\lambda}_{s1} = \frac{a + n_1 + 1}{a + b + nm + 2} \tag{9.139}$$

A uniform prior corresponds to zero parameter values, $a = b = 0$:

$$\hat{\lambda}_{s1} = \frac{n_1 + 1}{nm + 2}, \text{ i.e.,} \qquad n = \frac{n_1 - 2\hat{\lambda}_{s1} + 1}{\hat{\lambda}_{s1} m} \tag{9.140}$$

This equation is used to estimate the number n of demands when the independent failure rate $\hat{\lambda}_{s1}$ is known.

The system run time T is estimated in a similar way.

$$\hat{\lambda}_{r1} = n_1/(mT), \text{ or } \quad \hat{\lambda}_{r1} = (n_1 + 1)/(mT + 2) \tag{9.141}$$

Example 11—Feedwater-system analysis. Consider a standby feedwater system involving trains of pumps, strainers, and valves [9]. Figure 9.11 is a three-train system. In the analysis, each train is regarded as a component. All failures collected so far can be interpreted as train failures on demand. There are no cascade failures such as a pump failed to start because of lack of water supply. The water supply tank is defined as being outside the system.

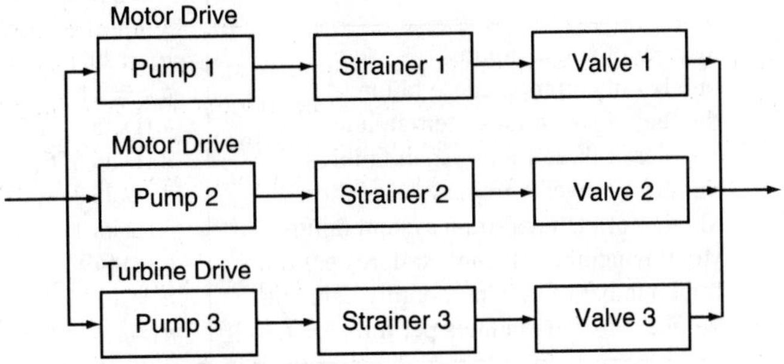

Figure 9.11. Standby feedwater system.

Table 9.4 identifies number of trains, number of failures, train types, and pump types (M: motor-driven, T: turbine-driven, D: diesel-driven). Table 9.5 summarizes run-time spans in calendar month and number of single- and multiple-failure instances.

TABLE 9.4. Multiple Failures in Standby Feedwater Systems

Data	Number of Failures and Train Types	Number of Trains	Pump Types M T D
1	2/T,T	2	0 2 0
2	2/T,T	2	0 2 0
3	2/T,D	2	0 1 1
4	2/T,D	2	0 1 1
5	3/M,M,T	3	2 1 0
6	3/T,T,T	3	0 3 0
7	2/M,M	3	2 1 0
8	2/M,T	3	2 1 0
9	2/M,M	3	2 1 0
10	2/M,M	3	2 1 0
11	2/T,T	3	0 3 0

Apply the beta-factor model to determine probabilities of feedwater system failure-to-start on demand. Consider one-out-of-two and one-out-of-three configurations. Consider also the cases of identical and diverse trains. Assume one system demand for each calendar month; the total number of demands is $n = 1641 \times 1 = 1641$ from Table 9.5.

Solution: Notice that the data involve both two- and three-train systems with identical or diverse pumps. Moreover, partial (rows 7 to 11) as well as complete system failures (rows 1 to 6) are included.

The beta-factor model assumes that the trains are identical. As shown by (9.129), determination of β_s requires n_1/m, the average number of single failures per train. This number is generic and less

TABLE 9.5. Number of Failures and Run Time Spans in Calendar Months

Description	Value
Two-train system run time	474
Three-train system run time	1167
System run time	$474 + 1167 = 1641$
Diverse-train system run time	1373
Identical-train system run time	268
Train run time	$2 \times 474 + 3 \times 1167 = 4449$
Number of single failures	$n_1 = 68$
Number of common-cause failures	$n_m = 11$
Number of two-train system failures	4 (Data 1, 2, 3, 4)
Number of three-train system failures	2 (Data 5, 6))
Number of diverse-train system failures	3 (Data 3, 4, 5)
Number of identical-train system failures	3 (Data 1, 2, 6)
Monthly number of single failures per train	$68/4449 = 0.0153$
Total number of system monthly demands	$n = 1641$
Number of single failures per train	$n_1/m = 0.0153 \times 1641 = 25$

dependent on the number of trains m. However, we only have a total number of single failures, $n_1 = 68$, during a system run time of 1641 months for systems with redundancy values $m = 2$ and 3. The total amount of train run time is 4449 months, as calculated in the sixth row of Table 9.5. Thus the monthly number of single failures per train is $68/4449 = 0.0153$. During the run time of 1641 months, $0.0153 \times 1641 = 25$ single failures occur per train, that is, $n_1/m = 25$.

The 11 common-cause events listed in Table 9.4 initiate the simultaneous failure of two or more trains. When we evaluate, for a particular system under investigation, that all 11 common-cause events would result in simultaneous failure of two trains, which is a conservative assumption, we have $n_m = 11$ for one-out-of-two systems and the parameter β_s is estimated as

$$\hat{\beta}_s = \frac{11}{11 + 25} = 0.3 \tag{9.142}$$

For the three-train system, only two common causes (rows 5 and 6) result in a total system failure. Assume that all 11 common-cause events would result in simultaneous failure of the three trains currently investigated. The same β_s value as for the two-train system is obtained.

We can also assign subjective weights to the partial failures due to common causes; if partial common-cause events are evaluated as partial, then zero weights are used, yielding $n_m = 2 + 0.0 \times 9 = 2$. The beta-factor becomes

$$\hat{\beta}_s = 2/(2 + 25) = 0.074 \tag{9.143}$$

These weights constitute an impact vector. By using the impact vector, we can quantify common-cause failures for an m-train system based on operating data collected for systems of different sizes.

A demand for each calendar month is assumed. A train fails 25 times by independent causes and 11 times (a conservative estimate) by common causes during the system run time of 1641 months. The overall demand-train-failure probability, $\hat{\lambda}_s$ in (9.130), is

$$\hat{\lambda}_s = \frac{11 + 25}{1641} = 0.022 \tag{9.144}$$

From (9.117), the failure probability of the one-out-of-two system is

$$Q_{1/2} = 0.3 \times 0.022 = 6.6 \times 10^{-3} \tag{9.145}$$

For a one-out-of-three system

$$Q_{1/3} = 0.3 \times 0.022 = 6.6 \times 10^{-3} = Q_{1/2}, \quad \text{for } \beta_s = 0.3 \tag{9.146}$$

$$Q_{1/3} = 0.074 \times 0.022 = 1.7 \times 10^{-3} < Q_{1/2}, \quad \text{for } \beta_s = 0.074 \tag{9.147}$$

Table 9.4 shows four instances of one-out-of-two system failures (data 1, 2, 3, and 4) during a run time of 474 months. This gives a point estimate of

$$Q_{1/2} = 4/474 = 8.4 \times 10^{-3} \tag{9.148}$$

Similarly, for the three-train system,

$$Q_{1/3} = 2/1167 = 1.7 \times 10^{-3} \tag{9.149}$$

As summarized in Table 9.6, the beta-factor model gives a slightly lower failure probability for the one-out-of-two configuration than the values directly calculated from the data. The conservative beta-factor $\beta_s = 0.3$ gives a comparatively higher failure probability for the one-out-of-three configuration, and a less conservative beta-factor $\beta_s = 0.074$ yields good agreement with the demand-failure probability calculated from the data.

TABLE 9.6. Summary of Beta-Factor and Data Estimation

System	β_s	β-Factor Model	Data
1/2	0.3	6.6×10^{-3}	8.4×10^{-3}
1/3	0.3	6.6×10^{-3}	1.7×10^{-3}
1/3	0.074	1.7×10^{-3}	1.7×10^{-3}
Diverse	0.125	2.8×10^{-3}	2.2×10^{-3}
Identical	0.428	9.4×10^{-3}	11×10^{-3}

Demand-failure probabilities for diverse and identical multiple-train systems are calculated as $3/1373 = 2.2 \times 10^{-3}$ and $3/268 = 11 \times 10^{-3}$, respectively (Table 9.5). The number of single failures per train for the diverse-train system during 1373 months of run time is $n_1/m = 0.0153 \times 1373 = 21$, yielding $\hat{\beta}_s = 3/(3+21) = 0.125$. Similarly, $n_1/m = 0.0153 \times 268 = 4$ for the identical-train system, yielding $\hat{\beta}_s = 3/(3+4) = 0.428$. Thus, $Q_{1/m} \simeq 0.125 \times 0.022 = 2.8 \times 10^{-3}$ for the diverse-train system ($m = 2$ or 3), and $Q_{1/m} \simeq 0.428 \times 0.022 = 9.4 \times 10^{-3}$ for identical-train system ($m = 2$ or 3), yielding good agreement with the failure probabilities calculated from the data (Table 9.6). ■

Example 12—Component-level analysis. The beta-factor model can be used at a component level, as well as on the multicomponent level just discussed.

Consider three components, a pump, a valve, and a strainer. From Table 9.7, the beta-factors for pumps (β_p), valves (β_v), and strainers (β_{st}) are

$$\hat{\beta}_p = 7/(7+15) = 0.32 \tag{9.150}$$

$$\hat{\beta}_v = 2/(2+10) = 0.17 \tag{9.151}$$

$$\hat{\beta}_{st} = 2/(2+0.3) = 0.87 \tag{9.152}$$

For simplicity of notation the demand-failure subscript s is not included.

The overall demand-failure probabilities of these components are

$$\hat{\lambda}_p = (7+15)/1641 = 0.013 \tag{9.153}$$

$$\hat{\lambda}_v = (2+10)/1641 = 0.0073 \tag{9.154}$$

$$\hat{\lambda}_{st} = (2+0.3)/1641 = 0.0014 \tag{9.155}$$

TABLE 9.7. Data at Component Level

Component	Single Failures	Multiple Failures	Monthly Single Failures per Component	Single Failures per Component
Pump	40	7	$40/4449 = 0.009$	$0.009 \times 1641 = 15$
Valve	26	2	$26/4449 = 0.006$	$0.006 \times 1641 = 10$
Strainer	1	2	$1/4449 = 0.0002$	$0.0002 \times 1641 = 0.3$

Consider a one-out-of-two train system, where each train consists of a valve, a pump, and a strainer. Denote the two valves by 1 and 2. Define

1. $VS1 \equiv$ single valve failure 1, where symbol V refers to valve, S to single failure, and 1 to the first valve.
2. $VG \equiv$ global common-cause failure of valves 1 and 2.

Then the valve 1 failure, $V1$, can be represented as

$$V1 = VS1 \vee VG \tag{9.156}$$

Similar notation is used for the two pumps and two strainers. The one-out-of-two train system failure, $T_{1/2}$, is

$$\begin{aligned} T_{1/2} &= (VS1 \vee PS1 \vee STS1 \vee VG \vee PG \vee STG) \wedge \\ &\quad (VS2 \vee PS2 \vee STS2 \vee VG \vee PG \vee STG) && (9.157) \\ &= VG \vee PG \vee STG \vee (VS1 \vee PS1 \vee STS1)(VS2 \vee PS2 \vee STS2) && (9.158) \end{aligned}$$

By symmetry, for the failure probability of the one-out-of-two system, we have

$$Q_{1/2} \simeq V_2 + P_2 + ST_2 + (V_1 + P_1 + ST_1)^2 \tag{9.159}$$

where V_j, for instance, signifies that all valves within a specific group of j valves fail simultaneously; $j = 1$ for an independent cause, and $j = 2$ for a common cause. The probability on the right-hand side, as estimated by the beta-factor model, is

$$\begin{aligned} Q_{1/2} &= \beta_p \lambda_p + \beta_v \lambda_v + \beta_{st} \lambda_{st} \\ &= 6.6 \times 10^{-3} \end{aligned} \tag{9.160}$$

As expected, the final numerical result is similar to that derived earlier with the beta-factor model at the train level [eq. (9.145)]. ■

9.3.3 Basic-Parameter Model

9.3.3.1 Model parameters. The basic-parameter (BP) model is similar to the Marshall-Olkin model [5] except that the BP model has time-based failure rates and demand-based failure probabilities while the Marshall-Olkin model is strictly time based.

For a group of m components in standby, which must start and run for t hours, there are $2m + 1$ different parameters of the form

λ_{sj} = failure-to-start-on-demand probability for a *particular* group of j components.
λ_{rj} = failure-to-operate rate for a *particular* group of j components.
t = common mission time.

In these definitions, the group is specified. For λ_{s2}, for example, components 1 and 2 form a group, and components 2 and 3 form another group. Each group has probability λ_{sj}. Thus for a three-component system, probability of failure involving exactly two components becomes 3 × λ_{s2} because there are three double-failure groups: (1,2), (1,3), (2,3). Figure 9.12 shows possible state transitions for a three-component system prior to a demand; Tables 9.8 and 9.9 show cases where component 1 failures are involved: one single failure, two double failures, and one triple failure for the three-component system; one single failure, three double failures, three triple failures, and one quadruple failure for the four-component system. Parameters λ_s and numerators and denominators of β, γ, and δ listed under "coverage" are described in Section 9.3.4.

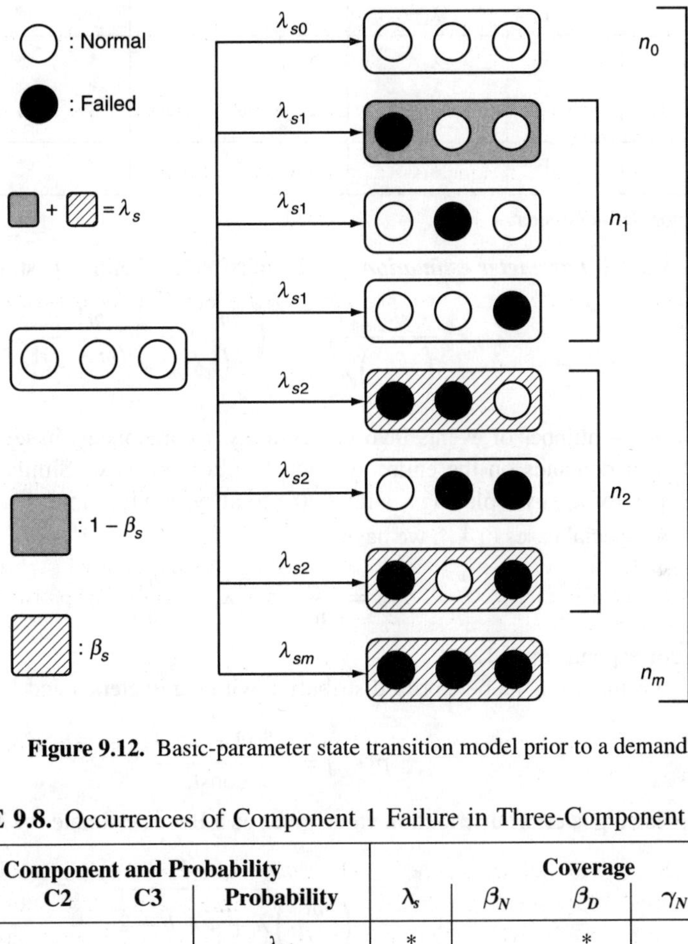

Figure 9.12. Basic-parameter state transition model prior to a demand.

TABLE 9.8. Occurrences of Component 1 Failure in Three-Component System

Component and Probability				Coverage				
C1	C2	C3	Probability	λ_s	β_N	β_D	γ_N	γ_D
F			λ_{s1}	*		*		
F	F		λ_{s2}	*	*	*		*
F		F	λ_{s2}	*	*	*		*
F	F	F	λ_{s3}	*	*	*	*	*

N: numerator, D: denominator

The BP model assumes that the probability or rate of a common-cause event depends only on the number j of components in a group. This is a symmetry assumption. The mission time t is usually known.

TABLE 9.9. Occurrences of Component 1 Failure in Four-Component System

Component and Probabilty					Coverage						
C1	**C2**	**C3**	**C4**	**Probability**	λ_s	β_N	β_D	γ_N	γ_D	δ_N	δ_D
F				λ_{s1}	*		*				
F	F			λ_{s2}	*	*	*		*		
F		F		λ_{s2}	*	*	*		*		
F			F	λ_{s2}	*	*	*		*		
F		F	F	λ_{s3}	*	*	*	*	*		*
F	F		F	λ_{s3}	*	*	*	*	*		*
F	F	F		λ_{s3}	*	*	*	*	*		*
F	F	F	F	λ_{s4}	*	*	*	*	*	*	*

N: numerator, D: denominator

9.3.3.2 Parameter estimation. The maximum-likelihood estimator for λ_{sj} is

$$\hat{\lambda}_{sj} = \frac{n_j}{\binom{m}{j} n}, \qquad \binom{m}{j} \equiv \frac{m!}{j!(m-j)!} \tag{9.161}$$

where $n_j \equiv$ number of events involving exactly j components in failed states, and $n \equiv$ number of demands on the entire system of m components. Similar estimators can be developed for λ_{rj} by replacing n with T, the total system run time.

As special cases of $\hat{\lambda}_{sj}$, we have

$$\hat{\lambda}_{sm} = \frac{n_m}{n}, \qquad \hat{\lambda}_{s1} = \frac{n_1}{mn} \tag{9.162}$$

This corresponds to (9.128).

Assume for λ_{sj} a beta prior distribution with parameters a and b:

$$p\{\lambda_{sj}\} = \frac{\lambda_{sj}^a (1 - \lambda_{sj})^b}{\text{const.}} \tag{9.163}$$

The mean a posteriori distribution value gives as a Bayes estimate for λ_{sj}:

$$\hat{\lambda}_{sj} = \frac{n_j + a + 1}{\binom{m}{j} n + a + b + 2} \tag{9.164}$$

A uniform prior corresponds to zero parameter values, $a = b = 0$.

Example 13—Two-out-of-three valve-system demand failure. Consider the hypothetical data in Table 9.10 for a two-out-of-three valve system (Figure 9.13). Calculate the demand-failure probability of this valve system.

Solution: Denote the valve failures by $V1$, $V2$, and $V3$, where failure $V1$ consists of independent and common-cause portions:

$$V1 = VS1 + (VD12 + VD13) + VG \tag{9.165}$$

TABLE 9.10. Data for Three-Component Valve Systems

Demands n	Single Failures n_1	Double Failures n_2	Triple Failures n_3
4449	30	2	1

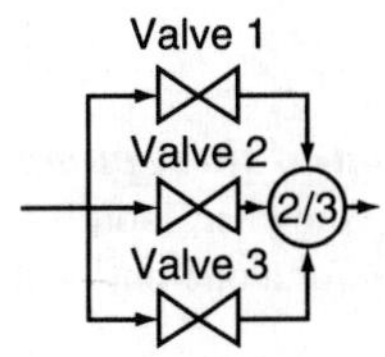

Figure 9.13. Two-out-of-three valve system.

where $VS1 \equiv$ single failure of valve 1
$VD12 \equiv$ double common-cause failure (CCF) of valves 1 and 2
$VD13 \equiv$ double CCF of valves 1 and 3
$VG \equiv$ global CCF of valves 1, 2, and 3 (9.166)

Similarly, we have

$$V2 = VS2 + (VD12 + VD23) + VG \tag{9.167}$$

$$V3 = VS3 + (VD13 + VD23) + VG \tag{9.168}$$

The simultaneous failure of valves 1 and 2 can be expressed as

$$V1V2 = (VS1 \vee VD12 \vee VD13 \vee VG)(VS2 \vee VD12 \vee VD23 \vee VG) \tag{9.169}$$

$$= VG \vee VD12 \vee (VS1 \vee VD13)(VS2 \vee VD23) \tag{9.170}$$

Thus the top event $V_{2/3}$ is

$$V_{2/3} = V1V2 \vee V1V3 \vee V2V3 \tag{9.171}$$

$$\begin{aligned} &= VG \vee VD12 \vee (VS1 \vee VD13)(VS2 \vee VD23) \vee VG \vee VD13 \vee \\ &\quad (VS1 \vee VD12)(VS3 \vee VD23) \vee VG \vee VD23 \vee \\ &\quad (VS2 \vee VD12)(VS3 \vee VD13) \end{aligned} \tag{9.172}$$

$$= VG \vee VD12 \vee VD13 \vee VD23 \vee VS1VS2 \vee VS1VS3 \vee VS2VS3 \tag{9.173}$$

Subcomponent-level failures are mutually independent. The probability of the top-event failure can be approximated by the first term of the inclusion-exclusion formula.

By symmetry, for the failure probability of the two-out-of-three valve system, we have

$$Q_{2/3} \equiv \Pr\{V_{2/3}\} \simeq V_3 + 3V_2 + 3V_1^2 \tag{9.174}$$

$$\simeq V_3 + 3V_2 \tag{9.175}$$

where V_j denotes that j valves in a specific group fail simultaneously.

The first term V_3 represents a contribution by global CCF; the second term $3V_2$ is a contribution by double CCF; the third term is a contribution by single failures.

From the definition of λ_{sj}, the following relations hold:

$$V_1 = \lambda_{s1}, \qquad V_2 = \lambda_{s2}, \qquad V_3 = \lambda_{s3} \tag{9.176}$$

The maximum-likelihood estimators ($m = 3$) of (9.161) are

$$\begin{aligned} V_1 &= \hat{\lambda}_{s1} = n_1/(3n) = 30/(3 \times 4449) = 2.2 \times 10^{-3} \\ V_2 &= \hat{\lambda}_{s2} = n_2/(3n) = 2/(3 \times 4449) = 1.5 \times 10^{-4} \\ V_3 &= \hat{\lambda}_{s3} = n_3/(n) = 1/4449 = 2.2 \times 10^{-4} \end{aligned} \quad (9.177)$$

Thus the demand-failure probability $Q_{2/3}$ is

$$Q_{2/3} = V_3 + 3V_2 = 0.00022 + 3 \times 0.00015 = 0.00067 \quad (9.178)$$

■

Example 14—One-out-of-three pump-system run failure. Data for a one-out-of-three pump system of Figure 9.14 are shown in Table 9.11, where symbol T denotes total run time. Calculate a failure-to-operate probability for a one-out-of-three pump system with mission time $t = 1$.

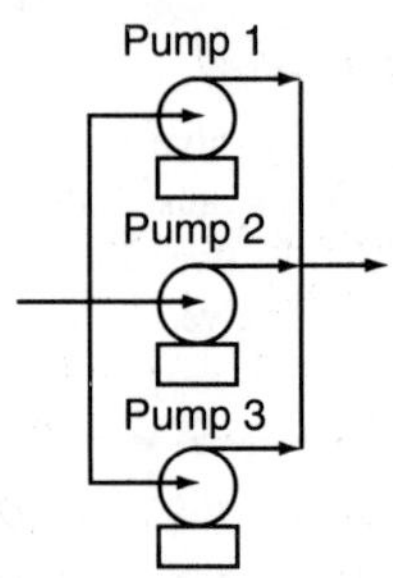

Figure 9.14. One-out-of-three pump system.

TABLE 9.11. Data for Three-Component Pump Systems

Exposure Time T	Single Failure n_1	Double Failures n_2	Triple Failures n_3	Mission Time t
4449	45	6	1	1

Solution: Denote by $P_{1/3}$ the failure of the one-out-of-three pump system. This can be expressed as

$$\begin{aligned} P_{1/3} &= (PS1 \vee PD12 \vee PD13 \vee PG) \wedge (PS2 \vee PD12 \vee PD23 \vee PG) \wedge \\ &\quad (PS3 \vee PD13 \vee PD23 \vee PG) && (9.179) \\ &= PG \vee PD12(PS3 \vee PD13 \vee PD23) \vee PD13(PS2 \vee PD23) \\ &\quad \vee PD23PS1 \vee PS1PS2PS3 && (9.180) \\ &= PG \vee PD12PD13 \vee PD12PD23 \vee PD13PD23 \vee PD12PS3 \\ &\quad \vee PD13PS2 \vee PD23PS1 \vee PS1PS2PS2 && (9.181) \end{aligned}$$

From symmetry, the system-failure probability is

$$Q_{1/3} \simeq P_3 + 3P_2^2 + 3P_1P_2 + P_1^3 \quad (9.182)$$

where P_j denotes that a particular group of j pumps fail simultaneously. The cases shown in Figure 9.12 are mutually exclusive, thus

$$Q_{1/3} \simeq P_3 \quad (9.183)$$

The definition of λ_{rj} and P_j yield the relations:

$$P_1 = \lambda_{r1}t, \qquad P_2 = \lambda_{r2}t, \qquad P_3 = \lambda_{r3}t \tag{9.184}$$

Similar to the maximum-likelihood estimators ($m = 3$) of (9.161), we have for $T = 4449$ and $t = 1$

$$\left.\begin{aligned} P_1 &= \hat{\lambda}_{s1}t = n_1 t/(3T) = 45/(3 \times 4449) = 0.0034 \\ P_2 &= \hat{\lambda}_{s2}t = n_2 t/(3T) = 6/(3 \times 4449) = 0.00045 \\ P_3 &= \hat{\lambda}_{s3}t = n_3 t/(T) = 1/4449 = 0.00022 \end{aligned}\right\} \tag{9.185}$$

Thus

$$Q_{1/3} \simeq P_3 = 2.2 \times 10^{-4} \tag{9.186}$$

■

9.3.4 Multiple Greek Letter Model

9.3.4.1 Model parameters. The multiple Greek letter (MGL) model is the most general extension of the beta-factor model. This model is also mathematically equivalent to the BP model; the principal difference is that a different set of parameters are used. For a group of m components in standby that must start and run for t hours, there would be, as with the BP model, $2m + 1$ different parameters of the form

λ_s = failure to start probability on demand for each component due to all independent and common causes. This corresponds to overall failure probability λ_s of the beta-factor model, equation (9.115). This probability is shown by the asterisks in Tables 9.8 and 9.9.

β_s = conditional probability that a component's failure to start is shared by one or more additional components, given that the former component fails. The numerator and denominator coverages are shown in Tables 9.8 and 9.9.

γ_s = conditional probability that a component's failure to start is shared by two or more additional components, given that the former component fails together with one or more additional components (see Tables 9.8 and 9.9).

δ_s = conditional probability that a component's failure to start is shared by three or more additional components, given that the former component fails together with two or more additional components (see Tables 9.8 and 9.9).

$\lambda_r, \beta_r, \gamma_r, \delta_r$ = same as λ_s, β_s, γ_s, and δ_s, respectively, except that the component-failure mode is failure to run instead of failure to start and parameters refer to rates rather than probabilities.

t = mission time

Tables 9.12 and 9.13 summarize demand-failure probability relationships among BP, MGL, and BFR models for three- and four-component systems. Similar relations hold for run-failure probabilities when suffix s is replaced by r.

The BP model is mathematically equivalent to the MGL model, while the beta-factor model is a special case of the MGL model, where $\gamma_s = \delta_s = 1$.

TABLE 9.12. Three-Component BP, Beta-Factor, MGL, and BFR Models

BP	Beta-Factor	MGL	BFR
λ_{s1}	$(1-\beta_s)\lambda_s$	$(1-\beta_s)\lambda_s$	$\lambda_{ic}+\mu P(1-P)^2$
λ_{s2}	0	$(1/2)(1-\gamma_s)\beta_s\lambda_s$	$\mu P^2(1-P)$
λ_{s3}	$\beta_s\lambda_s$	$\gamma_s\beta_s\lambda_s$	$\mu P^3+\omega$
$\hat{\lambda}_{s1}=\dfrac{n_1}{3n}$	$\hat{\lambda}_s=\dfrac{n_1+2n_2+3n_3}{3n}$	$\hat{\lambda}_s=\dfrac{n_1+3n_3}{3n}$	$\hat{\lambda}_{ic}=\dfrac{n_{ic}}{3n}$
$\hat{\lambda}_{s2}=\dfrac{n_2}{3n}$	$\hat{\beta}_s=\dfrac{3n_3}{n_1+3n_3}$	$\hat{\beta}_s=\dfrac{2n_2+3n_3}{n_1+2n_2+3n_3}$	$[\hat{P}^2-3\hat{P}+3]s=3n_+$
$\hat{\lambda}_{s3}=\dfrac{n_3}{n}$	$\hat{\gamma}_s=1$	$\hat{\gamma}_s=\dfrac{3n_3}{2n_2+3n_3}$	$\hat{\mu}=\dfrac{n_+/n}{1-(1-\hat{P})^3}$, $\quad\hat{\omega}=n_L/n$

TABLE 9.13. Four-Component BP, Beta-Factor, MGL, and BFR Models

BP	Beta-Factor	MGL	BFR
λ_{s1}	$(1-\beta_s)\lambda_s$	$(1-\beta_s)\lambda_s$	$\lambda_{ic}+\mu P(1-P)^3$
λ_{s2}	0	$(1/3)(1-\gamma_s)\beta_s\lambda_s$	$\mu P^2(1-P)^2$
λ_{s3}	0	$(1/3)(1-\delta_s)\gamma_s\beta_s\lambda_s$	$\mu P^3(1-P)$
λ_{s4}	$\beta_s\lambda_s$	$\delta_s\gamma_s\beta_s\lambda_s$	$\mu P^4+\omega$
$\hat{\lambda}_{s1}=\dfrac{n_1}{4n}$	$\hat{\lambda}_s=\dfrac{n_1+4n_4}{4n}$	$\hat{\lambda}_s=\dfrac{n_1+2n_2+3n_3+4n_4}{4n}$	$\hat{\lambda}_{ic}=\dfrac{n_{ic}}{4n}$
$\hat{\lambda}_{s2}=\dfrac{n_2}{6n}$	$\hat{\beta}_s=\dfrac{4n_4}{n_1+4n_4}$	$\hat{\beta}_s=\dfrac{2n_2+3n_3+4n_4}{n_1+2n_2+3n_3+4n_4}$	$[1-(1-\hat{P})^4]s=4\hat{P}n_+$
$\hat{\lambda}_{s3}=\dfrac{n_3}{4n}$	$\hat{\gamma}_s=1$	$\hat{\gamma}_s=\dfrac{3n_3+4n_4}{2n_2+3n_3+4n_4}$	$\hat{\mu}=\dfrac{n_+/n}{1-(1-\hat{P})^4}$
$\hat{\lambda}_{s4}=\dfrac{n_4}{n}$	$\hat{\delta}_s=1$	$\hat{\delta}_s=\dfrac{4n_4}{3n_3+4n_4}$	$\hat{\omega}=n_L/n$

9.3.4.2 Relations between BP and MGL models. For a group of three similar components, the MGL model parameters are defined in terms of the BP model parameters as follows (see Tables 9.8 and 9.9, which enumerate exclusive cases for three- and four-component systems based on rare-event assumptions):

$$\lambda_s = \lambda_{s1}+2\lambda_{s2}+\lambda_{s3} \tag{9.187}$$

$$\beta_s = \frac{2\lambda_{s2}+\lambda_{s3}}{\lambda_{s1}+2\lambda_{s2}+\lambda_{s3}} = \frac{2\lambda_{s2}+\lambda_{s3}}{\lambda_s} \tag{9.188}$$

$$\gamma_s = \frac{\lambda_{s3}}{2\lambda_{s2}+\lambda_{s3}} = \frac{\lambda_{s3}}{\beta_s\lambda_s} \tag{9.189}$$

Similarly, for a group of four similar components,

$$\lambda_s = \lambda_{s1}+3\lambda_{s2}+3\lambda_{s3}+\lambda_{s4} \tag{9.190}$$

$$\beta_s = \frac{3\lambda_{s2}+3\lambda_{s3}+\lambda_{s4}}{\lambda_{s1}+3\lambda_{s2}+3\lambda_{s3}+3\lambda_{s4}} = \frac{3\lambda_{s2}+3\lambda_{s3}+\lambda_{s4}}{\lambda_s} \tag{9.191}$$

$$\gamma_s = \frac{3\lambda_{s3} + \lambda_{s4}}{3\lambda_{s2} + 3\lambda_{s3} + 3\lambda_{s4}} = \frac{3\lambda_{s3} + \lambda_{s4}}{\beta_s \lambda_s} \tag{9.192}$$

$$\delta_s = \frac{\lambda_{s4}}{3\lambda_{s3} + 3\lambda_{s4}} = \frac{\lambda_{s4}}{\gamma_s \beta_s \lambda_s} \tag{9.193}$$

These relations can be generalized to m-component systems.

$$\left.\begin{aligned} \lambda_s &= \sum_{j=1}^{m} \binom{m-1}{j-1} \lambda_{sj} \\ \beta_s &= \frac{1}{\lambda_s} \sum_{j=2}^{m} \binom{m-1}{j-1} \lambda_{sj} \\ \gamma_s &= \frac{1}{\beta_s \lambda_s} \sum_{j=3}^{m} \binom{m-1}{j-1} \lambda_{sj} \\ \delta_s &= \frac{1}{\gamma_s \beta_s \lambda_s} \sum_{j=4}^{m} \binom{m-1}{j-1} \lambda_{sj} \end{aligned}\right. \tag{9.194}$$

The inverse relations for the BP and MGL models hold for three-component systems:

$$\left.\begin{aligned} \lambda_{s1} &= (1 - \beta_s)\lambda_s \\ \lambda_{s2} &= (1/2)(1 - \gamma_s)\beta_s \lambda_s \\ \lambda_{s3} &= \gamma_s \beta_s \lambda_s \end{aligned}\right\} \tag{9.195}$$

Similarly, for a four-component system,

$$\left.\begin{aligned} \lambda_{s1} &= (1 - \beta_s)\lambda_s \\ \lambda_{s2} &= (1/3)(1 - \gamma_s)\beta_s \lambda_s \\ \lambda_{s3} &= (1/3)(1 - \delta_s)\gamma_s \beta_s \lambda_s \\ \lambda_{s4} &= \delta \gamma \beta \lambda_s \end{aligned}\right\} \tag{9.196}$$

9.3.4.3 Parameter estimation. Using the BP model estimators of (9.161) and (9.194), we obtain

$$\hat{\lambda}_s = \frac{1}{mn} \sum_{j=1}^{m} j n_j \tag{9.197}$$

$$\hat{\beta}_s = \sum_{j=2}^{m} j n_j / \sum_{j=1}^{m} j n_j \tag{9.198}$$

$$\hat{\gamma}_s = \sum_{j=3}^{m} j n_j / \sum_{j=2}^{m} j n_j \tag{9.199}$$

$$\hat{\delta}_s = \sum_{j=4}^{m} j n_j / \sum_{j=3}^{m} j n_j \tag{9.200}$$

Equation (9.197) for the component overall-failure probability λ_s coincides with (9.130) when $n_2 = \cdots = n_{m-1} = 0$.

$$\hat{\lambda}_s = \frac{n_1 + m n_m}{mn} = \frac{n_m + (n_1/m)}{n} \tag{9.201}$$

For a three-component system, we have

$$\left.\begin{aligned}\hat{\lambda}_s &= (n_1 + 2n_2 + 3n_3)/(3n)\\ \hat{\beta}_s &= (2n_2 + 3n_3)/(n_1 + 2n_2 + 3n_3)\\ \hat{\gamma}_s &= (3n_3)/(2n_2 + 3n_3)\end{aligned}\right\} \quad (9.202)$$

The Bayes estimator for β_s using a beta prior distribution with parameters a and b is

$$\beta_s^* = \frac{2n_2 + 3n_3 + a}{n_1 + 2n_2 + 3n_3 + a + b} \quad (9.203)$$

Similarly, for a beta prior distribution with parameters c and d,

$$\gamma_s^* = \frac{3n_3 + c}{2n_2 + 3n_3 + c + d} \quad (9.204)$$

The parameter $\hat{\beta}_s$ coincides with the beta-factor β of (9.129) when $n_j = 0,\ 1 < j < m$:

$$\hat{\beta}_s = \frac{mn_m}{n_1 + mn_m} = \frac{n_m}{n_m + (n_1/m)} \quad (9.205)$$

The relationships for the failure-to-operate mode remain the same with the subscript r exchanged for s.

Example 15—Two-out-of-three valve-system demand failure. Consider the valve data in Table 9.10. Calculate the demand-failure probability for a two-out-of-three valve system.

Solution: Equation (9.202) gives

$$\left.\begin{aligned}\hat{\lambda}_s &= (30 + 2 \times 2 + 3 \times 1)/(3 \times 4449) = 0.00277\\ \hat{\beta}_s &= (2 \times 2 + 3 \times 1)/(30 + 2 \times 2 + 3 \times 1) = 0.189\\ \hat{\gamma}_s &= 3/(2 \times 2 + 3 \times 1) = 0.429\end{aligned}\right\} \quad (9.206)$$

From (9.195) we have

$$\begin{aligned}V_1 &= \lambda_{s1} = (1 - \beta_s)\lambda_s\\ &= (1 - 0.189) \times 0.00277 = 2.2 \times 10^{-3} \quad (9.207)\\ V_2 &= \lambda_{s2} = \frac{1}{2}(1 - \gamma_s)\beta_s\lambda_s\\ &= 0.5 \times (1 - 0.429) \times 0.189 \times 0.00277 = 1.5 \times 10^{-4} \quad (9.208)\\ V_3 &= \lambda_{s3} = \gamma_s\beta_s\lambda_s\\ &= 0.429 \times 0.189 \times 0.00277 = 2.2 \times 10^{-4} \quad (9.209)\end{aligned}$$

Equations (9.177) and (9.209) show the equivalence between BP and MGL models. ■

9.3.5 Binomial Failure-Rate Model

9.3.5.1 Model parameters. The original binomial failure-rate (BFR) model developed by Vesely [7] included two types of failures.

1. Independent failures.
2. Nonlethal shocks that act on the system as a Poisson process with rate μ and that challenge all components in the system simultaneously. Upon each nonlethal shock, each component has a constant and independent failure probability P.

The name of the model arises from the fact that the failed component distribution resulting from a shock occurrence is a binomial distribution.

A more recent version of the BFR model developed by Atwood [8] includes a lethal shock with rate ω. When this shock occurs, all components fail with a conditional probability of 1.

The BFR model for failures during operation requires use of the following set of five parameters, irrespective of the number of components (Figure 9.15).

λ_{ic} = independent failure rate for each component. Subscript ic stands for independent cause.
μ = occurrence rate for nonlethal shocks.
P = conditional probability of failure of each component, given a nonlethal shock.
ω = occurrence rate for lethal shocks.
$t\ (\leq T)$ = mission time.

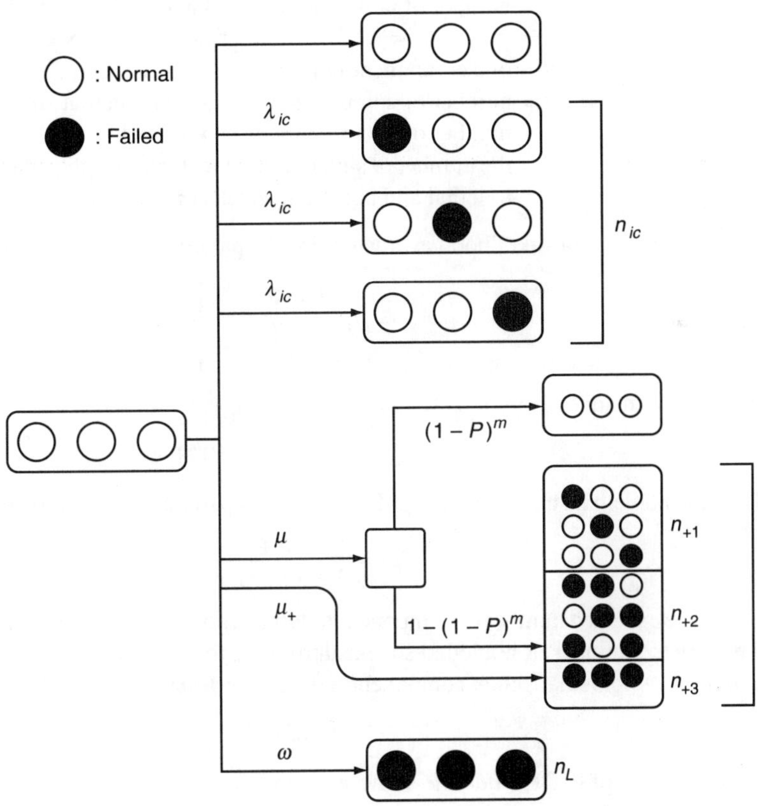

Figure 9.15. BFR state transition model during mission.

This model can easily be extended to failure-on-demand problems; thus two sets of parameters apply; one set for failures on demand, and the other for failure in operation. The BFR model is not equivalent to the BP model nor to the MGL model; in the BFR model, common-cause failures occur either by a binomial impact or a global impact. The total number of BFR parameters remains constant regardless of the number of components. The

BFR model treats each event as a lethal or nonlethal shock, and single failures are classified as independent or nonlethal. The beta-factor model, on the other hand, only describes lethal-shock common-cause events.

For a three-component system, for example, the following relations hold between BP and BFR models (t: mission time).

$$\left.\begin{aligned} \lambda_{r1}t &= \lambda_{ic}t + \mu t P(1-P)^2 \\ \lambda_{r2}t &= \mu t P^2(1-P) \\ \lambda_{r3}t &= \mu t P^3 + \omega t \end{aligned}\right\} \tag{9.210}$$

The BFR model includes the beta-factor model as a special case when $\mu = 0$.

9.3.5.2 Parameter estimation. To develop estimators for the parameters, additional quantities are used.

T = run time for the system.
μ_+ = rate of nonlethal shocks that cause at least one component failure.
n_{+i} = number of nonlethal shocks that cause i simultaneous failures.
$n_+ = \sum_{i=1}^{m} n_{+i}$ = total number of nonlethal shocks that cause at least one component failure.
$s = \sum_{i=1}^{m} i n_{+i}$ = number of component failures by nonlethal shocks.
n_L = number of occurrences of lethal shocks.
n_{ic} = the number of single-component failures not counting failures due to lethal and nonlethal shocks ($n_{ic} + n_{+1} = n_1$).

The maximum-likelihood estimators for the parameters λ_{ic}, μ_+, and ω are

$$\left.\begin{aligned} \lambda_{ic} &= n_{ic}/(mT) \\ \mu_+ &= n_+/T \\ \omega &= n_L/T \end{aligned}\right\} \tag{9.211}$$

From the definition of μ_+ and μ

$$\mu_+ = \mu[1 - (1-P)^m] \tag{9.212}$$

Thus the nonlethal shock rate μ is calculated when parameter P is known.

$$\mu = \frac{\mu_+}{1 - (1-P)^m} \tag{9.213}$$

The expected number of component failures per nonlethal shock is mP. Furthermore, the expected number of nonlethal shocks during the total run time T is μT. Thus the total number s of nonlethal shock component failures is estimated as

$$s = \mu T m P \tag{9.214}$$

Substituting μ of (9.213) into the above equation,

$$s = \frac{\mu_+ T m P}{1-(1-P)^m} = \frac{n_+ m P}{1-(1-P)^m} \tag{9.215}$$

Parameter P is the solution of this equation, and rate μ is now calculatable from (9.213).

Example 16—One-out-of-three pump-system run failure. Consider the data in Table 9.14, which is a modified version of Table 9.11. Note that all single failures are due to independent causes ($n_{ic} = 45, n_{+1} = 0$); the simultaneous failure of three pumps is due to the lethal

TABLE 9.14. Data for BFR Model

Exposure Time T	Single Random n_{ic}	Single Nonlethal n_{+1}	Double Nonlethal n_{+2}	Triple Nonlethal n_{+3}	Lethal n_L	Mission Time t	Positive Nonlethal n_+	Weighted Sum s
4449	45	0	6	0	1	1	6	12

shock; the nonlethal shocks result in six cases of simultaneous failures of two pumps. Calculate the run-failure probability of the one-out-of-three system for mission time $t = 1$.

Solution: From (9.211),

$$\lambda_{ic} = \frac{45}{3 \times 4449} = 0.00337 \tag{9.216}$$

$$\mu_+ = 6/4449 = 0.00135 \tag{9.217}$$

$$\omega = 1/4449 = 0.000225 \tag{9.218}$$

Equation (9.215) yields the equality

$$2P^2 - 6P + 3 = 0 \tag{9.219}$$

or

$$P = 0.634, \qquad 1 - P = 0.366 \tag{9.220}$$

The nonlethal shock rate μ is calculated from (9.213):

$$\mu = \frac{0.00135}{1 - 0.366^3} = 0.00142 \tag{9.221}$$

Thus from (9.210)

$$\left.\begin{aligned} P_1 &= \lambda_{ic} t + \mu t P(1-P)^2 \\ &= 0.00337 + 0.00142 \times 0.634 \times 0.366^2 = 0.0035 \\ P_2 &= \mu t P^2 (1-P) \\ &= 0.00142 \times 0.634^2 \times 0.366 = 0.00021 \\ P_3 &= \mu t P^3 + \omega t \\ &= 0.00142 \times 0.634^3 + 0.000225 = 0.00059 \end{aligned}\right\} \tag{9.222}$$

The run-failure probability of the one-out-of-three pump system is

$$Q_{1/3} \simeq P_3 = 0.00059 \tag{9.223}$$

A comparison between (9.185) and (9.222) is shown in Table 9.15. This indicates the following.

1. The single-failure probabilities are approximately equal.
2. The BFR model yields a smaller double-failure probability because it assumes a binomial failure mechanism, given a nonlethal shock.
3. The BFR model yields a larger triple-failure probability because it considers as causes both lethal and nonlethal shocks.

9.3.6 Markov Model

The common-cause models described so far assume that systems are nonrepairable; for repairable systems, Markov transition diagrams can be used, where transition rates are estimated by appropriate parametric models. Consider a one-out-of-two system. Assume

TABLE 9.15. BP and BFR for 1/3 Pump System Run Probability

	BP	BFR
P_1	0.0034	0.0035
P_2	0.00045	0.00021
P_3	0.00022	0.00059

■

that the system is subject to a common cause C that occurs with rate λ_{r2}, and that each component has an independent failure rate λ_{r1} and repair rate μ. Then the behavior of the cut set can be expressed by the Markov transition diagram of Figure 9.16, where the indicator variable 1 denotes the existence of component failure, and the variable 0 the nonexistence. A cut set fails when it falls into state (1, 1). Common cause C creates the multiple-component transition from state (0, 0) to (1, 1).

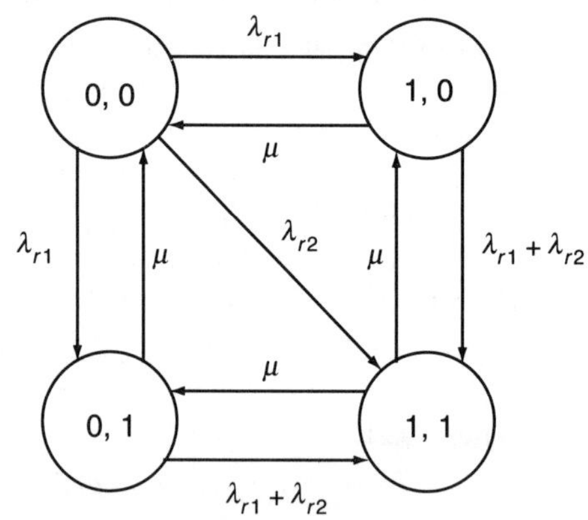

Figure 9.16. Transition diagram for 1/2 system subject to common cause.

The beta-factor model shows that rates λ_{r2} and λ_{r1} can be calculated from the overall component failure rate λ_r and parameter β_r:

$$\lambda_{r2} = \beta_r \lambda_r, \qquad \lambda_{r1} = (1 - \beta_r)\lambda_r \tag{9.224}$$

Denote by P_{ij} the probability of state (i, j). The following equation holds.

$$\begin{pmatrix} \dot{P}_{00} \\ \dot{P}_{01} \\ \dot{P}_{10} \\ \dot{P}_{11} \end{pmatrix} = \begin{pmatrix} -(2\lambda_{r1} + \lambda_{r2}) & \mu & \mu & 0 \\ \lambda_{r1} & -(\lambda_{r1} + \lambda_{r2} + \mu) & 0 & \mu \\ \lambda_{r1} & 0 & -(\lambda_{r1} + \lambda_{r2} + \mu) & \mu \\ \lambda_{r2} & \lambda_{r1} + \lambda_{r2} & \lambda_{r1} + \lambda_{r2} & -2\mu \end{pmatrix} \begin{pmatrix} P_{00} \\ P_{01} \\ P_{10} \\ P_{11} \end{pmatrix} \tag{9.225}$$

Let P_j be the probability of the state where j components are failed: $P_0 = P_{00}$, $P_1 = P_{01} + P_{10}$, and $P_2 = P_{11}$. Equation (9.225) can be rewritten as a three-state differential equation (Figure 9.17).

$$\begin{pmatrix} \dot{P}_0 \\ \dot{P}_1 \\ \dot{P}_2 \end{pmatrix} = \begin{pmatrix} -(2\lambda_{r1} + \lambda_{r2}) & \mu & 0 \\ 2\lambda_{r1} & -(\lambda_{r1} + \lambda_{r2} + \mu) & 2\mu \\ \lambda_{r2} & \lambda_{r1} + \lambda_{r2} & -2\mu \end{pmatrix} \begin{pmatrix} P_0 \\ P_1 \\ P_2 \end{pmatrix} \tag{9.226}$$

The failed-state probability P_2 can be calculated numerically.

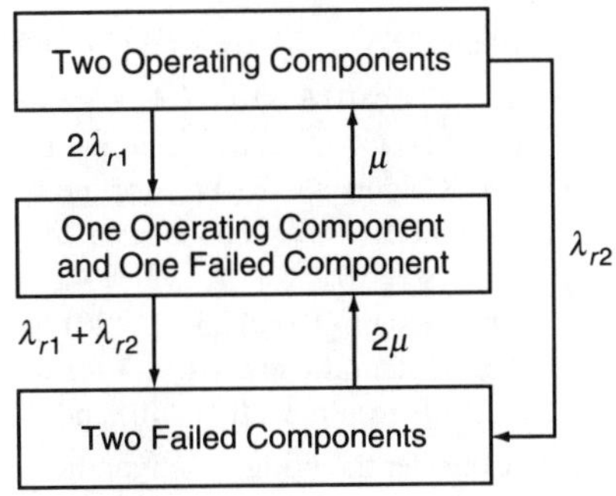

Figure 9.17. Simplified common-cause diagram.

REFERENCES

[1] Fleming, K. N., A. Mosleh, and R. K. Deremer. "A systematic procedure for the incorporation of common cause events into risk and reliability models," *Nuclear Engineering and Design*, vol. 93, pp. 245–273, 1986.

[2] Dyer, D. "Unification of reliability/availability/repairability models for Markov systems," *IEEE Trans. on Reliability*, vol. 38, no. 2, pp. 246–252, 1989.

[3] Fleming, K. N. "A reliability model for common mode failure in redundant safety systems." In *Proc. of the Sixth Annual Pittsburgh Conference on Modeling and Simulation*. General Atomic Report GA-A13284, April, pp. 23–25, 1975.

[4] Pickard, Lowe and Garrick, Inc. "Seabrook station probabilistic safety assessment." Prepared for Public Service Company of New Hampshire and Yankee Atomic Electric Company, PLG-0300, December 1983.

[5] Marshall, A. W., and I. Olkin. "A multivariate exponential distribution," *J. of the American Statistical Association*, vol. 62, pp. 30–44, 1967.

[6] Fleming, K. N., et al. "Classification and analysis of reactor operating experience involving dependent events." Pickard, Lowe and Garrick, Inc., PLG-0400, prepared for EPRI, February 1985.

[7] Vesely, W. E. "Estimating common cause failure probabilities in reliability and risk analyses: Marshall-Olkin specializations." In *Proc. of the Int. Conf. on Nuclear Systems Reliability Engineering and Risk Assessment*, pp. 314–341, 1977.

[8] Steverson, J. A., and C. L. Atwood. "Common cause fault rates for valves." USNRC, NUREG/CR-2770, February 1983.

[9] USNRC. "PRA procedures guide: A guide to the performance of probabilistic risk assessments for nuclear power plants." USNRC, NUREG/CR-2300, 1983, Appendix B.

PROBLEMS

9.1. Let $\boldsymbol{P}(t)$ and $\boldsymbol{A}$ be an n-vector and an $n \times n$ matrix. It can be shown that the differential equation

$$\dot{\boldsymbol{P}}(t) = \boldsymbol{A}\boldsymbol{P}(t)$$

can be solved sequentially as

$$\begin{aligned}\boldsymbol{P}(\Delta) &= \exp(\boldsymbol{A}\Delta)\boldsymbol{P}(0)\\ \boldsymbol{P}(k\Delta) &= \exp(\boldsymbol{A}\Delta)\boldsymbol{P}([k-1]\Delta)\end{aligned}$$

where Δ = small length of time

$\exp(\boldsymbol{A}\Delta) = \boldsymbol{I} + \boldsymbol{A}\Delta + \frac{A^2\Delta^2}{2!} + \frac{A^3\Delta^3}{3!} + \frac{A^4\Delta^4}{4!} + \cdots$

$\boldsymbol{I}$ = unit matrix

(a) Calculate $\exp(\boldsymbol{A}\Delta)$ for the warm standby differential equation of (9.12) with $\lambda = 0.001$, $\bar{\lambda} = 0.0005$, and $\mu = 0.01$, considering up to the second-order terms of $\Delta = 10$.

(b) Obtain $Q_r(10)$ and $Q_r(20)$ for the warm standby, using $\exp(\boldsymbol{A}\Delta)$.

(c) Obtain the exact $Q_r(t)$ for the warm standby, using Laplace transforms. Compare the results with $Q_r(10)$ and $Q_r(20)$ of (b).

9.2. Consider the bridge configuration of Figure P9.2. Assume steady-state probabilities:

$$Q_1 = \Pr\{1\} = 0.03, \qquad Q_2 = \Pr\{2\} = 0.02$$
$$Q_r = \Pr\{1 \cap 2\} = 0.0003, \qquad Q_3 = \Pr\{3\} = Q_4 = \Pr\{4\} = 0.02$$
$$Q_5 = \Pr\{5\} = 0.0002$$

Calculate the system unavailability Q_s.

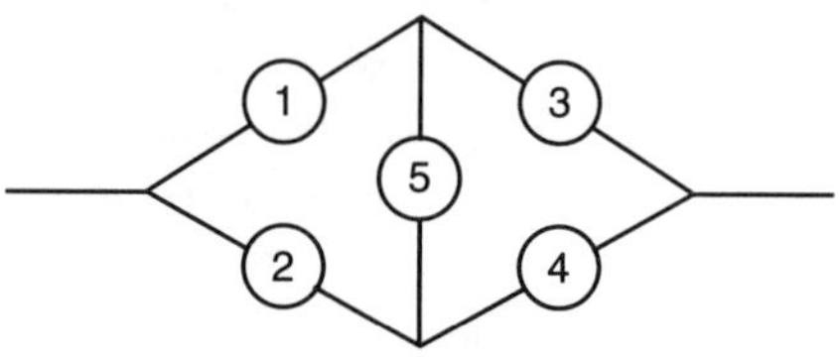

Figure P9.2. A bridge-circuit reliability block diagram.

9.3. **(a)** Determine a differential equation for the two-out-of-three standby redundancy with three pumps and one repair crew, using as data

$$\lambda = 0.001, \qquad \bar{\lambda} = 0.0001, \qquad \mu = 0.1$$

(b) Obtain the matrix $\exp(\boldsymbol{A}\Delta) \simeq \boldsymbol{I} + \boldsymbol{A}\Delta$ for a small time length Δ as well. Calculate $P_{(i)}(t)$, $(i = 0, 1, 2, 3)$ at $t = 3$ by setting $\Delta = 1$.

(c) Determine a differential equation for reliability calculation.

(d) Determine a differential equation for repairability calculation.

9.4. A standby redundancy consists of five identical components and has two principal components and two repair crews.

(a) Obtain the differential equation for the redundant configuration, using as data $\lambda = 0.001$, $\bar{\lambda} = 0.0005$, $\mu = 0.01$.

(b) Calculate the steady-state unavailability $Q_r(\infty)$.

(c) Calculate the steady-state unconditional failure intensity $w_r(\infty)$.

9.5. **(a)** Perform a subcomponent-level analysis when the three-train pump system of Figure 9.9 has a three-out-of-three configuration.

(b) Perform a subcomponent-level analysis for a two-out-of-three configuration of the pump system.

9.6. Develop a beta-factor state transition model for a four-component system prior to a demand.

9.7. Develop a basic-parameter state transition model for a four-component system prior to a demand.

9.8. Develop the BFR state transition model for a four-component system during mission.

10

Human Reliability

10.1 INTRODUCTION

Humans design, manufacture, install reliable and safe systems, and function as indispensable working elements in systems where monitoring, detection, diagnosis, control, manipulation, maintenance, calibration, or test activities are not automated. We can operate plants manually when automatic control fails.

However, to quote Alexander Pope, "to err is human." Human errors in thinking and rote tasks occur, and these errors can destroy aircraft, chemical plants, and nuclear power plants. Our behavior is both beneficial and detrimental to modern engineering systems. The reliability and safety analyst must consider the human; otherwise, the analysis is not creditable.

It is difficult to provide a unified, quantitative description of the positive and negative aspects of human beings in terms of reliability and safety parameters. However, a unified view is necessary if we are to analyze and evaluate. As a first approximation, the human is viewed as a computer system or electronic robot consisting of a main CPU, memory units, I/O devices, and peripheral CPUs. This view is, of course, too simple. Differences among humans, computer systems, and robots must be clarified [1].

We begin in Section 10.2 with a human-error classification scheme suitable for PRAs. Section 10.3 compares human beings with hardware systems supported by computers. The comparison is useful in understanding humans; we are not machines to the extent that some machines behave like us; machines are only tools to simulate and extend human functions. Sections 10.4 and 10.5 describe how various factors influence human performance. Examples of human errors are presented in Section 10.6. A general process for human-error PRA quantification is given in Section 10.7. This process is called SHARP (systematic human action reliability procedure [2,3].

Section 10.8 presents a quantification approach suitable to maintenance and testing prior to an accident. An event-tree–based model to quantify human-error events that appear in event and fault trees is developed. This methodology is called THERP (technique for human-error rate prediction) [4–6]. Although THERP is a systematic and powerful technique for quantifying routine or procedure-following human tasks, it has limitations in dealing with thought processes like accident diagnosis. The remaining two sections deal with the thought process. Section 10.9 describes the HCR (human cognitive reliability) model [7, 3] to quantify nonresponse error probabilities under time stress during an accident. Unfortunately, the nonresponse error is not the only failure mode during an accident; human behavior is unpredictable, and wrong actions that cause hazardous consequences are often performed. Section 10.10 deals with wrong actions.

10.2 CLASSIFYING HUMAN ERRORS FOR PRA

Event and fault trees should include human-error events taking place before and after initiating events. These can then be analyzed by human reliability analysts using the error types proposed by SHARP.

10.2.1 Before an Initiating Event

This is called a pre-initiator error (see Chapter 3). There can be at least two types of human errors prior to an initiating event [3]:

1. Test and Maintenance Errors: These occur under controlled conditions (e.g., no accident, little or no time pressure) before an initiating event. A typical example is failure to return safety equipment to its working state after a test, thus causing a latent failure of the safety system. Most test and maintenance activities are routine, procedure-following tasks. These types of human errors must be included in fault trees, and quantification is based on direct data, expert judgment, and/or THERP.
2. Initiating-Event Causation: An accident may be initiated by human error, particularly during start-ups or shutdowns, when there is a maximum of human intervention. The initiating events, of course, appear as the first heading in any event tree, and human errors are included in the appropriate fault trees describing initiating-event occurrences. This type of error can be assessed similarly to the test and maintenance errors; the PRA assessments are traditionally based on initiating-event frequency data such as, for example, that 40 to 50% of unnecessary nuclear power plant trips are caused by human error.

10.2.2 During an Accident

This is a post-initiator human error containing accident-procedure errors and recovery errors (see Chapter 3). Wakefield [8] gives typical human response activities during accidents.

1. Manual backup to automatic plant response.
2. Change of normal plant safety response.
3. Recovery and repair of failed system.
4. Total shift to manual operation.

The tree shown in Figure 10.1 represents generalized action sequences taken during an accident [3]. This is an operator action tree (OAT), as proposed by Wreathall [9]. The event-tree headings are arranged in the following order.

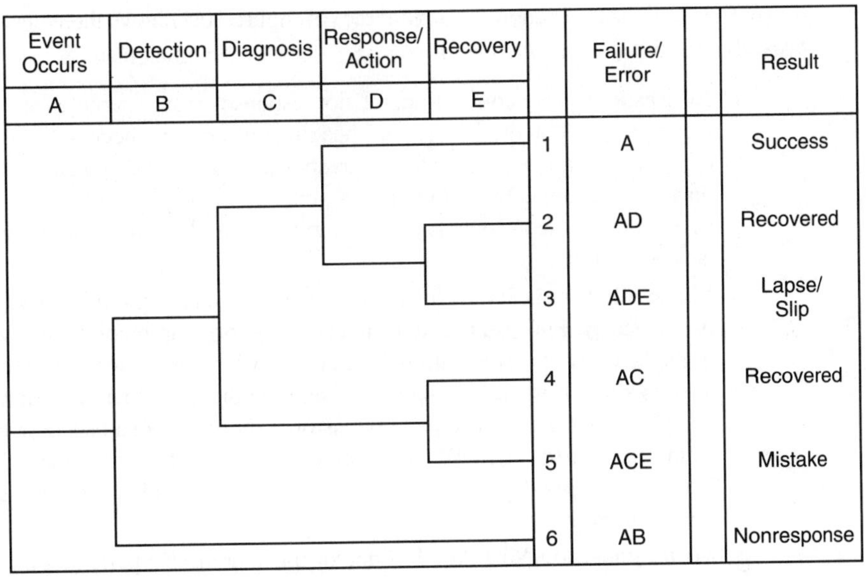

Figure 10.1. Operator action tree.

1. **Abnormal Event Occurrence:** An abnormal event such as a power transformer failure or loss of water to a heat exchanger.
2. **Detection:** Abnormal events are detected through deviant instrument readings.
3. **Diagnosis:** Engineers assess the situation, identify plant response, and determine actions to be taken to implement the response.
4. **Response/Action:** The engineers or technicians execute the actions determined in the diagnostic phase.
5. **Recovery:** Engineers rediagnose the situation, correct previous errors, and establish a course of action as additional plant symptoms and/or support personnel become available.

The detection-diagnosis-response (D-D-R) model is similar to the stimulus-organism-response (S-O-R) model used by psychologists since 1929. Engineers must detect abnormalities, diagnose the plant to determine viable actions, and execute them under high stress within a given period of time. The time constraints becomes a crucial factor in predicting human performance: nobody can run one hundred meters in less than nine seconds.

The diagnosis phase is a holistic thought process; it is difficult to decompose diagnostic processes into sequences of basic tasks, but when such a decomposition is feasible, the diagnosis becomes much simpler, similar to maintenance and test processes.

Woods et al. [10] describe three error-prone problem-solver types.

1. **Garden path:** This fixation-prone problem solver shows excessive persistence on a single explanation and fails to consider revisions in face of discrepant evidence.
2. **Vagabond:** This problem solver tends to jump from one explanation to another, leading from one response action to another.
3. **Hamlet:** This problem solver considers so many possible explanations that his response is slow.

The OAT (or EAT: engineer action tree) of Figure 10.1 shows three classes of unsuccessful responses.

1. **Nonresponse:** By convention, the nonresponse error is depicted as sequence 6 in the OAT; note that the "Detection" heading failure is not necessarily the only cause of the nonresponse; rather the nonresponse is an overall result of detection and diagnosis failures. Even if engineers generate incorrect solutions, this is regarded as a nonresponse as long as these solutions yield the same consequence as a total lack of response.
2. **Lapse/Slip (Omission):** No actions are taken even if remediations were generated (sequence 3). For instance, a technician may forget to manipulate a valve in spite of the fact that the remediation called for valve manipulation. The technician may also be slow in manipulating the valve, thus the valve manipulation may not be completed in time. This type of omission error results in a lack of action different from the nonresponse. When a technician forgets to do a remedial action, this is called a *lapse*-type *omission* error; the slow technician commits a *slip*-type *omission* error.
3. **Misdiagnosis or Mistake:** If a doctor misdiagnoses a patient, a hazardous drug worse than "no drug" may be prescribed. Wrong remedial actions more hazardous than no action are undertaken when engineers misdiagnose problems. These fixes are often not correctable if recovery fails. This is sequence 5 in the OAT, which is caused by "Diagnosis" failures followed by a "Recovery" failure. Wrong prescriptions and wrong diagnoses are mistakes or logic errors.
4. **Lapse/Slip (Commission):** Hazardous, wrong actions will occur even if correct solutions have been determined. For instance, a technician may manipulate the wrong switch or erroneously take the wrong action even though the correct course of action was formulated. This is sequence 3 in the OAT, which is caused by "Response" failures. Incorrect recall and execution are called *lapse* and *slip commission* errors, respectively.

Sequence 1 is a case where "Detection," "Diagnosis," and "Response" are all performed correctly; errors in "Action" and "Diagnosis" phases are corrected in the "Recovery" phase in sequences 2 and 4, respectively.

The nonresponse, lapse/slip-type omission, misdiagnosis, and lapse/slip-type commission after accident initiation are typically included in an event tree. Recovery, when considered, modifies accident-sequence cut sets in the same way that successful application of the emergency brake could, theoretically, avoid an accident if the foot brake fails.

10.3 HUMAN AND COMPUTER HARDWARE SYSTEM

10.3.1 The Human Computer

Human and machine. Hardware systems are more reliable, precise, consistent, and quicker than humans [11]. Hardware systems, although inflexible, are ideal for routine and repetitive tasks. People are less reliable, less precise, less consistent, and slower but more flexible than hardware; we are weak in computation, negation logic, normative treatment, and concurrent processing but strong in pattern recognition and heuristics. We are flexible in manipulation, data sensing, and data processing where the same purpose can be accomplished by different approaches. Hardware is predictable, but human behavior is unpredictable; we can commit all types of misdiagnosis and wrong actions. People frequently lie to absolve themselves from blame. Human beings are far superior in self-correction capability than machines. Humans are purposeful; they form a solution and act accordingly, searching for relevant information and performing necessary actions along the way. This goal-oriented behavior is good as long as the solution is correct; otherwise, the wrong solution becomes a dominant source of common-cause failures. We can anticipate. We have strong intuitive survival instincts.

Two-level computer configuration. A typical computer hardware system for controlling a manufacturing plant is configured in two levels; it has a main CPU and peripheral CPUs. Input devices such as pressure or temperature sensors gather data about plant states. The input CPUs at the periphery of the computer system process the raw input data and send filtered information to the main CPU. The main CPU processes the information and sends commands to the output CPUs, which control the output devices. Simple or routine controls can be performed by the I/O CPUs, which may bypass the main CPU. The peripheral CPUs have some autonomy.

Life-support ability. Figure 10.2 is a simplistic view of the human being as a computer system. A major difference between Figure 10.2 and the usual computer configuration is the existence of a life-support unit consisting of the "old CPU" and internal organs. The life-support unit is common to all animals. The old CPU is a computer that controls the internal organs and involuntary functions such as respiration, blood circulation, hormone secretion, and body temperature. We usually consume less energy than hardware of similar size and ability. The old CPU senses instinctively and, in the case of a normal human being, instructs it to seek pleasant sensations and avoid unpleasant ones. For example, if a plant operator is instructed to monitor displays located far apart in a large control room, the operator tends to look at the displays from far away to minimize walk-around [4]. This instinctive response prompts reading errors.

Sensing ability. The input devices in Figure 10.2 are sense organs such as eyes, ears, nose, and skin proprioceptors. Each device is not linked directly to the new CPU; each sense organ has its own CPU linked with the new CPU. This is similar to a two-level computer configuration. A visual signal, for instance, is processed by its own CPU, which differs from the one that processes audible signals. The multi-CPU configuration at the periphery of sensory organs enables input devices to function concurrently; we can see and hear simultaneously.

Manipulative ability. Human output devices are motor organs such as hands, feet, mouth, and vocal chords. These motor organs are individually controlled by efferent nerve impulses from the brain. The sophisticated output CPU servomechanism controls each motor organ to yield voice or body movement. An experienced operator can function as a near-optimal PID controller with a time lag of about 0.3 s. However, even an experienced typist commits typing errors. Computer systems stand still, but the human ambulates. This mobility can be a source of trouble; it facilitates the type of deliberate nullification of essential safety systems that occurred at Three Mile Island and Chernobyl.

Memorizing ability. The "new CPU" in the brain has associated with it a memory unit of about 10^{12} bits. Some memory cells are devoted to long-term memory and others

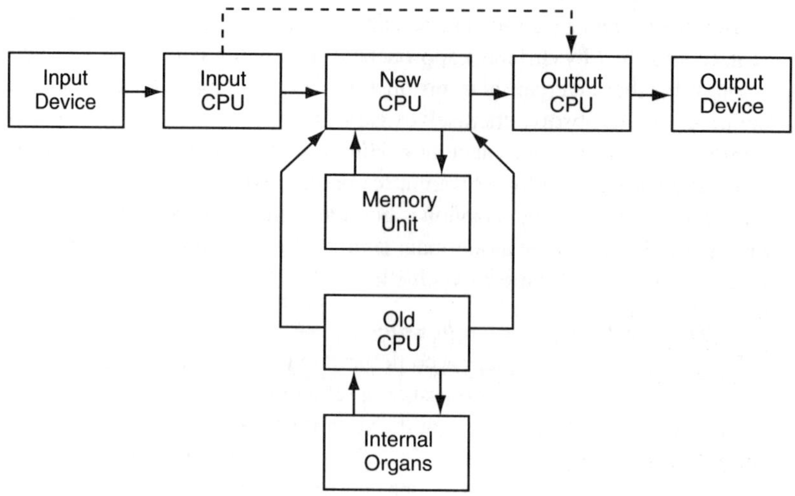

Figure 10.2. Humans as computer systems.

to short-term memory or registers. The human memory is not as reliable as LSI memory. New information relevant to a task (e.g., meter readings and procedural statements) is first fed into the short-term memory, where it may be lost after a certain period of time; a task that requires short-term memory of seven-digit numbers is obviously subject to error. The short-term memory is very limited in its capacity. During an accident, it is possible for items stored in short-term memory to be lost in the course of gathering more information [9]. The fragility of human short-term memory is a source of lapse error when a task is suddenly interrupted; coffee breaks or telephone calls trigger lapse-type errors.

The long-term memory houses constants, rules, principles, strategies, procedures, cookbook recipes, and problem-solving capabilities called *knowledge*. A computer program can be coded in such a way that it memorizes necessary and sufficient data for a particular task. The human brain, on the other hand, is full of things irrelevant to the task; a plant operator may be thinking about last night's quarrel with his wife. The behavior of the computer is specified uniquely by the program, but the human computer is a trashbox of programs, some of which can be dangerous; the operator, for example, may assume that a valve is still open because it used to be open. Long-term memory also decays.

A computer program starts its execution with a reset operation that cancels all extraneous factors. It is impossible, on the other hand, to reset the human computer. The past conditions the future and can trigger human errors, including malevolent ones.

Thinking ability. The new CPU, surrounded by long- and short-term memory and peripheral CPUs, generates plans, and orders relevant peripheral CPUs to implement them; purposefulness is one of the major differences between human beings and machines. These plans are formed consciously and unconsciously. Conscious plan formation is observed typically in the diagnosis phase that assesses current situations and decides on actions consistent with the assessment. Thus planned, goal-oriented activity in the new CPU ranges from unconscious stimulus-responses, to conscious rule-based procedures characterized by IF-THEN-ELSE logic, to serious knowledge-based thought processes. Human behavior is a repetition of action formulation and implementation. Some plans are implemented automatically without any interference from the new CPU and others are implemented consciously, as by a novice golf player. Humans can cope with unexpected events. We can also anticipate. We are very good at pattern recognition.

The processing speed of the new CPU is less than 100 bits per second—far slower than a computer, which typically executes several millions of instructions a second: The human being can read only several words a second. The sense organs receive a huge amount of information per second. Although the raw input data are preprocessed by the peripheral input CPUs, this amount of inflowing information is far larger than the processing speed of the new CPU. This slow processing speed poses difficulties, as will be described in Section 10.3.2. The new CPU resolves this problem by, for instance, "scan and sample by priority," and "like-to-like matching." The new CPU is also weak in handling negation logic; AND or OR logic is processed more easily than NAND or NOR; this suggests that we should avoid negative sentences in written procedures. A normative approach such as game theory is not to be expected.

10.3.2 Brain Bottlenecks

As stated in Section 10.3.1, the new CPU processing speed is slow and the short-term memory capacity is small. The long-term memory capacity is huge and the sense organs receive a tremendous amount of information from external stimuli. Because of its slow processing speed, the new CPU is the bottleneck in the Figure 10.2 computer configuration and is responsible for most errors, so it is quite natural that considerable attention has been paid to human-error rates for tasks involving the new CPU, especially for time-limited diagnostic thought processes during accidents.

The human computer system is an unbalanced time-sharing system consisting of a slow main computer linked to a large number of terminals. Considering the large discrepancy in performance, it is amazing that, historically, the human being has functioned as an indispensable element of all systems. It is also not surprising that most designers of space-vehicles, nuclear plants, complex weapons systems, and high-speed aircraft would like to replace humans with hardware; because of improvements in hardware, human errors have become important contributors to accidents. Human evolution is slower than machine evolution. Let us now briefly discuss how the new CPU bottleneck manifests itself.

1. **Shortcut:** People tend to simplify things to minimize work loads. Procedural steps or system elements irrelevant to the execution of current tasks are discarded. This tendency is dangerous when protection devices are nullified or safety-related procedures are neglected.
2. **Perseverance:** When an explanation fits the current situation, there is a tendency to believe that this explanation is the only one that is correct. Other explanations may well fit the situation, but these are automatically rejected.
3. **Task fixation:** The input information is scanned and sampled by priority, as is memory access. The prioritization leads to task-fixation errors, which occur when people become preoccupied with one particular task (usually a trivial one) to the exclusion of other tasks that are usually more important. People tend to concentrate on particular indicators and operations, while neglecting other, possibly critical, items.
4. **Alternation:** This occurs when an engineer constantly changes a decision while basic information is not changing [9]. Systematic responses become unavailable.

5. **Dependence:** People tend to depend on one another. Excessive dependence on other personnel, written procedures, automatic controllers, and indicators are sometimes harmful.
6. **Naivety:** Once trained, humans tend to perform tasks by rote and to bypass the new CPU. Simple stimulus-response manipulations that yield unsafe results occur. Naivety is characterized by thought processes typified by inductive logic or probability; this logic assumes that things repeat themselves in a stationary world. Inductive logic often fails in nonstationary situations and plant emergencies.
7. **Queuing and escape:** This phenomenon typically occurs when the work load is too high.
8. **Gross discrimination:** Details are neglected. Both scanning range and speed increase; qualitative rather than quantitative information is collected.
9. **Cheating and lying:** When the human thinks it is to its advantage, it will lie and cheat. In America, over 85% of all college students admit to cheating on their school work.

Reason [12] lists basic error tendencies. From a diagnosis point of view, these include the following.

1. **Similarity bias:** People tend to choose diagnostic explanations based on like-to-like matching.
2. **Frequency bias:** People tend to choose diagnostic explanations with a high frequency of past success.
3. **Bounded rationality:** People have only limited mental resources for diagnosis.
4. **Imperfect rationality:** People rarely make diagnoses according to optimal or normative theories (e.g., logic, statistical decision theory, subjective expected utility, etc.).
5. **Reluctant rationality:** People perform diagnoses that minimize conscious thinking. According to Henry Ford, the average worker wants a job in which he does not have to think.
6. **Incomplete/incorrect knowledge:** Human knowledge is only an approximation of external reality. We have only a limited number of models about the external world.

Human-machine systems should be designed in such a way that machines help people achieve their potential by giving them support where they are weakest [11,13], and vice versa. For instance, carefully designed warning systems are required to relieve human beings of unnecessary thought processes and guide human beings according to appropriate priorities. A good procedure manual may present several candidate scenarios and suggest which one is most likely. Displays with hierarchical arrangements save scanning time and decrease the work load. The human computer has a very unbalanced configuration and thus requires a good operating system and peripheral engineering intelligence to mitigate new CPU bottlenecks.

10.3.3 Human Performance Variations

Determinism and indeterminism. Electronic computers, which are deterministic machines, have internal clocks that tick several million times a second, and programs are executed in exact accordance with the clock. Each memory cell has a fixed bit capacity and stores an exact amount of data, and the arithmetic unit always performs calculations to a fixed precision. The processing speed and program execution results remain constant over many trials, given the same initial condition and the same input data. Human computers, on the other hand, have indeterministic, variable performance and yield different results over many trials.

Five performance phases. The following five phases of human performance typify the new CPU [14].

1. **Unconscious phase:** This occurs in deep sleep or during brain paroxysms or seizures. The new CPU intelligence stops completely.
2. **Vacant phase:** Excessive fatigue, monotony, drugs, or liquor can induce a vacant phase. The new CPU functions slowly.
3. **Passive phase:** This is observed during routine activities. The new CPU functions passively. Display-panel monitoring during normal situations is often done in this phase.
4. **Active phase:** The brain is clear and the new CPU functions actively at its best performance level, searching for new evidence and solutions. This phase does not last long, and a passive phase follows shortly.
5. **Panic phase:** Excessive tension, fear, or work load bring on this phase. The new CPU stresses, overheats, lacks cool judgment, and loses rationality.

Visceral causes of performance variation. Diverse mechanisms characterize the human computer performance variation. We now describe one mechanism specific to the human being as an animal, namely, the performance variation occurs because the new CPU is controlled by the old CPU, the visceral function system. The following three control modes are typical [14].

1. **Activity versus rest rhythm:** Excessive fatigue, be it mental or physiological, is harmful. Given that fatigue occurs, the old CPU commands the new CPU to rest. This phenomenon occurs typically with a one-day cycle. Figure 10.3 shows a frequency profile of traffic accidents caused by overfatigued drivers on a Japanese highway. The horizontal axis denotes hours of the day. We observe that the number of accidents involving asleep-at-the-wheel drivers is a maximum in the early morning when the one-day rhythm commands the new CPU to sleep. It is also interesting that the TMI accident started at 4 A.M.; the operators in the control room were most likely in a vacant phase when they failed to correctly interpret the 85 alarms set off during the first 30 s of the accident.
2. **Instinct and emotion:** The old CPU senses pleasant and unpleasant feelings, whether they are emotional or rational. When pleasant sensations occur, the old CPU activates the new CPU. This is a cost/benefit mechanism related to human motivation. Certain types of unpleasant feelings inactivate the new CPU. Other types of unpleasant feelings such as excessive fear, agony, or anxiety tend to overheat the new CPU and drive it into the panic phase.
3. **Defense of life:** When the new CPU detects or predicts a situation critical to human life, this information is fed back to the old CPU. A life crisis is a most unpleasant sensation; the old CPU commands the new CPU to fight aggressively or run from

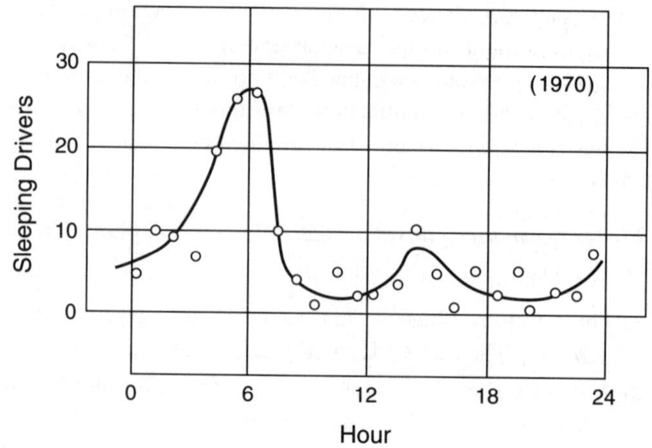

Figure 10.3. Frequency profile of traffic accidents on a highway.

danger and panic ensues. The defense-of-life instinct frequently causes people to deny and/or hide dangerous situations created by their own mistakes.

Characteristics during panic. Typical characteristics of the human in its defense-of-life phase are summarized below [15]. These are based on investigations of the behavior of pilots in critical situations before airplane crashes.

1. Input channels
   - **(a)** Abnormal concentration: Abnormal indications and warnings are monitored with the highest priority. Normal information is neglected.
   - **(b)** Illusion: Colors and shapes are perceived incorrectly. Size and movement are amplified.
   - **(c)** Gross perception: People try to extract as much information as possible in the time available. The speed and range of scanning increase and data input precision degrades.
   - **(d)** Passive perception: Excessive fatigue and stress decrease desire for more information. The eyes look but do not see.
   - **(e)** Paralysis: Input channels are cut off completely.
2. Processing at the new CPU
   - **(a)** Local judgment: Global judgment becomes difficult. A solution is searched for, using only that part of the information that is easily or directly discernible.
   - **(b)** Incorrect priority: Capability to select important information decreases.
   - **(c)** Degraded matching: It becomes difficult to compare things with patterns stored in memory.
   - **(d)** Poor accessibility: Failures of memory access occurs. Irrelevant facts are recalled.
   - **(e)** Qualitative judgment: Quantitative judgment becomes difficult: All judgment is qualitative.
   - **(f)** Pessimism: The action time remaining is underestimated and thought processes are oversimplified; important steps are neglected.
   - **(g)** Proofs: Decisions are not verified.
   - **(h)** Complete paralysis: Information processing at the new CPU stops completely.
   - **(i)** Escape: Completely irrelevant data are processed.

3. Output channels
   (a) Routine response: Habitual or skilled actions are performed unconsciously.
   (b) Poor choice: Switches and levers are selected incorrectly.
   (c) Excessive manipulation: Excessive force is applied to switches, buttons, levers, and so on. Muscle tensions and lack of feedback make smooth manipulations difficult. Overshooting and abrupt manipulations result.
   (d) Poor coordination: It becomes difficult to coordinate manipulation of two things.
   (e) Complete irrelevance: A sequence of irrelevant manipulations occurs.
   (f) Escape: No manipulation is performed.

We see that most of these characteristics are extreme manifestations of bottlenecks in the new CPU together with survival responses specific to animal life.

10.4 PERFORMANCE-SHAPING FACTORS

Any factor that influences human performance is called a PSF (performance-shaping factor). The PSFs from Handbook [4] are shown in Table 10.1. These PSFs are divided into three classes: internal PSFs operating within the individual, external PSFs existing outside the individual, and stressors. The external factors are divided into situational characteristics, job and task instructions, and task and equipment characteristics, while the stressors are psychological and physiological. The internal PSFs are organismic factors and represent internal states of the individual. Psychological and physiological stress levels of an individual vary according to discrepancies between the external PSFs, such as complexity, and internal PSFs, including previous training and experience; for instance, experienced drivers do not mind driving in traffic, whereas novices do.

10.4.1 Internal PSFs

Internal PSFs are divided into three types: hardware, psychological, and cognitive.

Hardware factors. These fall into four categories: physiological, physical, pathological, and pharmaceutical.

1. Physiological factors: Humans are organisms whose performance depends on, for example, physiological factors caused by fatigue, insufficient sleep, hangovers, hunger, 24-hour rhythms, and hypoxia. These factors are also related to environmental conditions such as low atmospheric pressure, work load, temperature, humidity, lighting, noise, and vibration.
2. Physical factors: These refer to the basic capabilities of the body as typified by size, force, strength, flexibility, eyesight, hearing, and quickness.
3. Pathological factors: These include diseases such as cardiac infarction and AIDs; mental diseases such as schizophrenia, epilepsy, and chronic alcoholism; and self-induced trauma.
4. Pharmaceutical factors: These refer to aberrant behavior caused by sleeping tablets, tranquilizers, antihistamines, and an extremely large variety of illegal drugs.

Psychological factors. These include fear, impatience, overachievement, overconfidence, motivation (or lack of it), anxiety, overdependence, introversion, or other emotional

TABLE 10.1. Performance-Shaping Factors

External PSFs	
Situational Characteristics: Those PSFs general to one or more jobs in a work situation	**Task and Equipment Characteristics**: Those PSFs specific to tasks in a job
1. Architectural features 2. Quality of environment (temperature, humidity, air quality, radiation, lighting, noise, vibration, degree of general cleanliness) 3. Work hours/work breaks 4. Shift rotation 5. Availability/adequacy of special equipment, tools, and supplies 6. Staffing parameters 7. Organizational structure (e.g., authority, responsibility, communication channels) 8. Actions by supervisors, coworkers, union representatives, and regulatory personnel 9. Rewards, recognition, benefits	1. Perceptual requirements 2. Motor requirements (speed, strength, precision) 3. Control-display relationships 4. Anticipatory requirements 5. Interpretation requirements 6. Decision-making requirements 7. Complexity (information load) 8. Narrowness of task 9. Frequency and repetitiveness 10. Task criticality 11. Long- and short-term memory 12. Calculational requirements 13. Feedback (knowledge of results) 14. Dynamic vs. step-by-step activities 15. Team structure and communication 16. Human–machine interface (design of prime equipment, test equipment, manufacturing equipment, job aids, tools, fixtures)
Job and Task Instructions: Single most important tool for most tasks	
1. Procedures required (written/not written) 2. Written or oral communications 3. Cautions and warning 4. Work methods 5. Plant policies (shop practices)	

TABLE 10.1. *Continued*

Stressor PSFs	
Psychological Stressors: PSFs that directly affect mental stress	**Physical Stressors**: PSFs that directly affect physical stress
1. Suddenness of onset 2. Duration of stress 3. Task speed 4. Task load 5. High jeopardy risk 6. Threats (of failure, loss of job) 7. Monotonous/degrading/meaningless work 8. Long, uneventful vigilance periods 9. Conflicts of motives about job performance 10. Reinforcement absent or negative 11. Sensory deprivation 12. Distractions (noise, glare, movement, flicker, color) 13. Inconsistent cueing	1. Duration of stress 2. Fatigue 3. Pain or discomfort 4. Hunger or thirst 5. Temperature extremes 6. Radiation 7. G-force extremes 8. Atmospheric pressure extremes 9. Oxygen insufficiency 10. Vibration 11. Movement constriction 12. Lack of physical exercise 13. Disruption of Circadian rhythm
Internal PSFs	
Organismic Factors:	
1. Previous training experience 2. State of current practice or skill 3. Personality and intelligence variables 4. Motivation and attitudes 5. Emotional state 6. Stress (mental or bodily tension)	7. Knowledge of required performance standards 8. Sex differences 9. Physical condition 10. Attitudes based on influence of family and other outside persons or agencies 11. Group identifications

instabilities. Overachievement, for instance, may cause a maintenance person to disconnect a protective device while making an unscheduled inspection of a machine, thus creating a hazard. Non-optimal workplace stress levels lead to abnormal psychological states. Psychological and physiological factors interact.

Cognitive factors. These are classified into skill-based abilities, rule-based abilities, and knowledge-based abilities.

1. Skill-based factors: These are concerned with levels of skill required to move hands or feet while performing routine activities. Practice improves these skills; thus routine activities are usually performed quickly and precisely. These skills are analogous to hard-wired software. Reflex-based mobility is especially important in crisis situations where time is a critical element. Reflex-based motor skills, however, are sometimes harmful because reflex actions can occur when they are not desired. The same can be said of routine thought processes.
2. Rule-based factors: These refer to the performance of sequential or branched tasks according to rules in manuals, checklists, or oral instructions. These rules are typified by IF-THEN-ELSE logic. Rule-based activities tend to become skill-based after many years of practice.
3. Knowledge-based factors: These refer to a level of knowledge relating to plant schematics, principles of operation, cause-consequence relations, and other intelligence. Knowledge utilized in problem solving is called *cues* [13]. The cues include interpreted, filtered, and selective stimuli or data; a series of rules; schemas; templates; lessons learned; and/or knowledge chunks for making a judgment or decision.

The physiological, physical, pathological, pharmaceutical, and psychological factors are called the six P's by Kuroda [15], who also considers psychosocial states. Although pathological or pharmaceutical factors are important, they could be neglected if we assume human quality control, or healthy people. This assumption, unfortunately, is frequently unjustified. An airplane crash occurred in Japan in 1981 when a pilot suffering from schizophrenia "maliciously" retrofired the jet engines just before landing. We could also neglect physical factors, provided that the human performing the task is basically capable of doing it. Then three factors remain: physiological, psychological, and cognitive. The first two factors are relatively short-term in nature, the third is long-term. In other words, the physiological and psychological factors may change from time to time, resulting in varying levels of physiological and psychological stresses.

In the following section we will discuss how the human computer in Figure 10.2 behaves when linked with external systems.

10.4.2 External PSFs

When linked with external systems, the human computer performance level varies dynamically with the characteristics of the external system and the individual person's internal states. Some PSFs apply to computer systems; others are specific to humans. The situational characteristics define background factors common to all human tasks; these characteristics form the environment under which tasks are performed.

The tasks consist of elementary activities such as selection, reading, manipulation, and diagnosis. The performance-shaping factors specific to each unit activity are called task and equipment characteristics in Table 10.1. The instructions associated with a sequence of unit activities go under the title of job and task instructions. The stressors are factors of psychological or physiological origin that decrease or increase stress levels.

Situational characteristics

1. **Architectural factors:** This refers to workplace characteristics, and includes such parameters as space, distance, layout, size, and number.
2. **Quality of environment:** Temperature, humidity, air quality, noise, vibration, cleanliness, and radiation are factors that influence hardware performance. The same is true for humans. Psychological stresses, however, are specific to people; technicians try to finish jobs quickly under poor environments such as noxious odors or high temperatures; this is specific to humans.
3. **Work hours/work breaks:** Hardware must be periodically maintained, and so must the human.
4. **Shift rotation:** Unfortunately, *après moi le déluge* attitudes are not uncommon.
5. **Availability/adequacy of special equipment, tools, and supplies:** Printers cannot print without paper or ribbon. Humans also require equipment, tools, and supplies. For better or worse, humans can do jobs without proper tools. A major accident at the Browns Ferry nuclear power plant was caused by a maintenance man who used a candle flame to check for air leaks.
6. **Staffing parameters:** In multicomputer systems it is important to allocate tasks optimally. The same is true of humans. Job dissatisfaction is a frequent cause of psychological stress and can engender uncooperative activities, and even sabotage.
7. **Organizational structure:** This includes authority, responsibility, and communication channels. These are typical of multicomputer systems in a hierarchical configuration, but psychological effects are specific to human beings.
8. **Actions by supervisors, coworkers, union representatives, and regulatory personnel:** The regulatory infrastructure of the workplace is very important (see Chapter 12). The human computer is subject to many influences. Occasionally, he or she is told to strike, or the government may declare the person's workplace to be unsafe.
9. **Rewards, recognition, benefits:** These are obviously specific to human beings.

Task and equipment characteristics. As described earlier, these characteristics refer to factors concerned with the degrees of difficulty of performing an activity.

1. **Perceptual requirements:** Visual indicators are more common than audible signals. Human eyesight, however, is limited; it may be difficult to read four digits from a strip-chart recorder. Some displays are easier to read than others.
2. **Motor requirements (speed, strength, precision):** Each engineering manipulator or actuator has limited speed, strength, or precision. The same is true for human motor organs.
3. **Control-display relationships:** Displays must be suggestive of control actions. If a display guides an operator toward an incorrect control mechanism, the probability of human error increases, especially under highly stressful situations; the stress factor is a psychological effect specific to human beings.
4. **Anticipatory requirements:** If an activity requires an operator to anticipate which display or control becomes important in the future, while performing a

current function, human error increases. Human computers are essentially in one-channel configurations and are not good at performing two or more procedures concurrently. The computer can execute several procedures concurrently in a time-sharing mode because of its high processing speeds and reliable memory.

5. **Interpretation requirement:** An activity requiring interpretation of information is more difficult than a routine activity because the interpretation itself is an additional, error-prone activity. Response times become longer and human error increases. The same is true for computer software. People interpret information in different ways, and this is a contributing factor to the high frequency of errors during shift changes; similar phenomena are observed when an operation is transformed from one computer system to another. The shift-change accidents occur because people lie. The last group does not want to tell the new group that anything is wrong: "Blame it on the next guy."
6. **Decision-making requirement:** A decision-making function makes an activity more attractive and increases volition. Absence of decision-making functions leads to boredom. These are psychological effects not generic to computers. Correct information must be provided if the decision maker is to select appropriate alternatives. This requirement applies also to an electronic computer. Decision-making functions must be consistent with the capability of each individual; similarly, a computer system requires software capable of making decisions. Decision-making increases stress levels.
7. **Complexity (information load):** The complexity of an activity is related to the amount of information to be processed and the complexity of the problem-solving algorithm. Error probability increases with complexity; this is common to both the human being and the computer.
8. **Narrowness of task:** General-purpose software is more difficult to design and more error-prone than special-purpose software. The latter, however, lacks flexibility.
9. **Frequency and repetitiveness:** Repetition increases both human and computer software reliability. Human beings, however, tend to be bored with repetitions. Rarely performed activities are error-prone. This corresponds to the burn-in phase for computer software. Just as an electronic system requires simulated tests for validation, human beings must be periodically trained for rarely performed activities. Fire and lifeboat drills are a necessity.
10. **Task criticality:** In a computer program with interrupt routines, critical tasks are executed with highest priority. Humans also have this capability, provided that activities are suitably prioritized. Psychological stress levels increase with the criticality of an activity; stress levels may be optimal, too high, or too low.
11. **Long- and short-term memory:** Human short-term memory is very fragile compared to electronic memory. Reliable secondary storage to assist humans is required.
12. **Calculational requirement:** Human beings are extremely low-reliability calculators compared to computers.
13. **Feedback (knowledge of results):** Suitable feedback improves performance for both human beings and computers; it is well known that closed-loop control is more reliable than open-loop control. Time lags degrade feedback-controller performance; for people, a time lag of more than several seconds is critical for

certain types of process control. Feedback is also related to motivation, and this is specific to human beings.

14. **Continuity (discrete versus continuous):** Continuity refers to correlation of variables in space and time. Dynamic multivariable problems are more difficult to solve than static, single-variable ones. The former are typified by the following.
    - **(a)** Some variables are not directly observable and must be estimated.
    - **(b)** Variables are correlated.
    - **(c)** The controlled process has a large time lag.
    - **(d)** Humans tend to rely on short-term memory because various display indicators should be interpreted collectively.
    - **(e)** Each unit process is complicated and difficult to visualize.
15. **Team structure and communication:** In some cases, an activity performed by one team member is verified by another. This resembles a mutual check provision in a two-computer system. Social aspects, such as collapse of infrastructure and conspiracy, are specific to human beings.
16. **Human–machine interface:** This refers to all interface factors between the human and machine. System designers usually pay considerable attention to interfaces between computers and machines. Similar efforts should be paid to the human–machine interfaces. The factors to be considered include the following.
    - **(a)** Design of display and control: functional modularization, layout, shape, size, slope, distance, number, number of digits, and color.
    - **(b)** Display labeling: symbol, letter, color, place, standardization, consistency, visibility, access, and content.
    - **(c)** Indication of plant state: clear and consistent correspondence between indicators and plant states, and consistent color coding.
    - **(d)** Amount of information displayed: necessary and sufficient warning signals, prioritized displays, hierarchical indications, and graphical display.
    - **(e)** Labeling and status indication of hardware: indication of hardware operating modes, visibility and clarity of labels.
    - **(f)** Protection provisions: fail-safe, foolproof, lock mechanisms, and warning devices.

Job and task instructions. In a computer, where menu-driven software is used, certain types of input data instruct the general-purpose software to run in a certain way. These data are indexed, paged, standardized, and modularized, especially when processing speed is a critical factor. Humans represent general-purpose software in the extreme. Instructions in the form of written or oral procedures, communications, cautions, and warnings should be correct and consistent with mental bottlenecks. For instance, a mixture of safety-related instructions and property damage descriptions on the same page of an emergency manual increase mental overload; column formats are more readable than narrative formats.

Stressors. The physiological and psychological stressors in Table 10.1 are specific to human beings. The TMI accident had a "suddenness of onset" factor because when it happened, few people believed it actually did.

10.4.3 Types of Mental Processes

Three types of mental processing are considered in the HCR model [7, 3]. Reference [3] defines the three types below.

1. **Skill-based behavior:** This behavior is characterized by a very close coupling between sensory input and response action. Skill-based behavior does not depend directly on the complexity of the task, but rather on the level of training and the degree of practice in performing the task. A highly trained worker performs skill-based tasks swiftly or even mechanically with a minimum of errors.
2. **Rule-based behavior:** Actions are governed by a set of rules or associations that are known and followed. A major difference between rule-based and skill-based behaviors stems from the degree of practice. If the rules are not well practiced, the human being has to recall consciously or check each rule to be followed. Under these conditions the human response is less timely and more prone to errors because additional cognitive processes must be called upon. The potential for error results from problems with memory, the lack of willingness to check each step in a procedure, or failure to perform each and every step in the procedure in the proper sequence.
3. **Knowledge-based behavior:** Suppose that symptoms are ambiguous or complex, the plant state is complicated by multiple failures or unusual events, or instruments give only indirect readings of the plant state. Then the engineer has to rely on personal knowledge, and behavior is determined by more complex cognitive processes. Rasmussen calls this knowledge based behavior [16,17]. Human performance in this type of behavior depends on knowledge of the plant and ability to use that knowledge. This type of behavior is expected to be more prone to error and to require more time.

Figure 10.4 shows a logic tree to determine the expected mental processing type. It is assumed that, for the routine task, the operator clearly understands the corresponding plant states. For the routine task, we see

1. If the routine task is so simple that it does not require a procedure, then the behavior is skill-based (sequence 1).
2. Even if the operator requires a procedure for the routine task, the behavior is skill-based when the operator is practiced in the procedure (sequence 2).
3. If the operator is not well practiced in the routine task procedure, then behavior is rule-based (sequence 3).
4. If a routine task procedure is unavailable, then behavior is rule-based because built-in rules must be used (sequence 4).

Consider next the nonroutine task. If the operator does not have a clear understanding of the corresponding plant state, then behavior is knowledge-based (sequence 9) because the plant must first be diagnosed. The following sequences consider the case when there is an understanding of the plant state, equivalent to a successful plant diagnosis.

1. If no procedures are available, then the behavior is knowledge-based (sequence 8) because the procedure itself must be invented.
2. If the procedure is not understood, then the behavior is knowledge-based (sequence 7) because it must first be understood.
3. If the procedure is well understood, behavior is rule-based (sequence 6) when the operator is not well practiced in the procedure.
4. With understanding and practice, behavior becomes skill-based.

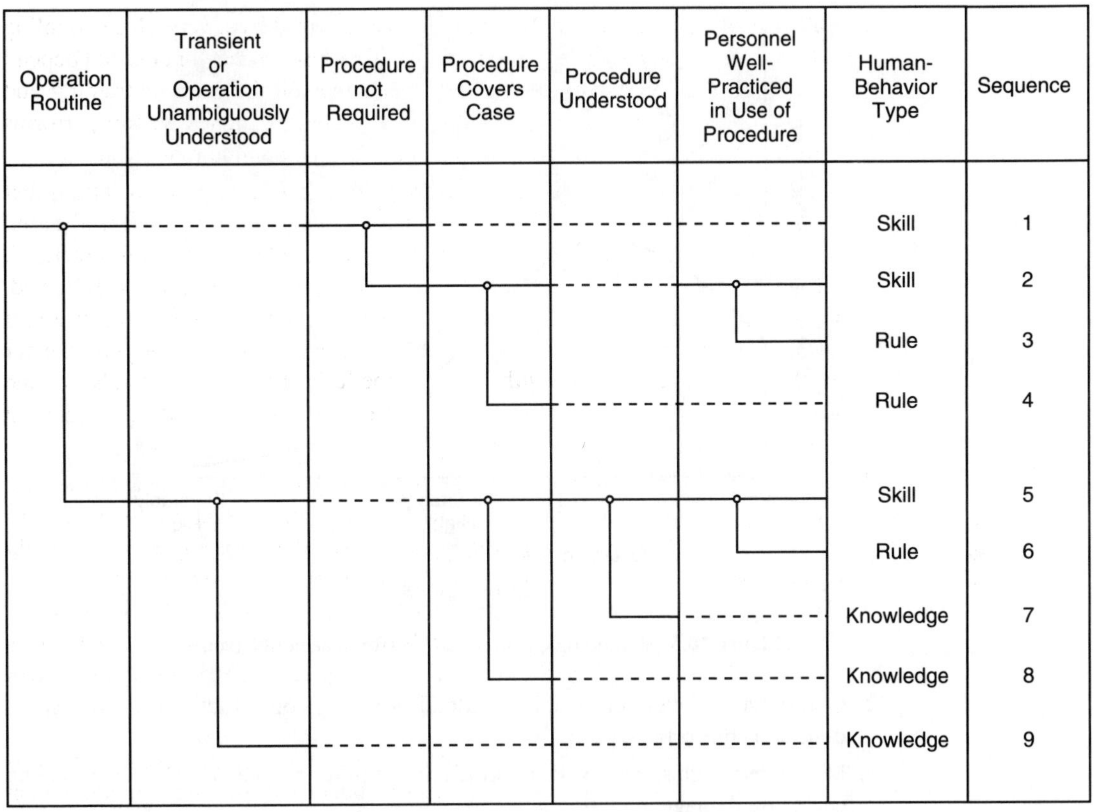

Figure 10.4. Logic tree to predict expected behavior.

10.5 HUMAN-PERFORMANCE QUANTIFICATION BY PSFS

10.5.1 Human-Error Rates and Stress Levels

A rote task is a sequence of unit activities such as selection, reading, interpretation, or manipulation. There are at least two types of human error: omission and commission. In a commission, a person performs an activity incorrectly. Omission of an activity, of course, is an omission error. An incorrectly timed sequence of activities is also a commission error.

Figure 10.5 shows a hypothetical relationship between psychological stresses and human performance [4]. The optimal stress level lies somewhere between low and moderately high levels of stress. Table 10.2 shows how human-error probabilities at the optimal stress level can be modified to reflect other non-optimal stresses. Uncertainty bounds are also adjusted. Notice that novices are more susceptible to stress than experienced personnel, except at extremely high stress levels. Discrete tasks are defined as tasks that only require essentially one well-defined action by the operator. Dynamic tasks are processes requiring a series of coordinated subtasks. The four levels of stress are characterized as follows [4]:

1. Very low stress level: lack of stimulus and low workload as exemplified by periodic scanning of indicators. No decisions are required.

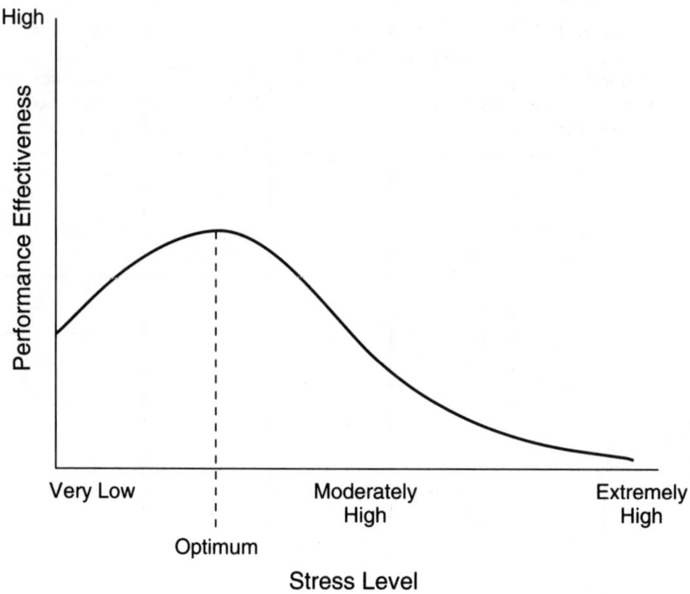

Figure 10.5. Psychological stress and performance effectiveness.

2. Optimal stress level: reasonable workload. Reading, control actions, and decisions done at a comfortable pace.
3. Moderately high stress level: workload that requires swift actions. Poor decisions can cause damage.
4. Extremely high stress level: imminent danger to life as posed by a fire or an airplane in uncontrolled descent.

Example 1—Wrong control selection. Consider an experienced worker whose task is to select a control from a group of identical controls identified only by labels. Assume that the selection-error probability (SEP) under the optimal stress level is 0.003 with a 90% confidence interval of (0.001 to 0.01). Calculate error probabilities for the other three levels of stress.

Solution: From Table 10.2 we have:

1. Extremely low stress level:

$$\begin{aligned} \text{SEP} &= 2 \times 0.003 = 0.006 \\ \text{Lower bound (LB)} &= 2 \times 0.001 = 0.002 \\ \text{Upper bound (UB)} &= 2 \times 0.01 = 0.02 \end{aligned}$$

2. Moderately high stress level: Use the formula for the step-by-step (discrete) tasks.

$$\begin{aligned} \text{SEP} &= 2 \times 0.003 = 0.006 \\ \text{LB} &= 2 \times 0.001 = 0.002 \\ \text{UB} &= 2 \times 0.01 = 0.02 \end{aligned}$$

3. Extremely high stress level:

$$\text{SEP} = 0.25, \qquad \text{LB} = 0.03, \qquad \text{UB} = 0.75 \tag{10.1}$$

■

TABLE 10.2. Probability of Error and Uncertainty Bounds for Stress Levels

Stress Level	HEP	Uncertainty Bounds
	Experienced Personnel	
Very low	2 × Table HEP	2 × Table Values
Optimum	Table HEP	Table Values
Moderately High		
Step-by-Step Tasks	2 × Table HEP	2 × Table Values
Dynamic Tasks	5 × Table HEP	5 × Table Values
Extremely High	0.25	0.03 to 0.75
	Novices	
Very low	2 × Table HEP	2 × Table Values
Optimum		
Step-by-Step Tasks	Table HEP	Table Values
Dynamic Tasks	2 × Table HEP	2 × Table Values
Moderately High		
Step-by-Step Tasks	4 × Table HEP	4 × Table Values
Dynamic Tasks	10 × Table HEP	10 × Table Values
Extremely High	0.25	0.03 to 0.75

More information about human error probability uncertainty bounds is given in Chapter 11.

10.5.2 Error Types, Screening Values

Assume that event and fault trees have been constructed by systems analysts. Human-reliability analysts then classify human errors into the types described in Section 10.2: type 1 (test and maintenance error), type 2 (initiating-event causation), type 3 (nonresponse), type 4 (wrong actions caused by misdiagnosis, slip, and lapse), and type 5 (recovery failure). The mental processes are then assessed for each error type. Thus there may be a large number of human errors in event and fault trees, and a screening process is required. In the SHARP procedure, the screening values listed in Tables 10.3 and 10.4 are used.

TABLE 10.3. Screening Values for Test and Maintenance Errors

Error	Remark	Skill	Rule	Knowledge
Test		0.0005–0.005	0.0005–0.05	0.005–0.5
Maintenance	Corrective	0.02	0.1	0.3
Maintenance	Preventive	0.003	0.03	0.1

Table 10.3 assumes the following.

1. No time pressure; multiply all values by two if less than 30 min are available
2. Nominal stress conditions
3. Average training

TABLE 10.4. Screening Values for Nonresponse and Wrong Actions

Error	Time	Skill	Rule	Knowledge
Nonresponse	Short	0.003	0.05	1.0
Nonresponse	Long	0.0005	0.005	0.1
Wrong action	15 min	0.001	0.03	0.3
Wrong action	5 min	0.1	1.0	1.0

4. If a systematic tagging/logging procedure is in place, reduce values by 10 to 30 (except for knowledge-based actions)

The following conditions are assumed for Table 10.4.

1. Human-error rates not in a database

2. Long time means longer than 1 hr

3. Short time means from 5 min to 1 hr

4. Screening values may be conservative by factors of 100 to 1000

For recovery errors, a screening-error probability of 1.0 is assumed; for initiating-event causation, values in abnormal event databases are assumed.

10.5.3 Response Time

A nominal median response time $\overline{T}_{1/2}$ is defined as the time corresponding to a probability of 0.5 that a required task has been successfully carried out under nominal conditions [3]. This time can be found from analyses of simulator data or from interviews with plant operating crews. In the HCR (human cognitive reliability) model [7,3], representative PSFs are defined as in Table 10.5 and their relations to the actual response time are formulated.

The actual median response time $T_{1/2}$ is calculated from the nominal median response time $\overline{T}_{1/2}$ by

$$T_{1/2} = (1 + K_1)(1 + K_2)(1 + K_3)\overline{T}_{1/2} \tag{10.2}$$

Example 2—Detection of automatic-shutdown failure. Consider the task of detecting that a failure of an automatic plant-shutdown system has occurred. The nominal median response time is $\overline{T}_{1/2} = 10$ s. Assume average operator ($K_1 = 0.00$) under potential emergency ($K_2 = 0.28$) with good operator/plant interface ($K_3 = 0.00$). The actual median response time $T_{1/2}$ is estimated to be

$$T_{1/2} = (1 + 0.00)(1 + 0.28)(1 + 0.00)(10) = 12.8 \text{ s} \tag{10.3}$$

Thus the potential emergency has lengthened the median response time by 2.8 s. Given the actual response time and a time limit, a nonresponse error probability can be estimated using a three-parameter Weibull reliability curve, as described in Section 10.9. ■

10.5.4 Integration of PSFs by Experts

The SLIM (success likelihood index methodology) [18] integrates various PSFs relevant to a task into a single number called a *success likelihood index* (SLI). The microcomputer implementation is called MAUD (multiattribute utility decomposition). For a given

TABLE 10.5. Definition of Typical PSFs

	PSFs	Coeff.	Criteria
	Operator Experience	K_1	
1	Expert	−0.22	Trained with more than five years experience
2	Average	0.00	Trained with more than six months experience
3	Novice	0.44	Trained with less than six months experience
	Stress Level	K_2	
1	Grave emergency	0.44	High stress situation, emergency with operator feeling threatened
2	High workload potential emergency	0.28	High stress situation, part-way through accident with high workload or equivalent
3	Optimal condition (normal)	0.00	Optimal situation, crew carrying out small load adjustments
4	Vigilance problem (low stress)	0.28	Problem with vigilance, unexpected transient with no precursors
	Operator/Plant Interface	K_3	
1	Excellent	−0.22	Advanced operator aids are available to help in accident situation
2	Good	0.00	Displays human-engineered with information integration
3	Fair	0.44	Displays human-engineered, but without information integration
4	Poor	0.78	Displays are available, but not human-engineered
5	Extremely poor	0.92	Displays are not directly visible to operator

SLI, the human-error probability (HEP) for a task is estimated by the formula

$$\log(\text{HEP}) = a \times \text{SLI} + b, \quad \text{or} \quad \text{HEP} = 10^{a\times\text{SLI}+b} \tag{10.4}$$

where a and b are constants determined from two or more tasks for which HEPs are known; if no data are available, they must be estimated by experts.

Consider, for instance, the PSFs: process diagnosis (0.25), stress level (0.16), time pressure (0.21), consequences (0.10), complexity (0.24), and teamwork (0.04) [19]. The number in the parentheses denotes the normalized importance (weight W_i) of a particular PSF for the task under consideration, as determined by experts.

The expert must select rating R_i from 0 to 1 for PSF i. Each PSF rating has an ideal value of 1 at which human performance is judged to be optimal. These ratings are based on diagnosis required, stress level, time pressure, consequences, complexity, and teamwork. The SLI is calculated by the following formula.

$$\text{SLI} = \sum_i W_i R_i \tag{10.5}$$

Example 3—SLIM quantification. Consider the weights and rating values in Table 10.6. The weights have already normalized, that is, $\sum W_i = 1$. The SLI is calculated as

TABLE 10.6. Normalized Weights and PSF Ratings for a Task

PSF	Normalized Weight	Rating
Process Diagnosis	0.25	0.40
Stress Level	0.16	0.43
Time Pressure	0.21	1.00
Consequences	0.10	0.33
Complexity	0.24	0.00
Teamwork	0.04	1.00

$$\mathrm{SLI} = (0.25)(0.40) + (0.16)(0.43) + (0.21)(1.00) + (0.10)(0.33) + (0.24)(0.00) + (0.04)(1.00) = 0.45 \qquad (10.6)$$

■

10.5.5 Recovery Actions

Some PSFs are important when quantifying recovery from failure. These include [8]:

1. Skill- or rule-based actions backed up by arrival of technical advisors
2. Knowledge-based actions backed up by arrival of offsite emergency response teams
3. New plant measurements or samples that prompt reassessments and diagnoses
4. Human/machine interface

10.6 EXAMPLES OF HUMAN ERROR

In this section we present typical documented examples of human errors [20–29].

10.6.1 Errors in Thought Processes

The accidents in this section are due to wrong solutions or faulty diagnoses, not lapse-/slip-type errors.

Example 4—Chemical reactor explosion. After lighting the pilot flame, the operator opened an air damper to permit 70% of maximum airflow to the burner. The air damper failed to open because it was locked, and the flame went out due to the shortage of air. The operator purged the air out of the reactor, and ignited the fuel again, and incomplete combustion with excess fuel in the reactor resulted. In the meantime, a coworker found that the air damper was locked, and released the lock. An explosive mixture of fuel and air formed and the reactor exploded.

The coworker's error was in thinking that unlatching the damper would resolve the system fault—a manifestation of frequency bias; removal of cause will frequently ensure a system's return to the normal state; an exceptional case is where the cause leaves irreversible effects on the system; in this example, excess fuel concentration in the reactor was an irreversible effect. The unlatching manipulation is an example of a wrong action due to a faulty solution. ■

Example 5—Electric shock. A worker used a defective voltage meter to verify that a 440-volt line was not carrying current prior to the start of his repair. The fact that the meter was defective was not discovered at the time, because he entered and repaired a switchboard box without receiving a shock—because of an electric power failure. Some time later he entered the box again.

He checked the voltage as before. By this time, however, the power failure had been repaired, and he was electrocuted.

The first successful entrance made him think that he had checked the voltage correctly. It was difficult for him to believe that the voltage measurement was incorrect and that an accidental power failure allowed him to enter the switchboard box without receiving a shock—a manifestation of frequency bias. ■

Example 6—Inadvertent switch closure. An electrical device needed repair, so the power supply was cut off. The repair took a long time and a shift change occurred. The foreman of the new shift ordered a worker to cut off the power supply to the device. However, the former shift had already opened the switch, so the worker actually closed it. He told the foreman that he had opened the switch, and the worker who started the repair was electrocuted.

It was quite natural for the worker to assume that the switch was closed because the foreman had ordered him to open it—frequency bias. Few people are skeptical enough to doubt a natural scenario—perseverance. This example also shows the importance of oral instructions, a performance-shaping factor in Table 10.1. ■

The following example shows human error caused by a predilection to take short-cuts.

Example 7—Warning buzzer. A buzzer that sounds whenever a red signal is encountered is located in the cab of a train. Traffic is heavy during commuter hours; the buzzer sounds almost continuously, so a motorman chose to run the train with the buzzer turned off because he was annoyed by the almost-continuous sound. One day he committed a rear-end collision. ■

Human errors caused by excessive dependence on other personnel or hardware devices are demonstrated by the following three examples.

Example 8—Excessive dependence on automatic devices. A veteran pilot aborted a landing because an indicator light showed that the front landing gear was stuck. He climbed to an altitude of 2000 ft, switched from manual navigation to autopilot, and inspected the indicator. The autopilot failed inadvertently and minutes later the airplane crashed. None of the crew had been monitoring the altimeter because they had confidence in the autopilot—this is a task-fixation error. ■

Example 9—Excessive dependence on protective devices. A veteran motorman in charge of yard operations for bullet trains failed to notice that the on-switches of the main and emergency brakes of a train were reversed on the train control panel. The yard operation was relatively easy-going and less stressful than driving a bullet train. The ex-motorman, in addition, had instinctive reliance on the "triplicate" braking system and neglected to follow basic procedural steps demanded of a professional. Neither the main nor the emergency brakes functioned, and the train ran away. This example also relates to performance-shaping factors such as "cautions and warnings" in Job and Task Instructions and "monotonous work" in Psychological Stresses in Table 10.1. ■

Example 10—Excessive dependence on supervisor. Figure 10.6 is a chemical plant that generates product by reaction of liquids X and Y. A runaway reaction occurs if feed rate Y becomes larger than X. In case of failure of the feed pump for liquid X, feed Y is automatically cut off, and a buffer tank supplies enough X to stabilize the reaction.

After a scheduled six-month maintenance, an operator inadvertently left valve 2 in the X-feed closed (commission error); this valve should have been open. Prior to start-up of the plant, operator B inspected the lines but failed to notice that valve 2 was closed (first omission error), and returned to the control room. Operator B and supervisor A started feeding X and Y. A deficiency of X developed because bypass valve 4 was also closed. The buffer tank, however, functioned properly and started to supply liquid X to the reactor. The operator stopped the start-up because a liquid-level indicator showed a decrease in the buffer tank level.

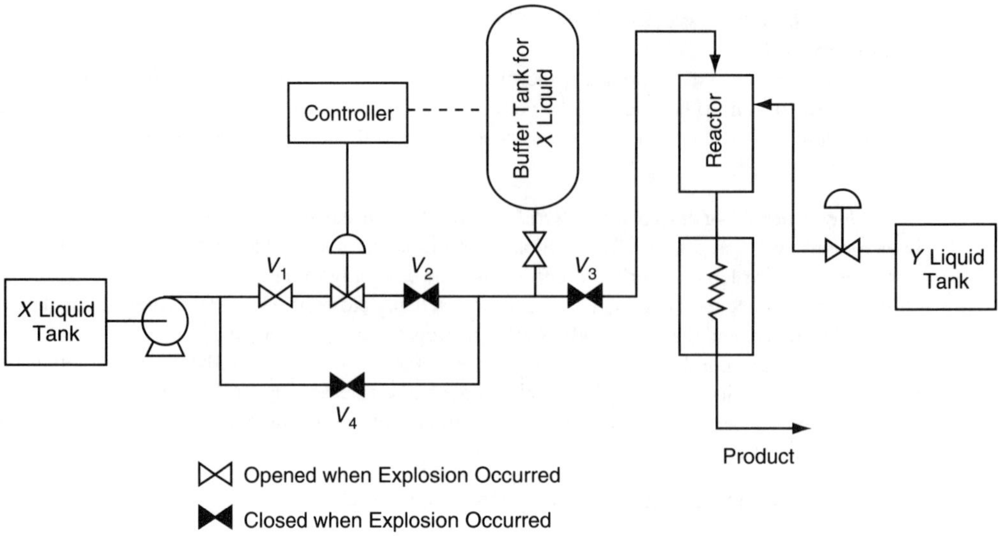

Figure 10.6. Diagram of a chemical plant.

Operator B went out to inspect the line again. He again failed to notice that valve 2 was closed (second omission error), and returned to the control room to resume the start-up. The level of the buffer tank began to decrease as before. The two operators stopped the operation and supervisor A went to check the line.

The supervisor also failed to notice that valve 2 was closed (third omission error) but saw that the level of the buffer tank would reach its normal level when he opened bypass valve 4 and that the level would decrease when he closed the bypass valve. He then closed valve 4 and then valve 3, and started a thorough inspection of the feed system.

At that time subordinate operator B in the control room was monitoring the buffer tank level. He noticed the normal level (because the supervisor had opened bypass valve 4). The subordinate had great faith in the supervisor and concluded that the supervisor had fixed everything—an error caused by excessive reliance on the supervisor. Because start-up operation was behind schedule (time pressure), he resumed the start-up. Unfortunately, by this time the supervisor had closed bypass valve 4 (valve 3 was still open). The level of the buffer tank began to decrease sharply and a low-level alarm went off. The subordinate initiated an emergency trip procedure but, unfortunately, valve 3 was being closed by the supervisor at that time. Lack of feed X caused a runaway reaction and an explosion occurred.

This example also shows the importance of performance-shaping factors such as "actions by supervisors and coworkers," "oral communications," "team structure," "status indication and labeling of valve," and "duration of stress," as well as "bad communication." ■

The next example illustrates sudden onset.

Example 11—Sudden onset. A line-of-sight landing of a commercial airplane was impossible because of rain and fog. The captain decided to go on autopilot until the airplane descended to an altitude where there was good visibility. He turned the autopilot on and then turned it off at 200 ft, where he started the visual landing. To this point the autopilot had been guiding the airplane along a normal trajectory with an angle of descent of 2.8 degrees. Figure 10.7 shows the distribution of wind speeds along a direction parallel to the flight path. The tailwind changed suddenly due to a headwind at 200 ft, which is where the captain switched from autopilot to manual landing. This type of wind distribution, which is known as *wind shear*, will make the airplane descend rapidly unless the pilot pulls the airplane up sharply and increases the thrust to prevent premature stall. He failed to do this and crashed. The captain failed to respond to the sudden onset of an unexpected event—a nonresponse failure occurred due to extreme time pressure. ■

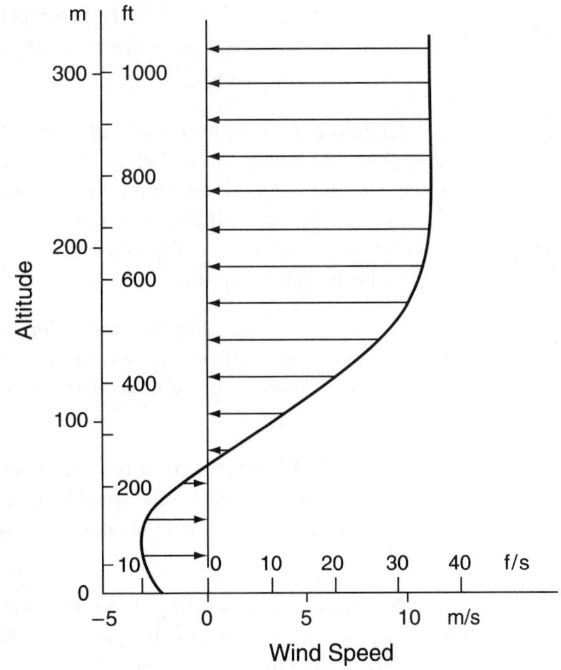

Figure 10.7. Distribution of wind parallel to runway.

The final example shows a decision-making error.

Example 12—Underestimated risk. A commercial airliner was landing in a storm, which the pilot underestimated. The airplane overran the runway and collided with a bank because of hydroplaning on the wet runway. ■

10.6.2 Lapse/Slip Errors

A simple slip-type selection error is illustrated by the following example, where the human–machine interface is a major performance factor.

Example 13—Human error at a hospital. A patient was to be put under anesthesia. A nurse connected the oxygen hose to the anesthesia supply and the anesthesia hose to the oxygen tank. The patient died. ■

Federal legislation enacted in the United States in 1976 has reduced the probability of this type of accident to zero. Human errors are often caused by reflex actions, as shown by the following example.

Example 14—Reflex response. In a machine that mixes and kneads polyester, a small lump of hard polymer jammed the rotating gears. Without thinking, a worker reached down to remove the polymer without first turning off the machine, thus injuring his hand. This is a slip error due to reflex response. ■

The next example is of a slip-type of omission error caused by the 24-hour body rhythm.

Example 15—Driving asleep. A motorman driving a train fell asleep very late at night, failed to notice a red signal, and the train crashed. ■

Human beings are especially error-prone when a normal sequence of activities is interrupted or disturbed. There are a variety of ways of interrupting a normal sequence, as shown by Examples 16 to 20.

Example 16—Interrupted activity. A temporary ladder was attached to a tank by two hooks. When the ladder was no longer needed, the supervisor ordered a worker to cut off the hooks and remove the ladder. The supervisor left the site, which is an interruption. The workman cut off the hooks and left for lunch, but did not remove the ladder, which still leaned against the tank wall. The supervisor returned to the site, climbed up the ladder, and fell. A lapse-type of commission error occurred due to an interruption. ■

Example 17—Leaving the scene for another task. A worker started filling a tank with LNG. He left the site to inspect some other devices and forgot about the liquified natural gas (LNG) tank. The tank was about to overflow when another worker shut off the feed. A lapse-type omission error occurred. ■

Example 18—A distraction. An operator was asked to open circuit breaker A. As he approached the switch box, he happened to notice that breaker B, which was adjacent to A, was dirty. He cleaned breaker B and then opened it in place of breaker A; a slip-type commission error occurred. ■

Example 19—Counting extra breakers. A device in circuit 2 of a four-circuit system failed, and a worker was ordered to open circuit breaker 2. He went to a switch box, where breakers 1, 2, 3, and 4 were located in a row. The breakers were numbered right to left, but he ignored the numbers and counted left to right. He opened breaker 3 instead of breaker 2 and damaged the system. A slip was induced by the unnecessary task of counting the breakers. ■

Example 20—A telephone call. An airport controller received a telephone call while controlling a complicated traffic pattern. He asked another controller to take over. A near miss occurred because the substitute operator was inexperienced. ■

10.7 SHARP: GENERAL FRAMEWORK

Human errors are diverse and no single model can deal with every possible aspect of human behaviors. SHARP provides a framework common to all human-reliability analysis models and suggests which model is best suited for a particular type of human error (for example, see Table 10.7); it also clarifies cooperative roles of systems and human-reliability analysts in performing a PRA.

SHARP consists of seven steps [3].

1. **Definition:** To ensure that all human errors are adequately considered and included in event and fault trees.
2. **Screening:** To identify the significant human interactions. Screening values in Section 10.5.2 are chosen; consequences of human errors are considered.
3. **Breakdown:** To clarify various attributes of human errors. These attributes include mental processes, available time, response time, stress level, and other PSFs.
4. **Representation:** To select and apply techniques for modeling human errors. These models include THERP, HCR, SLIM-MAUD, and confusion matrix.

TABLE 10.7. Error Types and Quantification Methods

Error Type	Quantification Method
Before Initiating Event	
Test and maintenance error	THERP
For Initiating Event	
Initiating-event causation	Experience Expert judgment, FT
During Accident	
Nonresponse Wrong actions Slip and lapse Recovery failure	HCR Confusion matrix THERP, SLIM-MAUD THERP, SLIM-MAUD, HCR

5. **Impact Assessment:** To explore the consequences of human errors in event and fault trees.
6. **Quantification:** To quantify human-error probabilities, to determine sensitivities, and to establish uncertainty ranges.
7. **Documentation:** To include all necessary information for the assessment to be traceable, understandable, and reproducible.

In the following sections, we describe the THERP model for routine and rule-based tasks typified by testing and maintenance before an accident, the HCR model for dealing with nonresponse errors under time stress, and the confusion matrix model [8] for wrong actions during an accident.

10.8 THERP: ROUTINE AND PROCEDURE-FOLLOWING ERRORS

10.8.1 Introduction

In this section we describe THERP. This technique, which was first developed and publicized by Swain, Rook, and coworkers at the Sandia Laboratory in 1962 for weapons-assembly tasks, was later used in the WASH-1400 study, and since then it has been improved to the point where it is regarded as the most powerful and systematic methodology for the quantification of human reliability for routine and procedure-following test and maintenance activities. THERP is relatively weak in analyzing time-stressed thought processes such as diagnosis during an accident, because a step-by-step analysis is frequently infeasible. This section is based primarily on papers by Swain, Guttmann, and Bell and the *PRA Procedures Guide* [4–6].

Human errors, defined as deviations from assigned tasks, often appear as basic events in fault trees. A THERP analysis begins by decomposing human tasks into a sequence of unit activities. Possible deviations are postulated for each unit activity. An event tree, called an HRA (human-reliability analysis) event tree to distinguish it from ordinary event trees, is then used to visualize the sequence of unit activities.

The HRA event tree is a collection of chronological scenarios associated with human tasks. Each limb of the event tree represents either a normal execution of a unit activity or an omission or commission error related to the activity. An intermediate hardware-failure status caused by a human error can be represented as a limb of an HRA tree. The human error appearing as a basic event in a fault tree or an ordinary event tree is defined by a subset of terminal nodes of the HRA event tree. The occurrence probability of the basic event is calculated after probabilities are assigned to the event tree limbs. Limb-probability estimates must reflect performance-shaping factors specific to the plant, personnel, and boundary conditions. Events described by limbs can be statistically dependent.

Before presenting a more detailed description of THERP, we first construct an illustrative event tree.

Example 21—HRA event tree for a calibration task. Assume that a technician is assigned the task of calibrating setpoints of three comparators that use OR logic to detect abnormal pressure [4]. The basic event in the fault tree is that OR detection logic fails due to a calibration error. The failed-dangerous (FD) failure occurs when all three comparators are miscalibrated.

The worker must first assemble the test equipment. If he sets up the equipment incorrectly, the three comparators are likely to be miscalibrated. The calibration task consists of four unit activities:

1. Set up test equipment
2. Calibrate comparator 1
3. Calibrate comparator 2
4. Calibrate comparator 3

Figure 10.8 shows the HRA event tree. We observe the following conventions.

1. A capital letter represents unit-activity failure or its probability. The corresponding lower-case letter represents unit-activity success or probability.
2. The same convention applies to Greek letters, which represent nonhuman events such as hardware-failure states caused by preceding human errors. In Figure 10.8 the hardware states are small test-equipment-setup error and large setup error.
3. The letters S and F are exceptions to the above rule in that they represent, respectively, human-task success and failure. Success in this example is that at least one comparator is calibrated correctly; failure is the simultaneous miscalibration of three comparators.
4. The two-limb branch represents unit-activity success and failure; each left limb expresses success and each right limb, failure. For hardware states, limbs are arranged from left to right in ascending order of severity of failure.
5. Limbs with zero or negligibly small probability of occurrence are removed from the event tree. The event tree can thus be truncated and simplified.

As shown in Figure 10.8, the technician fails to correctly set up the test equipment with probability 0.01. If she succeeds in the setup, she will correctly calibrate at least one comparator. Assume that miscalibration of each of the three comparators occurs independently with probability 0.01; then simultaneous miscalibration occurs with probability $(0.01)^3 = 10^{-6}$, which is negligibly small. The success limb $a = 0.99$ can therefore be truncated by success node S_1, which implies that one or more comparators are calibrated correctly.

Setup error A results in a small or a large test-equipment error with equal probability, 0.5 for each. We assume that the technician sets up comparator 1 without noticing a small setup error. This is shown by the unit-failure probability $B = 1.0$. While calibrating the second comparator, however, she would probably notice the small setup error because it would seem strange that the two comparators happen to require identical adjustment simultaneously. Probability $c = 0.9$ is assigned to the successful discovery of a small setup error. Success node S_2 implies the same event as S_1. If the technician neglects the small setup error during the first two calibrations, a third calibration error

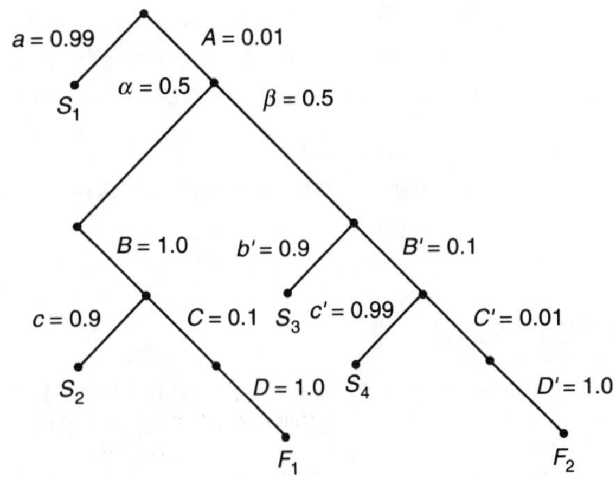

A = failure to set up equipment

α = small test-equipment-setup error
B = small setup error/failure to detect first calibration error
C = small setup error/failure to detect second calibration error
D = small setup error/failure to detect third calibration error

β = large test-equipment-setup error
B' = large setup error/failure to detect first calibration error
C' = large setup error/failure to detect second calibration error
D' = large setup error/failure to detect third calibration error

Figure 10.8. Probability tree diagram for hypothetical calibration.

is almost certain. This is shown by unit probability $D = 1.0$. Failure node F_1 implies sequential miscalibration of three comparators.

A large test-equipment-setup error would probably be noticed during the first calibration because it would seem strange that the first comparator required such a large adjustment. This is indicated by success probability $b' = 0.9$ of finding the setup error. Success node S_3 results because the technician would almost surely correct the setup error and calibrate at least one comparator correctly. Even if the large setup error at the first calibration is neglected, it would almost surely be noticed during the second calibration, thus yielding success node S_4 with probability $c' = 0.99$. The technician would assuredly fail to find the setup error at the third calibration if the error was neglected during the first and second calibrations. This is evidenced by unit-failure probability $D' = 1.0$. Failure node F_2 also implies sequential miscalibration (simultaneous failure) of the three comparators.

The probability of a success or failure node can be calculated by multiplying the appropriate probabilities along the path to the node.*

$$\begin{aligned}
\Pr\{S_1\} &= 0.99 \\
\Pr\{S_2\} &= (0.01)(0.5)(1.0)(0.9) = 0.0045 \\
\Pr\{S_3\} &= (0.01)(0.5)(0.9) = 0.0045 \\
\Pr\{S_4\} &= (0.01)(0.5)(0.1)(0.99) = 0.000495 \\
\Pr\{F_1\} &= (0.01)(0.5)(1.0)(0.1)(1.0) = 0.0005 \\
\Pr\{F_2\} &= (0.01)(0.5)(0.1)(0.01)(1.0) = 0.000005
\end{aligned}$$

Because the basic event in question is simultaneous miscalibration of three comparators, probability $\Pr\{F\}$ of occurrence of the basic event is the sum of failure-node probabilities:

---

*Nonsignificant numbers are carried simply for identification purposes.

$$\Pr\{F\} = \Pr\{F_1\} + \Pr\{F_2\}$$
$$= 0.0005 + 0.000005 = 0.000505$$

Probability $\Pr\{S\}$ of non-occurrence of the basic event is simply the complement of $\Pr\{F\}$:

$$\Pr\{S\} = \Pr\{S_1\} + \Pr\{S_2\} + \Pr\{S_3\} + \Pr\{S_4\}$$
$$= 0.99 + 0.0045 + 0.0045 + 0.0000495$$
$$= 0.999495 = 1 - \Pr\{F\}$$

■

10.8.2 General THERP Procedure

Steps in a human reliability analysis are depicted in Figure 10.9.

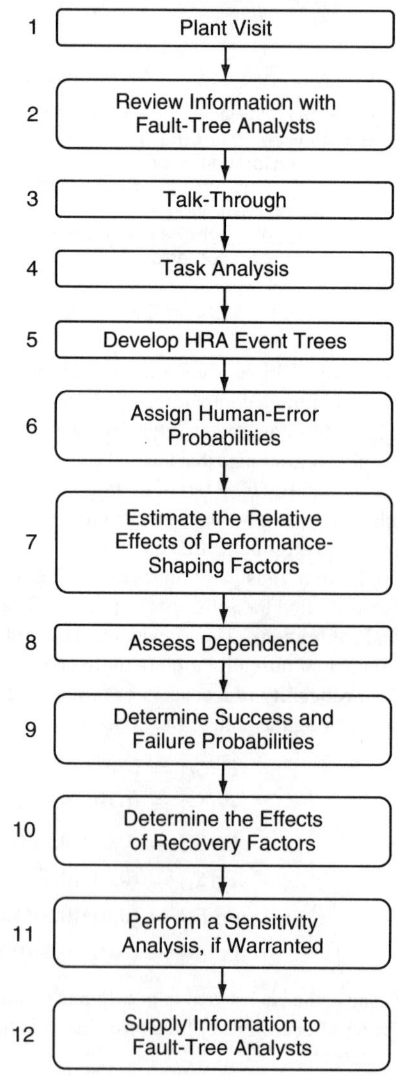

Figure 10.9. Overview of a human-reliability analysis.

Steps 1 to 3: Plant visit to talk-through. The first three procedural steps should extract the following intelligence.

1. Human-error-related events in the fault or event trees
2. Human tasks related to the event
3. Boundary conditions under which the tasks are performed. These include control room aspects, general plant layout, administrative system, time requirements, personnel assignments, skill requirements, alerting cues, and recovery factors from an error after it occurs.

Step 4: Task analysis. The fourth step, task analysis, clarifies each human task and decomposes it into a sequence of unit activities. For each unit activity, the following aspects must be clarified.

1. The piece of equipment in question
2. Human action required
3. Potential human errors
4. Location of controls, displays, and so on.

If different tasks or activities are performed by different personnel, staffing parameters must be identified during the task analysis.

Step 5: Developing HRA event trees. The fifth step, HRA-event-tree development, is essentially a dichotomous classification. The size of the event tree is large if many unit activities are involved; however, its size can be reduced if the event tree is truncated, using the following simplifications.

1. **Combining dependent events:** The occurrence of an event sometimes specifies a sequence of events. For instance, omission failure to close the first valve usually leads to omission failures for the remaining valves if the valves are perceived as a group.
2. **Neglecting small probabilities:** If the occurrence probability in a limb of the event tree is negligibly small, that limb and all successors can be removed from the tree.
3. **Failure or success node:** If a path in an event tree is identified as a success or a failure node of the task being analyzed, further development of the event tree from that node is not required.
4. **Neglecting recovery factors:** If one notices an error (commission or omission) after performing a unit activity and resumes the process, such a resumption conceptually constitutes a loop in the event tree and increases its size and complexity. Recovery factors such as cues given by annunciator displays facilitate resumption of normalcy. It is often better, however, to postpone consideration of recovery factors until after total system success and failure probabilities have been determined [6]. Estimated failure probabilities for a given sequence in an HRA event tree may be so low, without considering the effects of recovery factors, that the sequence will not be a dominant failure mode. In this case recovery can be dropped from further consideration. As a matter of fact, "neglecting recovery factors" is analogous to "neglecting small probabilities": a rule that helps guide human-reliability analyses toward dominant failure modes.

Step 6: Assigning human-error probabilities. The sixth step in Figure 10.9 is the assignment of estimated *Handbook* [4] or database probabilities to event-tree failure limbs. The data estimates are usually based on the following limiting assumptions [6].

1. The plant is operating under normal conditions. There is no emergency or other state that produces abnormal operator stress.
2. The operator need not wear protective clothing. If protective clothing is necessary, we must assume that the operator will attempt to complete the task quickly because of the poor working environment. This increases human-error probability.
3. A level of administrative control roughly equal to industry-wide averages.
4. The tasks are performed by licensed, qualified plant personnel.
5. The working environment is adequate to optimal.

A reliability analyst should be familiar with the organization of the HEPs (human-error probabilities) in Chapter 20 of Swain and Guttmann's *Handbook of Human Reliability Analysis* [4]. The description that most closely approximates the situation under consideration should be identified, and if there are discrepancies between the scenario in the *Handbook* and the one under consideration, the HEP should be modified to reflect actual performance conditions. Usually, this is done during assessment of the performance-shaping factors (i.e., Step 7 in Figure 10.9). Tables A10.6 to A10.13 in the Appendix list some of the HEPs in the *Handbook*. These are the BHEPs (basic human-error probabilities) used in the next step.

Step 7: Evaluating PSFs. Some of the PSFs affect the whole task, whereas others affect only certain types of errors. Table 10.2 indicates how BHEPs are modified by the stress level, a typical PSF.

Step 8: Assessing dependence. THERP considers five types of dependence: complete dependence (CD), high-level dependence (HD), moderate-level dependence (MD), low-level dependence (LD), and zero dependence (ZD), that is, independence.

Consider the labeled part of the event tree in Figure 10.10; unit activity B follows activity A. Assume that preceding activity A fails, and let BHEP denote unconditional failure probability of activity B (i.e., failure probability when activity B occurs alone). The conditional failure probability given failure of A is obtained by the following equations, which reflect five levels of dependence.

1. CD:

$$B = 1.0 \tag{10.7}$$

Unit activity B always fails upon failure of activity A.

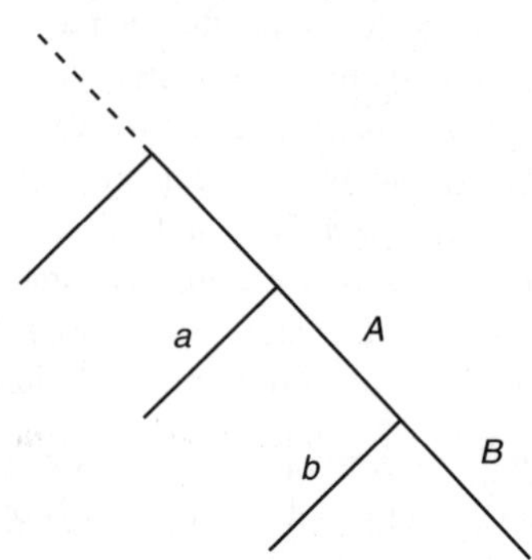

Figure 10.10. Event tree to illustrate dependency.

2. HD:

$$B = \frac{1 + \text{BHEP}}{2} \tag{10.8}$$

3. MD:

$$B = \frac{[1 + 6(\text{BHEP})]}{7} \tag{10.9}$$

4. LD:

$$B = \frac{[1 + 19(\text{BHEP})]}{20} \tag{10.10}$$

5. ZD:

$$B = \text{BHEP} \tag{10.11}$$

Equations (10.8) to (10.11) are depicted in Figure 10.11. For small values of BHEP, the conditional failure probability converges to 0.5, 0.15, and 0.05 for HD, MD, and LD, respectively.

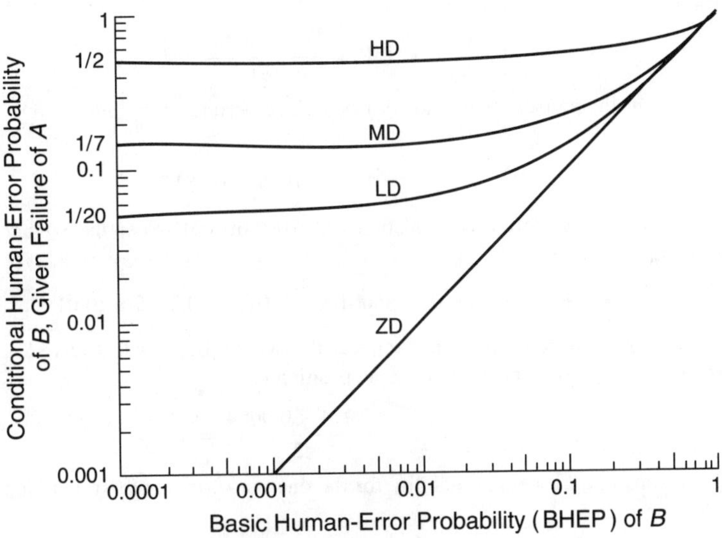

Figure 10.11. Modification of BHEP by HD, MD, and LD.

Step 9: Success and failure probabilities. The ninth step is to calculate basic-event success and failure probabilities.

Recovery factors are considered at the tenth step for failure limbs that have relatively large probabilities and contribute to the occurrence of basic events. A sensitivity analysis is carried out if necessary, and results of the human-reliability analysis are then transmitted to fault-tree analysts.

A detailed THERP example for errors during a plant upset is given in Appendix A.1. The following example shows a THERP application to test and maintenance.

Example 22—Scheduled test and unscheduled maintenance. Consider a parallel system of two trains consisting of valves $V1$ and $V2$ and pumps $P1$ and $P2$ (Figure 10.12). These two valves could be unintentionally closed after monthly pump maintenance or unscheduled maintenance to repair pump failures; assume that both trains are subject to unscheduled maintenance when a pump fails. Pump failure occurs with a monthly probability 0.09. Thus maintenance (scheduled or unscheduled) is performed 1.09 times per month, or once every four weeks. Evaluate the HEP that the one-out-of-two system fails by the human error of leaving the valves closed [3].

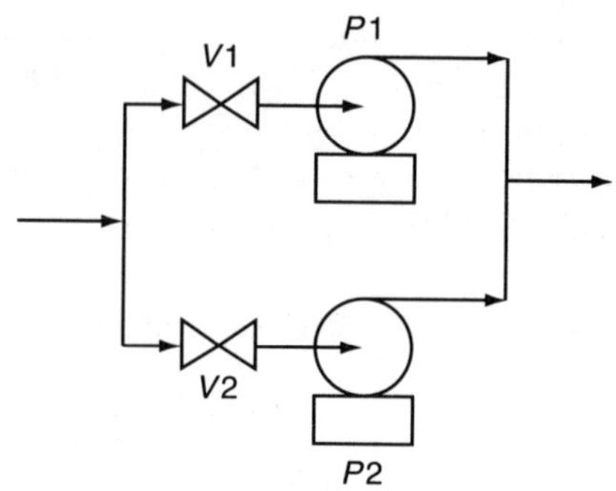

Figure 10.12. Parallel train-cooling system with valves and pumps.

Assume that the HEP for leaving the valve closed is 0.01; a control-room-failure probability to detect the failure is 0.1. A low dependency between these failure probabilities results in a conditional HEP of:

$$\text{HEP} = \frac{1 + 19 \times 0.1}{20} = 0.15 \tag{10.12}$$

Thus the probability of valve $V1$ being in closed position immediately after test/maintenance is

$$0.01 \times 0.15 = 0.0015 \tag{10.13}$$

Assume a weekly flow validation with HEP of 0.01. Then the average HEP during the four weeks is

$$(0.0015 \times 1 + 0.0015 \times 0.01 + 0.0015 \times (0.01)^2 + 0.0015 \times (0.01)^3)/4 \simeq 0.0004 \tag{10.14}$$

If there is a high dependence between the two trains, given that valve 1 is closed, the dependent probability for valve 2 being in the same position is

$$\frac{1 + 4 \times 0.0004}{2} = 0.5 \tag{10.15}$$

This results in a mean unavailability for the one-out-of-two train system due to both valves in the closed position of:

$$0.0004 \times 0.5 = 0.0002 \tag{10.16}$$

■

10.9 HCR: NONRESPONSE PROBABILITY

Denote by $\Pr\{t\}$ the nonresponse probability within a given time window t. The HCR model states that this probability follows a three-parameter Weibull reliability.

$$\Pr\{t\} = \exp\left[-\left\{\frac{(t/T_{1/2}) - B}{A}\right\}^C\right] \tag{10.17}$$

where t is the time available to complete a given action or a set of actions following a stimulus;
$T_{1/2}$ is the estimated median time to complete the action(s);
A, B, C are correlation coefficients associated with the type of mental processing, i.e., skill, rule or knowledge;

The time window t is estimated from analysis of the event sequence following the stimulus. Given the PSFs in Section 10.5.3, the median time $T_{1/2}$ is estimated from the nominal median time by (10.2). Values in Table 10.8 are recommended for the parameters A, B, and C. Three mental-processing types are shown in Figure 10.4, and curves of the Weibull reliability for the three types are given in Figure 10.13.

TABLE 10.8. HCR Correlation Parameters

Mental Processing	A	B	C
Skill	0.407	0.7	1.2
Rule	0.601	0.6	0.9
Knowledge	0.791	0.5	0.8

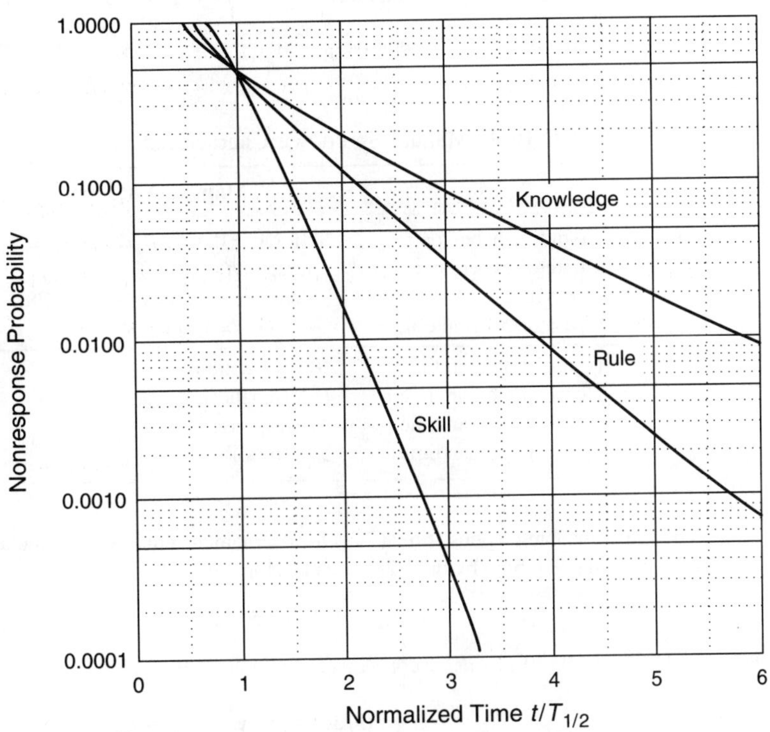

Figure 10.13. HCR model curves.

The normalized time ($t/T_{1/2}$) in (10.17) is the available time divided by the median time. The HCR model assumes the median time is affected by the PSFs in Section 10.5.3, the HCR model curves' shapes vary according to the mental-processing type, and the nonresponse probability decreases in proportion to the normalized time $(t/T_{1/2})$.

The following example describes an HCR application involving a single operator response, that is, manual shutdown. Appendix A.2 presents a case with two responses in series.

Example 23—Manual plant shutdown. A reactor is cooled by a heat exchanger. Consider as an initiating event loss of feedwater to the heat exchanger. This calls for a manual plant shutdown by the control room crew if the automatic-shutdown system fails. Suppose that the crew must complete the plant shutdown within 79 s from the start of the initiating event. We have the following information about the detection, diagnosis, and action phases.

1. Detection: The control panel information interface is good. The crew can easily see or hear the feedwater-pump trip indicator, plant shutdown alarm, and automatic-shutdown failure annunciator. The nominal median time for detection is 10 s.
2. Diagnosis: The instrumentation is such that the control room personnel can easily diagnose the loss-of-feedwater accident and the automatic-shutdown failure, so a misdiagnosis is not a contributing statistical likelihood. The nominal median diagnosis time is 15 s.
3. Response: The control panel interface is good, so slip errors for the manual shutdown are judged negligible. The nominal median response time is also negligible.

Table 10.9 summarizes the cognitive-processing type, PSFs, and nominal median time for manual shutdown.

TABLE 10.9. Manual Shutdown Characteristics

Task	**Manual shutdown**
Cognitive behavior	Skill ($A = 0.407$, $B = 0.7$, $C = 1.2$)
Operator experience	Average ($K_1 = 0.00$)
Stress level	Potential emergency ($K_2 = 0.28$)
Operator/plant interface	Good ($K_3 = 0.00$)
Nominal median time	10 s (detection)
Nominal median time	15 s (diagnosis)
Nominal median time	0 s (response)
Nominal median time	25 s (total)

The actual median response time ($T_{1/2}$) for the manual shutdown is calculated by multiplying the 25-s nominal median time by the 1.28 stress level in Table 10.9:

$$T_{1/2} = 1.28 \times 25 = 32 \text{ s} \tag{10.18}$$

From the HCR model (10.17), using constants from Table 10.9:

$$\Pr\{79\} = \exp\left[-\left\{\frac{(79/32) - 0.7}{0.407}\right\}^{1.2}\right] = 0.0029/\text{demand} \tag{10.19}$$

If the stress is changed to its optimal level (e.g., $K_2 = 0$), the nonresponse probability becomes 0.00017/demand; if knowledge-based mental processing is required and the corresponding constants are taken from Table 10.9, the HCR model yields 0.028/demand. In this example, only nonresponse probability is considered. If lapse/slip errors during the response phase cannot be neglected, these should also be quantified by an appropriate method such as THERP. ■

10.10 WRONG ACTIONS DUE TO MISDIAGNOSIS

If a doctor does not prescribe an appropriate drug for a seriously hypertensive patient, he makes a nonresponse failure; if the doctor prescribes a hypotensive drug for the wrong patient, he commits an incorrect action. When unsuitable plans are formed during the diagnosis phase, the resultant actions are inevitably wrong. For a chess master, an incorrect plan results in a wrong move. The typical cause of a wrong action is misdiagnosis.

Because event trees are based on a binary logic, the failure branch frequently implies a nonresponse. Because human behavior is unpredictable, there are an almost countless number of wrong actions. Their inclusion makes the event-tree analysis far more complex because tree branches increase significantly. However, if we can identify typical wrong actions caused by initiating-event or procedure confusions, then event-tree analysis is simplified. In this section, the Wakefield [8] approach to misdiagnosis is described.

10.10.1 Initiating-Event Confusion

An approach to misdiagnosis based on confusion matrices is shown in Table 10.10. Each row or column represents an initiating event; a total of five initiating events are considered. Symbol L in row i and column j represents a likelihood that the row i initiating event is misdiagnosed as the column j initiating event; symbol C denotes the severity or impact of this misdiagnosis. The likelihood and severity are usually expressed qualitatively as high, medium, low, negligible, and so forth.

TABLE 10.10. Confusion Matrix

	I1	I2	I3	I4	I5
I1		L12,C12	L13,C13	L14,C14	L15,C15
I2	L21,C21		L23,C23	L24,C24	L25,C25
I3	L31,C31	L32,C32		L34,C34	L35,C35
I4	L41,C41	L42,C42	L43,C43		L45,C45
I5	L51,C51	L52,C52	L53,C53	L54,C54	

Plant-response matrix. Information required for constructing the confusion matrix is the plant-response matrix shown in Table 10.11. Each row denotes an initiating event; each column represents a plant indicator such as a shutdown alarm. The symbols used are ON: initiation of alarm; OFF: termination of signal; U: increase; D: decrease; X: increase or decrease; 0: zero level. From this matrix, we can evaluate the likelihood of misdiagnosing initiating events.

TABLE 10.11. Plant Response Matrix

	R1	R2	R3	R4	R5	R6
I1	ON	OFF	U	D	X	0
I2	ON	ON	X	U	D	D
I3	ON	OFF	D	D	0	U
I4	OFF	ON	0	X	0	0
I5	OFF	OFF	D	X	U	D

Initiating-event procedure matrix. This matrix shows, for each initiating event, procedures to be followed, and in what order. In Table 10.12 each row represents an initiating event and each column a procedure. The entry number denotes a procedure execution order. This matrix clarifies which procedure could be mistakenly followed when initiating events are misdiagnosed.

TABLE 10.12. Initiating-Event Procedure Matrix

	P1	P2	P3	P4	P5	P6	P7
I1	1	2	3				
I2	1						
I3	1			2	3		5
I4	1		2		3	4	
I5	1	2		3			

10.10.2 Procedure Confusion

Plant response, along with the initiating event, plays a key role in procedure selection in the event of a plant upset.

Procedure-entry matrix. The matrix of Table 10.13 shows, in terms of plant response, when a particular procedure must be initiated. Each row denotes a procedure and each column a plant indicator. The entry symbols enclosed in parentheses denote that no other symptom is needed for the operator to initiate the procedure. This matrix is useful for identifying the likelihood of using incorrect procedures, especially when procedures are selected by symptoms. From the plant-response and procedure-entry matrices, we can evaluate procedures that may be confused.

TABLE 10.13. Procedure Entry Matrix

	R1	R2	R3	R4	R5	R6
P1	ON	OFF				
P2	ON		U			
P3	ON	(OFF)		(D)	0	
P4	ON	ON				
P5		OFF	D		0	
P6	OFF	ON				0
P7	OFF	OFF		X		D

10.10.3 Wrong Actions Due to Confusion

Initiating-event confusion or procedure confusion eventually leads to wrong actions. Some actions are related to event-tree headings. If a procedure calls for turning off a coolant pump, this action negates an event-tree heading calling for coolant pump operation.

Procedure-action matrix. The procedure-action matrix of Table 10.14 shows, for each procedure, actions related to the event-tree headings. Each row and column represents a procedure and an action, respectively. The E entry denotes a safety-function execution or verification at the event-tree heading. The O entry is a nullification of the heading function. When an initiating-event confusion is identified, the actions in the correct procedure in Table 10.12 are compared with those in the incorrectly selected procedure to assess the impact of misdiagnosis; similar assessment is performed for the procedure confusion depicted in Table 10.13. If the incorrect procedure affects only one event-tree heading, the frequency of the corresponding action is added to the existing failure modes for the heading. If multiple headings are affected, a new heading is introduced to represent this dependency.

TABLE 10.14. Procedure Action Matrix

	A1	A2	A3	A4	A5	A6
P1	E			O	E	O
P2	E	O			O	E
P3	O	E	E	E		E
P4		O	E			
P5		E	O	E	E	
P6	E				E	E
P7	O			E	E	E

REFERENCES

[1] Price, H. E., R. E. Maisano, and H. P. Van Cott. "The allocation of functions in man-machine systems: A perspective and literature review." USNRC, NUREG/CR-2623, 1982.

[2] Hannaman, G. W., and A. J. Spurgin. "Systematic human action reliability procedure." Electric Power Research Institute, EPRI NP-3583, 1984.

[3] IAEA. "Case study on the use of PSA methods: Human reliability analysis." IAEA, IAEA-TECDOC-592, 1991.

[4] Swain A. D., and H. E. Guttmann. "Handbook of human reliability analysis with emphasis on nuclear power plant applications." USNRC, NUREG/CR-1278, 1980.

[5] Bell B. J., and A. D. Swain. "A procedure for conducting a human reliability analysis for nuclear power plants." USNRC, NUREG/CR-2254, 1981.

[6] USNRC. "PRA procedures guide: A guide to the performance of probabilistic risk assessments for nuclear power plants." USNRC, NUREG/CR-2300, 1983.

[7] Hannaman, G. W., A. J. Spurgin, and Y. D. Lukic. "Human cognitive reliability model for PRA analysis." Electric Power Research Institute, NUS-4531, 1984.

[8] Wakefield, D. J. "Application of the human cognitive reliability model and confusion matrix approach in a probabilistic risk assessment," *Reliability Engineering and System Safety*, vol. 22, pp. 295–312, 1988.

[9] Wreathall, J. "Operator action trees: An approach to quantifying operator error probability during accident sequences." NUS Rep. No. 4159, 1982 (NUS Corporation, 910 Clopper Road, Gaithersburg, Maryland 20878).

[10] Woods, D. D., E. M. Roth, and H. Pople, Jr. "Modeling human intention formation for human reliability assessment," *Reliability Engineering and System Safety*, vol. 22, pp. 169–200, 1988.

[11] Hancock, P. A. "On the future of hybrid human-machine systems." In *Verification and Validation of Complex Systems: Human Factors Issues*, edited by Wise et al. Berlin: Springer-Verlag, 1993, pp. 61–85.

[12] Reason, J. "Modeling the basic error tendencies of human operators," *Reliability Engineering and System Safety*, vol. 22, pp. 137–153, 1988.

[13] Silverman, B. G. *Critiquing Human Error—A Knowledge Based Human-Computer Collaboration Approach*. London: Academic Press, 1992.

[14] Hashimoto, K. "Human characteristics and error in man-machine systems," *J. Society of Instrument and Control Engineers*, vol. 19, no. 9, pp. 836–844, 1980 (in Japanese).

[15] Kuroda, I. "Humans under critical situations," *Safety Engineering*, vol. 18, no. 6, pp. 383–385, 1979 (in Japanese).

[16] Rasmussen, J. *Information Processing and Human-Machine Interaction: An Approach to Cognitive Engineering*. New York: North-Holland Series in System Science and Engineering, 1986.

[17] Hollnagel, E. *Human Reliability Analysis: Context and Control*. New York: Academic Press, 1993.

[18] Embrey, D. E. et al. "SLIM-MAUD: An approach to assessing human error probabilities using structured expert judgment." USNRC, NUREG/CR-3518, 1984.

[19] Apostolakis, G. E., V. M. Bier, and A. Mosleh. "A critique of recent models for human error rate assessment," *Reliability Engineering and System Safety*, vol. 22, pp. 201–217, 1988.

[20] Hayashi, Y. "System safety," *Safety Engineering*, vol. 18, no. 6, pp. 315–321, 1979 (in Japanese).

[21] Nakamura, S. "On human errors," *Safety Engineering*, vol. 18, no. 4, pp. 391–394, 1979 (in Japanese).

[22] Kano, H. "Human errors in work," *Safety Engineering*, vol. 18, no. 4, pp. 186–191, 1979 (in Japanese).

[23] Hashimoto, K. "Biotechnology and industrial society," *Safety Engineering*, vol. 18, no. 6, pp. 306–314, 1979 (in Japanese).

[24] Aoki, M. "Biotechnology and chemical plant accidents caused by operator error and its safety program (2)," *Safety Engineering*, vol. 21, no. 3, pp. 164–171, 1982 (in Japanese).

[25] Iiyama, Y. "A note on the safety of Shinkansen (JNR's high-speed railway)," *Safety Engineering*, vol. 18, no. 6, pp. 360–366, 1979 (in Japanese).

[26] Kato, K. "Man-machine system and safety in aircraft operations," *J. Society of Instrument and Control Engineers*, vol. 19, no. 9, pp. 859–865, 1980 (in Japanese).

[27] *Aviation Week & Space Technology*, April 7, 1975, pp. 54–59.

[28] *Aviation Week & Space Technology*, April 14, 1975, pp. 53–56.

[29] Furuta, H. "Safety and reliability of man-machine systems in medical fields," *J. Society of Instrument and Control Engineers*, vol. 19, no. 9, pp. 866–874, 1980 (in Japanese).

CHAPTER TEN APPENDICES

A.1 THERP FOR ERRORS DURING A PLANT UPSET

The following example shows THERP can be applied to defined-procedure tasks during plant upsets where diagnosis and time-pressure elements are relatively insignificant. THERP can also be extended to cases where time is limited; the techniques of Winslow Taylor may be modified to quantify human errors for defined-procedure tasks under time stress. The nonresponse HCR model in Section 10.9 considers the detection-diagnosis-response as a holistic process when a task analysis is infeasible.

Consider four tasks described in a procedure manual for responding to a small LOCA (loss of coolant accident) at a heat-generating reactor involving hazardous materials. The reactor vessel is housed in a containment. The reactor pressure was high during the early accident period, and the HPI (high-pressure injection) pumps have successfully started and supplied coolant to the reactor.

Tasks in manual

1. Task 1. Monitor RC (reactor-coolant) pressure and temperature. Maintain at least a 50°F margin to saturation by holding RC pressure near the maximum allowable pressure of the cooldown pressure-temperature curve. The pressure can be controlled by manipulating heater switches for a pressurizer.
2. Task 2. When the RC margin to saturation becomes > 50°F, throttle HPI MOVs (motor-operated valves) to hold pressurizer water level at the setpoint. Initiate plant cooldown by Tasks 3 and 4 below at a rate that allows RC pressure to be maintained within the cooldown pressure-temperature envelope.
3. Task 3. Switch from short-term HPI pumps to long-term LPI (low-pressure injection) pumps.
   - **3.1.** Verify that HPI tank outlet valve MU-13 for HPI is closed.
   - **3.2.** Open valves DH-7A and DH-7B for LPI discharge to HPI pump suction, verify that HPI suction crossover valves MU-14, MU-15, MU-16, and MU-17 are open, and verify that HPI discharge crossover valves MU-23, MU-24, MU-25, and MU-26 are open.
   - **3.3.** Go to basement 4 to close floor drain valves ABS-13 and ABS-14 and watertight doors. Go to the third floor to close ventilation room purge dampers CV-7621, CV-7622, CV-7637, and CV-7638 from ventilation control panel (east wall of the ventilation room).
   - **3.4.** Verify that both LPI pumps are operating and LPI MOVs are open (MOV-1400 and MOV-1401).
4. Task 4. Monitor the level in water storage tank (WST) that supplies water to the LPI pumps. When the WST level has fallen to 6 ft or when the corresponding low-level alarm is received, transfer the LPI pump suction to containment basement sump by verifying that the sump suction valves inside containment MOV-1414 and MOV-1415 are open. Open sump suction valves outside containment MOV-1405 and MOV-1406, and then close both WST outlets MOV-1407 and MOV-1408. Close catalyst tank outlets MOV-1616 and MOV-1617, which supply water to another safety system.

As stated in the procedure manual, verify all actions and, if necessary, correct the status of a given item of equipment. For example, if the operator verifies that a valve should be open and, on checking its status, finds it closed, it is opened manually.

Boundary conditions. In the talk-through (Step 3) in Figure 10.9, some general information is gathered that relates to the performance of the four tasks.

1. The plant follows an emergency procedure in dealing with the small LOCA. It is assumed that the situation has been diagnosed correctly and that the operators have correctly completed the required precursor actions. The level of stress experienced by the operators will be higher if they have already made prior mistakes. Task 1 will start approximately 1 hr after start of the LOCA.
2. At least three licensed operators are available to deal with the situation. One of them is the shift supervisor.
3. Tasks 1, 2, 3.4, and 4 are performed in the control room, while Tasks 3.1, 3.2, and 3.3 take place outside the control room.
4. Allocation of controls and displays are shown in Figure A10.1. The tasks are performed on five different building levels—F3, F1, B2, B3, and B4.

Task analysis. In the task-analysis step depicted in Figure 10.9, we decompose the four tasks into the unit activities shown in Table A10.1. The symbols CB and ESFP in the location column denote a control board and emergency safety features panel, respectively. The O and C columns represent omission and commission errors, respectively. The error labels underlined in these two columns are the more serious ones.

In the human-reliability analysis that follows, we assume that three operators are involved: supervisory operator I, senior operator II, and junior operator III. Operator I performs activities required at the ESFP in the control room on the first floor. An exception is unit task 6 at CB. Operator II carries out the activities at the CB in the control room and also goes to the ventilation room on the third floor to perform Task 3.3, activity 12. Operator III is in charge of activities on the basement levels; protective clothing must be worn. The allocation of operators to the unit activities are:

I: 5, 6, 14, 16, 17, 18, 19
II: 1, 2, 3, 4, 12, 15
III: 7, 8, 9, 10, 11, 13

The functions performed by operators I and II are summarized in the event tree of Figure A10.2, and those performed by operator III are modeled by Figure A10.3.

Assigning BHEP. *A*—Omit monitoring: Activities 1 to 4 form a task group, thus probability of an omission error applies to the entire task, and only by forgetting to perform Task 1 will the operator forget to perform any element of it (see column O in Table A10.1).

Because we are dealing with the operator's following a set of written procedures, we use an error estimate from Table A10.6 (see page 530). This table presents estimates of errors of omission made by operators using written procedures. These estimates reflect the probability, under conditions stated, of an operator's omitting any one item from a set of written procedures. Because the procedures in this example are emergency procedures that do not require any step check-off by the operator, we use the section of Table A10.6 that deals with procedures having no check-off provision. Given that "omit monitoring" applies to a

F3	**Ventilation Room** Switches for CV-7621, 7622, 7637, 7638
F2	
F1	**Control Room** (see below)
B1	
B2	**HPI Pump Room** MU-13
B3	**LPI Pump Room** MU-14, 15, 16, 17 MU-23, 24, 25, 26 DH-7A, DH-7B
B4	**B4 Rooms** ABS-13, ABS-14 Watertight Doors

Control Room

Control Board	ESF Panel
RC Pressure Chart Recorder	Switches for 4 HPI MOVs
RC Temperature Digital Indicator	Indicators for LPI Pumps
Cool-Down Curve	Indicators for MOV-1400, 1401
Heater Switches	Switches for MOV-1400, 1401
WST-Level Indicator	Indicators for MOV-1414, 1415
	Switches for MOV-1414, 1415
	Switches for MOV-1405, 1406
	Switches for MOV-1407, 1408
	Switches for MOV-1616, 1617

Equipment	Description
CV-7621, CV-7622, CV-7637, CV-7638	Purge Dampers in Ventilation Room
MOV-1400, MOV-1401	LPI MOVs
MOV-1414, MOV-1415	Sump Suction Valves Inside Containment
MOV-1405, MOV-1406	Sump Suction Valves Outside Containment
MOV-1407, MOV-1408	WST Outlets
MOV-1616, MOV-1617	Catalyst Tank Outlets
ABS-13, ABS-14	B4 Floor Drain Valves
DH-7A, DH-7B	LPI Discharge Valves to HPI Pump Suction
MU-14, MU-15, MU-16, MU-17	HPI Pump Suction Crossover Valves
MU-23, MU-24, MU-25, MU-26	HPI Pump Discharge Crossover Valves
MU-13	HPI Tank Outlet

Figure A10.1. Allocation of controls and displays.

long list of written procedures, its estimated HEP is 0.01 (0.005 to 0.05), as in item 5 of Table A10.6. The significance of the statistical error bounds is discussed in Chapter 11.

B—Pressure-reading error: The operator reads a number from a chart recorder. Table A10.7 (see page 530) presents estimated HEPs for errors made in reading quantitative information from different types of display. For the chart recorder in question, item 3 from the table is used, 0.006 (0.002 to 0.02).

C—Temperature-reading error: This error involves reading an exact value from a digital readout; therefore, item 2 from Table A10.7 applies, 0.001 (0.0005 to 0.005).

D—Curve-reading error: This applies to activity 3. The HEP for errors made in reading quantitative information from a graph is used, item 4 from Table A10.7, 0.01 (0.005 to 0.05).

Because feedback from manipulating heater switches incorrectly is almost immediate, the probability of making a reversal error during activity 4 is not considered.

TABLE A10.1. A Task Analysis Table

Task	Unit Task	Description	Location	Operator	O	C
Task 1	1	Read RC pressure chart (analog)	F1, CB	II	$\underline{A}$	$\underline{B}$
	2	Read RC temperature (digital)	F1, CB	II	$\underline{A}$	$\underline{C}$
	3	Read pressure-temperature cooldown curve on a tape	F1, CB	II	$\underline{A}$	$\underline{D}$
	4	Manipulate pressurizer heater switches to control the pressure and temperature	F1, CB	II	$\underline{A}$	
Task 2	5	Throttle four HPI MOVs	F1, ESFP	I	E	G
	6	Initiate cooldown (Tasks 3 and 4) following written procedures	F1, CB	I	$\underline{H}$	
Task 3.1	7	Verify MU-13 (closed)	B2	III	$\underline{T,U}$	
Task 3.2	8	Open DH-7A and DH-7B	B3	III	$\underline{T,V}$	
	9	Verify MU-14, MU-15, MU-16, and MU-17 (open)	B3	III	$\underline{T,V}$	
	10	Verify MU-23, MU-24, MU-25, and MU-26 (open)	B3	III	$\underline{T,V}$	
Task 3.3	11	Close ABS-13 and ABS-14	B4	III	$\underline{T,W}$	
	12	Close CV-7621, CV-7622, CV-7637, and CV-7638	F3	II	I	J_1-J_4
	13	Close watertight doors	B4	III	$\underline{T,W}$	
Task 3.4	14	Verify that both LPI pumps are on and that	F1, ESFP	I	K	L_1, M_1
		MOV-1400 and MOV-1401 are open	F1, ESFP	I	K	L_2, M_2
Task 4	15	Monitor WST level	F1, CB	II	$\underline{N}$	$\underline{O}$
	16	Verify MOV-1414 and MOV-1415 (open)	F1, ESFP	I	$\underline{N}$	P_1, Q
	17	Open MOV-1405 and MOV 1406	F1, ESFP	I	$\underline{N}$	$\underline{P_2}, \underline{R_2}$
	18	Close MOV-1407 and MOV-1408	F1, ESFP	I	$\underline{N}$	P_3, R_3
	19	Close MOV-1616 and MOV-1617	F1, ESFP	I	$\underline{N}$	P_4, R_4

E—Omit throttling HPI MOVs: There are four switches for four HPI MOVs on the vertical ESFP on the first floor control room. For the operator, throttling four HPI MOVs is a unit activity. Therefore, probability of an omission error applies to them all. The same HEP used for omission error *A*, 0.01 (0.005 to 0.05), is used.

G—Incorrectly select fourth MOV: The four HPI MOVs on the panel are delineated with colored tape; therefore, a group selection error is very unlikely. However, it is known that a similar switch is next to the last HPI MOV control on the panel. Instead of MOVs 1, 2, 3, and 4, the operator may err, and throttle MOVs 1, 2, 3, and the similar switch. Table A10.8 (see page 531) contains HEPs for errors of commission in changing or restoring valves. Because item 7 most closely approximates the situation described here, an HEP of 0.003 (0.001 to 0.01) applies.

H—Omit initiating cooldown: This applies to unit activity 6. The error is one of omission of a single step in a set of written procedures, so 0.01 (0.005 to 0.05) in Table A10.6 is used. Activities 7 to 11 are performed on basement levels by operator III, so we next consider activity 12 as performed by operator II on the third floor.

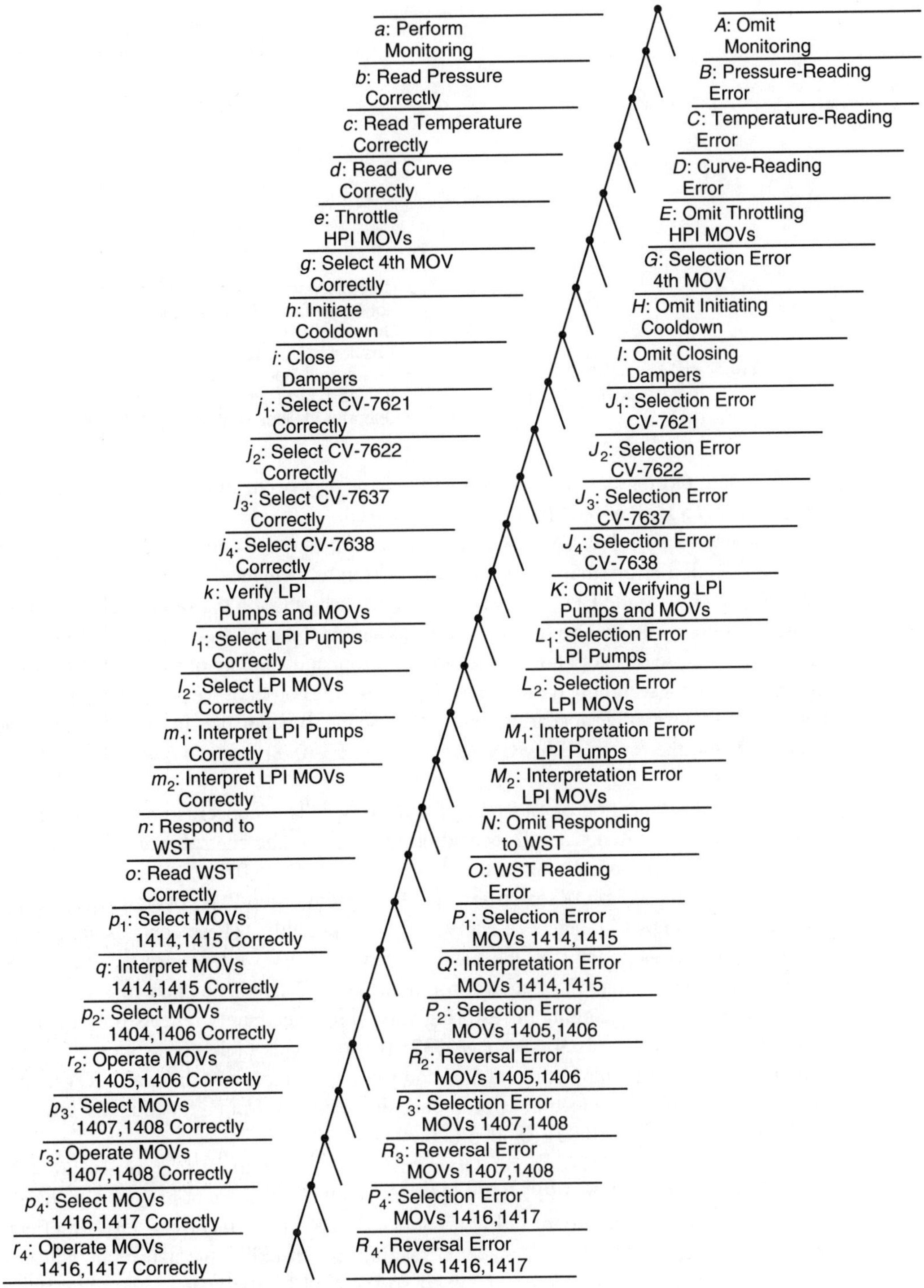

Figure A10.2. HRA event tree for operators I and II in the control room.

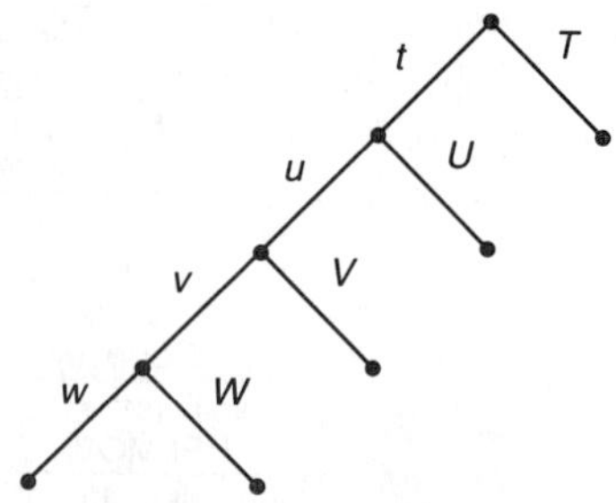

T = Control Room Operator (I or II) Does not Order Tasks for Operator III
U = Operator III Does not Verify Position of MU_13 in HPI Pump Room
V = Operator III Does not Verify/Open Valves in LPI Pump Room
W = Operator III Does Not Isolate B4 Rooms

Figure A10.3. HRA event tree for operator III outside the control room.

I—Omit closing dampers: An omission error may occur in unit activity 12 in Task 3.3. As in *H*, an HEP of 0.01 (0.005 to 0.05) is used.

J—Incorrectly select CVs: A commission error may arise in unit activity 12. Four possible selection errors may occur in manipulation of switches for CV-7621, CV-7622, CV-7637, and CV-7638. The switches are close to each other on the ventilation room wall on the third floor, but we have no specific information about ease or difficulty of locating the group. Because it is not known whether the layout and labeling of the switches help or hinder the operator searching for the controls, we take the conservative position of assuming them to be among similar-appearing items. We use the same HEP as in the selection error associated with the fourth HPI MOV (error *G*), 0.003 (0.001 to 0.01), for each of these MOVs (J_1–J_4).

K—Omit verification of LPI pumps and MOVs: This concerns unit activity 14 in Task 3.4. Equipment items are all located on the ESFP in the control room. The error is one of omitting a procedural step, so the HEP is 0.01 (0.005 to 0.05).

L—LPI pump and MOV selection error: If procedural step 14 is not omitted, selection errors for LPI pumps (L_1) and LPI MOVs (L_2) are possible. These controls are part of groups arranged functionally on the panel. They are very well delineated and can be identified more easily than most control room switches. There is no entry in Table A10.8 (commission errors in changing or restoring valves) that accurately reflects this situation, so an HEP from Table A10.9 (see page 532) is used. This table consists of HEPs for commission errors in manipulating manual controls (e.g., a hand switch for an MOV). Item 2 in this table involves a selection error in choosing a control from a functionally grouped set of controls; its HEP is 0.001 (0.0005 to 0.005).

M—LPI pump and MOV interpretation error: Errors of interpretation are also possible for LPI pumps (M_1) and the LPI MOVs (M_2). Given that the operator has located correct switches, there is a possibility of failing to notice they are in an incorrect state. In effect, this constitutes a reading error, one made in "reading" (or checking) the state of an indicator lamp. No quantitative information is involved, so Table A10.10 (see page 532), which deals with commission errors in checking displays, is used. The last item in the table describes an error of interpretation made on an indicator lamp, so 0.001 (0.0005 to 0.005) is used.

N—Omit responding WST: This applies to unit activities 15 to 19 in Task 4. If the operator omits responding to (or monitoring) the WST level, other activities in Task 4 will not be performed. The same omission HEP used previously, 0.01 (0.005 to 0.05), applies.

O—WST reading error: An error in reading the WST meter could be made without the omission error in *N*. If it is read incorrectly, other activities in Task 4 will not be performed. Going back to Table A10.7 for commission errors made in reading quantitative information, the HEP to use in reading an analog meter is 0.003 (0.001 to 0.01), the first item in the table.

P—MOV selection error: This applies to unit activities 16 to 19. Errors P_1, P_2, P_3, and P_4 involve selecting a wrong set of MOV switches from sets of functionally grouped switches on the ESFP. As in *L*, this HEP is from Table A10.9, 0.001 (0.0005 to 0.005).

Q—MOVs 1414, 1415 interpretation error: This concerns unit activity 16 in Task 4. An interpretation error could be made in checking the status of an indicator lamp. An HEP of 0.001 (0.0005 to 0.005) is assigned.

R—MOV reversal error: There are three possible errors, R_2, R_3, and R_4, for unit activities 17, 18, and 19, respectively. Instead of opening valves, the operator might close them or vice versa. The switches are on the ESFP. Because errors of commission for valve-switch manipulations are involved, Table A10.9 is used. Item 7 most closely describes this error; hence an HEP of 0.001 (0.0001 to 0.1).

Let us next consider the event tree for the task performed by operator III. The unit activities are 7 to 11 and 13. Figure A10.3 shows the event tree.

T—Control room operator omits ordering task: Activities 7 to 11 and 13 are performed outside the control room. If operator I forgets to order operator III to perform this set of activities, this constitutes failure to carry out plant policy. An HEP of 0.01 (0.005 to 0.05) from Table A11.11 (see page 532), item 1, is used.

U—Omit verifying MU-13: This involves unit activity 7 in Task 3.1. As shown in Figure A10.1 and Table A10.1, activity 7 is performed on the second-floor basement; activities 8, 9, and 10 are carried out on basement 3; and activities 11 and 13 on basement 4. Operator III sees these as three distinct unit tasks, one on each of three levels. We assume that the operator will not be working from a set of written procedures but from oral instructions from supervisory operator I in the control room. Data for this model are found in Table A10.12 (see page 533). Operator III must recall three tasks, so we use item 3 in the table, which shows an HEP of 0.01 (0.005 to 0.05) for each task.

Valve MU-13 is a manual valve on basement 2 and no selection error is possible. It is not deemed likely that the operator will make a reversal error in this situation.

V—Omit to verify/open valves in LPI pump room: This involves unit activities 8, 9, and 10, which are viewed as a unit task performed in the LPI pump room of basement 3. As stated in *A*, an HEP of 0.01 (0.005 to 0.05) is used. Neither a selection error nor a reversal error is deemed likely.

W—Omit isolating B4 rooms: These are omission errors for unit activities 11 and 13. An HEP of 0.01 (0.005 to 0.05) was assumed, as in *U* and *V*. Valves ABS-13 and ABS-14 are large, locally operated valves in basement 4. They are the only valves there. Similarly, there is only one set of watertight doors. Again, neither selection nor reversal errors are considered likely.

Evaluating PSFs. As described in Section 10.8.2, global PSFs affect the entire task, whereas local PSFs affect only certain types of errors. Nominal HEPs in *Handbook* tables consider these local PSFs. We next consider the effect of global PSFs—those that will affect all HEPs. As stated in the original assumptions, the operators are experienced, and because they are following an emergency procedure, they are under a moderately high level of stress. We see from Table 10.2 that the HEPs for experienced personnel operating under a moderately high stress level should be doubled for discrete tasks and multiplied by 5 for dynamic tasks.

Figure A10.2 is the HRA event tree for control room actions for which the nominal HEPs in Table A10.2 apply. The only dynamic tasks in this table are those calling for monitoring activities: the monitoring of the RC temperature and pressure indicators (unit activities 1 and 2), the interpretation of these values (activities 3 and 4), and the WST level monitoring (activity 15). Hence nominal HEPs, B, C, D, and O in Table A10.2 are multiplied by 5 to yield new HEPs; those for other events in the table are doubled.

Another overriding PSF that must be considered is the effect of operator III's having to wear protective clothing. The first error T takes place in the control room. The HEPs T, U, V, and W must be doubled to reflect effects of moderately high stress levels. HEPs U, V, and W must be doubled again to reflect the effects of the protective clothing. The new HEPs are shown in Table A10.3.

Assessing dependence. Several cases of dependence have already been accounted for (see Table A10.1).

1. Omission error A: This omission applies to tasks consisting of activities 1 to 4.
2. Omission error E: For errors of omission, the four HPI MOVs are completely dependent.
3. Commission error G: The first three HPI MOVs are free of selection errors, while the fourth is susceptible.
4. Omission error H: For errors of omission, steps in the cooldown procedures are completely dependent.
5. Omission error I: The four CVs are completely dependent with respect to the omission error.
6. Omission error N: Unit activities 15 to 19 are completely dependent.
7. Commission error O: The same dependence as in case 6 exists for this reading error.
8. Omission error T: The omission applies to the task consisting of activities 7 to 11 and 13.
9. Omission errors U, V, and W: Each set of activities performed on a plant level is completely dependent with respect to omission.

The presence of operators I and II in the control room constitutes a recovery (or redundancy) factor with a high dependence between the two operators. Equation (10.8) indicates that an error is caught by another operator about half the time; this is a form of human redundancy.

Table A10.2 shows the HEPs as modified to reflect the effects of dependence. Probabilities of error for the two operators have been collapsed into a single limb for each type of error. For instance, HEP A is modified in the following way.

$$\text{new } A = \frac{(\text{old } A)[1 + (\text{old } A)]}{2} = \frac{(0.02)(1 + 0.02)}{2} = 0.0102 \tag{A.1}$$

TABLE A10.2. Quantification of Human Error for Operators I and II Tasks

Symbol	Description	BHEP	Modified by PSFs	Modified by HD
A:	Omit monitoring	0.01(0.005 to 0.05)	0.02	0.0102
$a = 1 - A$:	Perform monitoring	0.99	0.98	0.9898
B:	Pressure-reading error	0.006(0.002 to 0.02)	0.03	0.0155
$b = 1 - B$:	Read pressure correctly	0.994	0.97	0.9845
C:	Temperature-reading error	0.001(0.0005 to 0.005)	0.005	0.0025
$c = 1 - C$:	Read temperature correctly	0.999	0.995	0.9975
D:	Curve-reading error	0.01(0.005 to 0.05)	0.05	0.0263
$d = 1 - D$:	Read curve correctly	0.99	0.95	0.9737
E:	Omit throttling HPI MOVs	0.01(0.005 to 0.05)	0.02	0.0102
$e = 1 - E$:	Throttle HPI MOVs	0.99	0.98	0.9898
G:	Selection error: 4th MOV	0.003(0.001 to 0.01)	0.006	0.003
$g = 1 - G$:	Select 4th MOV correctly	0.997	0.94	0.997
H:	Omit initiating cooldown	0.01(0.005 to 0.05)	0.02	0.0102
$h = 1 - H$:	Initiate cooldown	0.99	0.98	0.9898
I:	Omit closing dampers	0.01(0.005 to 0.05)	0.02	0.0102
$i = 1 - I$:	Close dampers	0.99	0.98	0.9898
J_1:	Selection error: CV-7621	0.003(0.001 to 0.01)	0.006	0.006
$j_1 = 1 - J_1$:	Select CV-7621 correctly	0.997	0.994	0.994
J_2:	Selection error: CV-7622	0.003(0.001 to 0.01)	0.006	0.006
$j_2 = 1 - J_2$:	Select CV-7622 correctly	0.997	0.994	0.994
J_3:	Selection error: CV-7637	0.003(0.001 to 0.01)	0.006	0.006
$j_3 = 1 - J_3$:	Select CV-7637 correctly	0.997	0.994	0.994
J_4:	Selection error: CV-7638	0.003(0.001 to 0.01)	0.006	0.006
$j_4 = 1 - J_4$:	Select CV-7638 correctly	0.997	0.994	0.994
K:	Omit verifying LPI pumps and MOVs	0.01(0.005 to 0.05)	0.02	0.0102
$k = 1 - K$:	Verify LPI pumps and MOVs	0.99	0.98	0.9898
L_1:	Selection error: LPI pumps	0.001(0.0005 to 0.005)	0.002	0.001
$l_1 = 1 - L_1$:	Select LPI pumps correctly	0.999	0.998	0.999
L_2:	Selection error: LPI MOVs	0.001(0.0005 to 0.005)	0.002	0.001
$l_2 = 1 - L_2$:	Select LPI MOVs correctly	0.999	0.998	0.999
M_1:	Interpretation error: LPI pumps	0.001(0.0005 to 0.005)	0.002	0.001
$m_1 = 1 - M_1$:	Interpret LPI pumps correctly	0.999	0.998	0.999
M_2:	Interpretation error: LPI MOVs	0.001(0.0005 to 0.005)	0.002	0.001
$m_2 = 1 - M_2$:	Interpret LPI MOVs correctly	0.999	0.998	0.999
N:	Omit responding: WST	0.01(0.005 to 0.05)	0.02	0.0102
$n = 1 - N$:	Respond to WST	0.99	0.98	0.9898
O:	WST reading error	0.003(0.001 to 0.01)	0.015	0.0076
$o = 1 - O$:	Read WST correctly	0.997	0.985	0.9924
P_1:	Selection error: MOVs 1414, 1415	0.001(0.0005 to 0.005)	0.002	0.001
$p_1 = 1 - P_1$:	Select MOVs 1414, 1415 correctly	0.999	0.998	0.999
Q:	Interpretation error: MOVs 1414, 1415	0.001(0.0005 to 0.005)	0.002	0.001
$q = 1 - Q$:	Interpret MOVs 1414, 1415 correctly	0.999	0.998	0.999
P_2:	Selection error: MOVs 1405, 1406	0.001(0.0005 to 0.005)	0.002	0.001
$p_2 = 1 - P_2$:	Select MOVs 1405, 1406 correctly	0.999	0.998	0.999
R_2:	Reversal error: MOVs 1405, 1406	0.001(0.0001 to 0.1)	0.002	0.001
$r_2 = 1 - R_2$:	Operate MOVs 1405, 1406 correctly	0.999	0.998	0.999
P_3:	Selection error: MOVs 1407, 1408	0.001(0.0005 to 0.005)	0.002	0.001
$p_3 = 1 - P_3$:	Select MOVs 1407, 1408 correctly	0.999	0.998	0.999
R_3:	Reversal error: MOVs 1407, 1408	0.001(0.0001 to 0.1)	0.002	0.001
$r_3 = 1 - R_3$:	Operate MOVs 1407, 1408 correctly	0.999	0.998	0.999
P_4:	Selection error: MOVs 1416, 1417	0.001(0.0005 to 0.005)	0.002	0.001
$p_4 = 1 - P_4$:	Select MOVs 1416, 1417 correctly	0.999	0.998	0.999
R_4:	Reversal error: MOVs 1416, 1417	0.001(0.0001 to 0.1)	0.002	0.001
$r_4 = 1 - R_4$:	Operate MOVs 1416, 1417 correctly	0.999	0.998	0.999

TABLE A10.3. Quantification of Human Error for Operators III Tasks

Symbol	Description	BHEP	Modified by PSFs	Modified by HD
T:	Omit ordering tasks	0.01(0.005 to 0.05)	0.02	0.0102
$t = 1 - T$:	Order tasks	0.99	0.98	0.9898
U:	Omit verifying MU-13 in HPI pump room	0.01(0.005 to 0.05)	0.04	0.04
$u = 1 - U$:	Verify MU-13 correctly	0.99	0.96	0.96
V:	Omit verifying/opening valves in LPI pump room	0.01(0.005 to 0.05)	0.04	0.04
$v = 1 - V$:	Verify/open valves in LPI pump room	0.99	0.96	0.96
W:	Omit isolating B4 rooms	0.01(0.005 to 0.05)	0.04	0.04
$w = 1 - W$:	Isolate B4 rooms correctly	0.99	0.96	0.96

Error J occurs in the third-floor ventilation room. In this case there is no dependence between the two operators because operator II goes to the room alone. The only event in Table A10.3 that is dependent is the first (i.e., T). If operator I forgets to order these tasks, operator II may prompt him:

$$\begin{aligned} \text{new } T &= \frac{(\text{old } T)[1 + (\text{old } T)]}{2} \\ &= \frac{(0.02)(1 + 0.02)}{2} = 0.0102 \end{aligned} \tag{A.2}$$

Determining success and failure probabilities. Once human-error events have been identified and individually quantified as in Tables A10.2 and A10.3, their contribution to the occurrence and non-occurrence of the basic event must be determined. Assume that, as indicated by underlined letters in Table A10.1, the paths ending in the nine error events A, B, C, D, H, N, O, P_2, R_2 are failure nodes. The event tree in Figure A10.2 can be simplified to Figure A10.4 if we collapse the limbs that do not contribute to system failure. The probability of each failure node can be calculated by multiplying the probabilities on the limbs of Figure A10.4. For instance, the path ending at node F_3 is

$$(0.9898)(0.98455)(0.0025) = 0.0024 \tag{A.3}$$

The occurrence probability of system failure is thus

$$\begin{aligned} \Pr\{F\} = 0.0102 + 0.0153 + 0.0024 + 0.0255 + 0.0097 + 0.0096 + 0.0070 \\ + 0.0009 + 0.0009 = 0.0815 \end{aligned} \tag{A.4}$$

Figure A10.4 is suitable for further analysis because it shows the relative contribution of events to system failure.

A similar decision was made with respect to the HRA event tree in Figure A10.3. It was decided that all paths terminating in human errors caused system failure.

Determining effects of recovery factors. Consider, for instance, omission error N. The operator should respond to the WST level's falling to 6 ft. Even if he forgets to monitor the level indicators, there is still a possibility that the low-level alarm (annunciator) will remind him of the need for follow-up actions. We will treat the alarm as an alerting cue and analyze its effect as a recovery factor. Table A10.13 (see page 533) lists HEPs for failing to respond to annunciating indicators. Assume that ten annunciators are alarming the accident. The probability of the operator's failing to respond to any one of these ten is 0.05 (0.005 to 0.5). Figure A10.5 shows the diagram for this recovery factor. Note that

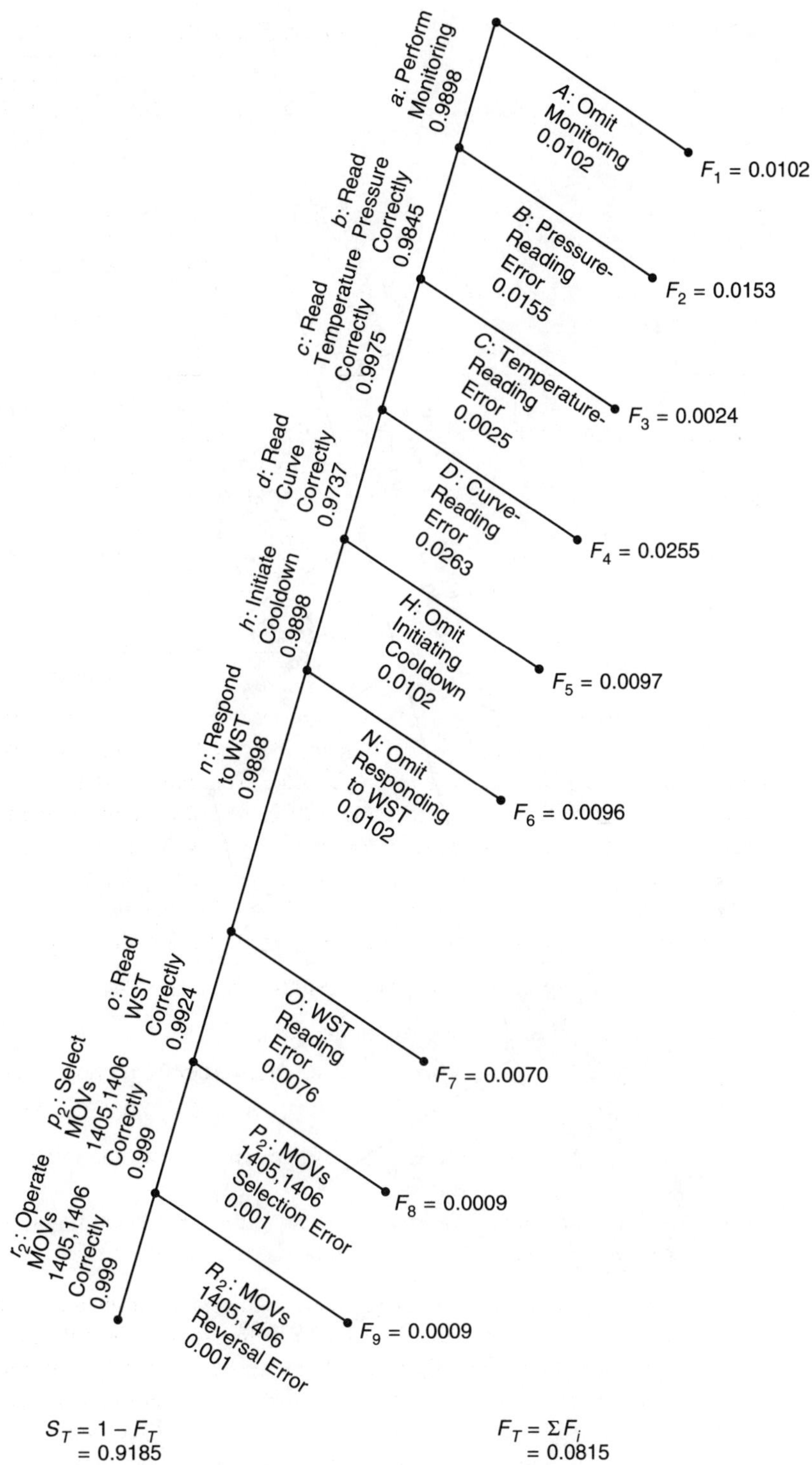

Figure A10.4. Truncated HRA event tree for control room actions.

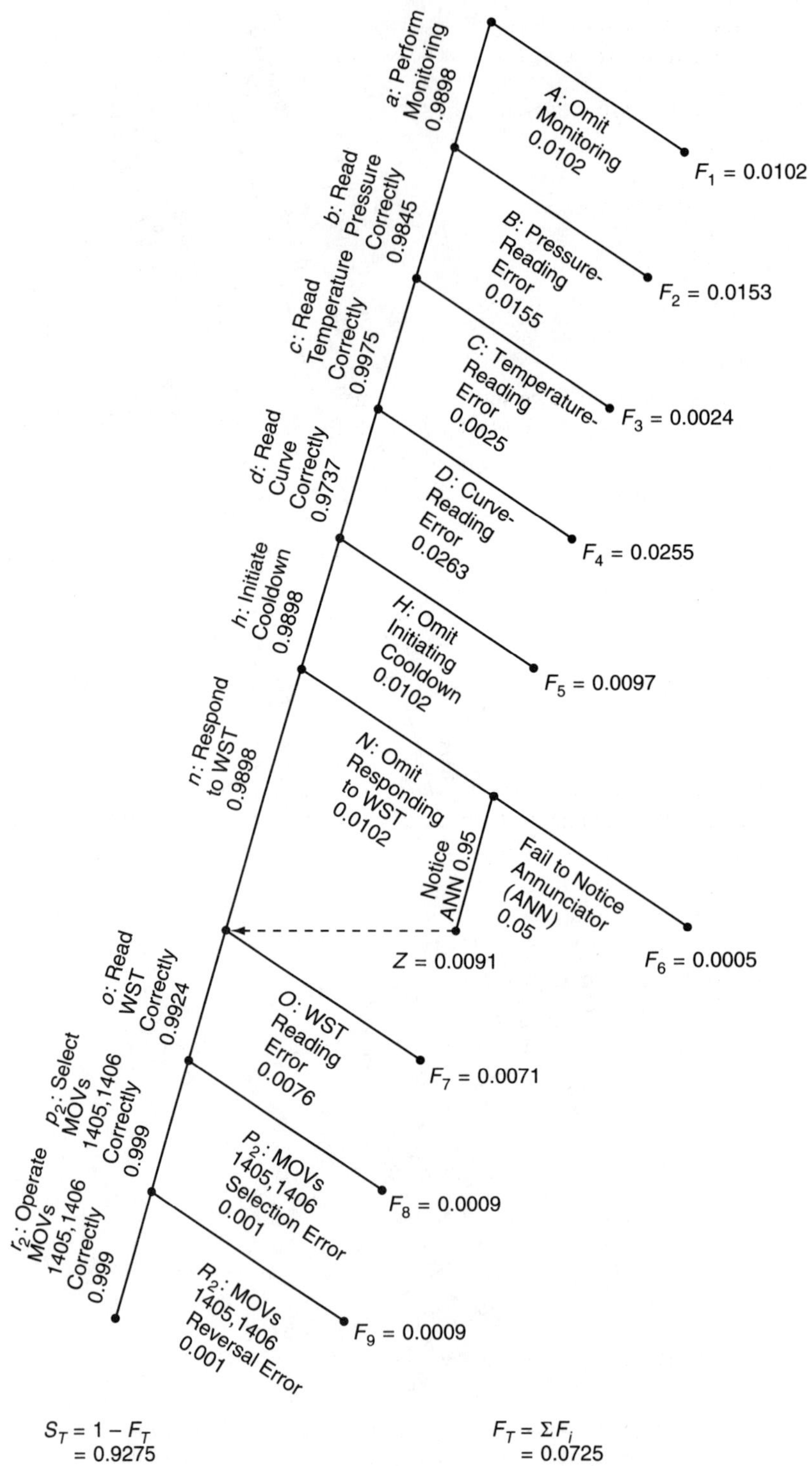

Figure A10.5. Control room HRA event tree including one recovery factor.

its inclusion in the analysis decreases the probability of total system failure from 0.0815 to 0.0725. If this is an adequate increase, no more recovery factors are considered.

Sensitivity analysis. In this problem the two most important errors, in terms of their high probability, are errors *B* and *D*—reading the RC pressure chart recorder and pressure-temperature curve. For RC pressure, if the display were a digital meter instead of a chart recorder, we see from Table A10.7 that this would change the basic HEP for that task from 0.006 (0.002 to 0.02) to 0.001 (0.0005 to 0.005). This new HEP must be modified to 0.005 (0.0025 to 0.025) to reflect effects of stress for dynamic tasks, and then modified again to reflect the effect of dependence, thus becoming 0.0025 (0.001 to 0.01). Using 0.0025 instead of 0.0155 results in a total-system-failure probability of 0.0604 as opposed to 0.0725.

To make the same sort of adjustment for error *D*, we redesign the graph so that it is comparatively easy to read. If we use the lower bound of the HEP in Table A10.7, item 4, instead of the nominal value, we have 0.005. This becomes 0.025 when modified for stress and 0.0128 when modified for human redundancy.

An HRA event tree with these new values is shown in Figure A10.6. Total-system-failure probability becomes 0.0475. Whether this new estimate of the probability of system failure is small enough to warrant incorporating both changes is a management decision.

A.2 HCR FOR TWO OPTIONAL PROCEDURES

Consider again the initiating event "loss of feedwater to a heat exchanger." Time data for relevant cues are given in Table A10.4. Assume that the plant has been shut down successfully, and that heat from the reactor must now be removed. Because of the loss of feedwater, the heat-exchanger water level continuously drops. The low-water-level alarms sound at 20 min after the start of the initiating event. Fortunately, a subcooling margin is maintained until the heat exchangers dry out; 40 min will elapse between the low-level alarms and the heat exchangers emptying. The operators have 60 min before damage to the reactor occurs. Operators have two options for coping with the accident.

TABLE A10.4. Time Data for Relevant Cues

Time	Remark
20 min	HEX alarm
40 min	From HEX alarm to dry-out
50 min	PORVs open
60 min	To fuel damage
1 min	Switch manipulation

1. Recovery of feedwater: The heat is removed by heat exchangers cooled by the feedwater. This is called a *secondary heat-removal recovery*.
2. Feed and bleed: The operators manually open reactor PORVs (pressure-operated relief valves) to exhaust heat to the reactor containment housing. Because the hot steam flows through the PORVs, the operators must activate the HPI to maintain the coolant inventory in the reactor. The combination of PORV open operation

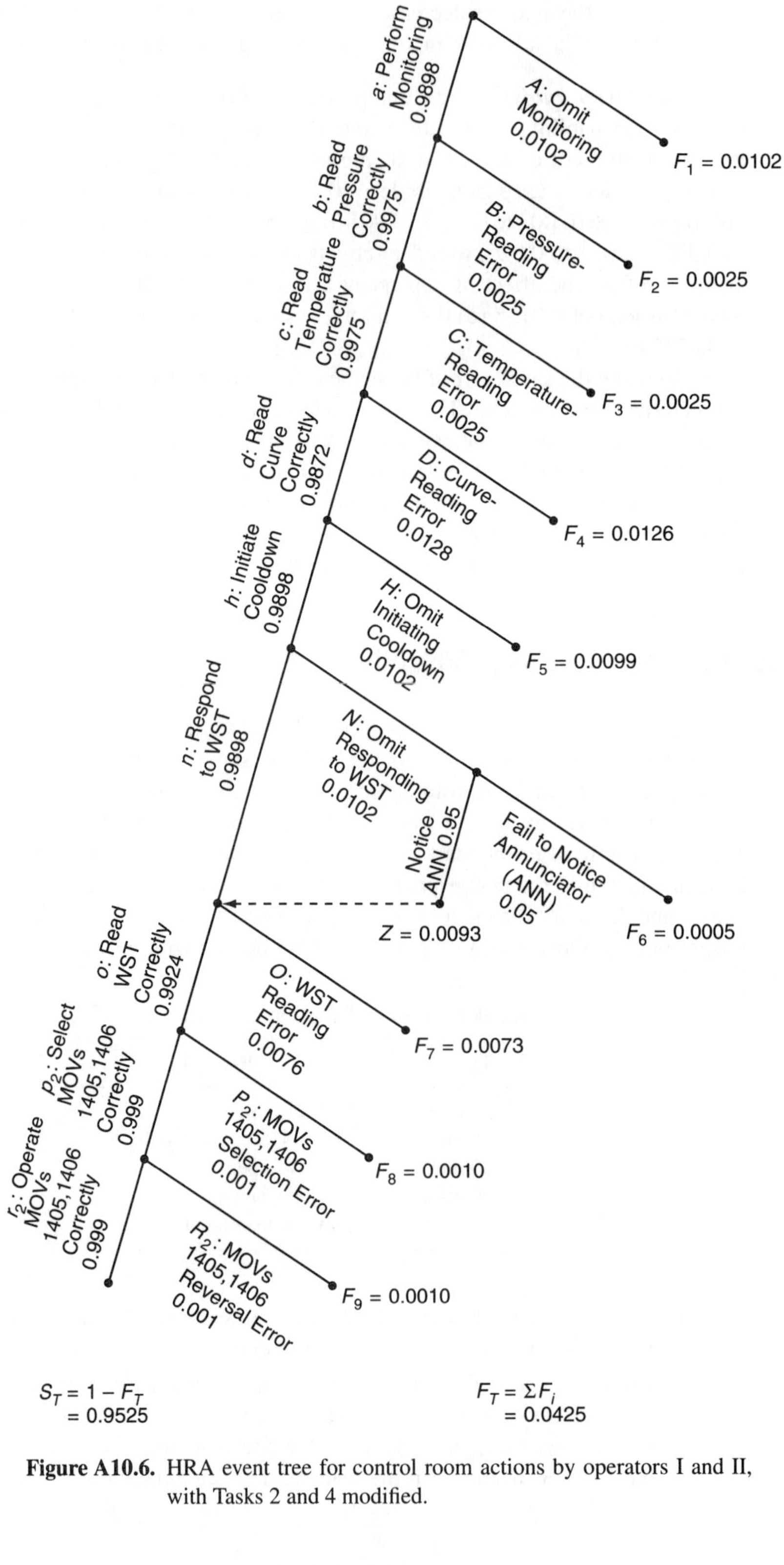

Figure A10.6. HRA event tree for control room actions by operators I and II, with Tasks 2 and 4 modified.

and HPI activation is called a *feed and bleed operation*. The implementation of this operation requires 1 min.

The HPI draws water from a storage tank. At some stage the HPI must be realigned to take suction from the containment sump because the storage tank capacity is limited; the sump collects the water lost through the PORVs. Once the realignment is carried out, the HPI system is referred to as being in the containment cooling mode.

There are three strategies for combining the two options.

1. Anticipatory: Engineers decide that the feedwater system recovery within the hour is impossible, and decide to establish feed and bleed as soon as possible. The time available to establish the feed and bleed operation is 60 min. The feed and bleed operation creates a grave emergency.
2. Procedure response: Plant engineers decide to first try feedwater system recovery, and then to establish feed and bleed when the low-water-level alarms from the heat exchangers sound.
3. Delayed response: It is decided to wait until the last possible moment to recover secondary heat removal. The engineers perceive recovery is imminent; they hesitate to perform the feed and bleed because it is a drastic emergency measure, it opens the coolant boundary, and it can result in damage to containment components. It is assumed that a PORV opens due to high pressure 50 min into the accident. This becomes a cue for the delayed response.

Anticipatory strategy. Anticipatory strategy characteristics are summarized in Table A10.5. Because 1 min is required for manipulating PORVs and HPI switches on the ESF panel, the time available to the operators is

$$60 - 1 = 59 \text{ min} \tag{A.5}$$

The median time from Table A10.5 modified by the PSFs is

$$T_{1/2} = (1 - 0.22)(1 + 0.44)(1 + 0.00)(8) = 9 \tag{A.6}$$

Application of the HCR Weibull model for knowledge-based mental processing gives

$$\Pr\{59\} = \exp\left[-\left\{\frac{(59/9) - 0.5}{0.791}\right\}^{0.8}\right] = 0.006 \tag{A.7}$$

TABLE A10.5. Characteristics of Anticipatory Strategy

Decision	Initiate feed and bleed
Cognitive behavior	Knowledge ($A = 0.791$, $B = 0.5$, $C = 0.8$)
Operator experience	Well-trained ($K_1 = -0.22$)
Stress level	Grave emergency ($K_2 = 0.44$)
O/P interface	Good ($K_3 = 0.00$)
Nominal median time	8 min
Manipulation time	1 min
Manipulation error rate	0.001 (omission)
Time to damage	60 min
Time window	60 − 1 = 59 min

Because the HEP for manipulation of PORVs and HPI is 0.001, the feed and bleed operation error becomes

$$0.006 + 0.001 = 0.007 \tag{A.8}$$

The successful feed and bleed (probability 0.993) must be followed by containment cooling mode realignment. Alignment failure is analyzed by the human-reliability fault tree of Figure A10.7. The leftmost basic event "screening value" denotes a recovery failure. The operator must close a suction valve at the storage tank to prevent the HPI pumps from sucking air into the system. The operator must open a new valve in a suction line from the containment sump. The realignment-failure probability is calculated to be 0.0005. Thus the total failure probability for the feed and bleed followed by the realignment consists of non-response probability, manipulation-failure probability, and realignment-failure probability when the preceding two failures do not occur:

$$\begin{aligned} \Pr\{\text{Anticipatory strategy failure}\} &= 0.006 + 0.001 + (1 - 0.007) \times 0.0005 \\ &= 0.0075 \end{aligned} \tag{A.9}$$

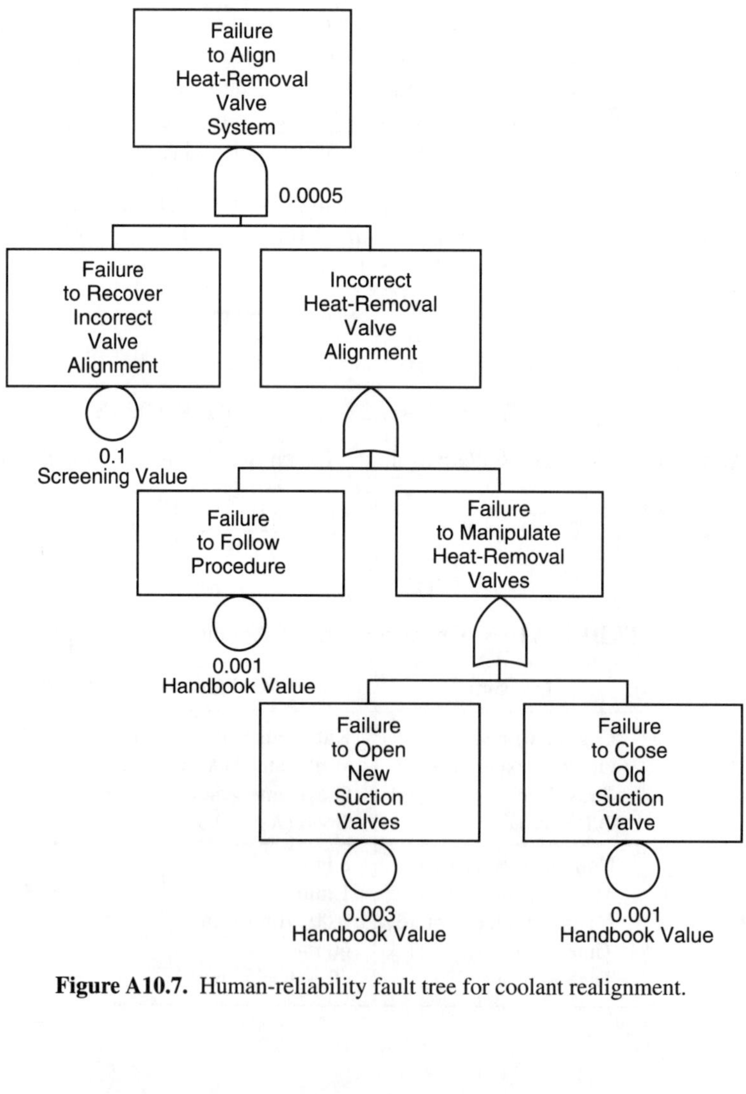

Figure A10.7. Human-reliability fault tree for coolant realignment.

Procedure-response strategy. The engineers first decide to recover the feedwater system. The feedwater-system recovery fails by hardware failures or human error, with probability 0.2. Because the operators try to recover the secondary cooling during the first 20 min until the heat exchanger low-water-level alarm, the time available for the feed and bleed operation is

$$A.1060 - 20 - 1 = 39 \tag{A.10}$$

With respect to the feed and bleed operation, only this time window is specific to the procedure response strategy; other characteristics remain the same as for the anticipatory strategy. Thus the nonresponse probability for the feed and bleed is

$$\Pr\{39\} = \exp\left[-\left\{\frac{(39/9) - 0.5}{0.791}\right\}^{0.8}\right] = 0.029 \tag{A.11}$$

Because the feed and bleed manipulation failure probability is 0.001, the failure probability of feed and bleed is 0.03.

This strategy fails when the following happens.

1. The feedwater recovery fails due to hardware failures or human error (probability 0.2), and the feed and bleed fails (probability 0.03).
2. The feedwater recovery fails (0.2), the feed and bleed succeeds ($1 - 0.03 = 0.97$), and the realignment activity fails (0.0005).

As a result, the procedure response strategy fails with probability

$$\begin{aligned}\Pr\{\text{Procedure-response strategy failure}\} &= (0.2)(0.03) + (0.2)(0.97)(0.0005) \\ &= 0.007\end{aligned} \tag{A.12}$$

Delayed-response strategy. The engineers first decide to recover the feedwater system. The feed and bleed cue is set off at 50 min when a PORV opens. Thus the engineers only have $10 - 1 = 9$ min for the feed and bleed decision. Assume rule-based mental processing and a nominal median time of 3 min. Then the actual median time becomes

$$T_{1/2} = 3 \times 1.44 \times 0.78 = 3.4 \tag{A.13}$$

The nonresponse probability is now

$$\Pr\{9\} = \exp\left[-\left\{\frac{(9/3.4) - 0.6}{0.601}\right\}^{0.9}\right] = 0.049 \tag{A.14}$$

Because the manual failure probability is 0.001, the feed and bleed failure probability is $0.049 + 0.001 \simeq 0.05$. This strategy fails in the following cases.

1. The feedwater system recovery fails due to hardware failures or human errors (estimated probability 0.05 because more time is available than in the procedure-response case), and the feed and bleed fails (probability 0.05).
2. The feedwater system recovery fails (0.05), the feed and bleed succeeds ($1-0.05 = 0.95$), and the realignment activity fails (0.0005).

As a result, the delayed-response strategy fails with probability

$$\Pr\{\text{Delayed-response strategy failure}\} = (0.05)(0.05) + (0.05)(0.95)(0.0005) = 0.0025 \tag{A.15}$$

Summation of results. Assume the three strategies occur with frequencies of 10%, 60%, and 30%. Then the overall failure probability, given the initiating event, is

$$0.0075 \times 0.1 + 0.007 \times 0.6 + 0.0025 \times 0.3 = 0.0057 \tag{A.16}$$

A.3 HUMAN-ERROR PROBABILITY TABLES FROM HANDBOOK

TABLE A10.6. Nonpassive Task Omission Errors in Written Procedures

Task	HEP	Interval
1. Procedures with checkoff provisions		
a. Short list $\leq$ 10 items	0.001	(0.0005 to 0.005)
b. Long list > 10 items	0.003	(0.001 to 0.01)
c. Checkoff provisions improperly used	0.5	(0.1 to 0.9)
2. Procedures with no checkoff provisions		
a. Short list $\leq$ 10 items	0.003	(0.001 to 0.01)
b. Long list > 10 items	0.01	(0.005 to 0.05)
3. Performance of simple arithmetic calculations	0.01	(0.005 to 0.05)
4. If two people use written procedures correctly—one reading and checking the other doing the work—assume HD between their performance		
5. Procedures available but not used		
a. Maintenance tasks	0.3	(0.05 to 0.9)
b. Valve change or restoration tasks	0.01	(0.005 to 0.05)

TABLE A10.7. Commission Errors in Reading Quantitative Information from Displays

Reading Task	HEP	Interval
1. Analog meter	0.003	(0.001 to 0.01)
2. Digital readout	0.001	(0.0005 to 0.005)
3. Printing recorder with large number of parameters	0.006	(0.002 to 0.02)
4. Graphs	0.01	(0.005 to 0.05)
5. Values from indicator lamps used as quantitative displays	0.001	(0.0005 to 0.005)
6. An instrument being read is broken, and there are no indicators to alert the user	0.1	(0.02 to 0.2)

TABLE A10.8. Commission Errors by Operator Changing or Restoring Valves

Task	HEP	Interval
1. Writing any one item when preparing a list of valves (or tags)	0.003	(0.001 to 0.01)
2. Change or tag wrong valve where the desired value is one of two-or-more adjacent, similar-appearing manual valves, and at least one other valve is in the same state as the desired valve, or the valves are MOVs of such type that valve status cannot be determined at the valve itself	0.005	(0.002 to 0.02)
3. Restore the wrong manual valve where the desired valve is one of two-or-more adjacent, similar-appearing valves, and at least two are tagged out for maintenance	0.005	(0.002 to 0.02)
4. Reversal error: change a valve, switch, or circuit breaker that has already been changed and tagged	0.0001	(0.00005 to 0.001)
5. Reversal error, as above, if the valve has been changed and NOT tagged	0.1	(0.01 to 0.5)
6. Note that there is more than one tag on a valve, switch, or circuit breaker that is being restored	0.0001	(0.00005 to 0.0005)
7. Change or restore wrong MOV switch or circuit breaker in a group of similar-appearing items (In case of restoration, at least two items are tagged)	0.003	(0.001 to 0.01)
8. Complete a change of state of an MOV of the type that requires the operator to hold the switch until the change is completed as indicated by a light	0.003	(0.001 to 0.01)
9. Given that a manual valve sticks, operator erroneously concludes that the valve is fully open (or closed)		
Rising-stem valves		
a. If the valve sticks at about three-fourths or more of its full travel (no provision indicator present)	0.005	(0.002 to 0.02)
b. If there is an indicator showing the full extent of travel	0.001	(0.0005 to 0.01)
All other valves		
a. If there is a position indicator on the valve	0.001	(0.0005 to 0.01)
b. If there is a position indicator located elsewhere (and extra effort is required to look at it)	0.002	(0.001 to 0.01)
c. If there is no position indicator	0.01	(0.003 to 0.1)

TABLE A10.9. Commission Errors in Operating Manual Controls

Task	HEP	Interval
1. Select wrong control from a group of identical controls identified by labels only	0.003	(0.001 to 0.01)
2. Select wrong control from a functionally grouped set of controls	0.001	(0.0005 to 0.005)
3. Select wrong control from a panel with clearly drawn lines	0.0005	(0.0001 to 0.001)
4. Turn control in wrong direction (no violation of habitual action)	0.0005	(0.0001 to 0.001)
5. Turn control in wrong direction under normal operating conditions (violation of habitual action)	0.05	(0.01 to 0.1)
6. Turn control in wrong direction under high stress (violation of a strong habitual action)	0.5	(0.1 to 0.9)
7. Set a multiposition selector switch to an incorrect setting	0.001	(0.0001 to 0.1)
8. Improperly mate a connector	0.01	(0.005 to 0.05)

TABLE A10.10. Commission Errors in Check-Reading Displays

Check-Reading Task	HEP	Interval
1. Digital indicators (these must be read, i.e., there is no true check-reading function for digital displays)	0.001	(0.0005 to 0.005)
2. Analog meters with easily seen limit marks	0.001	(0.0005 to 0.005)
3. Analog meters with difficult-to-use limit marks, such as scribe lines	0.002	(0.001 to 0.01)
4. Analog meters without limit marks	0.003	(0.001 to 0.01)
5. Analog-type chart recorders with limits	0.002	(0.001 to 0.01)
6. Analog-type chart recorders without limit marks	0.006	(0.002 to 0.02)
7. Confirming a status change on a status lamp	Negligible	
8. Checking the wrong indicator lamp (in an array of lamps)	0.003	(0.001 to 0.01)
9. Misinterpreting the indication on the indicator lamps	0.001	(0.0005 to 0.005)

TABLE A10.11. HEPs Related to Administrative Control Failure

Operation	HEP	Interval
1. Carry out a plant policy when there is no check on a person	0.01	(0.005 to 0.05)
2. Initiate a checking function	0.001	(0.0005 to 0.005)
3. Use control room written procedures under the following operating conditions		
a. Normal	0.01	(0.005 to 0.05)
b. Abnormal	No basis for estimate	
4. Use a valve-restoration list	0.01	(0.005 to 0.05)
5. Use written maintenance procedure when available	0.3	(0.05 to 0.9)
6. Use a checklist properly (i.e., perform one step and check it off before proceeding to next step)	0.5	(0.1 to 0.9)

TABLE A10.12. Errors in Recalling Special Oral Instruction Items

Task	HEP	Interval
Items Not Written Down by Recipient		
1. Recall any given item, given the following number of items to remember		
a. 1 (same as failure to initiate task)	0.001	(0.0005 to 0.005)
b. 2	0.003	(0.001 to 0.01)
c. 3	0.01	(0.005 to 0.05)
d. 4	0.03	(0.01 to 0.1)
e. 5	0.1	(0.05 to 0.5)
2. Recall any item if supervisor checks to see that the task was done	Negligible	
Items Written Down by Recipient		
1. Recall any item (exclusive of errors in writing)	0.001	(0.0005 to 0.005)

TABLE A10.13. Failure to Respond to One Randomly Selected Annunciator

Number of Annunciators	HEP	Interval
1	0.0001	(0.00005 to 0.001)
2	0.0006	(0.00006 to 0.006)
3	0.001	(0.0001 to 0.01)
4	0.002	(0.0002 to 0.02)
5	0.003	(0.0003 to 0.03)
6	0.005	(0.0005 to 0.05)
7	0.009	(0.0009 to 0.09)
8	0.02	(0.002 to 0.2)
9	0.03	(0.003 to 0.3)
10	0.05	(0.005 to 0.5)
11–15	0.10	(0.01 to 0.999)
16–20	0.15	(0.015 to 0.999)
21–40	0.20	(0.02 to 0.999)
> 40	0.25	(0.025 to 0.999)

PROBLEMS

10.1. What category of human error(s) would you say was (were) typical of the following scenario:

> The safety system for a hydrogeneration reactor had safety interlocks that would automatically shut down the reactor if 1) reactor temperature was high, 2) reactor pressure was high, 3) hydrogen feed rate was high, 4) hydrogen pressure was high, or 5) hydrogen concentration in the reactor was too high. The reliability of the sensors was low, so there was about one unnecessary shutdown every week. The operators were disturbed by this, so they disabled the relays in the safety circuits by inserting matches in the contacts. One day, the reactor exploded.

10.2. Pictorialize a human being as a computer system.

10.3. Enumerate human characteristics during panic.

10.4. List performance-shaping factors.

10.5. Consider a novice operator whose task is to select a valve and turn it off when an appropriate light flashes. Assume that the selection error under optimal stress level is 0.005 with a 90% confidence interval of (0.002 to 0.01). Calculate error probabilities for the other three levels of stress.

10.6. Four redundant electromagnets that control a safety system are all calibrated by one electrician. The failed-dangerous situation occurs if all four magnets are miscalibrated. Construct an HRA event tree, following the procedure leading to Figure 10.8.

10.7. Three identical thermocouple temperature sensors are used to monitor a reaction. All three are calibrated by the same worker. Because they activate a two-out-of-three logic shutdown circuit, a failed-dangerous situation occurs if all three, or two out of three, are miscalibrated. Construct an HRA event tree, following the procedure leading to Figure 10.8.

10.8. **(a)** Enumerate twelve steps for a THERP procedure.

(b) Explain five types of dependency formulae for THERP to calculate a failure probability of activity B, given failure of preceding activity A.

10.9. The tasks described in a procedure manual for dealing with a temperature excursion in a chemical reactor are as follows.

Task 1: Monitor reactor pressure and temperature. If the pressure or temperature continue to rise, initiate tasks 2 and 3.

Task 2: Override the electronically operated feed valve and shut the feed valve manually.

Task 3: Override the electronically controlled cooling water valve, and open valve manually. If the cooling water supply has failed, turn on the emergency (water tower) supply.

Task 1 is done in the control room. Tasks 2 and 3 are carried out at separate locations by different operators who receive instructions by walkie-talkies from the control room. Further details for the tasks are as follows.

1.1. Read pressure (P).

1.2. Read temperature (T).

2.1. Open relay RE-6.

2.2. Shut feed valve VA-2 manually.

3.1. Verify that cooling water pump P-3 is operating.

3.2. Open relay RE-7.

3.3. Open cooling water valve VA-3 fully.

3.3. Verify cooling water flow to reactor by feeling pipe. If no flow, open emergency water supply VA-4.

(a) Construct an HRA event tree for each operator.

(b) Quantify the human errors using appropriate HEPs.

10.10. **(a)** Give performance-shaping factors used in the HCR model.

(b) Describe a formula for determining an actual response time from a nominal median response time.

(c) Explain an HCR model equation for determining a nonresponse probability.

11

Uncertainty Quantification

11.1 INTRODUCTION

11.1.1 Risk-Curve Uncertainty

Uncertainty quantifications should precede final decision making based on PRA-established risk curves of losses and their frequency. Consider a set of points on a particular risk curve: $\{(F_1, L_1), \ldots, (F_m, L_m)\}$, where L_i is a loss caused by accident scenario i and F_i is the scenario frequency (or probability). There are m points for m scenarios. The occurrence likelihood of each scenario is predicted probabilistically by its frequency. We will see in this chapter that the risk curve is far from exact because the scenario frequency is a random variable with significant uncertainty. Risk-curve variability is important because it influences the decision maker, and gives reliability analysts a chance to achieve uncertainty reductions.

A particular scenario i and its initiating event is represented by a path on an event tree, while basic causes of this scenario are analyzed by fault trees. Thus the frequencies of these basic causes (or events) ultimately determine the frequency F_i of scenario i. In other words, the scenario frequency (or probability) is a function of the basic cause frequencies:

$$F_i = F_i(\lambda_1, \ldots, \lambda_n) \tag{11.1}$$

A hardware component failure is a typical basic cause; other causes include human errors and external disturbances. The failure frequency λ_j of component j is estimated from generic failure data, plant-specific failure data, expert evaluation of component design and fabrication, and so on. This frequency estimate takes on a range of values rather than a single exact value, and some values are more likely to occur than others. The component-failure frequency can only be estimated probabilistically, and the frequency itself is a random variable. As a consequence, the scenario frequency F_i is also a random variable.

11.1.2 Parametric Uncertainty and Modeling Uncertainty

The uncertainty in component-failure frequency is a *parametric uncertainty* because the frequency is a basic variable of the scenario frequency function F_i, and because the component-level uncertainty stems from uncertainties in the component-lifetime distribution parameters. The parametric uncertainty can be due to factors such as statistical uncertainty because of finite component test data, or data evaluation uncertainty caused by subjective interpretations of failure data. The data evaluation uncertainty is greater than the statistical uncertainty, which can be obtained using a variety of traditional, theoretical approaches.

Unfortunately, parametric uncertainty is not the only cause of the risk-curve variability. The scenario frequency function F_i itself may not be realistic because of various approximations made during event-tree and fault-tree construction and evaluation, and assumptions about types of component-lifetime distributions, and because the scenarios are not exhaustive, with important initiating events being missed. These three sources of risk-curve variability are *modeling uncertainties*. Elaborate sensitivity analyses and independent PRAs for the same plant must be performed to evaluate modeling uncertainty, and scenario completeness can be facilitated by systematic approaches such as a master logic diagram to enumerate initiating events; however, there is no method for ensuring scenario completeness.

11.1.3 Propagation of Parametric Uncertainty

In this chapter, we describe the transformation of component-level parametric uncertainties to system-level uncertainties. Viable approaches include Monte Carlo methods, analytical moment methods, and discrete probability algebra. The Monte Carlo method is widely applicable, but it requires a mathematical model for the system and a large amount of computer time to reduce statistical fluctuations due to finite simulation trials. The moment method is a deterministic calculation, and requires less computation time, but the system-level output function F_i must be approximated to make the calculation feasible. Discrete probability algebra is efficient for output functions with simple structures, but it requires a large amount of computer memory for complicated functions with many repeated variables. Before describing these propagation approaches, let us first consider the parametric uncertainty from the point of view of statistical confidence intervals, failure data interpretation, and expert opinions.

11.2 PARAMETRIC UNCERTAINTY

11.2.1 Statistical Uncertainty

Statistical uncertainty can be evaluated by classical probability or Bayesian probability; both yield component reliability confidence intervals, as described in Chapter 7. The component-level uncertainty decreases as more failure and success data become available.

Another important aspect of statistical uncertainty is common-cause analysis [1]. The multiple Greek letter model described in Chapter 9 treats common-cause analysis of dependent-component failures. The Greek parameters β and γ are subject to statistical uncertainty as is the component overall failure rate. Denote by n_j the number of common-cause events involving exactly j component failures. Suppose we observe n_1, $2n_2$, and $3n_3$ component failures, thus the total number of failures is $n_1 + 2n_2 + 3n_3$.

Consider a situation where this total number is fixed. For Greek parameters β and γ, the likelihood of observing n_1, $2n_2$, and $3n_3$ is a multinomial distribution:

$$\Pr\{n_1, 2n_2, 3n_3|\beta, \gamma\} = (1-\beta)^{n_1}[\beta(1-\gamma)]^{2n_2}[\beta\gamma]^{3n_3}/\text{const.} \quad (11.2)$$

$$= \beta^{2n_2+3n_3}(1-\beta)^{n_1}\gamma^{3n_3}(1-\gamma)^{2n_2}/\text{const.} \quad (11.3)$$

where the constant is a normalizing factor for the probability:

$$\text{const.} = \sum_{n_1+2n_2+3n_3=\text{fixed}} [\text{numerator}] \quad (11.4)$$

Assume a uniform a priori probability density for β and γ.

$$p\{\beta, \gamma\} = \beta^0(1-\beta)^0\gamma^0(1-\gamma)^0/\text{const.} \quad (11.5)$$

From the Bayes theorem, we have the multinomial posterior probability density of β and γ,

$$p\{\beta, \gamma|n_1, 2n_2, 3n_3\} = \beta^A(1-\beta)^B\gamma^C(1-\gamma)^D/\text{const.} \quad (11.6)$$

where constants A, B, C, and D are

$$A = 2n_2 + 3n_3 \quad (11.7)$$

$$B = n_1 \quad (11.8)$$

$$C = 3n_3 \quad (11.9)$$

$$D = 2n_2 \quad (11.10)$$

The modes, means, and variances of the posterior density are summarized in Table 11.1. The variances decrease as the total number of component failures, $n_1+2n_2+3n_3$, increases. The uncertainties in the Greek parameters can be propagated to the system level to reflect basic-event dependencies by methods to be described shortly.

TABLE 11.1. Mode, Mean, and Variance of Common-Cause Parameters β and γ

	β	γ
Mode	$\dfrac{A}{A+B}$	$\dfrac{C}{C+D}$
Mean	$\dfrac{A+1}{A+B+2}$	$\dfrac{C+1}{C+D+2}$
Variance	$\dfrac{(A+1)(B+1)}{(A+B+2)^2(A+B+3)}$	$\dfrac{(C+1)(D+1)}{(C+D+2)^2(C+D+3)}$

11.2.2 Data Evaluation Uncertainty

Component-failure data analysis is not completely objective; there are many subjective factors. Typical data include number of component failures m, number of demands n, and component exposure time interval T. The statistical uncertainty assumes that m, n, and T are given constants. In practice, these data must be derived from plant and test data, which involves subjective interpretation. The resultant uncertainties in m, n, and T have significant effects on the parametric uncertainty, especially for highly reliable components; one failure per 100 demands gives a failure frequency significantly different from zero failures per 100 demands.

11.2.2.1 Number of failures. Data classification and counting processes are subject to uncertainty. To determine the number of failures, we must first identify the component, its failure mode or success criteria, and causes of failure.

Failure mode and success criteria. Component failures are frequently difficult to define precisely. A small amount of leakage current may be tolerable, but at some higher level it can propagate system failure. In some cases plant data yield questionable information about component-success or -failure states. Suppose the design criteria state that a standby pump must be able to operate continuously for 24 hours after startup. In the plant, however, the standby pump was used for only two hours before being taken off-line; the two hours of successful operation do not ensure 24 hours of continuous operation.

Failure causes. Double counting must be avoided. If a failure due to maintenance error is included as a basic event in a fault tree, then the maintenance failure should not be included as a hardware failure event. Functionally unavailable failures and other cascade failures are often represented by event and fault trees. A common-cause analysis must focus on residual dependencies.

11.2.2.2 Number of demands and exposure time. For a system containing r redundant components, one system demand results in r demands on a component level. The redundancy parameter r is often unavailable, however, especially in generic databases, so we must estimate the average number of components per system. The number of system demands also depends on estimated test frequencies; exposure time T varies according to the number of tests and test duration.

11.2.3 Expert-Evaluated Uncertainty

In some cases the component-failure frequency is estimated solely by expert judgment based on engineering knowledge and experience. This is an extreme case of data uncertainty. The IEEE Std-500 [2] is a catalogue of component-failure rates based on expert evaluation. Each expert provided four estimates for each failure rate: low, recommended, high and maximum; then a consensus value was formed for each category (low, recommended, etc.) by geometric averaging,

$$\lambda = \left[\prod_{i=1}^{n} \lambda_i\right]^{1/n} \tag{11.11}$$

where λ_i is expert i value, and n is the number of experts (about 200). The a priori distribution for the failure rate or the component unavailability is then modified by plant-specific data via the Bayes theorem [3]. Human-error rates are estimated similarly.

Apostolakis et al. [4] found that expert opinions were biased toward low failure frequencies. Mosleh and Apostolakis [3,5] showed that the geometric averaging of expert opinions is based on three debatable assumptions: the experts are independent, they are equally competent, and they have no systematic biases. This aspect is discussed again in Section 11.4.6.

11.3 PLANT-SPECIFIC DATA

In this section, we describe how to combine expert opinion and generic plant data into plant-specific data to evaluate component-unavailability uncertainty.

11.3.1 Incorporating Expert Evaluation as a Prior

Suppose that m_1 fuse failures are observed during n_1 demands at plant 1. This information constitutes plant-specific data D_1 about the fuse failures. These data must be combined with expert opinions EX.

Denote by Q_1 the fuse-failure probability at plant 1. Assume a priori probability density $p\{Q_1\}$. This density is derived from expert knowledge EX. From the Bayes theorem, the posterior probability density of the fuse-failure probability Q_1, given the plant-specific data D_1, becomes

$$p\{Q_1|D_1\} = \Pr\{D_1|Q_1\}p\{Q_1\}/\text{const.} \tag{11.12}$$

$$= \Pr\{m_1, n_1|Q_1\}p\{Q_1\}/\text{const.} \tag{11.13}$$

$$= p\{Q_1\}Q_1^{m_1}(1-Q_1)^{n_1-m_1}/\text{const.} \tag{11.14}$$

where the constants are normalizing factors for $p\{Q_1|D_1\}$. The posterior density represents the uncertainty in the fuse-failure probability. This uncertainty reflects the plant-specific data and expert opinion. This is a single-stage Bayesian approach, and is similar to the Bayes formula in Chapter 7.

11.3.2 Incorporating Generic Plant Data as a Prior

11.3.2.1 Generic and plant-specific data. Component-failure data from one plant cannot be applied directly to another plant because of differences in design, operating procedures, maintenance strategies, or working conditions. Denote by $D_k, k \geq 2$, the similar fuse data in other plants. We now combine plant-specific data D_1, generic plant data D_2 to D_{N+1}, and expert opinion EX to derive a probability density for the fuse-failure probability Q_1 of plant 1.

Consider a total of $N + 1$ plants. Plant 1 is the plant for which the fuse failure probability Q_1 is to be evaluated. Suppose that the experience of generic plant k has been m_k failures out of n_k demands. Then the generic data are

$$D_k = (m_k, n_k), \qquad k = 2, \ldots, N+1 \tag{11.15}$$

11.3.2.2 Single-stage Bayes formula. A single-stage Bayes formula for combining the plant-specific and generic data is

$$p\{Q_1|D_1, \ldots, D_{N+1}\} = \Pr\{D_1, \ldots, D_{N+1}|Q_1\}p\{Q_1\}/\text{const.} \tag{11.16}$$

In this formula, the likelihood $\Pr\{D_1, \ldots, D_{N+1}|Q_1\}$ is the probability of obtaining the plant-specific and generic data when fuse-failure probability Q_1 is assumed for our plant. However, generic plants have different failure probabilities from Q_1 and the likelihood of generic plant data cannot be determined, which is the reason for using a two-stage Bayes approach, where each plant has its own fuse-failure probability.

11.3.2.3 Two-stage Bayes formula

Second-stage Bayes formula. Denote by $\boldsymbol{G} = (D_2, \ldots, D_{N+1})$ the generic plant data. The Bayes formula (11.14) is rewritten to include generic data $D_2, \ldots, D_{N+1}$ as a condition:

$$p\{Q_1|D_1, \mathbf{G}\} = \Pr\{D_1|Q_1, \mathbf{G}\}p\{Q_1|\mathbf{G}\}/\text{const.} \tag{11.17}$$

Because the plant-specific data are obtained independently of the generic plant data,

$$\Pr\{D_1|Q_1, \mathbf{G}\} = \Pr\{D_1|Q_1\} = \Pr\{m_1, n_1|Q_1\} \tag{11.18}$$

Thus

$$p\{Q_1|D_1, \mathbf{G}\} = \Pr\{m_1, n_1|Q_1\}p\{Q_1|\mathbf{G}\}/\text{const.} \tag{11.19}$$

$$= p\{Q_1|\mathbf{G}\}Q_1^{m_1}(1 - Q_1)^{n_1 - m_1}/\text{const.} \tag{11.20}$$

The a priori density $p\{Q_1|\mathbf{G}\}$ in (11.20) is obtained by the first-stage Bayes formula described in the next section. This approach is called a two-stage Bayes approach because two Bayes equations are used [4]; the first stage yields the a priori density $p\{Q_1|\mathbf{G}\}$, and the second stage the a posteriori density $p\{Q_1|D_1, \mathbf{G}\}$ by (11.20).

First-stage Bayes formula. Imagine that fuse-failure probabilities are $N + 1$ samples taken at random from a population. We do not know the exact fuse-failure probability population, however, and we consider r candidate populations. Denote by ϕ the indicator variable of these populations. From expert knowledge EX, we only know a priori that population 1 is likely with probability $\Pr\{\phi = 1\}$, population 2 with probability $\Pr\{\phi = 2\}$, and so on:

$$\Pr\{\phi = j\}, \qquad j = 1, \ldots, r, \qquad (r \geq 1) \tag{11.21}$$

Denote by $\phi_j(Q)$ the density for population j. In terms of the populations, the a priori density is

$$p\{Q_1|\mathbf{G}\} = \sum_{j=1}^{r} p\{Q_1|\phi = j, \mathbf{G}\}\Pr\{\phi = j|\mathbf{G}\} \tag{11.22}$$

$$= \sum_{j=1}^{r} p\{Q_1|\phi = j\}\Pr\{\phi = j|\mathbf{G}\} \tag{11.23}$$

Note in (11.22) that Q_1 is sampled from population j independently of generic data $\mathbf{G}$, given population j. Thus

$$p\{Q_1|\phi = j, \mathbf{G}\} = p\{Q_1|\phi_j = j\} \tag{11.24}$$

Consider the conditional probability density $p\{Q_1|\phi = j\}$. In this expression, the fuse-failure probability Q_1 is a random sample from population j. Because the population has unavailability distribution $\phi_j(Q)$, we have

$$p\{Q_1|\phi = j\} = \phi_j(Q_1) \tag{11.25}$$

Thus the a priori density is

$$p\{Q_1|\mathbf{G}\} = \sum_{j=1}^{r} \phi_j(Q_1)\Pr\{\phi = j|\mathbf{G}\} \tag{11.26}$$

This shows that the a priori density is a weighted sum of populations, where probability $\Pr\{\phi = j|\mathbf{G}\}$ is a weighting factor.

Using the Bayes theorem, the weighting factor can be expressed as

$$\Pr\{\phi = j|\mathbf{G}\} = \Pr\{\phi = j\}\Pr\{\mathbf{G}|\phi = j\}/\text{const.} \tag{11.27}$$

Because the N generic failure probabilities are sampled at random from given population j, we obtain

$$\Pr\{\boldsymbol{G}|\phi = j\} = \prod_{k=2}^{N+1} \Pr\{m_k, n_k|\phi = j\} \tag{11.28}$$

where

$$\Pr\{m_k, n_k|\phi = j\} = \int_0^1 \phi_j(Q_k)\binom{m_k}{n_k} Q_k^{m_k}(1 - Q_k)^{n_k - m_k} dQ_k, \quad k = 2, \ldots, N+1 \tag{11.29}$$

Two-stage Bayes approach. The two-stage Bayes approach proceeds as follows (see Problem 11.2 for populations of discrete Q values).

1. The likelihood of generic plant data D_k, given population j, is obtained from (11.29).
2. The likelihood of N generic plants data $\boldsymbol{G}$, given population j, is obtained from the product expression (11.28).
3. The a priori probability of population j is given by $\Pr\{\phi = j\}$, which is based on expert knowledge EX. This distribution is modified by the first-stage Bayes formula (11.27) to reflect the generic data for N plants.
4. The new a priori density $p\{Q_1|\boldsymbol{G}\}$ is obtained by the weighted sum (11.26).
5. The a posteriori probability density is evaluated using the second-stage Bayes formula (11.14).

11.4 LOG-NORMAL DISTRIBUTION

11.4.1 Introduction

The log-normal distribution plays an important role in uncertainty propagation because reliability parameter confidence intervals such as unavailability and failure rates are often expressed by multiplicative error factors, an AND gate output becomes a log-normal random variable when input variables are log-normal, and log-normal random variables can be used to represent multiplicative dependencies among experts or components. Unfortunately, the OR gate output is not a log-normal variable even if input variables are log-normal. This section describes the log-normal distribution, its relation to confidence intervals, AND gate output characteristics, and a multiplicative dependency model.

11.4.2 Distribution Characteristics

Because a random variable can be viewed as having a range of values, a probability distribution, such as the log-normal, can be assigned this range to obtain the likelihood of occurrence of any one particular value.

When the range or the confidence interval of a variable is expressed as a multiplicative rather than additive error factor, the log-normal is the proper distribution to describe the variable.

Variable Q has a log-normal distribution if its natural logarithm $X = \ln Q$ has a normal distribution with mean μ and variance σ^2. Characteristics of this distribution are summarized in Table 11.2. The density function is shown in Figure 11.1. Because parameter

μ is the median of $\ln Q$, the median $\tilde{Q}$ of Q is

$$\tilde{Q} = \exp(\mu) \tag{11.30}$$

The mode, mean, and variance can be calculated from the median. The mode is smaller than the median, while the mean $\overline{Q}$ is larger than the median; these differences become more significant as parameter σ^2 becomes larger:

$$\text{Mode} = \tilde{Q}\exp(-\sigma^2) < \text{Median} = \tilde{Q} < \text{Mean} \equiv \overline{Q} = \tilde{Q}\exp(0.5\sigma^2) \tag{11.31}$$

The variance is

$$V\{Q\} = \exp(\sigma^2)\exp(2\mu)\left[\exp(\sigma^2) - 1\right] = (\overline{Q})^2\left[(\overline{Q}/\tilde{Q})^2 - 1\right] \tag{11.32}$$

TABLE 11.2. Log-Normal Distribution

Symbol	$\log-\text{gau}^*(\mu, \sigma^2)$
Variable	$0 < Q$
Location Parameter	$-\infty < \mu < \infty$
Scale Parameter	$0 < \sigma$
Density	$\frac{1}{\sqrt{2\pi}\sigma Q}\exp\left[-\frac{1}{2}\left(\frac{\ln Q-\mu}{\sigma}\right)^2\right]$
$1 - 2\alpha$ Error Factor	K
$1 - 2\alpha$ Interval	$[Q_L \equiv \tilde{Q}/K, \quad Q_U \equiv \tilde{Q}K]$
Median $\tilde{Q}$	$\sqrt{Q_U Q_L}$
Parameter μ	$\ln \tilde{Q}$
α point L	$\Pr\{x \geq L\} = \alpha, \quad x \sim \text{gau}^*(0, 1)$
Parameter σ	$(\ln K)/L$
Median $\tilde{Q}$	$\exp(\mu)$
Mode	$\tilde{Q}\exp(-\sigma^2)$
Mean $\overline{Q}$	$\tilde{Q}\exp(0.5\sigma^2)$
Variance $V\{Q\}$	$(\overline{Q})^2[(\overline{Q}/\tilde{Q})^2 - 1]$
$Q_s = Q_1 \cdots Q_n$	$\sim \log-\text{gau}^*(\sum_{i=1}^n \mu_i, \sum_{i=1}^n \sigma_i^2)$
$\tilde{Q}_s$	$\tilde{Q}_1 \cdots \tilde{Q}_n$
$\overline{Q}_s$	$\overline{Q}_1 \cdots \overline{Q}_n$
$V\{Q_s\}$	$(\overline{Q}_s)^2[(\overline{Q}_s/\tilde{Q}_s)^2 - 1]$

11.4.3 Log-Normal Determination

Suppose that a random variable Q has a $1 - 2\alpha$ confidence interval between $Q_L \equiv \tilde{Q}/K$ and $Q_U \equiv \tilde{Q}K$, where $\tilde{Q}$ is the median and K is a multiplicative error factor constant greater than one. In other words, let Q_L and Q_U be the $1 - \alpha$ and α points, respectively.*

$$\Pr\{Q \geq Q_L\} = 1 - \alpha, \qquad \Pr\{Q \geq Q_U\} = \alpha \tag{11.33}$$

---

*Q_L and Q_U are also called 100αth and $100(1-\alpha)$th percentiles, respectively.

$$\Pr\{Q \leq Q_L\} = \alpha, \quad \Pr\{Q \leq Q_U\} = 1 - \alpha$$

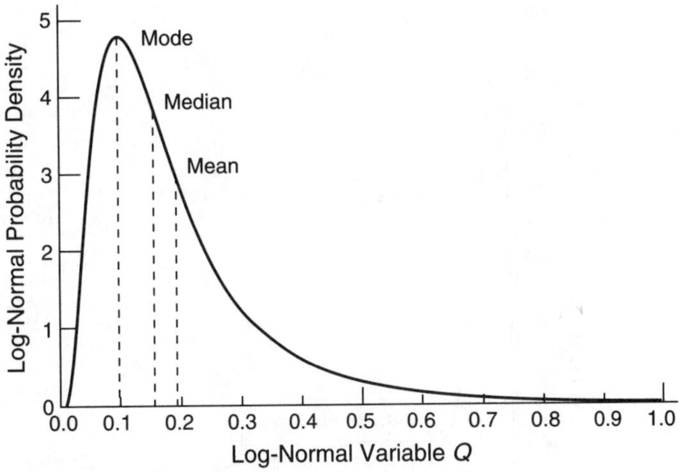

Figure 11.1. Log-normal density.

Variable Q falls in the range $[\tilde{Q}/K, \tilde{Q}K]$ with a probability of $1 - 2\alpha$.

$$\Pr\{Q \in [\tilde{Q}/K, \tilde{Q}K]\} = 1 - 2\alpha \tag{11.34}$$

Because $\tilde{Q}$ is a median, parameter μ is

$$\mu = \ln \tilde{Q} \tag{11.35}$$

It is seen that $[(\ln Q) - \mu]/\sigma$ is a zero mean and unit-variance normal random variable with confidence interval:

$$\Pr\{[(\ln Q) - \mu]/\sigma \in [-(\ln K)/\sigma, \quad (\ln K)/\sigma]\} = 1 - 2\alpha \tag{11.36}$$

Denote by L the $100(1 - \alpha)$th percentile (or α point) of the normal distribution with zero mean and unit variance.

$$\Pr\{x \le L\} = 1 - \alpha, \qquad x \sim \text{gau}^*(0, 1) \tag{11.37}$$

The log-normal distribution parameters for variable Q are determined by the following formulas:

$$(\ln K)/\sigma = L, \qquad \text{or} \quad \sigma = (\ln K)/L \tag{11.38}$$

Example 1—Log-normal parameters μ and σ. Consider the three components in Table 11.3; three median unavailabilities and a common 90% error factor $K = 3.0$ are given. The parameters μ and σ for these three components are given in the table. The three log-normal densities are shown in Figure 11.2. Figure 11.3 shows how component 1 log-normal density varies according to different error factors. ■

Example 2—Mean, variance, and mode. Consider the components in Table 11.3. Using the formulas of Table 11.2, the means, variances, and modes of component unavailabilities are as given in Table 11.4. ■

11.4.4 Human-Error-Rate Confidence Intervals

According to Apostolakis et al. [6], the authors of the *Handbook of Human Reliability* [7] suggest that for HEPs (human error probabilities) the uncertainty bounds in Table 10.2 be

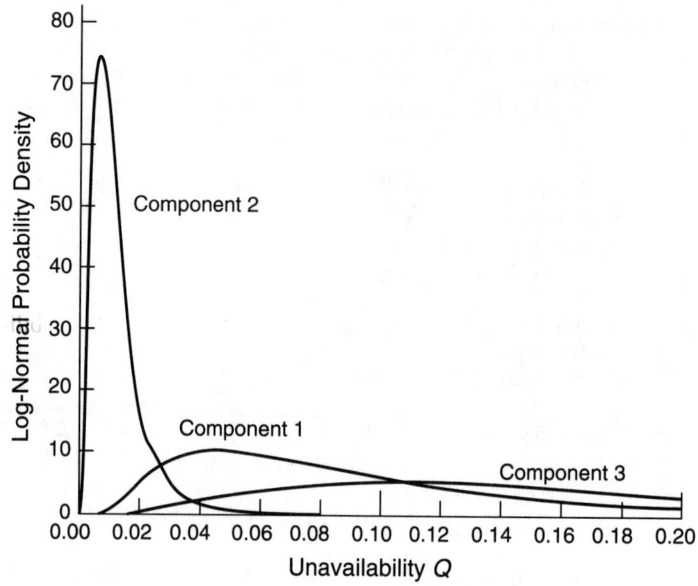

Figure 11.2. Log-normal densities for the three components.

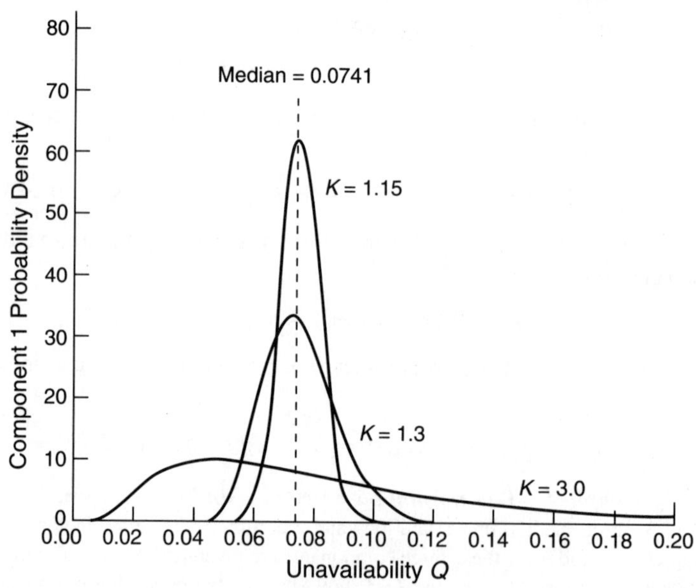

Figure 11.3. Component 1 log-normal density with different error factors.

used as the 0.95 and 0.05 points (i.e., 5th and 95th percentiles) of a log-normal distribution. Others use these bounds as 0.9 and 0.1 points because experts tend to be overconfident in their assessment of HEP distributions. Swain and Guttmann do not appear to object to this practice.

For HEPs greater or equal to 0.1, reference [8] recommends a beta density to describe HEP uncertainty.

$$\Pr\{Q \le \text{HEP} < Q + dQ\} = \frac{1}{\text{const.}} Q^r (1 - Q)^s dQ, \qquad 0 \le Q \le 1 \tag{11.39}$$

TABLE 11.3. Log-Normal Characteristics for Example Components

Component	Median Unavailability $\tilde{Q}$	90% Error Factor K	Location Parameter $\mu = \ln \tilde{Q}$	0.05 point = 95th Percentile L	Scale Parameter $\sigma = (\ln K)/L$
1	7.41×10^{-2}	3.0	−2.602	1.605	0.6845
2	9.90×10^{-3}	3.0	−4.615	1.605	0.6845
3	1.53×10^{-1}	3.0	−1.877	1.605	0.6845

TABLE 11.4. Mean, Median, Mode, and Variance of Component Availabilities

Component	Location μ	Scale σ	Median $\tilde{Q} = \exp(\mu)$	Mean $\overline{Q} = \tilde{Q} \exp(0.5\,\sigma^2)$	Variance $V\{Q\} = \overline{Q}^2[(\overline{Q}/\tilde{Q})^2 - 1]$	Mode $\tilde{Q} \exp(-\sigma^2)$
1	−2.602	0.6845	7.41×10^{-2}	9.37×10^{-2}	5.24×10^{-3}	4.64×10^{-2}
2	−4.615	0.6845	9.90×10^{-3}	1.25×10^{-2}	9.28×10^{-5}	6.20×10^{-3}
3	−1.877	0.6845	1.53×10^{-1}	1.93×10^{-1}	2.20×10^{-2}	9.58×10^{-2}

where const. is a normalization factor, r and s are both greater than zero, and the mean $\overline{Q}$ is given by $\overline{Q} = (r+1)/(r+s+2)$.

The choice of r and s generally involves a process of choosing the smallest integers larger than zero that give an appropriate $\overline{Q}$ point estimate. For example, if $\overline{Q} = 0.1$, then $r = 1$ and $s = 17$; if $\overline{Q} = 0.7$, then $r = 6$ and $s = 2$.

For HEPs less than 0.1, the guidelines stated in [7] can be used to assign a log-normal density to the HEP.

$$\Pr\{Q \le \text{HEP} < Q + dQ\} = \frac{1}{\sqrt{2\pi}\sigma Q} \exp\left[\frac{-(\ln Q - \mu)^2}{2\sigma^2}\right] dQ, \qquad Q > 0 \tag{11.40}$$

where the mean $\overline{Q}$ and the median $\tilde{Q}$ are given by

$$\overline{Q} = \tilde{Q}\exp(0.5\sigma^2), \qquad \tilde{Q} = \exp(\mu) \tag{11.41}$$

Denote by $Q_{0.05}$ and $Q_{0.95}$ the 0.05 and 0.95 points, respectively ($Q_{0.05} > Q_{0.95}$). If the range is estimated to be 100 (i.e., $Q_{0.05}/Q_{0.95} = 100$), then error factor K is 10, and σ is $\ln(10)/1.605 = 1.4$. Suppose that the mean HEP is $\overline{Q}$. The HEP is considered to be log-normally distributed about a median, $\tilde{Q} = \overline{Q}\exp(-0.5\sigma^2) = 0.38\overline{Q}$, with the 0.05 point being $Q_{0.05} = 10\tilde{Q} = 3.8\overline{Q}$ and the 0.95 point $Q_{0.95} = \tilde{Q}/10 = 0.038\overline{Q}$.

11.4.5 Product of Log-Normal Variables

Consider a parallel system with n statistically independent components where the failure can be expressed as an AND gate output, and the system corresponds to a minimal cut set of a fault tree. Assume that unavailability of component i is distributed with a log-normal distribution with parameters μ_i and σ_i. Then the parallel system unavailability $Q_s = Q_1 \cdots Q_n$ is also distributed with a log-normal distribution because $\ln Q_s$ is a sum of the normal random variable $\ln Q_i$. As shown in Table 11.2, log-normal parameters μ_s and σ_s for the AND gate unavailability Q_s are given by the sum of the component parameters.

$$Q_i \sim \log -\text{gau}^*(\mu_i, \sigma_i^2) \tag{11.42}$$

$$Q_s = \prod_{i=1}^{n} Q_i \sim \log -\text{gau}^*(\mu_s, \sigma_s^2) \tag{11.43}$$

$$\mu_s = \sum_{i=1}^{n} \mu_i \tag{11.44}$$

$$\sigma_s^2 = \sum_{i=1}^{n} \sigma_i^2 \tag{11.45}$$

Median $\tilde{Q}_s$ and mean $\overline{Q_s}$ of Q_s are given by products of component medians and means, respectively:

$$\tilde{Q}_s = \exp(\mu_s) = \exp(\sum_{i=1}^{n} \mu_i) = \prod_{i=1}^{n} \tilde{Q}_i \tag{11.46}$$

$$\overline{Q_s} = E\{\prod_{i=1}^{n} Q_i\} = \prod_{i=1}^{n} \overline{Q_i} \tag{11.47}$$

Because variable Q_s is log-normally distributed, its variance $V\{Q_s\}$ is

$$V\{Q_s\} = (\overline{Q_s})^2[(\overline{Q_s}/\tilde{Q}_s)^2 - 1] \tag{11.48}$$

This variance can also be expressed in terms of component medians and means:

$$V\{Q_s\} = \left[\prod_{i=1}^{n} (\overline{Q_i})^2\right]\left[\prod_{i=1}^{n} \left(\overline{Q_i}/\tilde{Q}_i\right)^2 - 1\right] \tag{11.49}$$

Example 3—AND gate. Consider a three-component parallel system consisting of the first component of Table 11.4. This is an AND gate, or cut set with three identical components. Calculate median $\tilde{Q}_s$, mean $\overline{Q_s}$, and variance $V\{Q_s\}$ of system unavailability Q_s from system log-normal parameters μ_s and σ_s, and from component mean $\overline{Q_i} = \overline{Q}$ and median $\tilde{Q}_i = \tilde{Q}$.

Solution: The system log-normal parameters are calculated as

$$\mu_s = -3 \times 2.602 = -7.806 \tag{11.50}$$

$$\sigma_s^2 = 3 \times 0.6845^2 = 1.406, \quad \text{or} \quad \sigma_s = 1.186 \tag{11.51}$$

Median $\tilde{Q}_s$, mean $\overline{Q_s}$, and variance $V\{Q_s\}$ are calculated from μ_s and σ_s as

$$\tilde{Q}_s = \exp(\mu_S) = \exp(-7.806) = 4.07 \times 10^{-4} \tag{11.52}$$

$$\overline{Q_s} = \tilde{Q}_s \exp(0.5\sigma_s^2) = 4.07 \times 10^{-4} \exp(0.5 \times 1.406) = 8.22 \times 10^{-4} \tag{11.53}$$

$$V\{Q_s\} = (\overline{Q_s})^2[(\overline{Q_s}/\tilde{Q}_s)^2 - 1] = 2.08 \times 10^{-6} \tag{11.54}$$

The system median, mean, and variance are obtained directly from the component mean $\overline{Q}$ and median $\tilde{Q}$.

$$\tilde{Q}_s = \tilde{Q}^3 = (7.41 \times 10^{-2})^3 = 4.07 \times 10^{-4} \tag{11.55}$$

$$\overline{Q_s} = \overline{Q}^3 = 8.22 \times 10^{-4} \tag{11.56}$$

$$V\{Q_s\} = (\overline{Q}^3)^2[(\overline{Q}^3/\tilde{Q}^3)^2 - 1] = 2.08 \times 10^{-6} \tag{11.57}$$

■

11.4.6 Bias and Dependence

In this section we first describe when the geometric mean formula (11.11) is justified. This formula is then applied to consensus estimates from expert evaluation of component-reliability parameters. A similar approach applies to components subject to operating conditions specific to a plant. These types of dependencies among reliability parameters sometimes become dominant in the uncertainty quantification of system unavailability estimates. This is similar to the dependencies among basic event occurrences yielding dominant effects on system unavailability point-value determinations.

11.4.6.1 Among experts. Consider a situation where a reliability parameter Y such as a component-failure rate or unavailability is evaluated by n experts. Denote by M the true value of Y. Introduce the following sum of normal random variable models for expert i:

$$\begin{aligned} \ln Y_i &= \ln M + \ln X_i + \ln Z \\ &\sim \text{gau}^*(\ln M + \mu_i + \mu_D, \sigma_i^2 + \sigma_D^2) \end{aligned} \tag{11.58}$$

where $\ln X_i$ and $\ln Z$ are independent normal random variables:

$$\ln X_i \sim \text{gau}^*(\mu_i, \sigma_i^2), \qquad \ln Z \sim \text{gau}^*(\mu_D, \sigma_D^2) \tag{11.59}$$

Common variable Z represents a statistical dependency among the experts, individual variable X_i represents an independent contribution to estimate Y_i from expert i, and means μ_i and μ_D are biases of $\ln Y_i$.

Equation (11.58) can be rewritten as:

$$\begin{aligned} Y_i &= M X_i Z \\ X_i &\sim \log-\text{gau}^*(\mu_i, \sigma_i^2) \\ Z &\sim \log-\text{gau}^*(\mu_D, \sigma_D^2) \\ M &= \text{ unknown true value} \end{aligned} \tag{11.60}$$

Variable Y_i has a log-normal distribution:

$$Y_i \sim \log-\text{gau}^*(\log M + \mu_i + \mu_D, \sigma_i^2 + \sigma_D^2) \tag{11.61}$$

with median

$$\tilde{Y}_i = M B_i, \qquad B_i \equiv \exp(\mu_i)\exp(\mu_D) \tag{11.62}$$

In other words, the expert i median value has bias B_i, which stems from nonzero means μ_i and μ_D in the log-scale representation.

Mean $\overline{Y}_i$ is given by

$$\overline{Y}_i = M B_i \exp(0.5\sigma_i^2 + 0.5\sigma_D^2) \tag{11.63}$$

Thus even if means μ_i and μ_D are zero, mean $\overline{Y}_i$ is biased due to variances σ_i^2 and σ_D^2.

Assume that the n experts are independent, that is, $Z \equiv 0$ or $\mu_D = \sigma_D = 0$; they are equally competent, that is, $\sigma_i \equiv \sigma$ and $\mu_i \equiv \mu$; and that they do not have any systematic bias, that is, $\mu_i = \mu = 0$. Then the probability density of obtaining expert data $Y_1, \ldots, Y_n$ can be expressed as

$$p\{Y_1, \ldots, Y_n\} = \prod_{i=1}^{n} \frac{1}{\sqrt{2\pi}\sigma Y_i} \exp\left[-\frac{1}{2}\left(\frac{\ln Y_i - \ln M}{\sigma}\right)^2\right]$$

Maximizing this density with respect to M gives the maximum-likelihood estimator of the unknown true value:

$$M = \left[\prod_{i=1}^{n} Y_i \right]^{1/n} \tag{11.64}$$

Thus under the dubious assumptions above, the geometric mean (11.11) is the best estimate of component-failure rate or unavailability. The maximum-likelihood estimator can be generalized to cases where the three assumptions do not hold.

11.4.6.2 Among components. If expert i is replaced by component i in the model of (11.60), it applies to the case where unavailabilities of n components have biases and statistical dependencies [9]. Such biases and dependencies represent, for instance, plant-specific operating conditions such as chemical corrosion. The resultant component-reliability parameter dependencies propagate to system levels by the methods described in the next section.

Example 4—Bias due to management deficiency. Assume the cooling system in Figure 11.4 with a principal pump that normally sends cooling water to a designated location [10]. A standby emergency pump sends water when the principal pump is down. A normally closed valve located upstream of the emergency pump must be opened on demand when the emergency pump is needed. The principal pump and emergency pump are of different type and manufacture. All three components are maintained by the same crew, however, and failure rates are affected by the quality of the maintenance team. This quality of maintenance, which is affected by plant organization and management policies, will influence all three components and raises or lowers their failure rate.

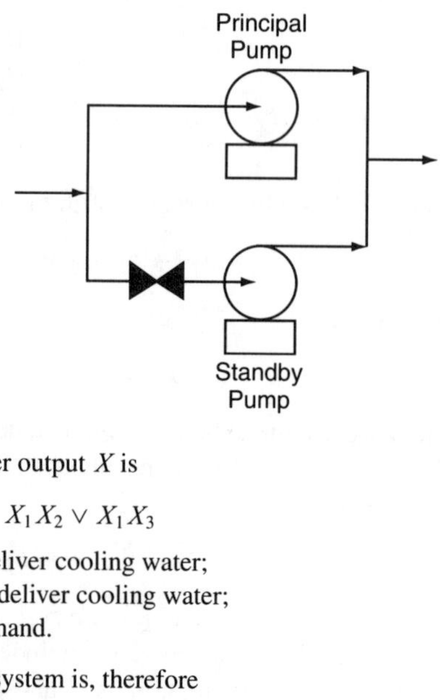

Figure 11.4. A cooling system with principal and standby pumps.

The event that there is no cooling water output X is

$$X = X_1X_2 \vee X_1X_3$$

where $X_1 =$ the principal pump fails to deliver cooling water;
$X_2 =$ the emergency pump fails to deliver cooling water;
$X_3 =$ the valve fails to open on demand.

The failure probability of the cooling system is, therefore

$$P\{X\} = P\{X_1X_2\} + P\{X_1X_3\} - P\{X_1X_2X_3\}$$

If the three events are independent with the same failure probability 0.1, then the cooling system fails about 1 in 50 demands.

$$P\{X\} = 0.1 \times 0.1 + 0.1 \times 0.1 - 0.1 \times 0.1 \times 0.1 = 0.019$$

Assume that the maintenance quality is so low that the principal pump fails with probability 0.2, and that the emergency pump and the valve fail with probability 0.8. These failures still occur independently, but failure probabilities have increased. The cooling-system failure probability becomes much larger (about one in five demands) than in the former case:

$$P\{X\} = 0.2 \times 0.8 + 0.2 \times 0.8 - 0.2 \times 0.8 \times 0.8 = 0.192$$

The high failure probability, 0.8, of the standby components may be due to latent failures prior to the principal pump failure. ■

11.5 UNCERTAINTY PROPAGATION

To facilitate the quantitative analysis of fault trees, it is convenient to represent fault trees in mathematical form: the structure functions and minimal cut set representations described in Chapter 8 are appropriate tools for this purpose. System unavailability $Q_s(t)$ may be obtained by methods such as complete expansion and partial pivotal decomposition of the structure function. For large and complex fault trees, the inclusion-exclusion principle based on minimal cut sets can be used to approximate $Q_s(t)$.

Figure 11.5 has the following structure function ψ and the corresponding system unavailability $Q_s(t)$.

$$\psi(Y) = 1 - (1 - Y_1)(1 - Y_2Y_3) \quad (11.65)$$

$$Q_s = 1 - (1 - Q_1)(1 - Q_2Q_3) \quad (11.66)$$

The inclusion and exclusion principle or an expansion of (11.66) gives the exact unavailability

$$Q_s = Q_1 + Q_2Q_3 - Q_1Q_2Q_3 \quad (11.67)$$

which is approximated by the first bracket

$$Q_s = Q_1 + Q_2Q_3 \quad (11.68)$$

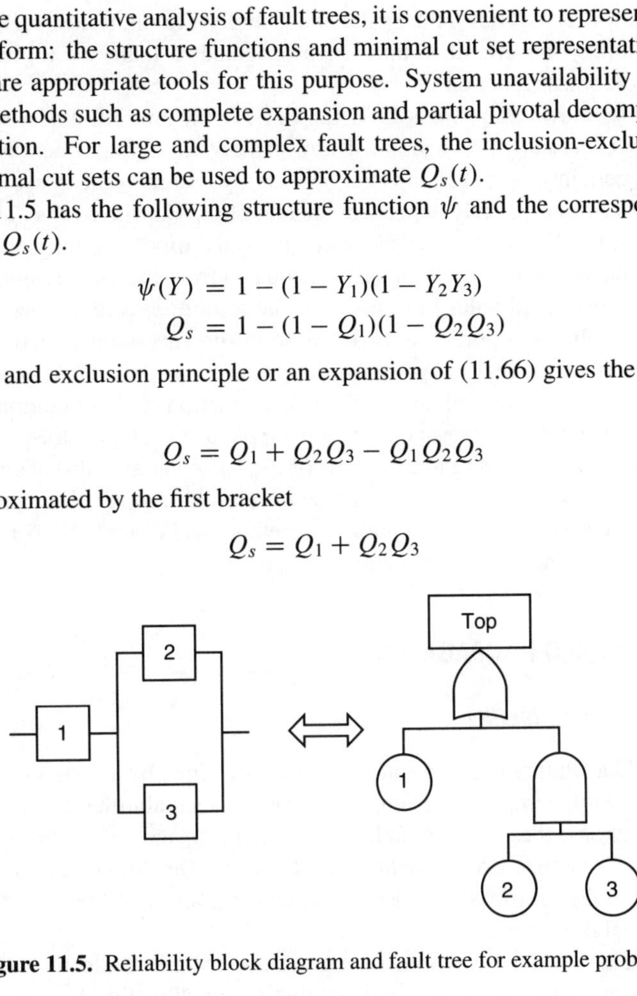

Figure 11.5. Reliability block diagram and fault tree for example problem.

For independent basic events, system unavailability Q_s is a multiple-linear polynomial function of component unavailabilities $Q_1, \ldots, Q_n$.

$$Q_s = \sum_{j=1}^{n} \left[\sum_{1 \le k_1 < \cdots < k_j \le n} \alpha_{k_1,\ldots,k_j} Q_{k_1} \cdots Q_{k_j} \right] \quad (11.69)$$

where each term in the sum is a product of j component unavailabilities. For the system unavailability expression (11.67),

$$Q_s = \underbrace{Q_1}_{j=1} + \underbrace{Q_2 Q_3}_{j=2} - \underbrace{Q_1 Q_2 Q_3}_{j=3} \tag{11.70}$$

For dependent basic events, consider a 2/3 valve system subject to a common cause. As shown in Chapter 9, the demand-failure probability V of the system is

$$V = V_3 + 3V_2 + 3V_1^2 \tag{11.71}$$

$$\simeq V_3 + 3V_2 = \gamma\beta\lambda + 3(1/2)(1-\gamma)\beta\lambda \tag{11.72}$$

$$= Y = F(\lambda, \beta, \gamma) \tag{11.73}$$

where λ is an overall failure rate, and β and γ are multiple Greek letter parameters. The λ, β, and γ uncertainties must be propagated to fault-tree top-event levels through the multiple-linear function F.

As shown in Sections 11.7.5 and 11.7.6, the multiple-linearity simplifies the unavailability-uncertainty propagation. Unfortunately, the output function $Y = F(X_1, \ldots, X_n)$ in the uncertainty propagation is not necessarily multiple-linear, especially when some basic events have statistically dependent uncertainties. Consider valve failures to be independent in (11.71): $V = 3V_1^2$. If the valve unavailability uncertainties are completely dependent, the uncertainty of V_1^2 must be evaluated from the uncertainty of V_1.

When fixed values are used for the failure rates and other parameters, the system unavailability is a point value. Because of the uncertainties and variations in the failure rates and parameters, however, these quantities are treated as random variables and, because the system unavailability $Q_s(t)$ is a function of these random variables, it is itself a random variable. The term *uncertainty propagation* refers to the process of determining the output variable distribution in terms of the basic variable distributions, given a functional relation $Y = F(X_1, \ldots, X_n)$. Three uncertainty propagation approaches are the Monte Carlo method, the analytical moment method, and discrete probability algebra: These are described in the next three sections.

11.6 MONTE CARLO PROPAGATION

11.6.1 Unavailability

Uncertainty propagation is conveniently done by a computerized Monte Carlo technique. In its simplest version, component unavailabilities are sampled from probability distributions, these unavailabilities are then propagated toward a top event, and a point value is calculated for system unavailability. The Monte Carlo sampling is repeated a large number of times, and the resultant point values are then used to evaluate the system unavailability uncertainty.

The SAMPLE computer program uses Monte Carlo to obtain the mean, standard deviation, probability range, and distribution for a function $Y = F(X_1, \ldots, X_n)$ [11]. This function can, for example, be system unavailability Q_s in terms of component unavailabilities $Q_1, \ldots, Q_n$. The function F could also be system reliability R_s, in terms of variable component-failure and -repair rates. Common-cause parameters such as those in (11.72) may be included as basic variables. Multiplicative dependency models such as (11.60) can also be simulated by Monte Carlo.

Given a function $Y = F(X_1, \ldots, X_n)$, values of the distribution parameters of the independent variables, and a specific input distribution, SAMPLE obtains a Monte Carlo sampling $x_1, \ldots, x_n$ from the input variable distributions and evaluates the corresponding $Y = F(x_1, \ldots, x_n)$. The sampling is repeated N (input parameter) times, and the resultant estimates of Y are ordered in ascending values $y_1 \leq y_2 \leq \cdots \leq y_N$ to obtain the percentiles of the Y distribution. The program has a choice of failure distributions as an input option (normal, log-normal, log-uniform, etc.).

Example 5—SAMPLE program. To illustrate the SAMPLE program and propagation technique we consider the system for which a reliability block diagram and fault tree are shown in Figure 11.5. The event data that contain the uncertainties in the above system are given in Table 11.3.

The system unavailability Q_s can be approximated as the first bracket of the inclusion-exclusion formula:

$$Q_s = Q_1 + Q_2 Q_3 \tag{11.74}$$

This function is included in the SAMPLE input as a function supplied by the user. The results of the computations are given in terms of probability confidence limits; the output is shown in Table 11.5.

TABLE 11.5. SAMPLE output

Distribution Confidence Limits	
Confidence (%)	Function Value
0.5	1.77×10^{-2}
1.0	1.88×10^{-2}
2.0	2.21×10^{-2}
5.0	2.66×10^{-2}
10.0	3.34×10^{-2}
20.0	4.47×10^{-2}
25.0	5.11×10^{-2}
30.0	5.69×10^{-2}
40.0	6.65×10^{-2}
50.0	7.67×10^{-2}
60.0	9.23×10^{-2}
70.0	1.09×10^{-1}
75.0	1.19×10^{-1}
80.0	1.31×10^{-1}
90.0	1.77×10^{-1}
95.0	2.22×10^{-1}
97.5	2.56×10^{-1}
99.0	3.15×10^{-1}
99.5	3.91×10^{-1}

Sample size: 1200
Mean: 9.48×10^{-2}
Variance: 4.53×10^{-3}
Standard deviation: 6.73×10^{-2}

Function values are the upper bounds of the indicated confidence limits. The 50% value is the median of the distribution, and the 95th and 5th percentiles are the upper and lower bounds of the 90% probability interval, respectively. ■

The SAMPLE program also generates frequency distribution functions like the histogram of Figure 11.6. The median point and the 90% confidence interval are indicated on the figure.

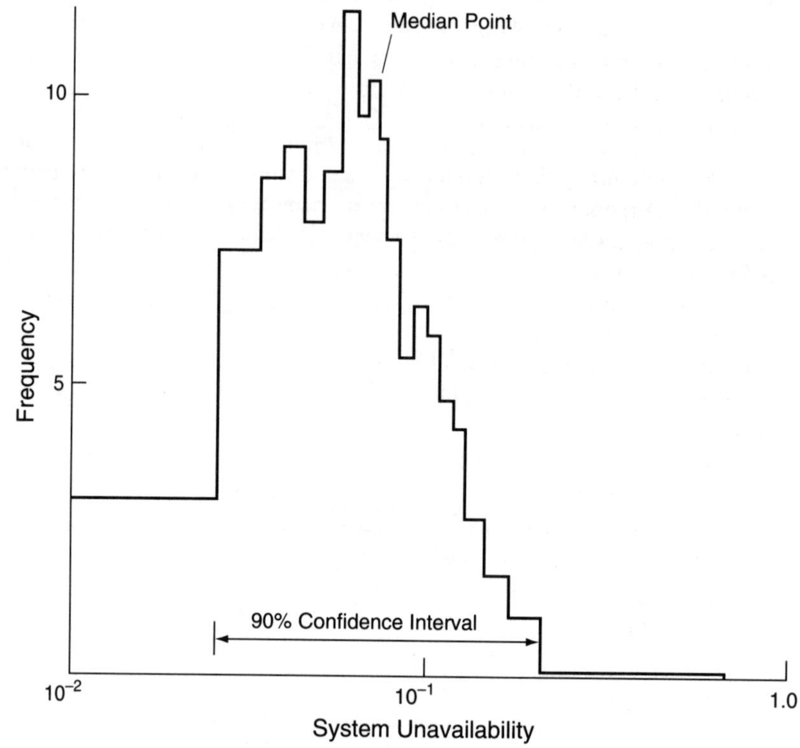

Figure 11.6. Confidence limits for top event by SAMPLE program.

11.6.2 Distribution Parameters

When component test data are available, we can propagate their values through component-lifetime distributions. Several techniques have been proposed; it should be noted, however, that the SAMPLE-type unavailability propagation based on the log-normal distributions is usually sufficient for practical purposes.

From a point of view of component testing, the distribution parameter propagation is classified into two types: binomial data and lifetime data.

Propagation of pass-fail or binomial data. Several methods are compared in reference [12]. Suppose that m failures are observed during a total of n tests. Denote by Q the component unavailability, and assume a priori probability density $p\{Q\}$. From the Bayes theorem, the posterior probability density of component reliability becomes

$$p\{Q|m,n\} = \Pr\{m,n|Q\}p\{Q\}/\text{const.} \tag{11.75}$$

$$= p\{Q\}Q^m(1-Q)^{n-m}/\text{const.} \tag{11.76}$$

Consider a prior such as a beta density with parameter values of 0.5:

$$p\{Q\} = Q^{0.5}(1-Q)^{0.5}/\text{const.} \tag{11.77}$$

This type of prior is one that contributes little prior information to the analysis relative to the binomial component test data. The component reliability is sampled from the posterior beta distribution with parameters $m + 0.5$ and $n - m + 0.5$. This technique is a Bayes method.

In a so-called *bootstrap method* [13], the component unavailability is first estimated from the binomial test data as $\hat{Q} = m/n$. Then the number of failures m^* is sampled by Monte Carlo from the binomial distribution $\hat{Q}^m(1 - \hat{Q})^{n-m}$. The unavailability estimate $Q^* = m^*/n$ is used as a component unavailability sample.

Propagation of lifetime data. Maximum-likelihood parameter estimations are summarized in Appendix A.1. This estimation starts with censored lifetime data that apply to time-terminated tests and failure-terminated tests. Equation (A.9) shows that a parameter estimator vector is asymptotically distributed and has a multidimension normal distribution. Furthermore, the component unavailability estimator, as shown in (A.11), is also asymptotically distributed with a normal distribution.

Parameter vector sampling from a multidimension normal distribution is called a *bivariate* s-*normal technique*, while reliability sampling from a single-dimension normal distribution is a *univariate* s-*normal technique* [14]. In the univariate beta technique, the normal distribution is replaced by a beta distribution; the beta distribution is used because, for values of unavailability smaller than 0.1, the component unavailability distribution is skewed; in addition, under the s-normal assumption, with the unavailability close to zero, a high percentage of the simulated reliability values are smaller than zero.

In the double Monte Carlo technique, a maximum-likelihood estimator (MLE) $\hat{\boldsymbol{\theta}}$ of unknown parameter vector $\boldsymbol{\theta}$ is first calculated from actual data. Artificial lifetime data are sampled randomly from the distribution determined by $\hat{\boldsymbol{\theta}}$. Another MLE is calculated from the simulation data, and used as a sample from the distribution parameter $\hat{\boldsymbol{\theta}}$. This is an extension of the bootstrap method for binomial test data.

11.6.3 Latin Hypercube Sampling

The direct Monte Carlo sampling is performed randomly and independently. Thus for a small sample size, there is a possibility that some regions of variable X_i are never sampled. This results in a large error, especially when there is a lack of sampling for variables that dominate output Y. The Latin hypercube sampling [15] is a mixture of random and systematic sampling to ensure that each interval or stratum of variable X_i is visited by exactly one Monte Carlo sample.

The range of variable X_i is divided into N strata of equal probability $1/N$. A value of X_i is sampled from each stratum according to a probability density proportional to $p\{X_i\}$, that is, the conditional probability of variable X_i, given that the variable takes on a value in the stratum. Denote by X_{ij}, $j = 1, \ldots, N$ the set of samples of variable X_i; X_{i1} sampled from the first stratum, and X_{iN} from the last stratum. Similar samples are generated for other variables. In a matrix form, we have the following input variable samples.

$$\begin{pmatrix} \text{stratum 1} & \cdots & \text{stratum } N \\ X_{11} & \cdots & X_{1N} \\ X_{21} & \cdots & X_{2N} \\ \vdots & \cdots & \vdots \\ X_{n1} & \cdots & X_{nN} \end{pmatrix} \begin{matrix} \\ \text{for variable } X_1 \\ \text{for variable } X_2 \\ \vdots \\ \text{for variable } X_n \end{matrix} \tag{11.78}$$

When these samples are randomly combined, we have ordinary Monte Carlo samples for n-dimension vector $(X_1, X_2, \ldots, X_n)$. In Latin hypercube sampling, row elements of the sampling matrix are randomly permuted within each row; this permutation is repeated independently for every row, and a new sampling matrix is obtained. Each column vector of the resultant sampling matrix becomes an n-dimension Latin hypercube sample. Thus we have a total of N samples. A value is sampled from each stratum, and this value appears exactly once in a column vector sample.

Denote by $(x_1, \ldots, x_n)$ a sample obtained by Latin hypercube sampling. This sample is distributed according to the original probability density:

$$p\{x_1, \ldots, x_n\} = p\{X_1 = x_1\} \cdots p\{X_n = x_n\} \tag{11.79}$$

Thus component values within a sample vector are independent. Different sample vectors are not independent any more, however, because a stratum component value appears only once in exactly one Latin hypercube sample.

Example 6—Latin hypercube sampling. Assume the following sampling data ($N = 3$ and $n = 2$):

$$\begin{pmatrix} -5 & 1 & 25 \\ -10 & 5 & 20 \end{pmatrix}, \quad \text{(2 dimension, 3 strata)} \tag{11.80}$$

Random permutations in each row may yield

$$\begin{pmatrix} 1 & -5 & 25 \\ 20 & 5 & -10 \end{pmatrix} \tag{11.81}$$

The two-dimension Latin hypercube samples become

$$\begin{pmatrix} 1 \\ 20 \end{pmatrix}, \begin{pmatrix} -5 \\ 5 \end{pmatrix}, \begin{pmatrix} 25 \\ -10 \end{pmatrix} \tag{11.82}$$

■

One advantage of Latin hypercube sampling appears when output Y is dominated by only a few input variables. The method ensures that each variable is represented in a fully stratified manner, no matter which component turns out to be important [15].

Consider a class of Monte Carlo estimators of the form

$$T(Y_1, \ldots, Y_N) = (1/N) \sum_{i=1}^{N} g(Y_i) \tag{11.83}$$

where Y_i is an output value from Monte Carlo trial i. If $g(Y) = Y$ then T represents the sample mean used to estimate $E\{Y\}$. If $g(Y) = Y^k$ we obtain the kth sample moment. By letting $g(Y) = 1$ for $Y \leq y$, and 0 otherwise, we obtain the usual empirical distribution function at point y. Denote by T_D and T_L estimators of direct Monte Carlo and Latin hypercube sampling, respectively.

The estimator takes different values when Monte Carlo trials of size N are repeated. The estimator variance is

$$V\{T\} = N^{-2} \left(\sum_{i=1}^{N} V\{g(Y_i)\} + \sum_{i \neq j} \mathrm{Cov}\{g(Y_i), g(Y_j)\} \right) \tag{11.84}$$

The covariance terms are zero for the direct Monte Carlo because the N trials are mutually independent. The two Monte Carlo methods yield the same variance terms $V\{g(Y_i)\}$ because basic variable samples in each trial i follow the same distribution. For the Latin hypercube sampling, the covariance terms are nonpositive if $Y = F(X_1, \ldots, X_n)$ is monotonic in each of its arguments, and $g(Y)$ is a monotonic function of Y. Thus under the monotonic assumption, the estimator variance $V\{T_L\}$ is no greater than estimator variance $V\{T_D\}$ [15].

11.7 ANALYTICAL MOMENT PROPAGATION

For an AND or OR gate output with independent inputs, mean and variance can be calculated analytically from the first and second input moments. As a consequence, fault-tree top-event probability mean and variance can be calculated recursively unless the tree has no repeated basic events. This type of moment propagation is described first.

For fault trees with repeated events, top-event unavailability expressions must be approximated to make the moment propagation feasible. Typical approximations include first bracket inclusion-exclusion, Taylor series expansion, orthogonal expansion, response surface methods, analysis of variance, and regression analysis. This section describes the first three approximations. References [16–18] describe the remaining three approximation methods.

11.7.1 AND gate

Equation (11.49) is a special case of variance propagation when component unavailabilities are log-normally distributed. We consider here how the mean and variance propagate through an AND gate with n input components having general distributions.

The top-event unavailability Q_s can be expressed as

$$Q_s = \prod_{i=1}^{n} Q_i \equiv Q_1 \wedge \cdots \wedge Q_n \tag{11.85}$$

The mean is

$$\overline{Q_s} = \prod_{i=1}^{n} \overline{Q_i} \tag{11.86}$$

Denote by an overbar an expected value operation. From the definition of variance,

$$\begin{aligned} V\{Q_1 \wedge \cdots \wedge Q_n\} &= \overline{Q_s^2} - (\overline{Q_s})^2 \\ &= \prod_{i=1}^{n} \overline{Q_i^2} - \prod_{i=1}^{n} (\overline{Q_i})^2 \end{aligned} \tag{11.87}$$

For identical input components,

$$V\{Q \wedge \cdots \wedge Q\} = (\overline{Q^2})^n - (\overline{Q})^{2n} \tag{11.88}$$

The first and second moments of Q_i are sufficient for calculating mean and variance propagation through an AND gate. These moments, on the component level, are listed in Table 11.6 for the log-normal components in Table 11.4.

Example 7—AND gate exact-moment propagation. Consider an AND gate with three identical components to which the data in the first row of Table 11.6 apply. The variance of the output event is

$$V\{Q \wedge Q \wedge Q\} = (\overline{Q^2})^3 - (\overline{Q})^6 = (1.40 \times 10^{-2})^3 - (9.37 \times 10^{-2})^6 = 2.07 \times 10^{-6} \tag{11.89}$$

yielding the same result as (11.57) except for round-off errors. ■

TABLE 11.6. First and Second Moments for Example Components

Component	$\overline{Q}$	$V\{Q\}$	$\overline{Q^2} = (\overline{Q})^4/(\tilde{Q})^2$	$\overline{A} = 1 - \overline{Q}$	$\overline{A^2} = V\{Q\} + (\overline{A})^2$
1	9.37×10^{-2}	5.24×10^{-3}	1.40×10^{-2}	9.063×10^{-1}	8.266×10^{-1}
2	1.25×10^{-2}	9.28×10^{-5}	2.49×10^{-4}	9.875×10^{-1}	9.752×10^{-1}
3	1.93×10^{-1}	2.20×10^{-2}	5.93×10^{-2}	8.070×10^{-1}	6.732×10^{-1}

11.7.2 OR gate

OR gate outputs are not log-normal random variables even if input variables are log-normally distributed. However, the first and second moments propagate in a similar way as for an AND gate. The exact-moment propagation formulas for the AND and OR gates are summarized in Table 11.7 together with formulas derived in Section 11.7.6.

TABLE 11.7. Exact and Approximate Moment Propagations for AND and OR

	AND Gate $V\{Q_1 \wedge \cdots \wedge Q_n\}$	OR Gate $V\{Q_1 \vee \cdots \vee Q_n\}$
Exact	$\prod_{i=1}^{n} \overline{Q_i^2} - \prod_{i=1}^{n} (\overline{Q_i})^2$	$\prod_{i=1}^{n} \overline{A_i^2} - \prod_{i=1}^{n} (\overline{A_i})^2$
Approximate	$\sum_{i=1}^{n} \left(\prod_{j \neq i}^{n} \overline{Q_i} \right)^2 V\{Q_j\}$	$\sum_{i=1}^{n} \left(\prod_{j \neq i}^{n} \overline{A_j} \right)^2 V\{A_i\}$
	$+ \sum_{i<j} \left(\prod_{k \neq i,j} \overline{Q_k} \right)^2 V\{Q_i\} V\{Q_j\}$	$+ \sum_{i<j} \left(\prod_{k \neq i,j} \overline{A_k} \right)^2 V\{A_i\} V\{A_j\}$

Consider an OR gate with n input components. Denote by $A_i = 1 - Q_i$ the availability of component i. The top-event unavailability is

$$Q_s = 1 - A_s = 1 - \prod_{i=1}^{n} A_i \equiv Q_1 \vee \cdots \vee Q_n \tag{11.90}$$

The mean of Q_s is given by

$$\overline{Q_s} = 1 - \prod_{i=1}^{n} \overline{A_i} \tag{11.91}$$

The variance of Q_s is equal to the variance of A_s:

$$A_s = \prod_{i=1}^{n} A_i \equiv A_1 \wedge \cdots \wedge A_n \tag{11.92}$$

yielding a variance formula that is dual with respect to (11.87).

$$V\{Q_1 \vee \cdots \vee Q_n\} = V\{A_1 \wedge \cdots \wedge A_n\} = \prod_{i=1}^{n} \overline{A_i^2} - \prod_{i=1}^{n} (\overline{A_i})^2 \tag{11.93}$$

For identical input components,

$$V\{Q \vee \cdots \vee Q\} = (\overline{A^2})^n - (\overline{A})^{2n} \tag{11.94}$$

The first and second moments of $A_i = 1 - Q_i$ are sufficient for calculating the propagation through OR gates. The component availability moments are given to four significant digits in Table 11.6 to avoid round-off errors due to the subtraction in (11.93).

Example 8—OR gate exact-moment propagation. Consider an OR gate with three identical components having the moment data in the first row of Table 11.6. The output event variance is

$$V\{Q \vee Q \vee Q\} = (\overline{A^2})^3 - (\overline{A})^6 = (8.266 \times 10^{-1})^3 - (9.063 \times 10^{-1})^6 = 1.06 \times 10^{-2} \tag{11.95}$$

Obviously, the OR gate variance is much larger than the AND gate variance. ■

11.7.3 AND and OR gates

The mean and variance propagations for AND and OR gates can be used recursively to propagate through a fault tree that has no repeated events.

Example 9—AND gate output to OR gate. Consider the fault tree of Figure 11.5 previously subject to Monte Carlo analysis. Relevant data for the three components are listed in Table 11.6. The top-event unavailability is

$$Q_s = Q_1 \vee Q_G, \qquad Q_G \equiv Q_2 \wedge Q_3 \tag{11.96}$$

The top-event variance becomes

$$V\{Q_s\} = V\{Q_1 \vee Q_G\} = \overline{A_1^2}\,\overline{A_G^2} - (\overline{A_1})^2(\overline{A_G})^2 \tag{11.97}$$

Thus the first and second moments of A_G and A_1 determine the variance.
The first moment of A_G is

$$\begin{aligned} \overline{A_G} &= 1 - \overline{Q_G} = 1 - \overline{Q_2}\,\overline{Q_3} \\ &= 1 - (1.25 \times 10^{-2})(1.93 \times 10^{-1}) = 9.9976 \times 10^{-2} \end{aligned} \tag{11.98}$$

Second moments of A_G are obtained from the first moment and the variance:

$$\begin{aligned} V\{Q_G\} &= V\{Q_2 \wedge Q_3\} = \overline{Q_2^2}\,\overline{Q_3^2} - (\overline{Q_2})^2(\overline{Q_3})^2 \\ &= (2.49 \times 10^{-4})(5.93 \times 10^{-2}) - (1.25 \times 10^{-2})^2(1.93 \times 1^{-1})^2 \\ &= 8.95 \times 1^{-6} \end{aligned} \tag{11.99}$$

$$\overline{A_G^2} = V\{Q_G\} + (\overline{A_G})^2 = 9.952 \times 10^{-1}$$

Substituting these first and second moments into (11.97), we have

$$V\{Q_s\} = (8.266 \times 10^{-1})(9.952 \times 10^{-1}) - (9.063 \times 10^{-1})^2(9.976 \times 10^{-1})^2 = 5.19 \times 10^{-3} \tag{11.100}$$

This exact variance is larger than the SAMPLE variance 4.53×10^{-3} in Table 11.5 by an insignificant amount. The difference stems from the statistical fluctuation due to the finite Monte Carlo trials, and approximation of the top-event unavailability by (11.74), the first inclusion and exclusion bracket. We will see in Section 11.7.6 that the statistical fluctuation dominates. ■

Example 10—OR gate output to AND gate. Consider the fault tree of Figure 11.7. All the components are identical and have the moment data of component 1 in Table 11.6. The top-event unavailability is

$$Q_s = Q_1 \wedge Q_G, \qquad Q_G \equiv Q_2 \vee Q_3 \tag{11.101}$$

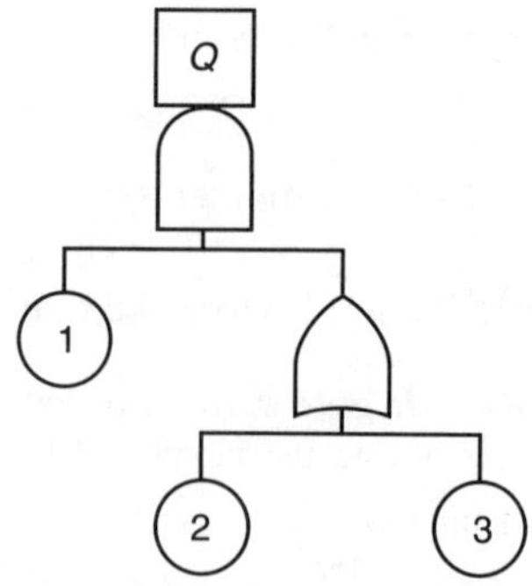

Figure 11.7. An AND/OR fault tree.

The top-event variance becomes

$$V\{Q_s\} = V\{Q_1 \wedge Q_G\} = \overline{Q_1^2}\,\overline{Q_G^2} - (\overline{Q_1})^2(\overline{Q_G})^2 \tag{11.102}$$

Again, the first and second moments of Q_G and Q_1 determine the variance.

The first moment of Q_G is

$$\begin{aligned}\overline{Q_G} &= 1 - \overline{A_2 A_3} = 1 - (\overline{A})^2 \\ &= 1 - (9.063 \times 10^{-1})^2 = 1.79 \times 10^{-1}\end{aligned} \tag{11.103}$$

Second moments of Q_G are obtained from the variance and the first moment:

$$\begin{aligned}V\{Q_G\} &= V\{A_2 \wedge A_3\} = \overline{A_2^2}\,\overline{A_3^2} - (\overline{A_2})^2(\overline{A_3})^2 = (\overline{A^2})^2 - (\overline{A})^4 \\ &= (8.266 \times 10^{-1})^2 - (9.063 \times 10^{-1})^4 = 8.60 \times 1^{-3} \\ \overline{Q_G^2} &= V\{Q_G\} + (\overline{Q_G})^2 = 4.06 \times 10^{-2}\end{aligned} \tag{11.104}$$

Substituting these first and second moments into (11.102), we have

$$V\{Q_s\} = (1.40 \times 10^{-2})(4.06 \times 10^{-2}) - (9.37 \times 10^{-2})^2(1.79 \times 10^{-1})^2 = 2.87 \times 10^{-4} \tag{11.105}$$

The AND/OR tree variance is smaller than that of the OR/AND tree because the former has only two-event cut sets, whereas the latter contains a single-event cut set. ■

11.7.4 Minimal Cut Sets

Because functions encountered in practical reliability and safety studies are complicated, it is impossible to analytically derive the mean $E\{Y\}$ and variance $V\{Y\} = E\{(Y - E\{Y\})^2\}$. Analytical calculation becomes feasible only when function F is approximated. One such approximation is a system-unavailability first-bracket approximation.

The exact-moment propagation cannot be used when the fault tree has repeated events because input events to some intermediate gates are no longer statistically independent, so approximation methods are required. We describe here a moment propagation using the sum of minimal cut set unavailabilities [19].

Assume that the fault tree has m minimal cut sets, $C_1, \ldots, C_m$. The first-bracket approximation of the system unavailability is

$$Q_s = \sum_{j=1}^{m} Q_j^* \tag{11.106}$$

where Q_j^* is the unavailability of minimal cut set C_j:

$$Q_j^* = \prod_{i \in C_j} Q_i \tag{11.107}$$

The mean system unavailability is now

$$\overline{Q_s} = \sum_{j=1}^{m} \overline{Q_j^*} \tag{11.108}$$

where $\overline{Q_j^*}$ is the mean unavailability of cut set C_j:

$$\overline{Q_j^*} = \prod_{i \in C_j} \overline{Q_i} \tag{11.109}$$

The system unavailability variance is expressed as a sum of cut set variances and covariances.

$$V\{Q_s\} = \sum_{j=1}^{m} V\{Q_j^*\} + 2\sum_{j<k} \mathrm{Cov}\{Q_j^*, Q_k^*\} \tag{11.110}$$

The cut set variance can be calculated from the first and second moments of component unavailabilities by the AND gate propagation formula (11.87). Denote by D_{jk} the set of basic events included both in cut set C_j and C_k; denote by S_{jk} the set of basic events included exclusively in C_j or C_k. As shown in Appendix A.2 of this chapter, the cut set covariance can be written as

$$\mathrm{Cov}\{Q_j^*, Q_k^*\} = \left[\prod_{i \in S_{jk}} \overline{Q_i}\right] V\{\prod_{i \in D_{jk}} Q_i\} \tag{11.111}$$

The variance term of the above equation can be evaluated by the AND gate propagation formula (11.87).

Example 11—OR gate output to AND gate. Consider again the fault tree of Figure 11.7. All the components are identical; they have the moment data of component 1 in Table 11.6. The fault tree has two minimal cut sets:

$$C_1 = \{1, 2\}, \qquad C_2 = \{1, 3\} \tag{11.112}$$

Only basic event 1 is common to both cut sets. Thus event sets D_{12} and S_{12} are

$$D_{12} = \{1\}, \qquad S_{12} = \{2, 3\} \tag{11.113}$$

Because the components are identical, equation (11.88) gives the cut set variance:

$$V\{Q_1^*\} = V\{Q_2^*\} = (\overline{Q^2})^2 - (\overline{Q})^4 \tag{11.114}$$

The cut set covariance is

$$\begin{aligned} \mathrm{Cov}\{Q_1^*, Q_2^*\} &= \overline{Q_2}\,\overline{Q_3} V\{Q_1\} \\ &= (\overline{Q})^2[(\overline{Q^2}) - (\overline{Q})^2] \end{aligned} \tag{11.115}$$

The system variance becomes

$$\begin{aligned} V\{Q_s\} &= V\{Q_1^*\} + V\{Q_2^*\} + 2\mathrm{Cov}\{Q_1^*, Q_2^*\} \\ &= 2(\overline{Q^2})^2 + 2\overline{Q^2}(\overline{Q})^2 - 4(\overline{Q})^4 = 6(\overline{Q})^2 V\{Q\} + 2[V\{Q\}]^2 \end{aligned} \tag{11.116}$$

Substituting the component 1 values in Table 11.6, we have

$$V\{Q_s\} = (6)(9.37 \times 10^{-2})^2(5.24 \times 10^{-3}) + (2)(5.24 \times 10^{-3})^2 = 3.31 \times 10^{-4} \tag{11.117}$$

This value is slightly different from the exact value of (11.105) because the system unavailability is approximated by the first bracket of the inclusion-exclusion formula. ■

11.7.5 Taylor Series Expansion

The Taylor series approximation applies to output functions other than system unavailability expressions with independent basic events. For instance, a common-cause equation such as (11.72) can be approximated by the expansion. Denote again by an overbar the operation of taking an expectation. One typical approach to simplifying the output function F is a second-order Taylor expansion around the variable means.

$$Y = Y_0 + \sum_{i=1}^{n} a_i(X_i - \overline{X_i}) + (1/2)\sum_{i=1}^{n}\sum_{j=1}^{n} a_{ij}(X_i - \overline{X_i})(X_j - \overline{X_j}) \tag{11.118}$$

where the constant term Y_0 is the function value evaluated at the variable means; coefficients a_i and a_{ij} are, respectively, first- and second-order partial derivatives of Y evaluated at the means:

$$\begin{aligned} Y_0 &\equiv F(\overline{X_1}, \ldots, \overline{X_n}) \\ a_i &\equiv \partial F(\overline{X_1}, \ldots, \overline{X_n})/\partial X_i \\ a_{ij} &\equiv \partial^2 F(\overline{X_1}, \ldots, \overline{X_n})/\partial X_i \partial X_j \end{aligned} \tag{11.119}$$

In a matrix form, the Taylor series expansion is

$$Y = Y_0 + \boldsymbol{a}^T(\boldsymbol{X} - \overline{\boldsymbol{X}}) + (1/2)(\boldsymbol{X} - \overline{\boldsymbol{X}})^T \boldsymbol{A}(\boldsymbol{X} - \overline{\boldsymbol{X}}) \tag{11.120}$$

where $\boldsymbol{X}$, $\overline{\boldsymbol{X}}$, and $\boldsymbol{a}$ are $n \times 1$ column vectors, and $\boldsymbol{A}$ is an $n \times n$ symmetric matrix. The superscript T denotes a vector transpose.

$$\boldsymbol{X} = \begin{pmatrix} X_1 \\ \vdots \\ X_n \end{pmatrix}, \quad \overline{\boldsymbol{X}} = \begin{pmatrix} \overline{X_1} \\ \vdots \\ \overline{X_n} \end{pmatrix}, \quad \boldsymbol{a} = \begin{pmatrix} a_1 \\ \vdots \\ a_n \end{pmatrix}, \quad \boldsymbol{A} = \begin{pmatrix} a_{11} & \ldots & a_{1n} \\ \vdots & \vdots & \vdots \\ a_{n1} & \ldots & a_{nn} \end{pmatrix} \tag{11.121}$$

Example 12—Expansion of OR gate. The (11.90) OR gate unavailability with $n = 3$ can be approximated by the following Taylor series expansion.

$$\begin{aligned} Q_s = 1 &- \overline{A_1}\,\overline{A_2}\,\overline{A_3} + \overline{A_2}\,\overline{A_3}(Q_1 - \overline{Q_1}) + \overline{A_1}\,\overline{A_3}(Q_2 - \overline{Q_2}) + \overline{A_1}\,\overline{A_2}(Q_3 - \overline{Q_3}) \\ &- \overline{A_3}(Q_1 - \overline{Q_1})(Q_2 - \overline{Q_2}) - \overline{A_2}(Q_1 - \overline{Q_1})(Q_3 - \overline{Q_3}) \\ &- \overline{A_1}(Q_2 - \overline{Q_2})(Q_3 - \overline{Q_3}), \qquad \overline{A_i} \equiv 1 - \overline{Q_i} \end{aligned} \tag{11.122}$$

Thus coefficient vector $\boldsymbol{a}$ and matrix $\boldsymbol{A}$ are

$$\boldsymbol{a} = \begin{pmatrix} \overline{A_2}\,\overline{A_3} \\ \overline{A_1}\,\overline{A_3} \\ \overline{A_1}\,\overline{A_2} \end{pmatrix}, \qquad \boldsymbol{A} = \begin{pmatrix} 0 & -\overline{A_3} & -\overline{A_2} \\ -\overline{A_3} & 0 & -\overline{A_1} \\ -\overline{A_2} & -\overline{A_1} & 0 \end{pmatrix} \tag{11.123}$$

Note that the diagonal elements of the coefficient matrix are all zero because the system unavailability is a multiple-linear function of component unavailabilities. ■

In the Taylor series expansion of (11.118), the second-order terms $(X_i - \overline{X_i})^2$ can be separated from the cross terms $(X_i - \overline{X_i})(X_j - \overline{X_j})$, $i \neq j$.

$$\begin{aligned} Y = Y_0 &+ \sum_{i=1}^{n} a_i(X_i - \overline{X_i}) + (1/2)\sum_{i=1}^{n} a_{ii}(X_i - \overline{X_i})^2 \\ &+ \sum_{1 \le i < j \le n} a_{ij}(X_i - \overline{X_i})(X_j - \overline{X_j}) \end{aligned} \tag{11.124}$$

When basic variables are statistically independent, mean $\overline{Y}$ becomes

$$\overline{Y} = Y_0 + (1/2) \sum_{i=1}^{n} V\{X_i\} \tag{11.125}$$

When the output function is multiple-linear, the second-order terms, except for the cross terms, do not exist, and we obtain simpler expressions.

$$\overline{Y} = Y_0 \tag{11.126}$$

$$V\{Y\} = \sum_{i=1}^{n} a_i^2 V\{X_i\} + \sum_{1 \le i < j \le n} a_{ij}^2 V\{X_i\} V\{X_j\} \tag{11.127}$$

Unfortunately, the general expression for variance $V\{Y\}$ becomes too complicated unless the function is multiple-linear. Jackson [20] developed a computer code to calculate the moment μ_k based on the formulas in Cox [21].

$$\mu_k \equiv \overline{(Y - \overline{Y})^k}, \qquad k = 1, 2, 3, 4 \tag{11.128}$$

The mean $\overline{Y}$, variance $V\{Y\}$, skewness, and kurtosis are determined, and these statistics are used to fit an empirical distribution to the calculated system moments.

The skewness and kurtosis are defined by

$$\sqrt{\beta} \equiv \mu_3 / \mu_2^{3/2}, \qquad \gamma \equiv \mu_4 / \mu_2^2 \tag{11.129}$$

The skewness $\sqrt{\beta}$ is positive if the probability density is biased left from the mean; it is negative if the bias is toward the right; the kurtosis is larger when the density has wide tails. The normal probability density, for instance, has a skewness of zero and kurtosis of three. As shown in the next section, mean, variance, skewness, and kurtosis of basic variables are required to calculate output variable mean and variance. These requirements are relaxed when the output function is multiple-linear.

11.7.6 Orthogonal Expansion

The variance of Y can be obtained analytically when the Taylor series approximation (11.124) is rewritten in terms of a sum of orthogonal functions [22]. As shown in Appendix A.3 of this chapter, the mean and variance now become

$$E\{Y\} = Y_0 + (1/2) \sum_{i=1}^{n} a_{ii} V\{X_i\} \tag{11.130}$$

$$\begin{aligned} V\{Y\} = & \sum_{i=1}^{n} \left[a_i \sqrt{V\{X_i\}} + (1/2)\sqrt{\beta_i} a_{ii} V\{X_i\} \right]^2 \\ & + (1/4) \sum_{i=1}^{n} a_{ii}^2 [V\{X_i\}]^2 (\gamma_i - \beta_i - 1) + \sum_{1 \le i < j \le n} a_{ij}^2 V\{X_i\} V\{X_j\} \end{aligned} \tag{11.131}$$

where a_i and a_{ij} are Taylor series coefficients and β_i and γ_i are the skewness and kurtosis of variable X_i:

$$\sqrt{\beta_i} = \overline{(X - \overline{X})^3} / [V\{X_i\}]^{3/2} \tag{11.132}$$

$$\gamma_i = \overline{(X - \overline{X})^4} / [V\{X_i\}]^2 \tag{11.133}$$

Variance $V\{Y\}$ increases monotonically when kurtosis γ_i increases, that is, when a basic variable density has a high peak and wide tails. Again, if the original function is multiple-linear, then we have the simpler expressions:

$$E\{Y\} = Y_0, \qquad V\{Y\} = \sum_{i=1}^{n} a_i^2 V\{X_i\} + \sum_{1\le i<j\le n} a_{ij}^2 V\{X_i\}V\{X_j\} \tag{11.134}$$

Note that variance $V\{Y\}$ is determined from component variances; higher order moments are not required.

For a three-component system, the (11.134) variance can be written in matrix form:

$$V\{Y\} = \begin{pmatrix} a_1^2 & a_2^2 & a_3^2 \end{pmatrix} \begin{pmatrix} V\{X_1\} \\ V\{X_2\} \\ V\{X_3\} \end{pmatrix} + (1/2)\begin{pmatrix} V\{X_1\} & V\{X_2\} & V\{X_3\} \end{pmatrix} \begin{pmatrix} 0 & a_{12}^2 & a_{13}^2 \\ a_{12}^2 & 0 & a_{23}^2 \\ a_{13}^2 & a_{23}^2 & 0 \end{pmatrix} \begin{pmatrix} V\{X_1\} \\ V\{X_2\} \\ V\{X_3\} \end{pmatrix} \tag{11.135}$$

Example 13—AND gate approximate propagation. Consider an AND gate with three input components. The top-event unavailability is

$$Q_s = Q_1 Q_2 Q_3 \tag{11.136}$$

The second-order Taylor series expansion is

$$Q_s = \overline{Q_1}\,\overline{Q_2}\,\overline{Q_3} + \underbrace{\begin{pmatrix} \overline{Q_2}\,\overline{Q_3} & \overline{Q_1}\,\overline{Q_3} & \overline{Q_1}\,\overline{Q_2} \end{pmatrix}}_{a^T} \begin{pmatrix} Q_1 - \overline{Q_1} \\ Q_2 - \overline{Q_2} \\ Q_3 - \overline{Q_3} \end{pmatrix} + (1/2)\begin{pmatrix} Q_1 - \overline{Q_1} & Q_2 - \overline{Q_2} & Q_3 - \overline{Q_3} \end{pmatrix} \underbrace{\begin{pmatrix} 0 & \overline{Q_3} & \overline{Q_2} \\ \overline{Q_3} & 0 & \overline{Q_1} \\ \overline{Q_2} & \overline{Q_1} & 0 \end{pmatrix}}_{A} \begin{pmatrix} Q_1 - \overline{Q_1} \\ Q_2 - \overline{Q_2} \\ Q_3 - \overline{Q_3} \end{pmatrix} \tag{11.137}$$

From (11.135), the variance of Q_s is given by

$$\begin{aligned} V\{Q_s\} &= (\overline{Q_2}\,\overline{Q_3})^2 V\{Q_1\} + (\overline{Q_1}\,\overline{Q_3})^2 V\{Q_2\} + (\overline{Q_1}\,\overline{Q_2})^2 V\{Q_3\} \\ &\quad + (\overline{Q_3})^2 V\{Q_1\}V\{Q_2\} + (\overline{Q_2})^2 V\{Q_1\}V\{Q_3\} + (\overline{Q_1})^2 V\{Q_2\}V\{Q_3\} \\ &= \sum_{i=1}^{3}\left(\prod_{j\ne i}^{3} \overline{Q_j}\right)^2 V\{Q_i\} + \sum_{i<j}^{3}\left(\prod_{k\ne i,j}^{3} \overline{Q_k}\right)^2 V\{Q_i\}V\{Q_j\} \end{aligned} \tag{11.138}$$

In case of the three identical components having unavailability Q, the variance simplifies to

$$V\{Q_s\} = 3(\overline{Q})^4 V\{Q\} + 3(\overline{Q})^2[V\{Q\}]^2 \tag{11.139}$$

Suppose that we have, as the identical component, the first component of Table 11.4, then the system variance is

$$\begin{aligned} V\{Q_s\} &= (3)(9.37 \times 10^{-2})^4(5.24 \times 10^{-3}) + (3)(9.37 \times 10^{-2})^2(5.24 \times 10^{-3})^2 \\ &= 1.93 \times 10^{-6} \end{aligned} \tag{11.140}$$

This variance is slightly smaller than the exact (11.54) variance 2.08×10^{-6} because the Taylor series expansion of (11.137) is a second-order approximation to the third-order equation (11.136). ■

Example 14—OR gate approximate propagation. For a three-input OR gate, (11.122) yields an expression similar to (11.138), where unavailability Q is replaced by availability A:

$$\begin{aligned} V\{Q_s\} &= (\overline{A_2}\,\overline{A_3})^2 V\{A_1\} + (\overline{A_1}\,\overline{A_3})^2 V\{A_2\} + (\overline{A_1}\,\overline{A_2})^2 V\{A_3\} \\ &\quad + (\overline{A_3})^2 V\{A_1\}V\{A_2\} + (\overline{A_2})^2 V\{A_1\}V\{A_3\} + (\overline{A_1})^2 V\{A_2\}V\{A_3\} \\ &= \sum_{i=1}^{3}\left(\prod_{j\neq i}^{3}\overline{A_i}\right)^2 V\{A_i\} + \sum_{i<j}^{3}\left(\prod_{k\neq i,j}^{3}\overline{A_k}\right)^2 V\{A_i\}V\{A_j\} \end{aligned} \tag{11.141}$$

Notice that the component availability variance is equal to the component unavailability variance, $V\{A_i\} = V\{Q_i\}$. This system unavailability variance is not exact because of the Taylor series approximation.

The variance is further simplified when the system unavailability expression is approximated by the first bracket of the inclusion-exclusion formula:

$$Q_s = Q_1 + Q_2 + Q_3$$

The Taylor series expansion becomes

$$Q_s = \overline{Q_1} + \overline{Q_2} + \overline{Q_3} + \underbrace{\begin{pmatrix} 1 & 1 & 1 \end{pmatrix}}_{a^T} \begin{pmatrix} Q_1 - \overline{Q_1} \\ Q_2 - \overline{Q_2} \\ Q_3 - \overline{Q_3} \end{pmatrix} \tag{11.142}$$

yielding the variance expression

$$V\{Q_s\} = V\{Q_1\} + V\{Q_2\} + V\{Q_3\} \tag{11.143}$$

Consider an OR gate with three identical input components whose component characteristics are those in the first row of Table 11.4. The approximation (11.141) gives the system variance

$$\begin{aligned} V\{Q_s\} &= 3(\overline{A})^4 V\{A\} + 3(\overline{A})^2[V\{A\}]^2 \\ &= (3)(1 - 9.37 \times 10^{-2})^4(5.24 \times 10^{-3}) + (3)(1 - 9.37 \times 10^{-2})^2(5.24 \times 10^{-3})^2 \\ &= 1.07 \times 10^{-2} \end{aligned} \tag{11.144}$$

while the first-bracket approximation of (11.143) yields

$$V\{Q_s\} = (3)(5.24 \times 10^{-3}) = 1.57 \times 10^{-2} \tag{11.145}$$

■

Example 15—SAMPLE tree approximate propagation. Consider the fault tree of Figure 11.5 previously analyzed using SAMPLE. The Taylor series system unavailability expansion of (11.74) is

$$\begin{aligned} Q_s &= \overline{Q_1} + \overline{Q_2}\,\overline{Q_3} + \underbrace{\begin{pmatrix} 1 & \overline{Q_3} & \overline{Q_2} \end{pmatrix}}_{a^T} \begin{pmatrix} Q_1 - \overline{Q_1} \\ Q_2 - \overline{Q_2} \\ Q_3 - \overline{Q_3} \end{pmatrix} \\ &\quad + (1/2)\begin{pmatrix} Q_1 - \overline{Q_1} & Q_2 - \overline{Q_2} & Q_3 - \overline{Q_3} \end{pmatrix} \underbrace{\begin{pmatrix} 0 & 0 & 0 \\ 0 & 0 & 1 \\ 0 & 1 & 0 \end{pmatrix}}_{A} \begin{pmatrix} Q_1 - \overline{Q_1} \\ Q_2 - \overline{Q_2} \\ Q_3 - \overline{Q_3} \end{pmatrix} \end{aligned} \tag{11.146}$$

yielding the variance expression

$$\begin{aligned} V\{Q_s\} &= V\{Q_1\} + (\overline{Q_3})^2 V\{Q_2\} + (\overline{Q_2})^2 V\{Q_3\} + V\{Q_2\}V\{Q_3\} \\ &= 5.24 \times 10^{-3} + (1.93 \times 10^{-1})^2(9.28 \times 10^{-5}) + (1.25 \times 10^{-2})^2(2.20 \times 10^{-2}) \\ &\quad + (9.28 \times 10^{-5})(2.20 \times 10^{-2}) = 5.24 \times 10^{-3} \end{aligned} \tag{11.147}$$

Although the top-event unavailability is approximated by the first inclusion-exclusion bracket, the result is in agreement with the exact variance (11.100). Notice that (11.146) is an exact Taylor series expansion of system unavailability approximation (11.74). Thus (11.147) is an exact value according to equation (11.74). We can conclude that the smaller SAMPLE variance in Table 11.5 stems from a statistical fluctuation due to a finite Monte Carlo sample size of 1200. ■

11.8 DISCRETE PROBABILITY ALGEBRA

When a continuous probability density is approximated by a set of discrete probabilities, the uncertainty propagation can be modeled by discrete arithmetic [23–26]. This approach can be regarded as a deterministic version of Monte Carlo, and is efficient for output functions with simple structures. Furthermore, the discrete probability approximation is free from the random fluctuations inherent in finite Monte Carlo trials. Denote by $\{(P_1, X_1), \ldots, (P_n, X_n)\}$ a discrete approximation where X_i is a discrete value of variable X and P_i is a discrete probability. The approximation is performed under the constraint

$$\sum_{i=1}^{n} P_i = 1 \tag{11.148}$$

Consider a function $Z = F(X, Y)$. Assume discrete approximations for variables X and Y: $\{(P_i, X_i)\}$ and $\{(Q_j, Y_j)\}$. If X and Y are statistically independent, then the discrete approximation for Z becomes

$$Z \sim \{[P_i Q_j, F(X_i, Y_j)]\} \tag{11.149}$$

The approximation for Z contains n^2 pairs, thus the number of pairs increases rapidly as the propagation proceeds, and pairs must be condensed or aggregated to avoid an exponential explosion.

Elementary operations among two different random variables include summation, difference, product, and ratio. Single variable operations include sum of a random variable and a constant, product of a random variable and a constant, product of the same random variable, and square root:

$$\begin{array}{cc} X+Y & X-Y \\ X\times Y & X/Y \\ X+C & C\times X \\ X^n & \sqrt{X} \end{array} \tag{11.150}$$

Consider the output function $Y = F(X_1, \ldots, X_n)$. Two situations arise. If each random variable appears only once in F, then the distribution for Y can be obtained by combining two random variables at a time.

Example 16—Discrete algebra for nonrepeated events. Consider the output equation

$$Y = X_1 X_2/(X_3 + X_4) \tag{11.151}$$

We first compute $V = X_1 X_2$ and $W = X_3 + X_4$, and then $Y = V/W$.

If at least one random variable appears more than once in F, then the expression for F has to be broken into two parts, a part without repeated random variables and one with the minimal expression containing repeated random variables. ■

Example 17—Discrete algebra for repeated events. Consider the output equation

$$Y = X_1 + (X_2 + X_3)(X_4 + X_5) + X_6 + X_3 X_5^{1/2} \tag{11.152}$$

This expression can be divided into two parts:

$$\begin{aligned} V &= X_1 + X_6 \\ W &= (X_2 + X_3)(X_4 + X_5) + X_3 X_5^{1/2} \end{aligned} \tag{11.153}$$

These parts are then combined, yielding $Y = V + W$. ■

Note that four variables must be combined to obtain W. For complicated fault trees, discrete probability algebra becomes difficult due to repeated events; however, for output functions with simpler structures, the discrete algebra, which is free from sampling errors, seems to be more efficient than Monte Carlo trials.

Colombo and Jaarsma [25] proposed discrete approximation by a histogram of equal probability intervals. This has the following advantages: the intervals are small where the density is high and large where the density is low and combinations of equal probability intervals form equal intervals, resulting in a regularly shaped histogram that facilitates the aggregation of intervals. Figure 11.8 shows a histogram obtained by discrete probability algebra with equal probability intervals [25].

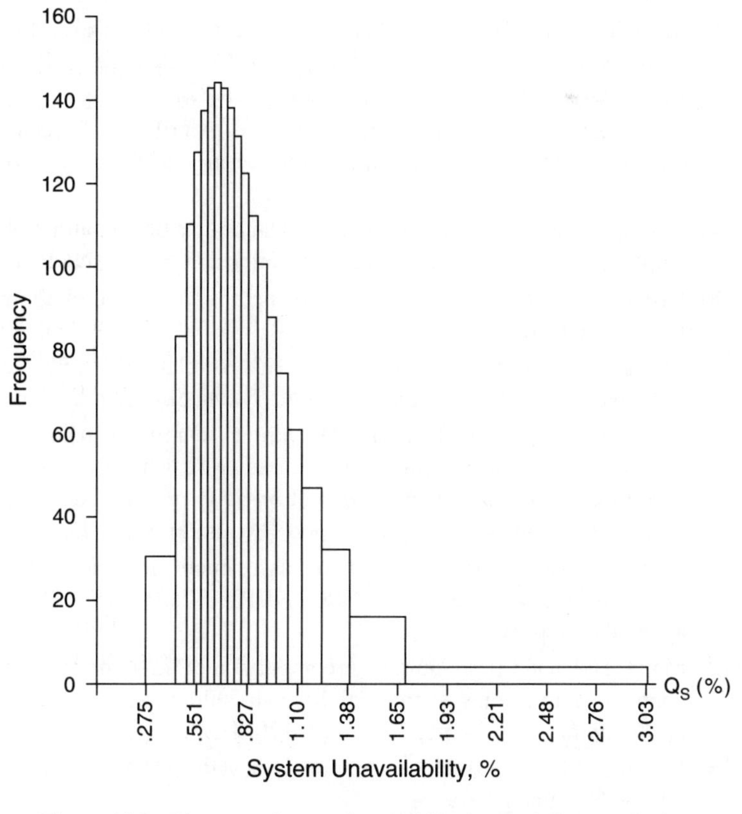

Figure 11.8. Histogram by equal probability interval discrete algebra.

11.9 SUMMARY

PRA engenders at least two sources of uncertainty: parametric uncertainty and modeling uncertainty. Parametric uncertainty involves statistical uncertainty and data evaluation uncertainty. Expert evaluation of component-reliability parameters results in extreme data evaluation uncertainty. The Bayes theorem and log-normal distribution are used to quantify component-level parametric uncertainty, which is propagated to the system level by methods such as Monte Carlo simulation, analytical moment calculation, and discrete probability algebra. The resultant risk-curve uncertainty is crucial to PRA decision making.

REFERENCES

[1] Mosleh, A. "Hidden sources of uncertainty: Judgment in the collection and analysis of data," *Nuclear Engineering and Design*, vol. 93, pp. 187–198, 1986.

[2] "IEEE guide to the collection and presentation of electrical, electronic and sensing component reliability data for nuclear power generating stations," New York: IEEE, IEEE Std-500, 1977.

[3] Apostolakis, G. "On the use of judgment in probabilistic risk analysis," *Nuclear Engineering and Design*, vol. 93, pp. 161–166, 1986.

[4] Apostolakis, G., S. Kaplan, B. J. Garrick, and R. J. Duphily. "Data specialization for plant specific risk studies," *Nuclear Engineering and Design*, vol. 56, p. 321–329, 1980.

[5] Mosleh, A., and G. Apostolakis. "Models for the use of expert opinions," presented at the Workshop on Low-Probability/High-Consequence Risk Analysis. Society for Risk Analysis, Arlington, VA, June 15–17, 1982.

[6] Apostolakis, G. E., V. M. Bier, A. Mosleh. "A critique of recent models for human error rate assessment," *Reliability Engineering and System Safety*, vol. 22, pp. 201–217, 1988.

[7] Swain, A. D., and H. E. Guttmann. "Handbook of human reliability analysis with emphasis on nuclear power plant applications." USNRC, NUREG/CR-1278, 1980.

[8] IAEA. "Case study on the use of PSA methods: Human reliability analysis." IAEA, IAEA-TECDOC-592, 1991.

[9] Zhang, Q. "A general method dealing with correlations in uncertainty propagation in fault trees," *Reliability Engineering and System Safety*, vol. 26, pp. 231–247, 1989.

[10] Wu, J. S., G. E. Apostolakis, and D. Okrent. "On the inclusion of organizational and managerial influences in probabilistic safety assessments of nuclear power plants." In *The Analysis, Communication, and Perception of Risk*, edited by B. J. Garrick and W. C. Gekler. pp. 429–439. New York: Plenum Press, 1991.

[11] USNRC. "Reactor safety study: An assessment of accident risk in U.S. commercial nuclear power plants." USNRC, NUREG-75/014 (WASH-1400), vol. 1, 1975, appendix III, p. 104.

[12] Martz, H. F., and B. S. Duran. "A comparison of three methods for calculating lower confidence limits on system reliability using binomial component data," *IEEE Trans. on Reliability*, vol. 34, no. 2, pp. 113–120, 1985.

[13] Efron, B. "Bootstrap method: Another look at the jacknife," *Annals of Statistics*, vol. 4, pp. 1–26, January 1979.

[14] Depuy, K. M., J. R. Hobbs, A. H. Moore, and J. W. Johnston, Jr. "Accuracy of univariate, bivariate, and a 'modified double Monte Carlo' technique for finding lower confidence limits of system reliability," *IEEE Trans. on Reliability*, vol. 31, no. 5, pp. 474–477, 1982.

[15] McKay, M. D., R. J. Beckman, and W. J. Conover. "A comparison of three methods for selecting values of input variables in the analysis of output from a computer code," *Technometrics*, vol. 21, no. 2, pp. 239–245, 1979.

[16] John, W. M. P. *Statistical Methods in Engineering and Quality Assurance*. New York: John Wiley & Sons, 1990.

[17] Meyers, R. H. *Response Surface Methodology*. Boston, MA: Allyn and Bacon, 1976.

[18] Kim, T. W., S. H. Chang, and B. H. Lee, "Comparative study on uncertainty and sensitivity analysis and application to LOCA model," *Reliability Engineering and System Safety*, vol. 21, pp. 1–26, 1988.

[19] Lee, Y. T., and G. E. Apostolakis. "Probability intervals for the top event unavailability of fault trees." University of California, Los Angeles, UCLA-ENG-7663, 1976.

[20] Jackson, P. S. "A second-order moments method for uncertainty analysis," *IEEE Trans. on Reliability*, vol. 31, no. 4, pp. 382–384, 1982.

[21] Cox, N. D., and C. F Miller. "User's description of second-order error propagation (SOERP) computer code for statistically independent variables." Idaho National Engineering Laboratory, TREE-1216, 1978. (Available from NTIS, Springfield, Virginia 22151 USA.)

[22] Cox, D. C., "An analytic method for uncertainty analysis of nonlinear output functions, with applications to fault-tree analysis," *IEEE Trans. on Reliability*, vol. 31, no. 5, pp. 465–468, 1982.

[23] Kaplan, S. "On the method of discrete probability distributions in risk and reliability calculation: Application to seismic risk assessment," *Risk Analysis*, vol. 1, no. 3, pp. 189–196, 1981.

[24] USNRC. "PRA procedures guide: A guide to the performance of probabilistic risk assessments for nuclear power plants." USNRC, NUREG/CR-2300, 1983.

[25] Colombo, A. G., and R. J. Jaarsma. "A powerful numerical method to combine random variables," *IEEE Trans. on Reliability*, vol. 29, no. 2, pp. 126–129, 1980.

[26] Ingrain, G. E., E. L. Welker, and C. R. Herrmann. "Designing for reliability based on probabilistic modeling using remote access computer systems." In *Proceedings of the 7th Reliability and Maintainability Conference*, San Francisco, July 1968.

CHAPTER ELEVEN APPENDICES

A.1 MAXIMUM-LIKELIHOOD ESTIMATOR

Consider lifetime test data for n identical components. The test for component i is terminated after time lapse c_i, which is a "censoring time" determined in advance. Some components fail before and others survive their censoring times. Denote by t_i the lifetime of component i. Define a new time x_i by:

$$x_i = \begin{cases} t_i, & \text{if } t_i \le c_i, \quad \text{i.e., failed components} \\ c_i, & \text{if } t_i > c_i, \quad \text{i.e., censored components} \end{cases} \tag{A.1}$$

Introduce the following component notations:

$f(t;\boldsymbol{\theta})$ probability density function
$r(t;\boldsymbol{\theta})$ failure rate
$R(t;\boldsymbol{\theta})$ reliability function

Denote by F and C the failed components and censored components, respectively. The likelihood L of the test data is defined as the probability density of obtaining the test results when the distribution parameter vector $\boldsymbol{\theta}$ is assumed.

$$L(\boldsymbol{\theta}) = \prod_{i\in F} f(x_i;\boldsymbol{\theta}) \prod_{i\in C} R(x_i;\boldsymbol{\theta}) \tag{A.2}$$

The logarithm of likelihood L is called a log-likelihood. The maximum-likelihood estimator of parameter vector $\boldsymbol{\theta}$ is the one that maximizes the likelihood or equivalently, the log-likelihood l. Because $f(t;\boldsymbol{\theta}) = r(t;\boldsymbol{\theta})R(t;\boldsymbol{\theta})$,

$$l(\boldsymbol{\theta}) = \ln L = \sum_{i\in F} \ln r(x_i;\boldsymbol{\theta}) + \sum_{i=1}^{n} \ln R(x_i;\boldsymbol{\theta}) \tag{A.3}$$

The Weibull distribution has the following failure rate and reliability function:

$$r(t;\boldsymbol{\theta}) = \lambda\beta(\lambda t)^{\beta-1}, \qquad R(t;\boldsymbol{\theta}) = \exp[-(\lambda t)^{\beta}], \qquad (\lambda \equiv 1/\sigma) \tag{A.4}$$

Denote by m the number of failed components in set F. The log-likelihood can be rewritten as

$$l(\lambda,\beta) = m\ln\beta + m\beta\ln\lambda + (\beta-1)\sum_{i\in F}\ln x_i - \lambda^{\beta}\sum_{i=1}^{n} x_i^{\beta} \tag{A.5}$$

The exponential distribution has the β-value of $\beta = 1$, thus

$$l(\lambda,1) = m\ln\lambda - \lambda\sum_{i=1}^{n} x_i \tag{A.6}$$

This log-likelihood is maximized at

$$\hat{\lambda} = \frac{m}{\sum_{i=1}^{n} x_i} \tag{A.7}$$

A so-called *Fisher information matrix* is defined by a Hessian at the maximum-likelihood estimator $\hat{\boldsymbol{\theta}}$.

$$\boldsymbol{I}(\boldsymbol{\theta}) = \begin{pmatrix} \partial^2 l/\partial\theta_1^2 & \cdots & \partial^2 l/\partial\theta_1\partial\theta_q \\ & \cdots & \\ \partial^2 l/\partial\theta_q\partial\theta_1 & \cdots & \partial^2 l/\partial\theta_q^2 \end{pmatrix} \tag{A.8}$$

It is known that the maximum-likelihood estimator is asymptotically distributed with a multidimensional normal distribution; the mean is the true parameter value, while the covariance is the inverse of the information matrix.

$$\hat{\boldsymbol{\theta}} \sim \text{gau}^*(\boldsymbol{\theta}, \boldsymbol{I}(\hat{\boldsymbol{\theta}})^{-1}) \tag{A.9}$$

The second-order partial derivatives can be obtained analytically for the Weibull distribution. The maximum-likelihood estimator is calculated by ordinary maximization algorithms. The covariance matrix is then obtained as

$$\begin{pmatrix} V\{\hat{\lambda}\} & \text{Cov}\{\hat{\lambda}, \hat{\beta}\} \\ \text{Cov}\{\hat{\lambda}, \hat{\beta}\} & V\{\hat{\beta}\} \end{pmatrix} \equiv \begin{pmatrix} V_{\lambda\lambda} & V_{\lambda\beta} \\ V_{\lambda\beta} & V_{\beta\beta} \end{pmatrix} = \boldsymbol{I}(\hat{\lambda}, \hat{\beta})^{-1} \tag{A.10}$$

The variance of unavailability $\hat{Q} = 1 - R(t;\ \hat{\lambda}, \hat{\beta})$ can be evaluated from

$$V\{\hat{Q}\} = \begin{pmatrix} \partial\hat{Q}/\partial\hat{\lambda} & \partial\hat{Q}/\partial\hat{\beta} \end{pmatrix} \begin{pmatrix} V_{\lambda\lambda} & V_{\lambda\beta} \\ V_{\lambda\beta} & V_{\beta\beta} \end{pmatrix} \begin{pmatrix} \partial\hat{Q}/\partial\hat{\lambda} \\ \partial\hat{Q}/\partial\hat{\beta} \end{pmatrix} \tag{A.11}$$

A.2 CUT SET COVARIANCE FORMULA

The cut set covariance can be expressed as

$$\text{Cov}\{Q_j^*, Q_k^*\} = \overline{Q_j^* Q_k^*} - \overline{Q_j^*}\ \overline{Q_k^*} \tag{A.12}$$

This covariance can be rewritten in terms of basic-event unavailabilities:

$$\begin{aligned} \text{Cov}\{Q_j^*, Q_k^*\} &= \left[\prod_{i \in D_{jk}} \overline{Q_i^2}\right]\left[\prod_{i \in S_{jk}} \overline{Q_i}\right] - \left[\prod_{i \in D_{jk}} (\overline{Q_i})^2\right]\left[\prod_{i \in S_{jk}} \overline{Q_i}\right] \\ &= \left[\prod_{i \in S_{jk}} \overline{Q_i}\right] V\left\{\prod_{i \in D_{jk}} Q_i\right\} \end{aligned} \tag{A.13}$$

A.3 MEAN AND VARIANCE BY ORTHOGONAL EXPANSION

Let Z be a random variable with probability density $p\{Z\}$. Denote by $\psi_k(Z)$ a kth order orthogonal polynomial defined by

$$\int \psi_k(Z)\psi_l(Z)p\{Z\}dZ = \begin{cases} 1, & \text{if } k = l \\ 0, & \text{if } k \neq l \end{cases} \tag{A.14}$$

The orthogonal polynomials up to the second order are given by

$$\psi_0(Z) = 1 \tag{A.15}$$

$$\psi_1(Z) = \frac{\begin{vmatrix} 1 & \overline{Z} \\ 1 & Z \end{vmatrix}}{\sqrt{\begin{vmatrix} 1 & \overline{Z} \\ \overline{Z} & \overline{Z^2} \end{vmatrix}}} \tag{A.16}$$

$$\psi_2(Z) = \frac{\begin{vmatrix} 1 & \overline{Z} & \overline{Z^2} \\ \overline{Z} & \overline{Z^2} & \overline{Z^3} \\ 1 & Z & Z^2 \end{vmatrix}}{\sqrt{\begin{vmatrix} 1 & \overline{Z} \\ \overline{Z} & \overline{Z^2} \end{vmatrix} \begin{vmatrix} 1 & \overline{Z} & \overline{Z^2} \\ \overline{Z} & \overline{Z^2} & \overline{Z^3} \\ \overline{Z^2} & \overline{Z^3} & \overline{Z^4} \end{vmatrix}}} \tag{A.17}$$

Introduce a normalized random variable Z_i:

$$Z_i \equiv (X_i - \overline{X_i})/\sqrt{V\{X_i\}} \tag{A.18}$$

Variable Z_i has a zero mean and a unit variance.

$$\overline{Z_i} = E\{Z_i\} = 0, \qquad \overline{Z_i^2} = V\{Z_i\} = 1 \tag{A.19}$$

Furthermore, the third- and fourth-order moments of Z_i are the skewness and kurtosis of the original variable X_i, respectively.

$$\overline{Z_i^3} = \sqrt{\beta_i} = \overline{(X - \overline{X})^3}/[V\{X_i\}]^{3/2} \tag{A.20}$$

$$\overline{Z_i^4} = \gamma_i = \overline{(X - \overline{X})^4}/[V\{X_i\}]^2 \tag{A.21}$$

The orthogonal polynomials for the normalized variable Z_i are much simpler because of the normalized characteristics of (A.19).

$$\psi_0(Z_i) = 1 \tag{A.22}$$

$$\psi_1(Z_i) = Z_i \tag{A.23}$$

$$\psi_2(Z_i) = \frac{Z_i^2 - \sqrt{\beta_i}Z_i - 1}{\sqrt{\gamma_i - \beta_i - 1}} \tag{A.24}$$

From the orthogonal property of (A.14), we have

$$\begin{aligned}
\overline{\psi_1(Z_i)} = \overline{\psi_2(Z_i)} &= 0, \quad \text{(zero mean)} \\
\overline{\psi_1(Z_i)^2} = \overline{\psi_2(Z_i)^2} &= 1, \quad \text{(unit variance)} \\
\overline{\psi_1(Z_i)\psi_2(Z_i)} &= 0, \quad \text{(zero covariance)} \\
\overline{\psi_1(Z_i)\psi_2(Z_j)} = \overline{\psi_1(Z_i)}\ \overline{\psi_2(Z_j)} &= 0, \qquad i \neq j, \quad \text{(zero covariance)}
\end{aligned} \tag{A.25}$$

The Taylor series expansion of (11.124) can be rewritten in terms of the normalized random variable Z_i.

$$Y = Y_0 + \sum_{i=1}^{n} b_i Z_i + (1/2)\sum_{i=1}^{n} b_{ii} Z_i^2 + \sum_{1 \le i < j \le n} b_{ij} Z_i Z_j \tag{A.26}$$

where coefficients b_i and b_{ij} are given by

$$b_i = a_i\sqrt{V\{X_i\}}, \qquad b_{ij} = a_{ij}\sqrt{V\{X_i\}V\{X_j\}} \tag{A.27}$$

The first-order terms Z_i and the cross terms $Z_i Z_j$ can be written in terms of $\psi_1(Z_i)$ and $\psi_1(Z_j)$; the second-order terms Z_i^2 can be rewritten in terms of $\psi_1(Z_i)$ and $\psi_2(Z_i)$.

$$\begin{aligned}
Z_i &= \psi_1(Z_i) \\
Z_i Z_j &= \psi_1(Z_i)\psi_1(Z_j), \qquad i \neq j \\
Z_i^2 &= \sqrt{\gamma_i - \beta_i - 1}\psi_2(Z_i) + \sqrt{\beta_i}\psi_1(Z_i) + 1
\end{aligned} \tag{A.28}$$

We have now an orthogonal expansion for (A.26):

$$\begin{aligned}
Y = {} & \left[Y_0 + (1/2)\sum_{i=1}^{n} b_{ii}\right] + \sum_{i=1}^{n}\left[b_i + (1/2)b_{ii}\sqrt{\beta_i}\right]\psi_1(Z_i) \\
& + (1/2)\sum_{i=1}^{n} b_{ii}\sqrt{\gamma_i - \beta_i - 1}\psi_2(Z_i) + \sum_{1 \le i < j \le n} b_{ij}\psi_1(Z_i)\psi_1(Z_j)
\end{aligned} \tag{A.29}$$

For a multiple-linear function, this expansion is simplified because the diagonal coefficients are all zero, that is, $b_{ii} = V\{X_i\}a_{ii} = 0$:

$$Y = Y_0 + \sum_{i=1}^{n} b_i\psi_1(Z_i) + \sum_{1\le i<j\le n} b_{ij}\psi_1(Z_i)\psi_2(Z_j) \tag{A.30}$$

From (A.25) the mean and variance of Y become

$$\begin{aligned} E\{Y\} &= Y_0 + (1/2)\sum_{i=1}^{n} b_{ii} \\ V\{Y\} &= \sum_{i=1}^{n}\left[b_i + (1/2)b_{ii}\sqrt{\beta_i}\right]^2 + (1/4)\sum_{i=1}^{n} b_{ii}^2(\gamma_i - \beta_i - 1) + \sum_{1\le i<j\le n} b_{ij}^2 \end{aligned} \tag{A.31}$$

Equation (11.131) is obtained when the above equation is rewritten in terms of the original coefficients a_i and a_{ij} of (11.118).

PROBLEMS

11.1. A multinomial posterior probability density is given by (11.6) for Greek parameters β and γ. Calculate Table 11.1 values when $n_1 = 12$, $n_2 = 6$, and $n_3 = 3$.

11.2. Consider two candidate populations for component unavailability Q.

Population $\phi = 1$		**Population $\phi = 2$**	
Q	Probability	Q	Probability
0.1	0.1	0.1	0.9
0.01	0.9	0.01	0.1

We know a priori that both populations are equally likely.

$$\Pr\{\phi = 1\} = \Pr\{\phi = 2\} = 0.5$$

Plant-specific and generic data are

$$\begin{aligned} D_1 &= (1, 50)\text{: Plant-specific data} \\ D_2 &= (1, 10) \equiv G\text{: Generic data} \end{aligned}$$

Show the following probability values.

(a) The likelihood of generic data G, given population j, is

$$\Pr\{G|\phi = 1\} = 0.12, \qquad \Pr\{G|\phi = 2\} = 0.36$$

(b) The probability of population j, given generic data G, is

$$\Pr\{\phi = 1|G\} = 0.25, \qquad \Pr\{\phi = 2|G\} = 0.75$$

(c) The a priori probability of plant 1 unavailability Q_1, given generic data G, is

$$\Pr\{Q_1 = 0.1|G\} = 0.7, \qquad \Pr\{Q_1 = 0.01|G\} = 0.3$$

(d) The a posteriori probability of plant 1 unavailability Q_1, given generic data G and plant-specific data D_1, is

$$\Pr\{Q_1 = 0.1|D_1, G\} = 0.18, \qquad \Pr\{Q_1 = 0.01|D_1, G\} = 0.82$$

11.3. Derive the mean and variance equations for log-normal random variable Q:

$$\begin{aligned} E\{Q\} &= \exp(\mu + 0.5\sigma^2) \\ V\{Q\} &= \exp(2\sigma^2 + 2\mu) - \exp(2\mu + \sigma^2) \end{aligned}$$

11.4. Prove the maximum-likelihood estimator (11.64).

11.5. Consider a three-out-of-three valve system. Obtain a demand-failure probability expression similar to (11.73).

11.6. Obtain two-dimensional Latin hypercube samples from the following sample data:

$$\begin{pmatrix} 6 & 2 & 4 & 2 \\ 1 & 3 & 1 & 5 \end{pmatrix}, \qquad \text{(2 dimension, 4 strata)}$$

11.7. Prove the inequality between AND and OR gate variance propagation.

$$V\{Q_1 \wedge Q_2\} < V\{Q_1 \vee Q_2\} \quad \text{if } \overline{Q_1}, \quad \overline{Q_2} < 0.5$$

11.8. Consider a two-out-of-three system. Evaluate system unavailability variance by moment propagation through minimal cut sets.

11.9. Derive (A.23) and (A.24), that is, orthogonal polynomials for a normalized random variable.

12

Legal and Regulatory Risks

12.1 INTRODUCTION

Multimillion-dollar regulatory agency fines and hundred-million-dollar jury verdicts make good headlines: here are recent samples stemming from product liability lawsuits and EPA, FDA, and OSHA (Occupational Safety and Health Administration) actions.

> "EPA Sues Celanese for $165,000,000 for Air Pollution"
> "Bard Medical Fined $63 Million by FDA"
> "Ford Assessed $128.5 Million in Pinto Crash"
> "EPA Fines Rockwell International $18.5 Million"
> "Jury Assesses Upjohn $127 Million—70-Year-Old Man Loses Use of Eye"
> "Chevron Hit with $127-Million Fine for Self-Reported Violation"
> "OSHA Fines Phillips $5.2 Million for Explosion"
> "Celotex to Pay $76 Million to Illinois 68-Year-Old in Asbestos Suit"

A plant shutdown due to an explosion or major failure is a catastrophe. A plant shutdown due to a lawsuit or a legal action taken by a government agency is an even more debilitating event. In 1993 the EPA collected $130 million in fines and brought 140 criminal charges, mostly against engineers. Currently, there are five to ten criminal charges against engineers every week by the EPA alone. The risks of a legal disaster are real. In the United States there have been many more plant stoppages for legal and regulatory matters than for accidents. There were 97,000 business bankruptcies in 1992. The number of Americans who lose jobs due to their firm's legal and regulatory problems is orders of magnitude higher than the number who lose their jobs due to industrial accidents. In 1992 the FDA commandeered 2922 product recalls and prosecuted 52 people for violating its dictates.

In addition to strongly influencing profitability, legal and regulatory practices influence product quality and plant safety. All countries have environmental and factory inspection agencies that mandate engineering design and manufacturing practices. In addition, all countries have labor laws. These labor laws strongly influence the manner in which safety and quality control programs are structured.

It is naive on the part of engineers and scientists to focus only on technical matters. What industry can and cannot do is mostly decided, in the United States, by politicians and lawyers. They run the legislatures, courts, and government agencies. It is incumbent, particularly on those who work in a field such as risk analysis—which has a large societal interface—to understand the legal and political processes that shape their companies' future, and to take an active role in influencing political decisions. Engineers must learn how to deal with government regulations and inspectors in order to reduce risks to themselves and their companies. Loss-prevention techniques should be developed.

12.2 LOSSES ARISING FROM LEGAL ACTIONS

In the United States, the risk of a company being crippled or closed down by lawsuits is far from negligible. Billion-dollar corporations such as Johns Manville, Robbins, and Dow Corning have been forced into bankruptcy by lawsuits. The light plane industry in America is heading for extinction; Cessna reported legal costs of over $20 million in 1993—enough to provide jobs for 300 engineers. The American machine tool industry is dead, and nobody with assets manufactures step ladders in the United States (if there are no assets, lawyer's don't sue: they only go after "deep pockets"). There are 1.24 million lawyers in the United States—a world record. It is estimated they take $\$1.00 \times 10^{12}$ (one trillion dollars) out of the American economy every year. This is money that, in other countries, is used for plant modernization, R&D, and for pay raises to workers. In 1992 liability awards and lawsuits amounted to $224 billion, or 4% of the gross national product, according to the Brookings Institute. This is about four times as much as the total salaries of all engineers in the United States.

To understand what industries can do to reduce the risk and losses from lawsuits, one must first understand the nature of the problem and how it arose: a good starting point is to read the book *Shark Tank: Greed, Politics and the Collapse of Finley Kumble, One of America's Largest Law Firms*, by Isaac Eisler. Kumble, who was head of the country's second largest law firm, had a favorite saying, "Praise the adversary lawyer; he is the catalyst by which you bill your client. Damn the client; he is your true enemy."

American attorneys are in the majority in the federal legislature, most federal agencies, and most state legislatures. Using slogans like "Consumer Protection," "Anti-Racketeering," and "Save the Environment," they have made it incredibly easy and profitable to launch lawsuits and to victimize corporations and rich individuals. Tort costs to the medical industry totaled $9.2 billion in 1994. Anyone doubting the fact that Congress makes laws that favor lawyers over industry and the public need only study the EPA's Superfund Program. Of the $20.4 billion spent thus far, according to the American Chemical Society, over $4 billion has been consumed in legal and filing fees. Almost nothing is being cleaned up. Consumer protection legislation has resulted in a similar mess. In the United States, litigious lawyers are paid not by their clients but by proceeds generated by suing the defendants ("contingency suits"), which give lawyers incentive to win suits by any means possible. In Houston, a law firm whose telephone number is INJ-URED pays for late-night TV advertisements directed at "employees who want to sue their employers... no fee charged."

An even greater abuse is that a company subject to an extortion-type lawsuit, and that wins in court, cannot recover its legal fees. Lawyers advertise widely and aggressively solicit clients. The situation is further exacerbated by the fact that lawyers "own" the courts, that is, the courts are run by lawyers for lawyers. Trials last for years, and sometimes decades, and cost from $50,000 to tens of millions: the average product liability lawsuit runs for 2.4 years. It is "against the law" for a person or a company to represent themselves in court, that is, judges force defendants to hire lawyers. It is a classic loss-prevention problem.

There are various types of lawsuits: although they pose greater and lesser risks to corporations, all cost money and resources. To quote R. J. Mahoney, president and CEO of Monsanto Chemical, "The legal system exacts a crushing cost on our way of life."

12.2.1 Nonproduct Liability Civil Lawsuits

This type of lawsuit arises from alleged mistakes made by company employees that cause damage. The $124-million award to a $93,000-a-year financial officer for wrongful discharge by a southwestern energy company was a civil lawsuit outcome. An automobile accident can bankrupt a medium-sized company if one of their trucks hits a school bus and hurts a number of children, because liability insurance, which typically is a few million dollars for a medium-sized company, will never be adequate. Furthermore, lawyers who specialize in automobile accident lawsuits will ask triple and punitive and exemplary damages because the company, according to the plaintiff's lawyer, failed to properly train and supervise and discipline their drivers. Exxon's multibillion-dollar Alaskan oil spill fine is a case in point. The captain was said to be drunk. The company is helpless to defend itself, even if it has an expensive training program; after all, an accident did happen.

It is noteworthy that the court papers and official charges served the defendant in a lawsuit, although signed by the court, are prepared by the plaintiff's lawyer for the judge's signature. The most outrageous charges are levied with no judicial review whatever. The problem this raises is that the judge, by signing these types of charges, has given the plaintiff's lawyer unlimited license to harass a company. For example, a plaintiff's lawyer can ask for financial, sales, personnel, and engineering records even though he or she is suing the company because their client slipped on the sidewalk and twisted an ankle. This is because included in the charges signed by the judge is the accusation of "willful neglect" and a request for "compensation" and "triple damages." The harassment is sanctioned by the judges on the grounds that the plaintiff's lawyer is entitled to know how much money the defendant has so it can be decided how much money to sue the company for. This type of harassment is called *discovery* and generates massive paperwork and legal fees.

Civil lawsuits, if properly handled, are usually not a major risk for a company because this type of lawsuit is usually not too costly and is customarily insured for. An exception, of course, is liability arising from the type of sabotage (accident) that befell Union Carbide at Bhopal, India. If this had happened in the United States, Union Carbide would surely now be in Chapter 11 bankruptcy. The utilities that ran the Three Mile Island reactor were not bankrupted because they have a statutory monopoly and can raise electricity rates.

12.2.2 Product Liability Lawsuits

Here is the ultimate nightmare. Johns Manville was bankrupted by asbestos lawsuits, and Robbins by lawsuits relating to intrauterine contraceptive devices. The onslaught of litigation in America relating to intrauterine contraceptive devices was such that, although they are still used and available everywhere else in the world, all American manufacturers were forced to discontinue production. The legislation relating to product liability lawsuits is so unfavorable to industry that entire industries that make products frequently involved in consumer or industrial accidents (ladders, machine tools, etc.) have not been able to survive the avalanche of lawsuits by people who use (or misuse) their products. Only one manufacturer of vaccines survives in the United States. An additional problem relating to product liability lawsuits is that of a product recall, which a company may decide to initiate voluntarily or may be forced to initiate by a government agency. FDA-mandated recalls of medical devices totaled nearly 3000 last year. Product liability insurance in the United States costs 20 times more than in Europe and 15 times more than in Japan. The GAO (Government Accounting Office) estimates that 60% of the product-liability awards go to attorneys.

It will be interesting to watch the trauma relating to the silicone (and saline) breast-implant controversy. In 1993 a Texas jury awarded one woman $27 million because the implant allegedly damaged her immune system and she became arthritic. Since then there have been eight scientific studies, including one large one sponsored by the PHS (Public Health Service) showing *no* relationship between breast implants and connective tissue diseases. So many lawsuits take place in Texas because it is the only state that permits civil charges to be filed irrespective of where the alleged act took place; and because Texas judges are elected, over 80% of their campaign contributions come from lawyers! Multiply the $27 million by four million, which is the total number of women who are said to be considering lawsuits (or who have already launched them in response to large newspaper, TV, and billboard advertisements by lawyers), and one cannot be too sanguine of the survival, in their present form, of premier corporations like Dow Chemical (Dow-Corning has already pleaded bankruptcy) and Bristol Myers Squibb. Pity their employees; both companies have recently announced large layoffs; a five-billion-dollar reserve fund was set up to cover losses.

12.2.3 Lawsuits by Government Agencies

In their zeal to further the cause of their back-home law partners, and at the behest of the strongest and richest of all lobby groups, the Trial Lawyers' Political Action Association, Congress—the majority of whom are lawyers—has given nearly all federal agencies (OSHA, FDA, NRC, EEOC, EPA, etc.) the right to level fines against industries and to launch lawsuits (including criminal proceedings) against companies and their employees. One result of these laws is that if a manufacturer has the bad luck to have an accident, it can be almost certain that one or more government agency will sue and/or level a large fine—always after the fact. Phillips Petroleum, CONOCO, and ARCO, for example, were fined millions by OSHA after they had plant explosions, despite the fact they easily passed OSHA inspections just prior to the accidents. Dr. Homsley, who was making artificial implants for over a decade in Houston, and who passed FDA manufacturing inspections yearly, suddenly was shut down and taken to court by the FDA for violating good manufacturing procedures after an implant failed. He closed his factory, declared bankruptcy, moved to Switzerland, and opened a new factory, after publicly denouncing the FDA for their Gestapo tactics. The authors' personal experience with OSHA, EPA, and FDA inspectors is that the fines and seizures are mostly the result of company employees reporting to inspectors that there was a product failure and that it had been voluntarily corrected. The government inspectors, by themselves, seldom find anything seriously wrong in routine inspections.

Government fines, even when they are as high as the $18.5-million fine levied against Rockwell International, traditionally are less than it would cost to defend the company in court against a federal lawsuit, so nearly everyone pleads innocent and then pays reduced fines. The net result, however, of this government prosecution of companies who have had the misfortune of experiencing a major accident or lawsuit is that the government aids and abets the cause of all the lawyers who—as a result of the accident—file legitimate (or fraudulent) civil lawsuits against the company because the government agencies, by their fines, have branded the company as criminal. An excellent example is the Superfund Program. In Riverside, California, an EPA lawsuit was followed by a civil suit on behalf of 3800 plaintiffs targeting 200 companies.

There is a misconception by a segment of the population that government inspectors and regulators are impartial servants of the people. This is most certainly not a universal truth. The pressure is on the inspector to find violations, whether they are justified or not.

Mendacity is a prevalent human trait; every survey taken shows that about 85% of college students and over 90% of high school students cheat at some time or another. The statistical distribution of people who are willing to stretch the truth is the same in the government as everywhere else. Company employees who deal with government inspectors must be made aware of this and be rigorously trained to do nothing other than answer questions laconically. The buddy-buddy approach is dangerous and puts the company at risk.

12.2.4 Workers' Compensation

Losses due to workers' compensation payments are so large they deserve special attention. In theory, workers' compensation insurance provides medical care and, if necessary, disability payments to workers who suffer job-related injuries. The fact that the company may or may not have generous health insurance policies and benefits for their workers is not pertinent: Workers' compensation is required in all states. In America, workers' compensation laws vary dramatically from state to state and can result in anything from a major to a moderate expense. In Texas, for example (where lawyers specializing in workers' compensation, according to legislative testimony, make yearly incomes in the $1 to $3 million category), an ex-employee can sue an employer for physical disability as long as one year after he or she worked for that employer. It is generally agreed that there is at least a 25% fraud factor in workers' compensation claims.

In most states, it is traditional for larger corporations to self-insure against the risk of workers' compensation lawsuits. The cost is high... about 1% of the sales in Texas in 1991: in the oil service business, premiums averaged $30 per $100 of payroll costs in 1990. The mechanism of self-insurance, by law in most states, is to pay the premium to an insurance company, who administers the program. The insurance companies invariably do safety compliance inspections and insist that the company have a full-time safety department, independent of size, thus generating further industry expense.

About half of workers' compensation payments are for medical costs, the rest for disability payments. Lower back claims, which, in a carefully rehearsed person, are impossible to refute, accounted for $11 billion (40%) of workers' compensation payment in 1993. The average cost of back pain is now $24,000, and the standard insurance company reserve is $80,000 per case. The National Center for Health Statistics tells us the two million carpal tunnel claims average $29,000 each!

In 1992, when a Houston company instituted company-wide drug tests the employees were given sixty days to clean up. Two days before the drug tests were to begin, five workers filed workers' compensation claims for back injuries. One of them had a traffic accident on the way to the workers' compensation office and was found by the police to be under the influence of drugs. Nevertheless, he, with the help of his lawyer, won their compensation/disability claim. Workers' compensation was originally created to benefit workers who were the victims of industrial accidents but, due to an onslaught of litigation, disability and medical payments are now being awarded for all types of personal aberrations (anxiety, depression, mental anguish, even obesity) because of alleged job-related stress above and beyond that related to domestic stress.

In most states workers' compensation cases involve quasi-judicial proceedings that do not end up in the courts. However, it is highly advisable to keep excellent employee health records and to contest all claims, particularly when the employee is represented by a lawyer. Company personnel should be trained to testify at workers' compensation hearings; the stakes are very high; loss prevention scenarios must be developed. Workers' compensation expenses exceed engineering budgets at many companies.

12.2.5 Lawsuit-Risk Mitigation

A naive viewpoint is to hypothesize that if a company does exhaustive manufacturing-risk and product-safety studies it will be immune from—or will win—liability lawsuits. A very contrary view was recently given by a high official of one of the most socially responsible of the large international companies. His hypothetical point was that, in an American court, a better defense than producing safety studies (which imply that the company made the studies because they felt the product or process was risky) is to deny any corporate knowledge that any safety problem ever existed. One can draw whatever conclusions one wants, but the consensus of experienced lawyers would be that if the only reason for doing a risk analysis is to generate paper and information that would be useful in a liability lawsuit, then this activity is a waste of time and money.

It is pitiful to note that testing and approval of products by government agencies such as the FDA, DOT, and PHS (Public Health Services), or the strongest of warning labels affixed to the product, are no deterrent to lawsuits. IUD devices and breast implants, for example, were FDA-approved for sale. Warning labels on cigarettes, which are monitored by the PHS, have not stopped lawsuits against tobacco companies. GM truck designs meet elaborate government safety requirements and DOT test standards, yet the company was tabbed by a jury for $99 million for willful negligence.

There is no geographical escape from lawsuits generated by federal agencies; however, product liability, general liability, and workers' compensation laws vary from state to state, so corporate location is important. In New Jersey, for example, workers' compensation laws are favorable to employers, and insurance costs are a small fraction of what they are in Texas. The difference in cost is because New Jersey has fixed schedules of payments and the process does not involve lawyers.

In the last five years, a number of states have passed tort reform laws to help companies survive product liability lawsuits. These laws, for example, do things such as limit the number of years, after sale, that a manufacturer is responsible for his products. Right now, in most states, manufacturers are unindemnified in perpetuity, even though the product has been repaired, rebuilt, and modified by users many times.

The ultimate—perhaps the only—way of avoiding the risk of American lawsuits is to become a truly international corporation. Dow Chemical, for example, which has half of their sales and manufacturing facilities outside the United States, reports that more than 90% of their total legal/insurance/lawsuit expenses arise in the United States. Increasingly, the chemical industry is moving overseas to lower, among other things, the risk of actions by government agencies and to avoid a costly, unfavorable legal climate. Employment in the U.S. chemical industry has dropped by more than 15% this decade, despite the fact that total worldwide employment by the industry increased almost by a factor of 1.5. The chemical industry has almost completely stopped all investment in new U.S. manufacturing plants.

The Robbins/Manville case and other such cases demonstrate that insurance cannot save a company from the thousands or tens of thousands lawsuits that might spring up—as they will in a product liability situation. For lawsuits other than massive product liability, risk mitigation is best practiced by settling out of court, that is, before the jury trial starts. Probably as many as 98% of all lawsuits that are filed are settled before they go to trial: over 90% of all lawyers in the United States have never been in a courtroom or tried a case. They rely on the fact that the defendant knows that a trial will be costly, so they customarily accept a payoff less than projected defense costs. Most lawsuits are settled out of court for $5000 to $10,000, even though the plaintiff initially asks for hundreds of thousands or millions of dollars and a jury trial. At best, lawsuits are an unsavory and unproductive activity for everyone except lawyers. At worst, they represent open and naked extortion by a group that controls the courts, and are able to force defendants into no-win situations.

12.2.6 Regulatory Agency Fines: Risk Reduction Strategies

The "fineiest" of all agencies, in the author's experience, is OSHA.... Their inspectors do not like to leave the premises with empty pockets. In 1983, the agency levied $4 million in fines, a number that avalanched to $120 million in 1994. Over half of the $120 million was for errant paperwork, not industrial safety violations. Like the EPA and FDA, the agency does not lack for personnel; one documented case involves a disruptive four-month visit to a chemical plant by a team of seven OSHA inspectors. In all, the federal regulatory bureaucracy employed 128,615 people in 1993.

In 1993, an OSHA inspector, unable to find anything else, fined our company $175 for not having an employee-signed Material Data Safety Sheet for a can of store-bought, WD-40 lubricant that the inspector spotted in a plumber's tool kit. It is pathetic that regulatory agency heads do not recognize that actions such as these promote hostility, not industrial safety. Small wonder that, in a recent survey by the Heritage Foundation, both employees and owners of businesses, by a two-to-one margin, viewed the government as an opponent rather than a partner in their pursuit of the American dream.

Although it is not immediately cost effective to fight a $175 regulatory agency fine, from a long-term risk management standpoint all violations should be contested, through at least one regulatory agency management level. The most effective course of action is to hire an in-state (not Washington) regulatory consultant to help prepare the appeal and accompany corporate technical people to the hearing, if there is one. Typically, these consultants are ex-agency employees who are on a first-name basis with the local field office employees and are familiar with agency politics and policies. It is a grave mistake to hire an attorney for a first-round appeal. Not only will the cost be much higher, but one is more likely to lose, because lower-level agency employees, who are likely to be engineers or science-degreed, don't like *any* lawyers, including their own agency's because, if nothing else, the lawyer's salaries are much higher than theirs. In dealing with the FDA, our company once made the naive mistake of hiring a Washington law firm to contest a product-recall violation. Two months and $15,000 in legal fees later, we had made no progress, so we fired the lawyer.

The agency people we were dealing with, who refused to talk with us as long as we had a lawyer, suddenly became very friendly, and settled the violation without a fine.

Once a matter is in the courts, one has no choice but to hire a lawyer. Although there appears to be no law against it, judges, in our experience, will not let a corporation represent itself in their courtrooms, even if it is abundantly clear that attorney costs will exceed any possible damage award. Some government agencies, the Commerce Department in particular, refuse to give information to anyone except an attorney. "Have your attorney call us," is what they tell you. In 1991, the Commerce Department levied an export/import ban on a small Dutch company, Delft Instruments, for allegedly selling bomb-sights to Saddam Hussein. It took over a year and $10,700,000 in fees to a gang of Washington attorneys to have the export/import ban lifted. By then, of course, the business was lost. Careful cost/benefit studies should precede all legal actions: that's the lesson here.

12.3 THE EFFECT OF GOVERNMENT REGULATIONS ON SAFETY AND QUALITY

The single most important goal of a government bureaucracy is to perpetuate itself and to annually convince the legislature to give it more: more people, more power, more money, and greater jurisdiction. A prime example is the U.S. Census Bureau, whose only legitimate mission is to do a head count so that congressional seats can be properly appointed. Over the years, ambitious directors of the census have convinced Congress to expand the scope of their operation to a point where the bureau spends $2 billion sending out, collecting, and tinkering with complicated questionnaires that are largely, if not mostly, not returned, or incorrectly filled out. Considering the fact that 22% of the population is functionally illiterate, the accuracy of the census bureau data can never be better than a guesstimate. The job could be done, just as accurately, by counting drivers' licenses and/or voter registrations, because a very large fraction of all census questionnaire answers are computer-synthesized. After every census, states, counties, and cities challenge the census results in court, charging that the information is incorrect.

The history of agencies created to hold industry's feet to the fire, vis-à-vis workplace safety, consumer protection, job discrimination, environmental protection, and restraint of trade, is not much different from the census bureau's. A case in point is the EEOC, the Equal Employment Opportunity Commission. Originally organized to enforce equal rights for minorities, the scope of the agency was then expanded to include women, and in 1992 expanded even more to assure equal rights in the workplace for disabled workers; in 1993 the Family Leave Bill was passed, which gives lawyers incredible powers to sue for damages above and beyond any personal loss. It is ironic that until 1995, Congress, which employs 12,000 people, has exempted itself from all equal opportunity and labor legislation, including the Family Leave Bill.

As the Census Bureau, which can't get the count right (they invariably "find" a much higher percentage of women than is known to exist), the EEOC has a great deal of difficulty "putting it together," so to speak, because "discrimination," "handicapped," and so on are subjective concepts that defy qualification. Nearly every alleged case is controversial and potentially represents a lawsuit because not only is the EEOC empowered to sue and fine a company, but so is the employee. A reasonable guess would be that about 5–10% of all people fired by industry end up suing their employer, and if the person is a minority, a female, handicapped or elderly, the risk of a lawsuit rises to 10–20%—except in the case of plant closing, mass layoffs due to retrenchment, or a prelawsuit settlement of some sort. Engineers, most of whom are in supervisory positions, must learn to protect their companies from this type of risk and subsequent losses.

12.3.1 Stifling of Initiative and Abrogation of Responsibility

There is another characteristic of government that has unfortunate consequences for industry. Government bureaucrats strive to compartmentalize and routinize everything. State air quality control boards, for example, use the same reporting and site approval and pollutant dispersion forms for chemical plants, breweries, and electronic assembly plants. If a company wants information on acceptable abatement technology, the standard agency approach is to give the applicant a list of registered and approved consultants and vendors. The people on the approved list always recommend standard technology. If a company needs to reduce ethylene oxide emission, for example, the agency will refer them to vendors who sell incinerators and acid absorption systems. The possibility of novel ideas and new solutions to old problems is thus greatly reduced. The safest, most prudent, and most economical course of action for any company is to say "yes, sir" and do anything that the government agency tells them to do. Appeal processes take so much time, money, and manpower that irreparable harm is done to the company.

Every government agency has a large legal staff. Reliance on the courts is hopeless; this takes years. If the FDA sends one of their infamous "15-day," comply-or-else letters, it would be suicide for a company to say "I won't comply. . . the violations cited by your agency are stupid and are the result of a plant inspection carried out by a semi-literate inspector who has no technical training whatsoever, and who has not the remotest understanding of my company's complex technology, business, products, or customers." The result of venting one's frustration in this impudent manner is a certain plant shutdown, no less costly than a major fire.

As organizations such as the FDA, NRC, OSHA, and EPA (all of whom are charged with regulating workplace safety) mature, they produce increasingly detailed reports, questionnaires, SOPs (standard operating procedures), and safety requirements. Permissible chemical and radiological exposure limits, as well as top-event risk standards, are set by government agencies. It would be unthinkable for anyone to apply for an air quality control board (AQCB) permit for a site expansion and not to categorically swear that every single agency requirement will be met. A company is no more than a collection of individuals: people, not companies, fill out site-application forms. When people make mistakes, the company pays dearly. As was pointed out earlier, 85% of college students admit to occasional or systematic cheating.

Given this natural state of the human being and the pressure of the workplace, is it any wonder that when the government issues technically or financially unattainable requirements, frequently one of two results occur? Marginal producers with minimal assets will meet the requirements on paper. They base future survival on the same set of premises as a driver who does 60 mph in a 55-mph speed zone; detection of the violation is uncertain, the penalty is manageable, and an excuse may work. Well-managed, technologically strong companies will locate new plants off-shore and run old ones as long as possible.

Totalitarian countries and welfare states are characterized by a lack of personal initiative and unwillingness by individuals to take responsibility for their own actions. Personal responsibility ends when what the government asks to be done has been done. As the governmental agencies become more and more specific in what they require in the way of safety studies, safe operation, and worker training, the safety engineer's attention and energies are diverted from creating an active safety program and become focused entirely on meeting government requirements and creating documents that satisfy armies of government inspectors.

When the NRC decrees that all reactor operators shall have five hours of training per month, the name of the game changes. Focus shifts from creating an active safety culture to one of creating, scheduling, and implementing a program that lasts for five hours per month, and is in passive compliance with NRC's training directives. If, because of a personnel department error, training-session attendance had not been recorded into an operator's personnel folder at the time of a government inspection, the company is subject to fines and court actions whether or not they have an excellent safety record and training program. When dealing with regulatory agencies, form invariably triumphs over substance. Emphasis is totally on the process—the product does not matter. In regulatory agencies run by lawyers, words are more important than actions.

12.3.2 Overregulation

The most lawless countries have the greatest number of laws. In 1964 the Brazilian government passed 300 major laws in one day. Clarity, purpose, and effectiveness were completely overshadowed by political posturing and enlightened self-interest. The laws were largely unenforceable and unenforced: as with the American prohibition, or "no spitting on the sidewalk." When the Brazilian government passed a law in 1965 that all professors at federal universities must be "tempo integral," that is, full-time professors, a tourist or naive citizen might have proclaimed "university reform is finally here." That was not the case at all. There had been three previous such laws, all unenforced and all unenforceable. The Congress of the United States has put an anti-business weapon in the hands of lawyers called the RICO (racketeering-influenced and corrupt organization) law. It is cited by plaintiff attorneys in tens of thousands of lawsuits against honest corporations and organizations. It is so vague that it has never been properly defined: the cases involving alleged violation of this law are won or lost on other, more substantive issues. Lawyers like to cite it because it has a triple-damage provision, which gives them enormous power to harass defendants. Interestingly enough, this racketeering law has been used successfully to sue anti-abortion groups who block women's access to abortion clinics.

The net result of overregulation is that nobody knows what the law really is and industry is at the mercy of judges and government inspectors. Company management must focus on sales and manufacturing if it is to survive in a worldwide, competitive business climate. When a fire inspector struts in and demands a complete reorganization of the company's warehouse because—he says—the code prohibits stacking closer than one foot from the ceiling, who knows whether he is right or wrong? There are different codes in every city and county. This also applies to the tax code. Companies doing business in all 50 states are inspected by revenue inspectors from each of these states (as well as the federal government) and are expected to know every one of the nation's millions of city, state, and county tax law regulations. This is the same situation a citizen faces when dealing with an IRS inspector. Nobody has read and understood the entire tax code. The IRS inspector pretends to know the code, so the citizen is wrong. Legal precedents are invariably too narrow or nonexistent. The IRS, when challenged in court, lost 70% of the cases, but few have enough money to fight the IRS.

Human beings and organizations do not function well under uncertainty. When it becomes impossible to know and understand the laws that pertain to your business, and when armies of government inspectors have the right to issue fines and summonses, and the corporation is immediately declared guilty as charged and must post fines until, at enormous expense and lost time, it proves itself innocent, then safety and reliability studies will not capture the attention of upper-level management, because they don't relate to immediate survival issues. The up-front investments in quality, safety, and reliability are high, and funds may not be available. The Wallace Corporation, which in 1990 won the Commerce Department's prestigious Malcom Baldridge National Quality Manufacturing Award, declared bankruptcy in 1991.

12.4 LABOR AND THE SAFE WORKPLACE

Consider what has happened in the public school system; probably the most regulated of the American workplaces. Magnetic weapons-inspection systems, barbed-wire fences, and security guards characterize many public schools in major cities. Undue focus and energy are put on dealing with the problems of system deviates. Management focuses on quelling disturbances rather than furthering the common good. The cost and manpower required to comply with government DOE (Department of Education) regulations is staggering. Each school district, by law, must retain professionally trained arbitrators assigned to mediate between parents of handicapped students and the district to assure complaining parents that the school has provided enough facilities and special programs to meet the needs of the child, the parents, and whatever advocacy group chooses to intervene. The school is mandated to provide the "least restrictive environment" for all disadvantaged students. Dyslexia and very low mental ability are considered handicaps, and such students are given special entitlements. Specialists in sight impairment, speech impairment, and general learning disabilities must, by law, be in place. All of this extracurricular effort requires extraordinary amounts of money and effort. School taxes have increased an average of 6.5% per year in the United States during the past 15 years, largely to pay for the costs of new programs mandated by the state and federal departments of education. Some of these increased expenditures have been used to pay attorneys who are suing the district on behalf of aggrieved parents or special interest groups. The city of Houston recently had a special election to raise $15 million to pay for unbudgeted legal bills. A quote attributed to Lee Iacocca, when he was the president of Chrysler, was "no matter what we budget for legal costs, it is never enough."

During the past two decades the educational community has witnessed an enormous effort on the part of the government to educate the population in civic tolerance—defined as the adoption of the viewpoint that no person is a liability to the community, regardless of their negative contributions to society. By implication, industry also is being pushed to "forgive and forget" and to automatically promote people in the same way the schools promote people, and pass students from grade to grade regardless of achievement.

The government has spent billions creating protected groups within the educational and public economic sectors. This enormous effort to create protected groups has failed both the majority and minority sectors of the population. In 1992, under the pseudo-idealistic guise that all people should have equal opportunity and access to employment, politicians seeking to strengthen and expand their political base extended the economically damaging concept of protected groups to private business, completely neglecting the fact that private industry, unlike public schools, cannot arbitrarily raise their prices 6.5% every year. Their European and Asian competitors are not forced to hire protected groups and are free to dismiss disloyal and unproductive employees without being brought to court by government agencies and contingency lawyers.

To use an analogy from athletics, the educational establishment and industry form a relay team. The baton that the educational establishment passes to the industry is the labor force. Twenty-two percent of this labor force is illiterate; in much of the country it has sprung from an environment where school absenteeism is as high as 25%, in which there is no punishment for poor performance or poor discipline, and people are trained to take advantage of protected-group and litigious advocacy situations. The baton being passed to industry consists of the most poorly educated work force (in terms of academic achievement) of all the industrialized countries in the world. The creation, under these conditions, of an effective, viable, corporate safety culture is a challenging task.

12.4.1 Shaping the Company's Safety Culture

Embedding a safety culture into the diverse ethnic and cultural group that comprises the American work force is a difficult, but certainly not impossible, task. It involves careful and patient management and realization that, from the standpoint of education, it involves both learning and unlearning. A new employee who has, in his 12 years of schooling, learned nothing but how to cheat and beat the system must be taught that now he *is* the system. If that cannot be done, and done very quickly, the employee should be terminated: there is no reasonable statistical hope of rehabilitation. This is a point repeatedly stressed by Joe Charbonneaux, one of America's most popular and successful management consultants. His seminars and courses on effective corporate management stress the concept that 27% of all company employees contribute negatively to productivity and have poor attitudes toward their work and their company, and that there is absolutely nothing that the company can do in the way of education or training that will change them or their behavior. The title of his most popular seminar is "Look Who's Wrecking Your Company."

The first step in setting a successful course is to recognize the obstacles ahead and to prepare to overcome them. This starts with the hiring process.

12.4.2 The Hiring Process

At the University of Houston, as at most universities, students are asked to comment on and rate all courses at the end of each semester. In the 1994 senior design course where the students worked in teams of four, one of the students offered the following comment: "What I learned in this course is that it is not possible to produce a good design when your coworkers are stupid and lazy." This may be the most valuable lesson he learned in his four years of college.

Considering the major responsibilities given risk, safety, and loss-prevention managers, it is very reasonable that they have a voice in the hiring process. Hiring decisions are too important to be left solely to the human resources (employment) departments. These departments are frequently more focused on avoiding EEOC fines and lawsuits (which would reflect badly on them) than on the risk taken by hiring someone who is dyslexic and might blow up the plant (which would reflect poorly on the risk manager).

A case in point is that the government, on the pretext of national security, is permitted to screen employees in a manner forbidden to industry. Under the 1990 Americans with

Disabilities Act (ADA) regulations, which Representative Richard Armey estimates will cost American industry $100 billion in the next five years, it is felony-level violation to ask any question relating to the job history of applicants (whether or not they fall into the protected group category).

Clearly, anyone with a learning disability that leads to impaired judgment or physical disabilities such as uncontrolled seizures or tremors puts all of his or her coworkers at risk in many job categories. The next point to note is the type of psychological mind-set or deviant behavior that makes people accident-prone. Among these are failure to understand, failure to read instructions, failure to seek advice, inability to make decisions under pressure, and losing ability under stress.

There are proven psychological stress tests used by the airline industry for testing pilots that provide excellent indicators of accident-proneness and inability to function under stress. Tests of this type should be given to operators of complex and dangerous plants and equipment. Drug testing must be compulsory. The rate of workplace drug abuse in 1992 (at companies that do drug testing) was 8.81%, with marijuana accounting for 39.5% of that amount.

Because of the high rate of (at least) one remission following drug rehabilitation (estimates as high as 65 percent have been published), the best drug policy, from a risk-aversion and cost-control standpoint, is universal, mandatory drug testing with immediate dismissal of *any* company employee failing a drug test. If uniformly applied, this policy is completely legal and less likely to engender costly lawsuits than vacillatory programs involving rehabilitation. Exxon, for example, has a policy allowing employees who fail drug tests to enter drug rehabilitation programs and continue to work, and is now fighting a class action lawsuit by "rehabilitated" employees who claim they were not promoted as quickly as people who did not have drug abuse histories. Engineers responsible for loss prevention and operations should demand their companies have strict, uncompromising, drug programs. Drugs distort judgment: drug abusers are as dangerous as drunken drivers and should not be tolerated in jobs where their actions can cause harm to others.

Poor judgment and mental instability have certain associated indicators such as poor driving and accident records, credit problems, and possibly a criminal record. Driver license records as well as school records should be examined by the risk and safety directors to establish whether or not errant tendencies, which put people and the plant at risk, can be detected.

Many employers ask job applicants to take the Wonderlic Personal Test. This test is internationally recognized as a standardized measurement of general cognitive ability. It requires no factual knowledge above what one learns by the sixth grade. Cognitive ability is, of course, a test prerequisite, but in most countries it is also a prerequisite for even the lowest-level industrial job. There are fifty questions; the average score for all job applicants is 21, which is also the average score for high school graduates. College graduates average 29; only 0.0034% of the people who take the test achieve perfect scores. The standard deviation of the Wonderlic is 7.12.

Because the Wonderlic test has been given to millions of people, it is possible to obtain precise correlations between scores on the test and age, ethnicity, schooling, and job function. The following observations can be made (source of the data is *User's Manual for the WPT and SLE*):

Table 12.1 shows that mental ability peaks early in life, a fact that is well established by other measures. Table 12.2, which is based on a sample of 116,977 people, is consistent throughout all educational levels and shows that, in a general mental ability test, there is no significant difference in test scores between women and men irrespective of race, and that whites outperform blacks at all educational levels by 30%. The 30% gap in cognitive skills widens to 40% in science and mathematics skills.

TABLE 12.1. Deterioration of Performance with Age Using Age 30 as a Base

Age	40–50	50–54	55–59	60+
Deterioration	10%	14%	19%	24%

TABLE 12.2. Relative Differences in Median Cognitive Test Scores by Race and Sex

Years of Education	**White**		**African-American**	
	Male	**Female**	**Male**	**Female**
9	100%	100%	71%	58%
12	100%	100%	70%	75%
15	100%	96%	76%	72%
18+	100%	93%	72%	66%
All (Avg.)	100%	97%	72%	68%

Clearly these test results pose a legal and moral problem. If a company wants to build a world-class business and beat the competition, it has to win the same way that a basketball team wins—by having better players on the average, and good match-ups at every position.

As with drug testing programs, a company's naive application of intelligence tests raises the risk of expensive litigation and regulatory agency fines. The Affirmative Action division of the Labor Department, which is responsible for seeing that all companies that sell to the government have acceptable Affirmative Action programs, has sued a number of companies using intelligence tests and/or has demanded that test scores be adjusted by race. Few companies fight with the Labor Department inspectors because, if the inspector does not like the company's Affirmative Action program, all government procurement contracts can be canceled, and that is a heavy stick indeed. In 1995, a company was applying the Wonderlic Test to screen out all job applicants who, according to the test results, did not have the equivalent of a sixth-grade education. The Department of Labor investigator sent to verify the company's Affirmative Action program decreed that the sixth-grade educational requirement was unnecessary and discriminatory because, of the thirty-eight people who failed the test, thirty-seven were black (one was Hispanic). A fine of $385,000 was levied and the possibility of a class action lawsuit was raised. This type of debacle could, possibly, have been avoided if the production engineers had written careful job descriptions (preferably verified by an outside consultant) justifying a sixth-grade educational level as a job requirement. In dealing with government bureaucracies, documentation is overwhelmingly important and becomes part and parcel of risk aversion.

It is much, much cheaper and less traumatic to pay an EEOC fine for not hiring members of their protected groups than to hire members and then to have to fire them because they don't perform on the job and/or cause accidents. The risk of a major loss due to fines and lawsuits is an order of magnitude higher in the case of an alleged discriminatory nonpromotion or firing than it is for nonhiring. In October of 1991, a California jury bludgeoned Texaco for $17.7 million, including a whopping $15 million in punitive damages, because a woman claimed she was twice passed over for promotion in favor of men. California, which has a reputation of having the strongest anti-industry (consumer-worker protection) legislation in the country, also permits compensatory damage for mental anguish, which is one of the reasons the award was so high. Under the new Civil Rights Act of 1991 (which, in 1993, was amended to remove all caps on punitive and compensatory damages), cases of the type described above are providing another feeding frenzy for attorneys.

The employee who does not want to be a team player is a serious safety risk. In the highest risk category is the sociopathetic loner, who is likely to do willful sabotage. Twelve willful acts of sabotage in American nuclear power plants were reported during the period 1981 to 1984. The most likely scenario for the Bhopal disaster is sabotage. Acts of willful sabotage are common, not rare. Of the 4899 acts of terrorism committed in the period January 1, 1970, to September 10, 1978, 39% were directed against business and commercial facilities. In the next highest risk category are people who are of less than average intelligence, emotional, and lacking in analytical skills. These, particularly if they are aggressive and permitted to do anything except rote tasks, will account for the overwhelming number of plant accidents. It is the risk manager's job to isolate or eliminate people who are potential safety risks. An accident-prone person will remain an accident-prone person for a lifetime. Too many people of this type, particularly if they are aggressive, end up in jobs where they have power to override automated safety systems, as at Three Mile Island. The smart, somewhat lazy person makes the best and safest plant operator.

12.5 EPILOGUE

Many electric devices, including those used in electrotherapy and patient monitoring, have accessories that are connected to them or to patients by pin connectors. In 1993 a nurse managed, somehow, to take two unattached electrode pin connectors and force them into a wall socket; a baby was injured. Obviously, this is a near-zero probability event that had never happened before and that, it is safe to say, will never happen again.

The FDA expressed the greatest of concern. They made this a high-profile event—they issued warning statements and press releases and sent express, registered, doomsday notices to every medical manufacturer in the country. In their zeal to protect the public and impress Congress, they have now issued dictums that every device manufacturer label all connectors, irrespective of size and shape, with warning labels to the effect that they should not be plugged into wall outlets. By actions such as these, the watchdog bureaucracy expands: The FDA budget has climbed to $764 million from $227 million in about five years. FDA regulations now occupy 4270 pages in the code of Federal Regulations. The head of the agency, David Kessler, was stamped a "Regulation Junkie" by columnist Tony Snow of *USA Today*. The cost and time involved in getting FDA approvals has increased an order of magnitude over this period without any proof whatsoever that medical devices have become safer. American medical device manufacturers, in a recent survey, reported overwhelmingly that the FDA was hindering the introduction of new and improved medical devices, and that their R&D programs have been curtailed. Most large medical-device companies, such as Baxter, have had major layoffs; others, such as Johnson & Johnson and Bristol-Meyers Squibb, have spun off their device divisions. William George, president of Medtronics, recently testified before Congress that he is moving a major research laboratory to Europe because of legal and regulatory problems in the United States. Many engineering jobs have been lost.

One sees this across the entire industrial sector. The chemical industry has curtailed R&D and the number of new chemicals put on the market has been drastically reduced. The latest EPA pronouncements on the dangers posed by chlorine and all chlorine-containing chemicals has paralyzed entire segments of the industry. Certainly, projected plant expansions have been canceled.

If one accepts the notion that many of the regulatory actions, such as the one mandating farm-product-based gasoline additives, are politically motivated, then they can only be countered by political action. It is quite clear that industry and industry associations do not have enough clout to defend themselves, nor do they have a political constituency that controls votes.

It is suggested that the engineering and scientific societies do what health professionals, lawyers, and others did decades ago: form political action committees. Political action is not un-American nor is it enlightened self-interest. There are about 1.5 million scientists and engineers in this country: if organized, they could make a difference. There is nothing un-American about engineering organizations demanding that OSHA and FDA factory inspectors be registered engineers. There is nothing un-American about the scientific societies asking that directors of agencies such as the EPA come from a scientific, rather than a legal/political, arena. It would appear that, at present, anyone who has ever worked in industry is automatically disqualified from working for a regulatory agency. The reverse should be the case.

In a recent lecture at the University of Delaware, one of the authors (E. J. Henley) distributed a questionnaire to the students asking if they favored their professional societies uniting and forming political action committees; the response was overwhelmingly "yes." The same affirmative response was given by a group of working chemical engineers that was posed the same question. Industries can be sued and regulated to death; the living proof is the nuclear industry, which has moved ahead in most countries and is moribund in America, due largely to the staggering burden posed by lawsuits and regulatory actions. Perhaps nuclear power, in the long run, will prove economically nonviable, but we will never know unless the assessment is made by engineers and scientists instead of politicians, regulators, and activist lawyers.

Index

A

B

C

F

G

Q

R